The Architecture of Imaging

Bill Rostenberg, AIA

CHRIS.
I ENJOYED PRESENTING AT HARVARD WITH YOU!
Best wishes
Bill Rostenberg

AHA

AHA books are published by American Hospital Publishing, Inc.,
an American Hospital Association company

The views expressed in this publication are strictly those of the author and do not represent official positions of the American Hospital Association.

Library of Congress Cataloging-in-Publication Data

Rostenberg, Bill.
The architecture of imaging / Bill Rostenberg.
p. cm.
Includes bibliographical references and index.
ISBN 1-55648-140-3
1. Hospitals—Radiological services—Design and construction. I. Title.
RA975.5.R3R67 1995
725'.5—dc20 95-17090
CIP

Catalog no. 043183

Printed in the USA

AHA is a service mark of the American Hospital Association used under license by American Hospital Publishing, Inc.

Text set in English Times
1M—09/95—0416

Cover graphics used with permission from Stone Marraccini Patterson, San Francisco. Images composed by D. Roger Hay.

Linda Conheady, Senior Editor
Anne Hermann, Editor
Dennis Spaag, Permissions Editor
Peggy DuMais, Production Coordinator
Cheryl Kusek, Cover Designer
Marcia Bottoms, Executive Editor
Brian Schenk, Books Division Director

For Nathan

Contents

List of Figures

List of Tables

About the Author

Bill Rostenberg, AIA, is senior medical planner with the San Francisco office of Stone Marraccini Patterson, Architecture—Planning—Interior Architecture. Mr. Rostenberg chairs the Technology Committee of the American Institute of Architects/Academy on Architecture for Health as well as the Health Facilities Committee of the American Institute of Architects' San Francisco chapter.

A recipient of the graduate fellowship in health facility design from the American Hospital Association and the American Institute of Architects in 1983, Mr. Rostenberg writes extensively on current issues in health facility design and planning. His book *Design Planning for Freestanding Ambulatory Care Facilities,* now out of print, was published in 1986 by American Hospital Publishing.

Mr. Rostenberg is an appointed member of the American Institute of Architects/Academy on Architecture for Health and serves as a liaison between that organization and both the Radiological Society of America and the American Healthcare Radiology Administrators. He is a member of the American Society for Hospital Engineering and is a registered architect in California and Arizona.

The author received a bachelor of arts degree in architecture from Washington University in St. Louis and bachelor and master degrees in architecture from the University of Arizona in Tucson.

Foreword

Medical imaging has undergone an explosive transformation in the past 20 years, becoming the most important diagnostic discipline in medicine. In addition to diagnostic imaging, a new branch also made its appearance—interventional radiology (image-guided and image-controlled surgical interventions). Lately, in order to combat the overwhelming oversaturation of image information, another new discipline has appeared on the scene—the picture archiving and communications system (PACS). The PACS has steadily advanced from infancy to become almost practical due to revolutionary advances in computer technology.

All these changes are occurring regularly, making many departments of radiology spatially obsolete. Even some departments designed in the past decade are becoming nonfunctional. New imaging procedures are expensive and therefore drive the need for efficiency in order to stay competitive in a managed care environment. Thus, it is imperative that health care architects, radiologists, radiological technicians, and hospital administrators understand each other's needs and develop imaging department designs that allow fast throughput, comfort, and privacy for patients; separation of stretcher patients from ambulatory patients; strategic locations for image processing; storage space for C-arm and other portable units; and flexibility for future developments. A must is to foresee the need for the communications systems of the future. This means installing cables for fiber optics, satellite dishes for microwave communication, and connections for high-speed telephone systems. An abundance of conduit must be introduced into all designs because retrofitting is extremely expensive, as are all modifications once the department begins to function. An imaging department that is properly designed also must blend outpatient and inpatient facilities without having the two collide. All these precepts are essential for the future because efficiency and full usage will be necessary for survival.

This book fulfills an important need and should become the bible for all professionals involved in the planning of imaging departments. It educates architects about equipment and the needs of the medical community and medical providers about architectural design concepts and planning issues. The book is up-to-date and even attempts to predict the needs of the future. Careful reading will save future headaches and unnecessary expenses.

Alexander R. Margulis, MD, DSc (HC)
San Francisco
1995

Preface

In 60 seconds, a healthy heart beats some 60 to 80 times. In 60 seconds, electron beam tomography records over a thousand views of cardiac activity. A thousand pictures in just a minute! A dozen images of every heartbeat! We acquire more information in a few seconds than we can examine in a day.

Medical imaging not only acquires information rapidly, but its technology changes almost as fast. In contrast, architecture is a slower and more deliberate process. Accommodation of rapid changes in equipment and technology can lead to costly changes in facility construction when flexibility is not incorporated into design. Because the building sciences probably will never evolve at the pace of the medical sciences, proactive planning coupled with an understanding of imaging's new role in medicine can reduce both the likelihood and the magnitude of costly construction mistakes.

The breadth of knowledge needed to develop even a simple imaging facility can easily overwhelm the inexperienced or misinformed. Furthermore, a misunderstanding of technology often compromises design opportunities that should not be sacrificed.

Armed with their own priorities and reasons for developing an imaging facility, architects and health care professionals sometimes approach problem solving differently. Often, they are unaware that each may be speaking a different language. One of the goals of *The Architecture of Imaging* is to provide designers and health care providers with a common language so that they can establish a team approach to creating quality through collaboration.

This book simplifies the design and planning process for both nonmedical and medical professionals. First, it equips architectural designers with a broad understanding of medical imaging as a basis for framing the proper questions that must be asked of facility users. Second, it provides a detailed, step-by-step explanation of design and planning activities to assist veteran and newly trained radiologists and health care administrators to work closely with architects.

The Architecture of Imaging is divided into six parts. Part 1 serves two functions: First, it explains the importance of high-quality design, and then it correlates various design approaches with both general changes in the health care industry and specific changes in medical imaging. This part provides an overview for both design professionals and medical practitioners.

Part 2 describes how to organize and manage an architectural project from the owner's perspective. Intended as a primer for health care professionals, it also will interest architects because it offers a comprehensive list of owner expectations. In addition, the chapter on equipment planning (chapter 5) is useful to both architects and health care professionals.

Part 3 explains the vast range of imaging techniques in use today, as well as newer modalities that are still in the research and development stages. Together, parts 1 through 3 establish the common language from which collaboration can grow and communication can be strengthened.

Part 4 builds on the idiom and explains important planning and design concepts for imaging facilities. This part is the heart of the book; it addresses both global and detailed concepts of facility design such as concept planning, department planning, and space planning. It also discusses the details of room layout and special utility needs.

Part 5 offers a vision of the future. This part discusses trends in health care and imaging and suggests how tomorrow's imaging projects may differ from today's.

Five useful appendixes and an index make up part 6. The appendixes include an examination of specific imaging facility projects, a list of data pertinent to radiation protect, a reprint of AIA construction guidelines for medical facilities, a glossary, a bibliography, and a detailed index.

The architecture of imaging is both changing and constant. Ever-changing equipment and procedures challenge the brightest and most focused professionals to establish future trends. With each new development, it becomes more apparent that imaging is here to stay as a superstar of modern health care.

Acknowledgments

The genesis of this book occurred in 1989 when the American Institute of Architects/Academy on Architecture for Health (then known as the Committee on Architecture for Health) began planning for a major symposium on medical technology and its impact on health care facility design. As vice-chair of the Technology Committee, the author of this book prepared what was intended to be a 5-page overview of medical imaging facilities. Some 60 pages later, after barely scratching the surface of the subject, he recognized both the challenge and the need for a detailed book-length discussion of the subject.

The symposium, also titled The Architecture of Imaging, took place in Charleston, South Carolina, in October 1990. It was hailed a success, and from it several significant events emerged. First, it marked the beginning of an important liaison among the American Institute of Architects, the Radiological Society of North America, and the American Healthcare Radiology Administrators. Second, it brought together architects, radiologists, administrators, and others interested in imaging facilities to examine the rapidly changing relationship between imaging technology and facility design. Third, it set the stage for future symposia to be presented by the Technology Committee. Fourth, for the author, it marked the beginning of several important professional relationships with individuals representing a spectrum of disciplines ranging from medicine to equipment manufacturing to architecture.

While writing *The Architecture of Imaging,* the author consulted many of those individuals. Heartfelt thanks go out to all of them, particularly the following people, without whom this book would never have been possible: Alexander Margulis, MD, DSc (HC); Thomas S. Harle, MD; Arthur Rosenbaum, MD; Steven Horri, MD; Carl Jansen, MD; Susanna Hoppszallern; John Campbell, FAHRA; Morris Stein, AIA; Scott Jenkins; Kim Hall, AIA; Annie Coull, AIA; Ray Brovold, AIA; William A. Foucher, AIA; Karen Terrill, RN; Elaine Campbell Dohms, FAHRA; Stewart Bushong, ScD, FACR, FACMP; Martha Bil Manevich, AIA; Joseph P. Readdy; Susan Becker; Henry C. Padgett, PhD; Brian Johnson; Mitchell Randall, MS; John Jay Clark; Tom Foyil; William P. Mazzetti Jr., PE; Walter N. Vernon IV, PE; John M. Pappas, PE; John S. Nelson, PE; Robert J. Bucci, PE; David S. Odegard, PE; Carl R. Grady; J. Richard Muirhead, PE; Carl J. Stumph, PE; Martin Ratner; and Barbara Denton, IIDA.

Special thanks go to the author's colleagues at Stone Marraccini Patterson: Michael Kelly; David L. Martino, AIA; Roger Hill, AIA; Rick Ottolino, AIA; D. Roger Hay; Paul Justison; Jenifer Altenoff; Kelly Fehr; Chase Young, AIA; Seema Gupta; Donald MacMillan, AIA; Robert Smith, AIA; and Stephen Friedland.

The author also wishes to recognize the following organizations for their assistance and encouragement: the American Institute of Architects/Academy on Architecture for Health, the Radiological Society of North America, and the American Healthcare Radiology Administrators.

Finally, the author extends thanks to the Books staff of American Hospital Publishing for recognizing the importance of a book on facility design during a time when health care reform occupied everyone's attention. Special recognition is deserved by Linda Conheady, Wayne Brown, and Anne Hermann, who edited the manuscript, and to Dennis Spaag, who managed the task of securing original artwork and permission to reprint materials from other architects, designers, and publishers.

How to Use This Book

A book devoted to a limited topic and intended for a singular audience can be difficult to write. Conceptualizing that same book for a diverse audience is even more challenging because both its content and its style are likely to be more appropriate, in some instances, for one audience than for another. Add to this a topic that is both broad and ever changing, and the difficult task of writing becomes a very difficult task indeed.

As mentioned in the foreword, *The Architecture of Imaging* was written for all the professionals involved in the planning of imaging departments. My intent is to provide a long-overdue resource on designing imaging facilities that will be of value to everyone involved in the process: architects, radiologists and other health care providers, administrators, and interior designers, regardless of whether they are seasoned specialists or newly practicing professionals.

For those readers whose interests include history, philosophy, management, medical science, design, systems analysis, regulation, and prophecy of imaging facilities, welcome to all that resides between the front and back covers of this book. For those who are decidedly more focused on a narrower range of issues rather than the entire spectrum, consider the following road map.

Begin with part 1, the overview, if you want to learn more about the context in which imaging has evolved. If you are familiar with project schedules and budgets but wish to learn more about magnetic resonance imaging, magnetic resonance spectroscopy, and magnetic resonance angiography, you might skim through part 2, "Development of an Imaging Facility," and then proceed to part 3, "Imaging Techniques."

If, however, you are more familiar with digital subtraction angiography and picture archiving and communications systems than with departmental gross square footage, schematic design, design development, and contract documents, you might concentrate on part 2 and only skim through part 3.

Some readers will head straight for part 4, "Design and Planning." This part provides both a broad and a detailed array of design and planning information. However, many of these data will be even more meaningful when read in conjunction with the preceding chapters. Certainly everyone will be interested in part 5, "The Future," and the appendixes that follow.

However, before you begin to read the book, please consider a word of caution. It is hoped that the information contained herein will be useful to all readers. However, because the subject matter is continuously changing, many of the topics and details may no longer apply to some facilities; they may have been accurate at the time of publication (summer 1995) but may have since been superseded, or they may be based on individual opinions rather than universally accepted rules. Because medical imaging and its architecture are both complex and ever changing, readers are encouraged to seek specific direction from design and planning professionals and from equipment manufacturers on particular projects. Therefore, the information contained in this book should not be considered to be more than general background information.

How to Use This Book

Part 1

Overview

Originally, man relied on magic to cure his ills, but then he began to worship technology. Of course the only difference between technology and magic is that we understand technology, but those things beyond our comprehension are magic. If my guess is right, we've just about maxed out on our ability to comprehend technology. . . . This year, I think we pass the comprehension barrier and to assimilate the new tools we will begin to accept them as magic.

S. Nowak, *Administrative Radiology,* Nov. 1991.

Chapter 1

Design Considerations for Imaging Facilities

Medicine is a science, but the practice of medicine is an art. This is especially true in the branch of medicine called *medical imaging*. The art of applying medical imaging requires high-technology equipment, tremendous care and patience, and a unique sensitivity, and all these requirements have implications for imaging facility design.

Medical imaging requires numerous architectural features that can accommodate equipment needs as well as human needs. Properly designed architecture in imaging facilities enables radiologists and radiology administrators to apply the art—and science—of their medicine in the most efficient way.

The architecture of an imaging facility also is a reflection of its medical providers, the neighborhood surrounding these providers, and the community of patients and families who come to the facility for medical care. (See figure 1-1.) A well-designed imaging facility—that is, an imaging facility that provides comfortable surroundings and convenient access—can create a positive impression that will benefit patients and the community. Good design also can facilitate work flow and interaction among health care employees. Thus, both health care and design professionals strive to make the architecture of imaging facilities the best it can be.

Like medicine, architecture embraces both science and art. Subject to the laws of gravity and the effects of weather, it must endure over time. Health care architecture, being additionally subject to the needs of patients, staff, and the general public, must set the stage for interaction among people, between people and machinery, and between people and their communities.

When applied to medical imaging, this comprehensive view of architecture sometimes is difficult to maintain as planners and designers wrestle with the myriad technical requirements that challenge them daily. Consequently, imaging facilities often are viewed simply as places for high-technology equipment. However, the fact that imaging equipment may cost considerably more than the enclosure surrounding it should not detract from the human aspects of the imaging environment. It is vital that design professionals not focus on technology requirements so closely that they forget the needs of the people who will use that technology.

Coordinating the technical demands of medical equipment often usurps precious design time that the designer originally allocated for less-technical tasks. When this happens, designers can become reactive instead of visionary. Often the result is architecture that merely solves immediate or short-term problems, rather than producing solutions that create opportunities for human interaction and support the healing process.

The human needs within the imaging facility, such as natural lighting, convenient circulation, and concise wayfinding, are not optional considerations. They must be incorporated into the facility design from the beginning stages of the project.

As imaging technology becomes more complex, so does the challenge of integrating form and function. As the functional requirements for any building type become more complex,

Figure 1-1. Design as a Reflection of Quality of Care

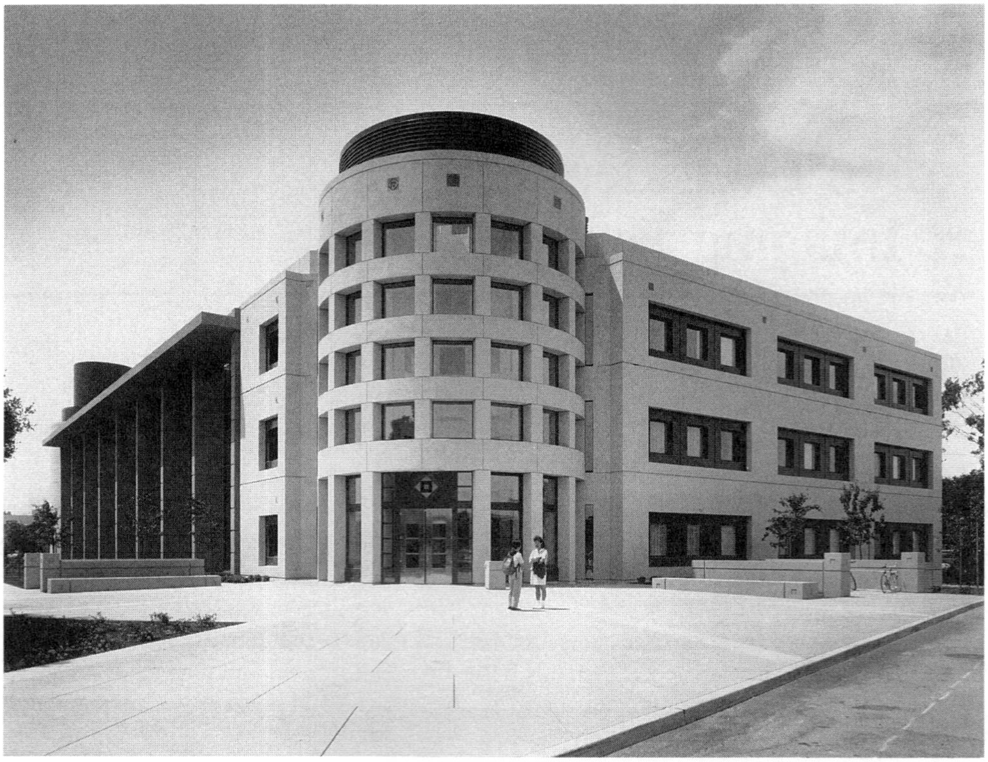

MSLS/MRS facility, Stanford University; design by Stone Marraccini Patterson, architects. Courtesy of SMP, San Francisco. Gregory Murphey, photographer. Used with permission.

so does the design process. One way to prevent technology from overpowering design is for the *architectural team* to thoroughly understand both the processes and the equipment used for medical imaging and for the *medical team* to understand how the design process will be orchestrated. With this approach, design professionals learn what questions to ask and when to ask them, and health professionals are better prepared to provide input into the design of their facility. Armed with this knowledge, the architectural and medical members of the project team can set the stage for high-quality health care architecture that meets the needs of both patients and staff. This chapter focuses on identifying those needs.

Special Needs of Imaging Facilities

How does the design of an imaging facility differ from that of other building types? It must accommodate the special needs of imaging patients and their families; the needs of the imaging staff including radiologists, technologists, other health care providers, administrators, clerical personnel, and housekeeping; and the needs of equipment in terms of its function, installation, maintenance, modification, and replacement.

The Needs of Patients

Patients and their families have many needs that can be addressed through effective imaging facility design. Some of these needs are for information, stress reduction, comfort, dignity, and privacy. If these needs can be addressed while patients are being treated at the imaging facility, patients will have a head start toward their ultimate goal of coping with their condition or attaining wellness.

Most patients come to an imaging facility to "solve a medical mystery." Ultrasound, magnetic resonance, computed tomography, or any one of a number of other imaging modalities offer special abilities to "see within" and visualize what otherwise would be "invisible" without their use. Because the information provided by these imaging modalities is used by the medical staff to determine a patient's course of treatment, it needs to be precise. In terms of facility design, this means that equipment has to be installed properly so that it can yield reliable and accurate results. It also means that user capacity must be considered to ensure that patients have access to the equipment they need in a timely manner.

In addition to accurate and timely information regarding their medical condition, patients have a great need for stress reduction. The diverse array of machinery, which enables radiologists and other physicians to diagnose and treat conditions, is foreign and even frightening to most patients. The odd postures patients must assume, the duration for which they must hold still, and the overall sense that their health and well-being may be determined in part by an electronically rendered illustration of their inner anatomy and physiology can be, at best, impersonal and intimidating. However, usually it is not the foreign instrumentation itself that patients are most frightened of but, rather, what it will tell about them.

Because patients already are under stress when they enter an imaging facility, the facility design should make it easy for them to find their way. A facility design that adds surprises—through circuitous circulation or unnecessarily long routes of travel—only heightens their level of anxiety.

Patients also need to be as comfortable as possible while waiting. Those undergoing nuclear medicine techniques may need to ingest radioactive substances before their scans, and those waiting for ultrasound scans may need to drink large quantities of water. Because patients often feel alienated in imaging facilities, waiting areas should be large enough to allow family members to be together (shown in figure 1-2) and comfortable enough to reduce patient stress, which can become a major obstacle to healing.

Patients also need to maintain a sense of dignity. When asked to remove clothing, patient dignity is taken away. However, when the surroundings are well designed, use quality finishes, and are adequately lighted, patients may feel less intimidated and more secure. Patient dignity is further assured when patients have a sense of privacy. They appreciate it when private offices and public spaces are acoustically treated with sound-absorbing materials that prevent their conversations from being overheard. Patient privacy also is enhanced when acoustic separation of patient and staff areas restricts the sounds of business within work areas.

The Needs of Staff

Imaging is an "information hub" of medicine. Staff members in an imaging facility have an even greater need than patients for precise, timely medical information. For example, imaging facilities must provide staff members with ready access to medical records, test results, scheduling and billing information, ancillary services information, and so on. Additionally, staff need adequate storage space.

To allow imaging facility staff members to perform their functions effectively, the flow of people, data, supplies, and equipment must be carefully planned. Each form of traffic moves with different characteristics and at different rates. Because facility design and layout influence work flow, they affect how well staff can conduct their business. Good design enables each type of work to proceed efficiently without restricting the flow of others.

Another factor in allowing staff members to perform their work effectively is that of ensuring that task lighting, the size and configuration of treatment rooms, and the many other elements that influence day-to-day job functions are matched to the type of work that staff will perform there and do not hinder staff efficiency. The needs of housekeeping and maintenance personnel also must be considered to ensure sanitary conditions.

In addition to timely, accurate information, good work flow, and appropriateness of design elements, staff members have other needs that affect imaging facility design. If based solely on the needs of equipment, for example, the enclosures for medical imaging services would be dark and monolithic. The weight of equipment and the requirements for radiation, radiofrequency, or magnetic shielding might suggest a windowless subterranean cave. However, staff members work long hours, often performing difficult tasks, and their work environment affects how they respond to and serve patients. They sometimes need break rooms and private areas to cope with the stresses of their jobs, and they appreciate pleasant surroundings as much as patients do. Thus, the needs of staff challenge designers to sculpt with color, lighting, and personality to improve the medical environment. Staff areas such as reading rooms and control rooms (shown in figure 1-3) deserve the same attention to detail and lighting as do public entries and waiting areas.

The Needs of Equipment

As imaging equipment becomes more computer based, the need for "clean" and uniform power and efficient air-conditioning systems is magnified. Therefore, infrastructure systems designed by engineers must be carefully coordinated with the architectural design.

Figure 1-2. A Large, Comfortable Waiting Area

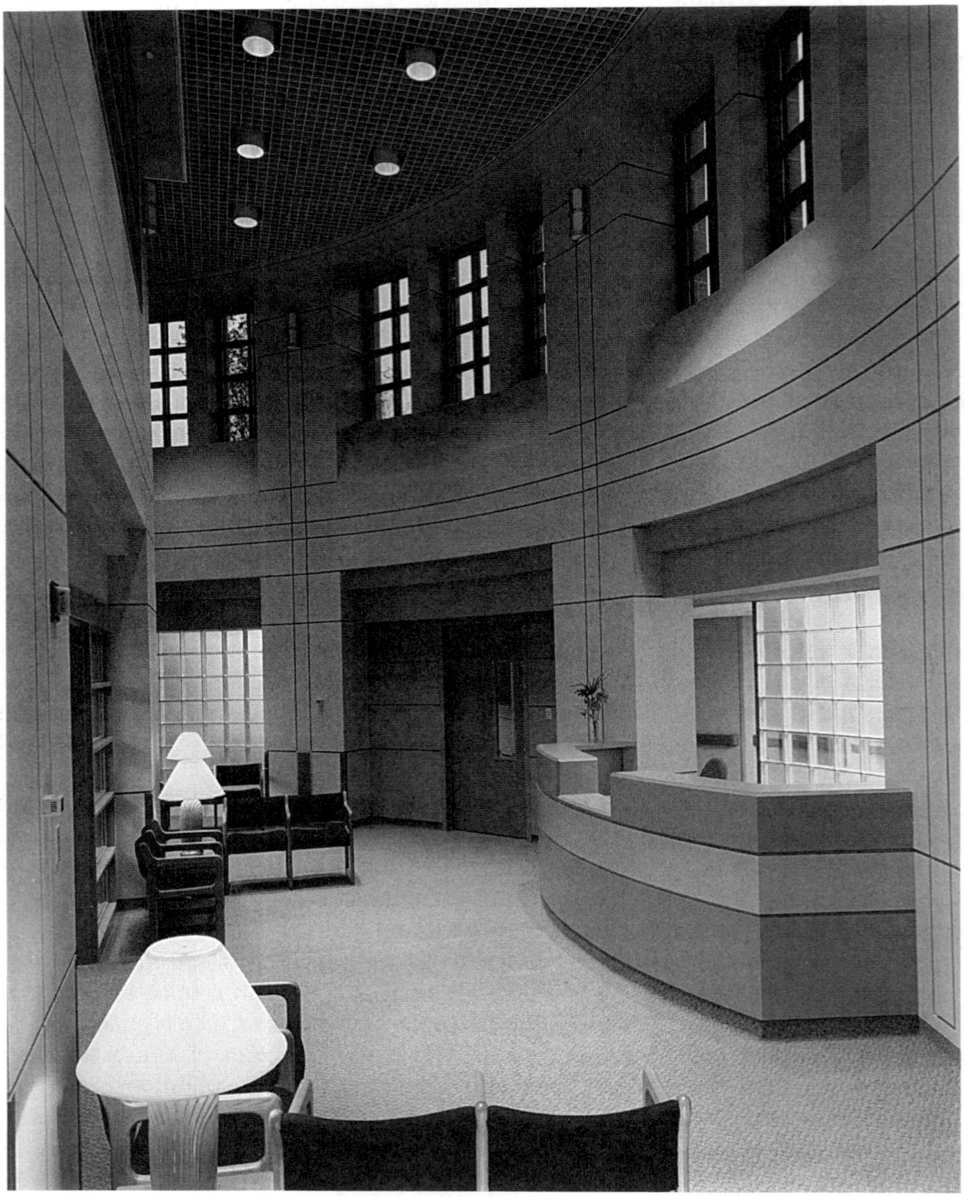

St. Louis University Medical Center; design by Stone Marraccini Patterson, architects. Courtesy of SMP, San Francisco. Alise O'Brien, photographer. Used with permission.

Figure 1-3. A Well-Designed Control Room

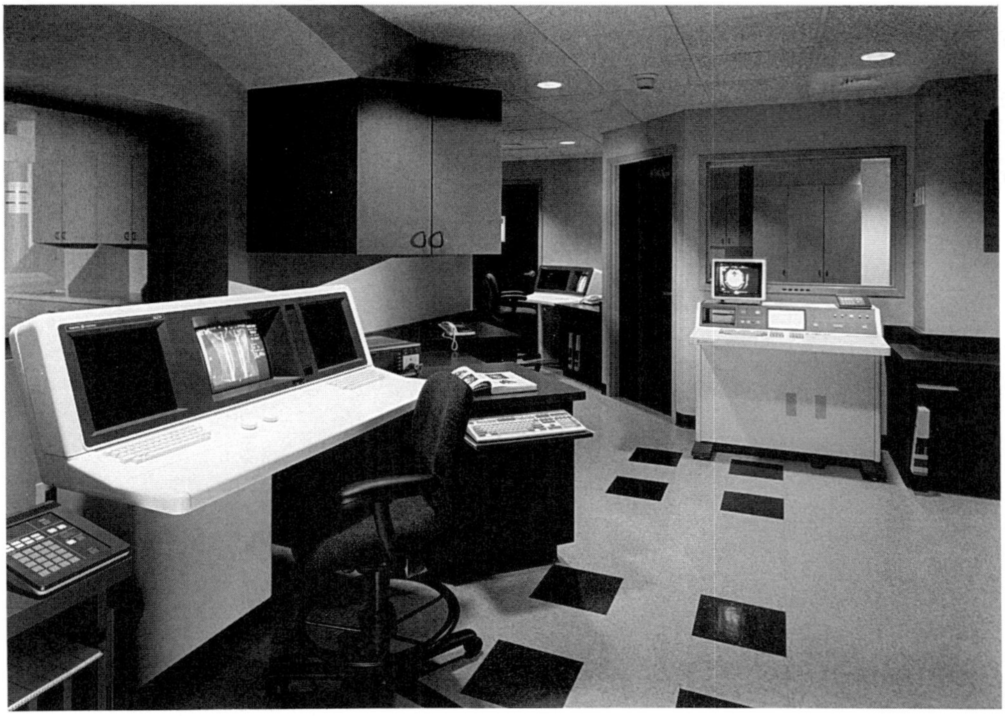

Courtesy of The Stein-Cox Group, Phoenix, Arizona. Photo by Mark Boisclair Photography, Phoenix, Arizona. Used with permission.

Because medical technology is changing at an increasingly rapid rate, the need for flexibility in every aspect of design becomes more crucial. Alternatives for future growth and modifications should be part of the initial design, not an afterthought.

Finally, although imaging equipment itself is shrinking in size, the capabilities of any single piece of equipment are expanding. As a result, multiple ancillary instruments may be used in the exam room. Therefore, the need for both examination space and support space (such as patient preparation areas and equipment storage rooms) may increase.

Implications

As we approach a new century—the second century of medical imaging—design, in its broadest definition, will continue to influence the quality of health care provided in many ways. Formal, functional, economic, and temporal aspects of the imaging environment determine how well the needs of medical imaging are met. Designers and health care providers who work closely together and understand the needs of patients, the needs of the health care staff, and the needs of equipment will be able to get maximum value from the architecture and technology in their imaging care facility.

Chapter 2

The Forces of Change in Imaging Facility Design

The 1990s have been a decade of unprecedented change for health care in the United States. Much of medical imaging is being reengineered, and the American health care system is being reshaped even more dramatically. Throughout the nation, health care is moving toward managed care in one form or another. Some regions of the country are leading this transformation; others are slowly following.

As a result, many of the incentives for providing imaging services and building imaging facilities present just a decade ago no longer apply. For example, in the past, fully occupied hospital nursing units and an abundance of heavily utilized imaging equipment meant more potential revenue. Today, under managed care systems, fewer occupied hospital beds mean lower expenses per covered life, and eliminating the unnecessary use of expensive diagnostic technology is a basic tenet of capitation. In the past, medical specialists had tremendous influence on the acquisition of technology. Today, and probably even more in the future, primary care providers are given greater responsibility for cost containment through controlled use of expensive technology. In addition, technology assessment is regularly performed by diverse committees and boards.

An awareness and understanding of the drivers that affect health care and imaging are important for anyone involved in the architecture of imaging facilities. Ironically, the wave of change is sometimes so rapid that new issues are likely to emerge within the course of planning and constructing a single project.

This chapter briefly reviews concurrent developments in health care and radiology throughout the past century. It also explores the present role of medical imaging and discusses factors that influence both imaging and architecture for imaging facilities. The chapter concludes with a set of challenges that architects and health care staff must address when planning a successful imaging facility.

Historical Developments in Health Care and Radiology

Following is a discussion of some of the major health care changes and developments that have taken place in the United States since the late 19th century. It is divided into four segments: the growth of American medical schools and hospitals and concurrent events in radiology (circa 1880–1910), the growth of cost accounting and imaging in hospitals (circa 1900–1920), the outpatient explosion (circa 1985), and the advent of managed care and information management (circa 1990).

The Growth of American Medical Schools and Hospitals and Concurrent Events in Radiology

Prior to 1880, fewer than 200 acute care hospitals and only 3 professional medical schools existed in the United States. However, by the first decade of the 20th century, there were more than 5,000 acute care hospitals and 1,000 medical schools. This 30-year period of explosive growth has been characterized by some as the first health care revolution in the United States.

This health care revolution coincided with Roentgen's discovery of X rays in 1895, Salvioni's description of the fluoroscopic "cryptoscope" in 1896,[1] and Edison's development of the fluoroscope, also in 1896. As described in figure 2-1, in the early years after these discoveries, not only was it difficult to obtain the electrical power to take X rays, but also physicians did not recognize their applications in patient care and regarded the findings as a curiosity.[2,3]

In the years following the first health care revolution, radiology slowly evolved from a curiosity into an interpretive function used to evaluate radiographic images that assisted other medical components of the hospital, such as the emergency (or accident) department and surgery. During this early period, X-ray services (for those institutions that had X-ray equipment) often depended on the hospital's general budget for funding and usually were given little financial support. This lack of funding was evident in the architecture of early imaging facilities. Frequently, they were small and dark and sometimes were situated below grade, that is, beneath the floors inhabited by most people.[4] Architect Edward F. Stevens depicted some diverse arrangements of X-ray facilities and in 1918 wrote about the growing interest in the use of "Roentgen-rays."

The Growth of Cost Accounting and Imaging in Hospitals

Fortunately, cost accounting began to be used in hospitals within a few decades following the discovery of X rays. Developed several years earlier, primarily for factories and manufacturing businesses, cost accounting enabled financial administrators to identify which products and services made or lost money.[5] Also during this period, American hospitals were being transformed from long-term homes for the chronically ill into "scientific-appearing facilities for acute intervention," growing rapidly in size and number. At the same time, they were beginning to draw middle-class paying patients.[6] The combination of cost accounting and patient revenues would do much to help boost the proliferation of imaging technology throughout the United States.

However, it was not until later that medical imaging advanced as a distinct branch of medicine, responsible initially for diagnosis and later for treatment of disease and injury. Eventually, imaging became a service essential to all aspects of the practice of medicine. As diagnostic and therapeutic radiology developed, imaging departments were reorganized as profit centers capable of generating considerable revenue.

The Outpatient Explosion

Beginning in the late 1970s and early 1980s and continuing to the present, a second health care revolution occurred. Fueled by economic concerns, technologic developments, and consumer education, the need for lengthy hospitalization was questioned. Insurance companies and regulators began to examine several alternatives to inpatient treatment. Additionally, federal

Figure 2-1. Some Interesting Events in the Early History of Radiology

1896 Dr. Harvey Cushing, a famous neurosurgeon, set up the X-ray department at Johns Hopkins Hospital in Baltimore. There he "exposed radiographic plates with the aid of a medical student who had to turn the crank of a static machine for 45 minutes to generate sufficient current."

1903 The first X-ray department at the Boston Children's Hospital was obliged to obtain its power from the Opera House nearby because the hospital had no electric current. When there was no music, there was no current. No opera, no X rays!

1912 Patients with broken bones severe enough to require surgery usually did not have an X ray taken before going to the operating room for repair.

cost-containment policies and diminishing reimbursement structures began to diminish the profit-generating potential of imaging departments.

In 1985, the prospective payment system through the use of diagnosis-related groups (DRGs), a national listing of diagnosis-related payments for medical services, first limited reimbursement for treatment provided to hospitalized patients. Suddenly health care delivery shifted its focus to outpatient treatment, which was not covered by DRGs.

As a result, patients who were hospitalized tended to be more acutely ill than had been the case with patients who had been hospitalized before that time. Patients with less-acute illnesses soon chose their place of diagnosis and treatment from among a number of outpatient settings. It was during this period that outpatient imaging centers first grew rapidly in number. The migration of imaging services to ambulatory care facilities, both freestanding and hospital based, continues today to some extent. (However, under managed care, construction of new imaging facilities in general has declined as most providers focus their efforts—and capital investment—on surviving in a challenging marketplace.)

Due to both the decline in inpatient length of stay and rapid advances in medical technology, the diagnostic and treatment components of many hospitals required expansion and revision during the changeover to outpatient services. The result was that construction of nursing units declined as imaging, surgery, and ancillary components of health care grew. Nonhospital health care facilities such as surgery centers, urgent care centers, and freestanding imaging centers flourished.

By the 1980s, imaging had developed a dual role. On the one hand, it was integral to centralized medical treatment within acute care hospitals. Yet it also was an important link in the referral network served by diverse, decentralized, and often independent outpatient settings. These settings included hospitals, clinics, and physicians' offices. In addition, imaging results were communicated to other settings, such as physicians' homes and remote reading centers, as needed.

By decade's end, the number of hospital beds relative to ancillary services had declined. This often involved the closure of independent hospitals and multihospital organizations. Many independent providers joined larger health maintenance organizations, managed care organizations, or preferred provider networks. By this time, electronic information systems had begun to connect a few hospitals with remote imaging sites. In some instances, digital images could travel electronically across the hall to complete a medical record or across the country to be interpreted by a radiology specialist.

The Era of Managed Care and Information Management

During the early 1990s, escalating health care costs dominated the nation's economic concerns and even affected the presidential elections. Proposed health care reform packages and moves toward increased managed care focused on providing universal health care coverage, promoting incentives throughout the health care system for cost reduction, and eliminating waste by improving methods of medical information management.

The impact of these initiatives on imaging is evident in three areas. First, utilization of many modalities has declined as insurance companies and other payers began requiring preauthorizations for the use of imaging procedures. Second, the preventive aspects of imaging (for example, early screening for suspected disease) have increased in importance as managed care shifts from an emphasis on disease treatment to an emphasis on health maintenance. Third, the perceived value of hospitalwide information systems (HISs), radiology information systems (RISs), and even picture archiving and communications systems (PACSs) and image management and communications systems (IMACSs) has increased. However, implementation of these systems has been slow because of the cost of implementing the systems and retraining personnel.

Coincidentally, the concepts behind health care reform began to take shape at a time when managed care was strong in some states but nonexistent in others and when much of the work force was composed of computer-literate workers. The proliferation of personal computers in the 1980s and 1990s quickly changed the magnitude of the impact that information now has on aspects of both the personal and professional lives of Americans. Computer networks, fax machines, and cellular phones make information immediately available 24 hours a day, fostering what some call "the information revolution." More important, personnel—both young and old—were expected to be, and in fact are now, capable of operating computers and many other types of information management tools. The increased reliance on electronic information management, coupled with computer-literate personnel, created the potential to restructure both the operational and the architectural aspects of health care in general—and medical imaging in particular.

As mentioned earlier, electronic information management has begun to affect health care and imaging services by enabling remote departments within hospitals and remote facilities across the country to be electronically linked. Financial, medical, and personal data, which previously had been delivered on paper, now pass through interconnecting cable networks that make them available electronically. Ideally, this results in more work being accomplished in less time, but it can also result in higher facility construction costs when sophisticated information management equipment and networks must be installed in new or renovated facilities.

Another result is that functional areas, which in the past had to be adjacent to certain activities, now can be located in remote locations. In fact, the physical organization of imaging departments is changing as image management and communications systems are slowly being incorporated into some daily routines. (See chapter 7, "Image Management and Film Processing.")

Although technology is now available for integrated electronic information management systems, implementation of such networks is not universal. Until digital image management systems become less expensive, and until more radiologists are comfortable diagnosing from computer monitors in place of film, the integration of electronic information systems into radiology departments will continue at its slow pace.

Yet there are compelling reasons to employ computers in radiology, especially considering some estimates that the entire body of medical knowledge doubles every five years. The ability to use new disease facts (information) and strategies for applying those facts (knowledge) could enable radiologists to give better care, if only they could remember it all.[7]

> Computers will become our new partners as we meet radiology's escalating demands, and they will keep us at the cutting edge of radiologic expertise. Intelligent radiologic workstations will not only retrieve and display images, but will also process them and provide "another set of eyes" to minimize the chances of missing important findings.[8]

Parallel Changes in Health Care and Medical Imaging

If a time line showing the milestones in medical imaging during the past century is compared to one showing key events in health care, a parallel pattern emerges. (See figure 2-2.) First, as stated earlier, the discovery of X rays coincided with the development of medical schools

Figure 2-2. Time Line Showing Major Events in Imaging and Health Care

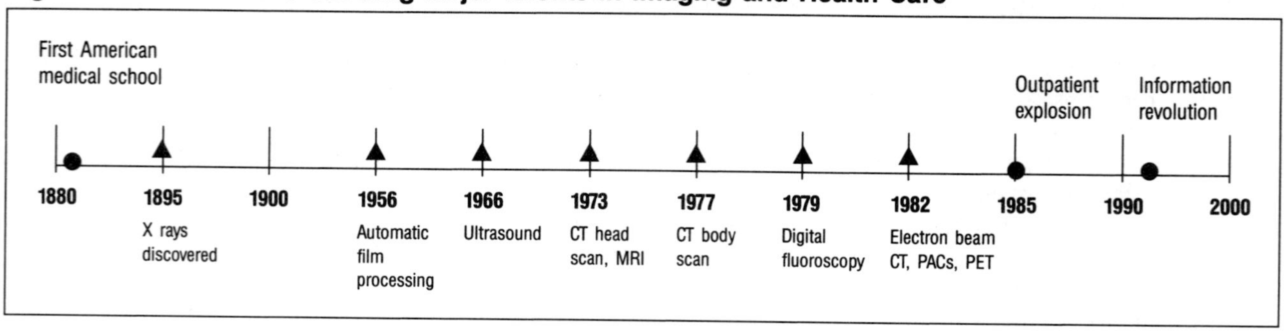

in the United States. Next, many of the new sophisticated imaging techniques such as computed tomography (CT) and magnetic resonance imaging (MRI) that make imaging so powerful were first introduced during, or just before, the explosion in outpatient services. Most are now appropriate for both inpatient and outpatient exams. Finally, the first large-scale installations of picture archiving and communications systems, information management and communication systems, radiology information systems, teleradiology, computed radiography, and other forms of digital medical image management coincide with the emergence of managed care and the information revolution. (A more detailed chronology of medical imaging milestones is shown in table 2-1.)

Just as they have in the past, developments in health care and technology will continue to influence the architecture of imaging facilities. Thus, an awareness of current trends in these fields is helpful for both health care and design professionals in approaching imaging projects.

The Role of Imaging Today

Recently, much attention has focused on imaging's preventive abilities. New techniques of viewing metabolic activity, combined with noninvasive procedures that provide exquisite detail of internal anatomy, now identify the potential for disease before it occurs. In this sense, medical imaging has developed from a reporting function, interpreting data about patients' past and present conditions, into a predicting and treating function, warning of and preventing physical deterioration beyond the early stages of involvement.

Additionally, health care cost-containment policies and a general trend toward noninvasive medical treatment have enabled imaging to replace surgery as the procedure of choice for diagnosing many, if not most, injuries and illnesses. The boundary between surgery and radiology has been further obscured by new interventional applications, allowing some imaging rooms to function as surgical suites. Such interventional suites have greater requirements for air handling, infection control, and preprocedural and postprocedural patient holding areas. In fact, many are located within the surgery department rather than within the radiology department. At the same time, imaging has become a significant component of surgical practice. (See chapter 14, "Imaging outside the Radiology Department.") Interventional radiology is less traumatic than surgery and thus requires less recovery time. For example, various cardiac procedures performed in the catheterization lab eliminate the need for open-heart surgery, which is more invasive and requires longer recuperation times for patients.

The extended role of medical imaging in diagnosis and treatment encourages researchers and equipment vendors to expand the limits of imaging technology. The cost of this research is significant, and yet the results have a considerable positive impact on patient outcome. As a result, medical imaging can be either one of the more cost-effective or one of the more costly health care services provided today, depending on how it is used.

Imaging's Complexity and Competitiveness among Specialties

Medical imaging is a highly complex blend of diagnostic and therapeutic subspecialties, which has implications for the role that imaging plays in health care. Questions regarding a given modality's appropriateness, its cost in relation to its results, and the most qualified type of specialist to administer it are constantly being debated. In addition, imaging referral patterns are shifting. In the past, referrals came primarily from surgical and medical specialists. In the future, more will come from primary care generalists and payer gatekeepers.

Many factors must be considered in determining which modality is best for a given condition. For example, will fast magnetic resonance techniques be able to reveal the same metabolic activity that single-photon emission computed tomography (SPECT) and positron emission tomography (PET) are so good at displaying? Does MRI provide a better image of the spine than CT? (See chapter 6, "Imaging Modalities.") Which modality is less expensive per procedure? Which is more cost-effective in terms of overall patient treatment?

Table 2-1. A Chronology of Medical Imaging Milestones

Imaging Technique	First Described	First Described by
X rays discovered	1895	Roentgen
Fluoroscopy	1896	Salvioni, Edison
Cineradiography	1896	Bleyer
Portable X ray	1901	Williams
Cardiac catheterization	1929[a]	Forssmann
Transverse axial tomography	1937, 1938[b]	Watson, Kieffer
Automatic film processor	1942[c]	
Principles of magnetic resonance	1946	Purcell, Bloch
Magnetic resonance spectroscopy	1946	
Diagnostic ultrasound: first described	1947–1948[d]	Dussik
Fluoroscopic image intensifier	1948[e]	Coltman
Scintillation scanner	1949[f]	Cassen
Multidirectional tomography	1951[g]	
Positron scanner	1953[h]	Brownell, Sweet
SPECT (single-photon emission computed tomography)	1963[i]	Kuhl, Edwards
Percutaneous transluminal angioplasty	1964[j]	Dotter, Judkins
Mass-produced dedicated mammography unit	1965[k]	CGR Company
Radionuclide multiplane tomographic scanner	1965[l]	Anger
Diagnostic ultrasound: first clinical use	1966[m]	
Computed tomographic head scan	1972[n]	Hounsfield
Computed tomographic body scan	1973[o]	
Magnetic resonance imaging: first image of a heterogeneous object	1973[p]	Lauterbur
Magnetic resonance imaging: first image of a live animal	1976[q]	
Magnetic resonance imaging: first human image	1977[r]	Damadian
Digital fluoroscopy/digital subtraction angiography	1979[s]	Mistretta
Commercial superconducting MR imager	1980[t]	
Magnetic resonance imaging: first routine clinical use	1981	
Picture archiving and communications systems	1982[u]	Boyd
Electron beam tomography	1982	
Photo-stimulable phosphors, computed radiography	1984[v]	Fuji
Biomagnetics/superconductive quantum interference device	1988[w]	
Magnetic resonance angiography	1990	

Sources:

a. Bushong, S. C. *Radiologic Science for Technologists: Physics, Biology, and Protection.* 5th ed. St. Louis: Mosby-Year Book, 1993, p. 12.
b. Eisenberg, R. L. *Radiology: An Illustrated History.* St. Louis: Mosby-Year Book, 1992, p. 435.
c. Bushong, 1993, p. 12.
d. Eisenberg, p. 454.
e. Bushong, 1993, p. 12.
f. Eisenberg, p. 417.
g. Bushong, 1993, p. 12.
h. Eisenberg, p. 420.
i. Bushong, 1993, p. 12.
j. Eisenberg, p. 527.
k. Eisenberg, p. 372.
l. Eisenberg, p. 421.
m. Bushong, 1993, p. 12.
n. Eisenberg, p. 473.
o. Eisenberg, p. 474.
p. Eisenberg, p. 474.
q. Eisenberg, p. 467.
r. Eisenberg, p. 469.
s. Bushong, S. C. *Radiologic Science for Technologists.* 3rd ed. St. Louis: Mosby-Year Book, 1984, p. 12.
t. Bushong, 1984, p. 12.
u. Bushong, 1984, p. 12.
v. Bushong, 1984, p. 12.
w. Bushong, 1984, p. 12.

The comprehensive nature of imaging often leads to different opinions about which specialist is best qualified to perform particular procedures. For example:

- Is interventional angiography (which was pioneered by radiologists) the realm of cardiovascular surgeons or interventional radiologists?
- With such interventional procedures, where does radiology end and surgery begin?
- Is a radiologist more qualified to interpret fetal ultrasound than an obstetrician?
- Will a miniature ultrasound stethoscope result in the demise of sonography as a radiologic subspecialty because all physicians will be trained in the technique and own their own equipment?[9]

Competition among imaging modalities sometimes leads to internal turf battles among those specialists who develop new techniques and those generalists who refer patients to them but might perform the procedures themselves instead.

The politics of medicine often complicate the planning process for imaging facilities, but they cannot be avoided. Territorialism is as fundamental to medical planning as the forces of gravity are to structural engineering. Therefore, a successful planning team must be trained in diplomacy as well as in facility planning.

The Forces of Change

Some of the conditions that began to change health care architecture during the explosion of outpatient services in the 1980s still exist today. In fact, patient-oriented design, economic concerns, and technological developments now shape the nature of health care delivery to a greater extent than ever before. These factors directly influence health insurance premiums, federal approval of new drugs and equipment, and even television advertisement. Indirectly, but in a very powerful way, they give form to a new health care architecture.

On careful analysis, medical imaging and the architecture of imaging facilities appear to be influenced in parallel. Depending on the point of view, the key forces shaping health care and health care architecture today can be seen as either being restrictive or creating new opportunities. In either case, they must be factored into the decision-making process for design and planning.

Patient-Oriented Design

One significant development influencing the architecture of imaging facilities is the change in attitude toward the needs of patients. Often, a delivery system that focuses on patients will allow the patients to use health care services more efficiently and therefore cost less to operate. In addition, many health care providers recognize that the physical environment of the health care facility affects the healing process. Within the often severe limitations of construction budgets, it is possible to provide natural lighting, clear wayfinding systems, and pleasant furnishings. For inpatients, a soothing environment can even hasten the recovery process. Faster recoveries obviously translate to cost savings.

Patient-Oriented Design and Imaging

One health care delivery concept, called *patient-focused care,* suggests that a drastic restructuring of the traditional health care delivery model (and thus the delivery of imaging services) can improve the patient's experience in the hospital as well as generate operational savings. Although a patient focus is not new to health care, this concept recently has been revisited in a way that modifies the traditional arrangement of hospital departments. Thus, it has broad implications on the form and function of health care facilities, especially imaging services.

Proponents of patient focusing suggest that the compartmentalization of services typical of the traditional hospital model requires an inordinate amount of inpatient movement to and from centralized departments with fixed equipment and specialized staffing.

> This compartmentalization, which establishes a narrow sense of what constitutes a job, can turn a simple task into an operational nightmare. Under this system, a routine X ray can require the involvement of 20 employees and the performance of 40 or more discrete tasks.[10]

In contrast, the revised patient-focused concept organizes the hospital around inpatient zones rather than medical disciplines. It promotes decentralization of a portion of many departments so that staff and equipment can come to the patient, instead of the patient being transported throughout the hospital. As a result, the number of distinct *patient encounters* is theoretically reduced, the number of staff full-time equivalents (FTEs) is cut, and the environment for staff to become cross-trained is enhanced.

> Hospitals employing a more progressive approach to operations can focus patient care while simultaneously simplifying workflows and achieving significant savings.[11]

One implication of patient focusing is that basic imaging services could be decentralized and repeated within distinct inpatient care areas. Under this approach, basic imaging services are provided adjacent to, or within, clusters of nursing units. The clusters generally consist of about 100 inpatient beds (subdivided into smaller nursing units); this arrangement is based on the assumption that the cost of additional imaging equipment will be outweighed by savings in the number of personnel needed to provide imaging services. (See figure 2-3.)

However, many observers doubt that the decentralized approach will result in cost savings. Critics of the patient-focused concept cite licensing restrictions and information management limitations as obstacles. Regardless of whether patient-focused care will become a new health care paradigm or simply a passing trend, more attention to the patient and increased productivity for health care workers are key issues to consider in the architecture of imaging facilities.

Figure 2-3. Patient-Focused Imaging Services

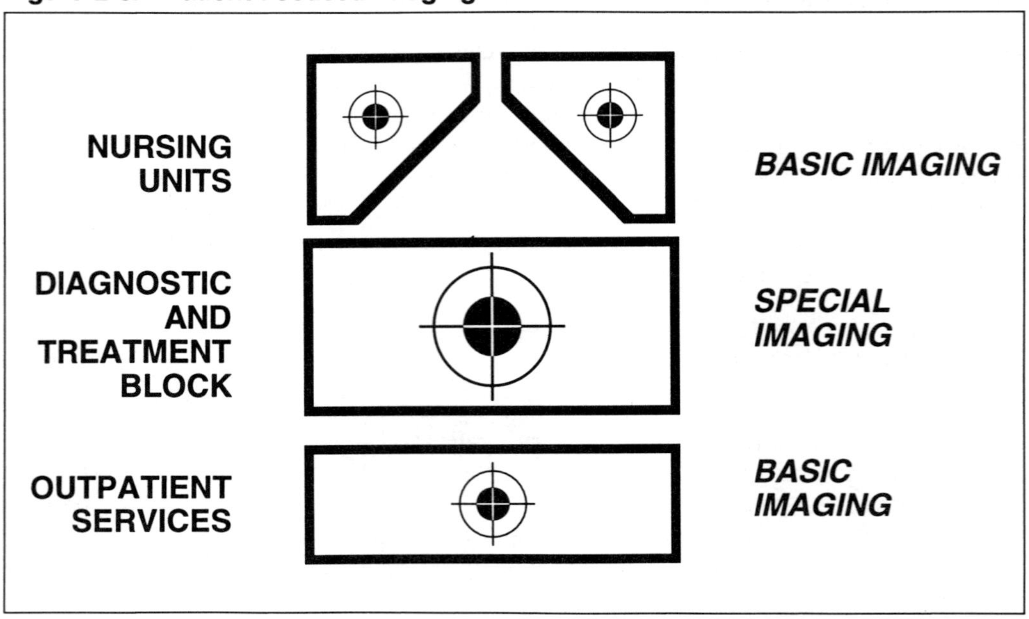

Patient-Oriented Design and Architectural Design

Because their perceptions about the architecture of an imaging facility influence how patients feel about the care provided there, special attention must be paid to design issues. For many people, the notion of health care architecture still brings to mind an image of large, impersonal institutional buildings, and the terms *hospital green* and *sterile environment* remain in the mind's eye as a carryover from past decades. Perhaps—because many hospitals from that era are still in operation—the "medical machine" stereotype will not easily disappear.

However, the notion that health care precludes dynamic design is changing. Patients prefer health care buildings to be user-friendly and unintimidating, and designers can do much to promote these qualities in imaging facilities. Imaging facilities—replete with technical complexity—now provide both the need and the opportunity for crafting a humane environment inside and out. Today, there is greater awareness of the healing environment's beneficial effect on patients and staff. Most designers recognize that patient recovery hastens and staff productivity increases in properly planned, well-lighted spaces.

Patients respond to environments that are designed to meet their specific needs. (See the section entitled Image in chapter 8, "Design Concepts.") They also respond to architectural packaging—the form and style that convey a facility's personality—as they develop first and lasting impressions of a facility. Like people, buildings have unique personalities. Some attract; others repel. All reflect on the quality of care provided within the facility. The strength of a facility's image depends on the clarity of the design concept and the skill by which it is articulated.

In today's changing medical environment, health care facilities need to maintain a positive image to reflect the quality of care they provide and to remain viable partners with other health care entities. The design and planning of an imaging facility can be an opportunity to promote a positive image if it takes into account patients' preferences and involves close collaboration between the medical staff and the architect.

Economics

Form follows financing! Economic variables have a profound influence on imaging facilities, affecting factors such as the ownership of facilities, staffing patterns, equipment acquisition, and the ability to acquire new technology. Because facility construction represents a relatively small part of total health care expenditures, the most significant savings come from the effective utilization of health care personnel. However, economic variables also influence how an imaging facility is designed. Design elements need to provide functional and aesthetic value. Design concepts need to allow for operational efficiency and provide a reasonable level of comfort.

Economics and Imaging

As the rules for medical reimbursement change, so do the referral patterns that affect imaging services. Because imaging services are so dependent on referrals from other physicians and because the reimbursement rates for imaging services are declining, not too long ago, many radiologists—in association with other health care providers—began opening their own imaging centers. Questions of self-referral and overreferral of imaging services soon led to legislation that places strict limitations on such joint ventures. Other legislation simply limits the profit-making potential of both hospital-based and freestanding imaging centers.

Ever since prospective pricing concepts were applied to health care reimbursement in the 1980s, insurers and legislators have been the ones who determine fees for service. DRGs are individual elements of a federally regulated price list that limit the dollar amount providers are reimbursed for treating specific medical conditions. Because each condition or DRG corresponds to a fixed-reimbursement price, rather than actual treatment costs, practitioners are given financial incentives to tighten their treatment budgets and to ensure that both staffing policies and equipment acquisitions are cost-effective.

Under managed care arrangements, cost control is even more aggressive. Capitation (the payment of an annual or monthly dollar amount per member or covered life) encourages providers to eliminate unnecessary medical treatment. To ensure efficient operations, it is essential to have proper facility layout. As the workload capacity of imaging equipment increases, the facility's ability to enable staff to work more efficiently also must increase. Medical planners should consider current departmental traffic patterns as well as how those patterns may be changing with the increased use of electronic image management and communications systems.

With regard to equipment, many facilities have responded to cost containment by seeking vendors that have developed "economy" equipment lines. These emphasize solid, dependable technology without the bells and whistles found in some of their more expensive models. For example, recent improvements in permanent magnet design suggest a cost-effective alternative (with some operational limitations) to higher-strength superconductive MRI equipment.

Much of the latest generation of equipment tries to minimize space and facility requirements. This may lower installation costs but not necessarily the price of the equipment itself. Some models of CT scanners now require less space than they did a few years ago in addition to requiring less-sophisticated air-conditioning and power supply equipment. (See figure 2-4.) However, a manufacturer's minimum dimensions are not necessarily conducive to optimal use of the space. (See chapter 12, "Space Requirements.")

Figure 2-4. Planning Guide Showing Minimal Requirements for Installation of Specific CT Equipment

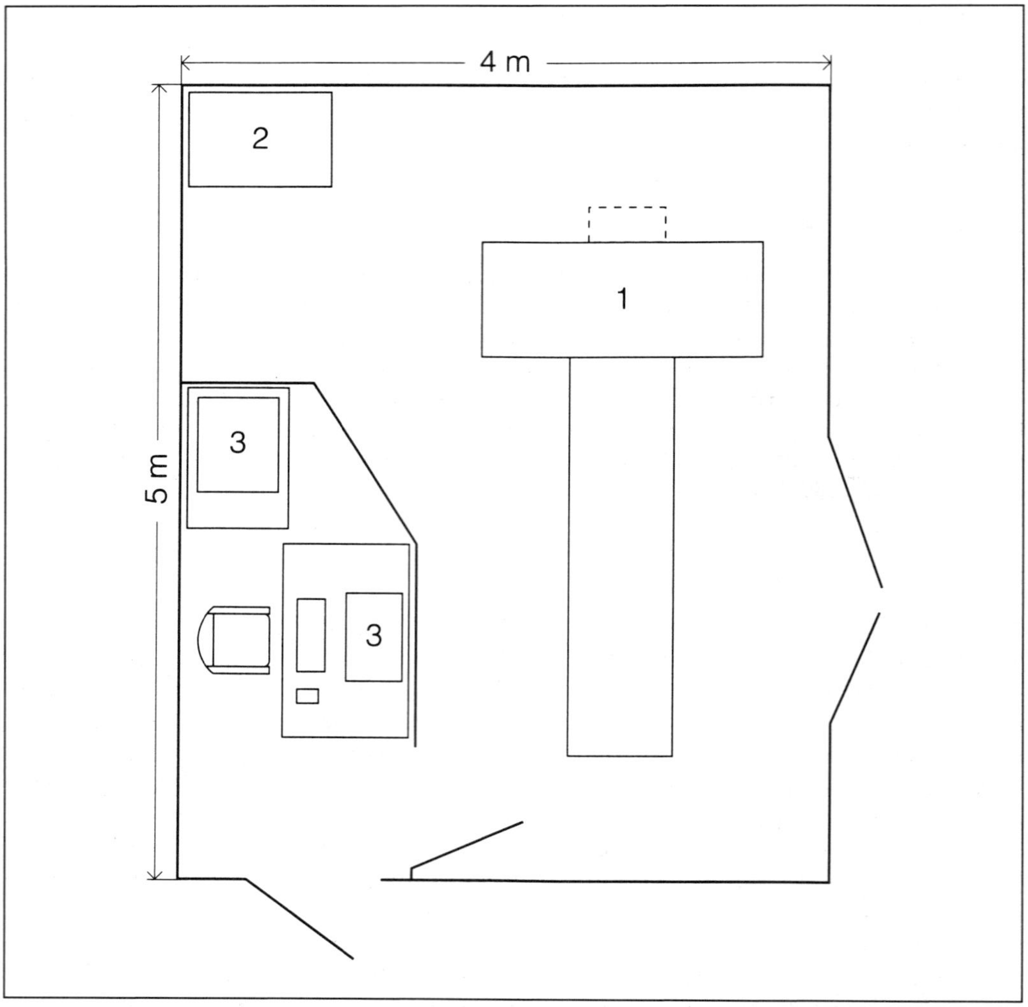

Note: Minimal dimensions do not generally yield optimal functional conditions. (1) Gantry with table, (2) power distribution system, (3) central console with imaging system and cassette camera.

Planning guide for CT courtesy of Siemens Medical Systems, Inc., Iselin, New Jersey. Used with permission.

Another way to increase operational efficiency and cut costs is to increase patient throughput, thereby enabling more patients to be examined with less equipment. Fast image acquisition and rapid film-processing techniques enable greater patient throughput and thus increase productivity. Each has been improved for most imaging modalities.

New imaging techniques raise larger economic questions about whether unrestricted medical treatment is a right or a privilege. Is it appropriate? Is it even a good idea? The debate continues. The current health care system in the United States is unaffordable for many. One view—held by Gail Wilensky, former Health Care Financing Administration (HCFA) administrator, as well as others—suggests that "the public's attraction to new medical technology is at least partly to blame for escalating medical-care costs. . . ."[12]

However, not everyone would agree that technology is to blame for rising health care costs. Another view, held by many medical outsiders as well as those within the profession, suggests that the high cost of health care is testimony to the overall success of modern medicine. Medical professionals can now treat so many diseases and illnesses because of the excellent knowledge base that enables them to know these conditions exist and to detect them early. Our aging population, another indicator of medicine's success, means people now live long enough to become affected by more chronic illness than previously. Some people feel that it is longevity and quality of life expectations that raise the cost of health care and not just technology.

With increased attention focused on economic forces in health care, many new technical improvements may never be brought to fruition. Recent legislation and a national mandate to lower health care costs and increase accessibility to services may hinder manufacturers' research and product development:

> A variety of methods to restrain these costs have been proposed and in some instances implemented; each one is likely to slow development of medical technology. These plans include outcomes research, development of practice guidelines, utilization reviews, a DRG-like payment system for outpatient services, and introduction of strict medical device legislation. But the most far-reaching policy is the new emphasis the government and third-party insurers are placing on cost-effectiveness.
>
> In deciding payment for health-care services by HCFA, when there are competing technologies available, we have the responsibility to examine the cost-effectiveness and to decide which technologies to cover, Wilensky said.
>
> New technologies will be at a disadvantage. They will have no track records, so conducting research to determine their effectiveness will be expensive. Manufacturers will have to obtain that information—and they will have to do it on their own.[13]

Another concept for cost containment is to ration medical care by limiting treatment. Care would be given only to those patients who have a high likelihood of showing a positive return on the initial financial investment. However, this approach raises serious fundamental ethical issues and questions the very basis of medicine itself.

Efforts to limit physician fees have had some effect. Cost containment of physician fees runs parallel to the regulatory efforts that already limit inpatient reimbursement. Federal legislation known as the resource-based relative value scale (RBRVS) became effective several years ago. Under RBRVS, radiologists' Medicare fees were cut by more than 30 percent. At the same time that Medicare reimbursement and radiologists' professional fees are being reduced, operational costs are escalating. "It's a fact of life that radiologists are going to get paid less. It's either going to be a whole lot less or just a lot less."[14]

Economics and the Quality of Architecture

With significant efforts under way to regulate the cost of health care—both medical and facility costs—the processes of delivering health care and designing health care architecture have become more complicated. Consequently, the price of architectural innovation (particularly in imaging facilities, where equipment costs are already high) now receives more scrutiny than before.

To preserve design quality in imaging facilities, two things must occur. First, image, ambiance, and aesthetics—those aspects of architecture that are difficult to quantify—need to support, rather than compromise, the delivery of imaging services. In this way, design amenities provide fundamental value and not additional expense. Second, communication between members of the project team needs to be clear and direct; miscommunication can lead to costly compromises in design and construction.

The Cost of Construction and the Value of High-Quality Design

Compared to the price of commercial or retail construction, the cost of building an imaging facility includes many additional premiums. Due to the heating, ventilating, and air-conditioning (HVAC) requirements of most imaging equipment and the vertical clearance of the equipment itself, floor-to-floor heights tend to be great, as illustrated in figure 2-5. (See chapter 12, "Space Requirements.") This means more materials and therefore higher cost. The weight of equipment also leads to increased cost due to the need for greater structural capacities and special mounting assemblies. (See chapter 15, "Physical Properties Influencing Design.") In addition, power requirements are high and special lighting usually is required. (See chapter 16, "Utility Requirements.")

Another consideration unique to imaging—radiation protection—also adds some expense. The cost of radio-frequency (RF) and magnetic shielding, where required, also adds up. (See chapter 15, "Physical Properties Influencing Design.") Finally, facilities designed to treat patients often are subject to more restrictive and thus more costly construction codes and regulations than other facility types. Despite the sum of all these special construction requirements, it is well recognized that imaging equipment is often more costly than the enclosure surrounding it.

If the preceding paragraphs describe *mandatory* construction features for imaging facilities, how much more will *good* or even *great* design cost? High-quality design in itself is not necessarily expensive; in fact, it should provide savings through effective use of space as well as interest and inspiration through innovation. Creative planning enables staffing and operational economies and allows for changes over time without disrupting present operations.

The human element of imaging facility design sometimes is overlooked but is crucial in design planning. The perceptions of staff, who spend much of their time within the space, and the emotions of patients, who are often terrified of the very events that necessitate their presence there, pose significant design opportunities. Sensitivity to the three dimensions of space and a judicious use of quality finishes can yield an exceptional environment without exceeding the realities and constraints of conservative budgets.

Figure 2-5. Section through an Imaging Room

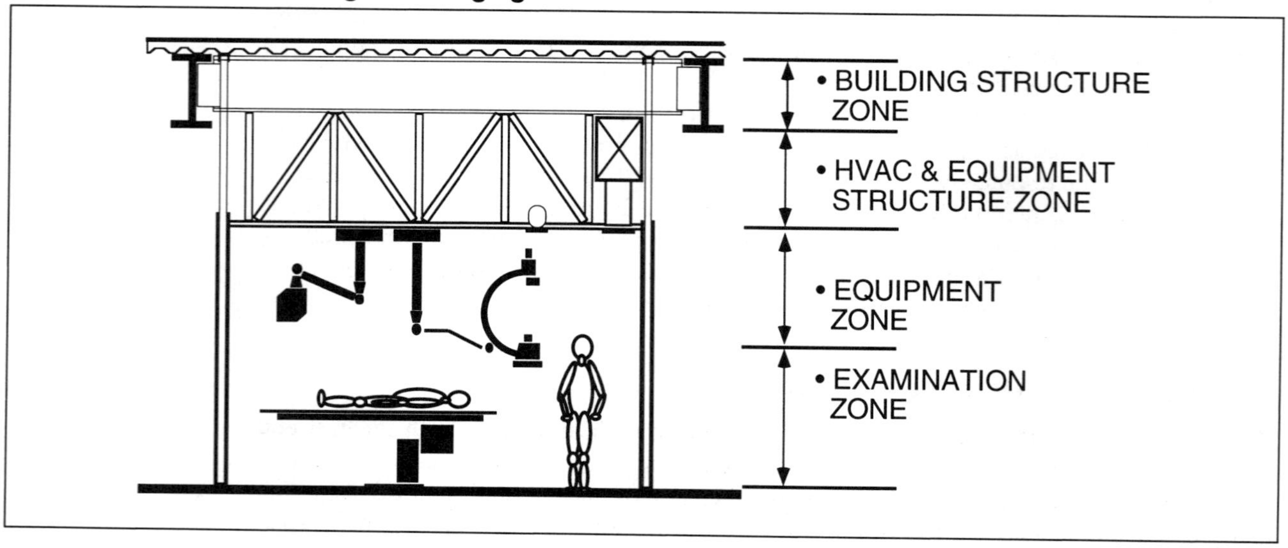

The Potential for Miscommunication in Complex Projects

The general concerns about clear communication among parties involved in any architectural project apply to the design of imaging facilities and have economic ramifications—that is, buildings are constructed by builders and not by architects. Builders rely on contract documents—drawings and specifications—prepared by architects to learn about the quality and nature of *what* the builder is to construct, and architects obtain information on user needs from their own experience and research and from the staff of the facility. Contract documents do not specify *how* to build a facility. They describe an end result, not means or methods. Therefore, all parties involved in the project need to share the same vision of the finished project. If they do not, the cost of constructing and managing the facility can exceed the project budget.

In addition, imaging projects often involve multiple decision makers: administrators, physicians, nursing staff, technologists, technicians, patient advocates, and so on. As the number of decision makers increases, so does the potential for miscommunication.

Medical projects that involve complex technology (such as imaging facilities) require a high degree of knowledge and coordination among various consultants and subcontractors. The most rapidly changing branches of technology (such as medical imaging) require an even greater degree of coordination. Whether it occurs through drawings, specifications, or written instructions, coordination relies on clear communication.

Technology

Advances in technology—largely computer based—bring new tools and opportunities to both the medical and architectural professions. These advances are changing the way both professions approach their work.

Technology and Imaging

With constant changes in the imaging field, it is surprising to realize that many dramatic advances have resulted from refinements of existing technology. "Although the x-ray equipment used today is quite sophisticated, there have not been many basic changes [in the principles of radiography] since Roentgen's time."[15]

In the shadow of varying regulatory restrictions, scientists and equipment developers succeeded in bringing the new imaging modalities of the sixties, seventies, and eighties to an astonishing level of sophistication and maturity. In fact, many current imaging marvels focus on improving these technologies by developing better software, improving equipment packaging, and reducing cost rather than dramatically changing the modalities and techniques themselves.

Compared to first-generation equipment, today's mature imaging technology is characterized by rapid image acquisition, ease of use, and increased powers of observation within small instrumentation. Most imaging modalities continue to be progressively less invasive. Moreover, imaging in general is being used more for intervention-based procedures, thus enhancing patient treatment. Perhaps the most significant development in imaging technology falls in the area of automated image and information management.

Rapid image acquisition enables better imaging of children, elderly, and severely injured patients who cannot hold still or be easily moved. It also improves equipment throughput capabilities. Important in this transition is the development of fast image acquisition techniques, such as ultrafast and spiral/helical CT and echoplanar and fast/turbo spin echo MR sequences, to visualize anatomy and physiology not detectable by slower methods. This increased ability gives medicine an extraordinary "new vision."[16]

Another technique that fosters rapid image acquisition is slip-ring technology. Slip-ring technology, a design feature enabling continuous rotation of the detectors within the CT gantry, has given rise to spiral and helical scanning techniques. Helical scanning, compared to conventional "slice-by-slice" imaging, decreases acquisition time dramatically and can yield volumetric rather than planar image data. A patient travels horizontally through the gantry while detectors trace a spiral region of interest. Such techniques have enabled "whole-body" imaging (for example, phased array imaging of the entire spine). MR also is capable of whole-body imaging.

Spiral imaging has improved the usefulness of three-dimensional (3-D) imaging and related reconstruction techniques. Ideal for surgical treatment planning, 3-D CT and MR enable remarkable noninvasive viewing of the head and brain and other body regions at various levels of depth. As digital image archiving, retrieval, and computer manipulation capabilities improve, 3-D imaging may become increasingly valuable. Current 3-D applications also include radiation treatment planning, vascular mapping of entire organs, and stereotactic robotically guided neurosurgery.

Greater image clarity is another benefit of new technology. Some branches of imaging, such as nuclear medicine, render images with lower spatial resolution but with exquisite metabolic clarity. Others, such as MR and CT, provide high contrast resolution depicting excellent anatomical data. Today, the two can be combined by merging data sets from different modalities. Complex MR acquisition and processing algorithms have brought about advances in MR angiography (MRA), an attractive alternative to diagnostic cerebral angiography in vascular imaging. (See chapter 6, "Imaging Modalities.")

Most equipment is getting smaller, and sometimes this can result in greater cost-effectiveness. Ultrasound, perhaps more than any other form of imaging, will see the greatest advances due to miniaturization. Today, tiny probes are used to guide neurosurgeons as they operate on delicate and hard-to-visualize sites within the brain. Other miniature ultrasound transducers allow vision from numerous locations within the body, including the interior of blood vessels examined by catheter angiography.

The development of cost-effective picture and image management systems (which are once again breathing new life after inauspicious beginnings) has the potential to revolutionize both the form and function of traditional radiology facilities. (These systems and their components are discussed further in chapter 7, "Image Management and Film Processing.") The ability to implement electronic image management systems begins with knowing how to justify the cost of various components of the system:

> The RIS [(radiology information system) can be] justified on lost charges. . . . The justification of remote viewing in the ICU is clinical speed and the elimination of lost film. The justification of the [archive] jukebox is reduction of film costs and storage.[17]

In summary, recent technical advances in medical imaging have focused on:

- Progressively reducing the duration of image acquisition
- Developing smaller, more cost-effective imaging instrumentation
- Improving spatial contrast and temporal resolution
- Developing image-guided interventional procedures
- Implementing automated and integrated image and information management
- Improving cost-effectiveness and patient outcomes

Mobile Technology

Most modalities, including MRI, CT, and PET, are capable of being installed inside relocatable or mobile trailers. (See figure 2-6, pp. 24–25.) This enables multiple users to share expensive equipment. Also, mobile units that remain at one site can reduce equipment and facility installation time and provide coverage when other equipment is not operational. Where modular construction or relocatable trailers are used, it is especially important that human factors and aesthetics be given adequate consideration within these confining spaces.

Somewhere during the process of planning an imaging facility, a technology dock should be considered. A *technology dock* is a structure where mobile trailers or other types of portable imaging enclosures can be incorporated into the facility. The technology dock has three distinct benefits:

1. *It enables the temporary use of imaging equipment during construction or renovation of more permanent facilities.* This is also beneficial for "short-lived" equipment. For example, if there is a need for a SPECT camera today, but it is likely that major improvements to SPECT equipment will be made in the next few years, a technology dock enables equipment to be replaced with minimal changes to the physical plant.
2. *It makes new technology accessible at less overall cost.* Because equipment can be shared (perhaps one mobile MRI trailer travels to three hospitals each week), equipment costs also can be shared.
3. *It is quick.* Compared to a permanent facility, which may take years to design and build, mobile equipment often is more readily available. In many states, mobile imaging installations are reviewed by the Department of Transportation and not the state planning agencies or building departments, although many state agencies are becoming more involved in regulating mobile health care structures.

Technology docks provide an additional advantage in seismically active locations or sites prone to other natural disasters. If provided with ample emergency power, water supply, sewage capabilities, and communications systems, mobile facilities may be able to be activated if the adjacent permanent structure becomes nonoperational or can be brought back on-line quickly once essential services are restored.

Although mobile imaging facilities might be appropriate in some instances where quick installation is the single most important factor or where sharing equipment among sites is necessary, it appears that mobile installations are more likely a temporary or partial solution than a long-term remedy. Usually support spaces, such as waiting, dressing, and clerical areas, are minimal. Also, access to the dock from the imaging department may be circuitous. Finally, adequate vehicular and pedestrian access must be provided. This can be difficult at some dense urban sites.

Technology and Architectural Services

It is not surprising that technological advances have a similar effect on the profession of architecture as they do on medicine. Both professions rely on translating and transmitting information, are visually oriented, specialize in pattern recognition, and rely heavily on the use of highly trained professional staff. Computer technology has consistently improved our ability to view and manipulate graphic data and has improved the productivity of both technical specialists and managers.

The initially slow evolution of computer use in architectural firms has paralleled that of similar systems in medical imaging departments. Computers originally were used in architectural offices on a limited basis; most early applications addressed database management and limited production of working drawings and construction details. At first, many designers and managers were reluctant to give up their traditional tools for a technology with which they were not entirely comfortable. However, many architects have now mastered computers as design tools, exploiting their power to rapidly manipulate 3-D volumes of space, exploring variations of shade and shadow, studying the effects of heat gain and loss, and comparing multiple window patterns of a building's exterior elevation without investing hours of drafting time.

Technology has brought to architecture a new ability to communicate ideas in early stages of development. Mathematical algorithms, similar to those that enable 3-D simulation of the brain for radiation treatment planning, are used to construct 3-D "fly-by" views representing what would be seen while approaching and walking through a building as if it had already been constructed.

Another advantage of computers in architecture is the ability to overlay drawings containing different types of information. This is similar to computer techniques used in imaging—for example, anatomical data from MR can be superimposed with functional data from nuclear medicine to provide a more complete picture of a patient's condition. Architectural drawings showing wall locations, ceiling patterns, and overhead equipment tracks are

Figure 2-6. Relocatable Imaging Facilities

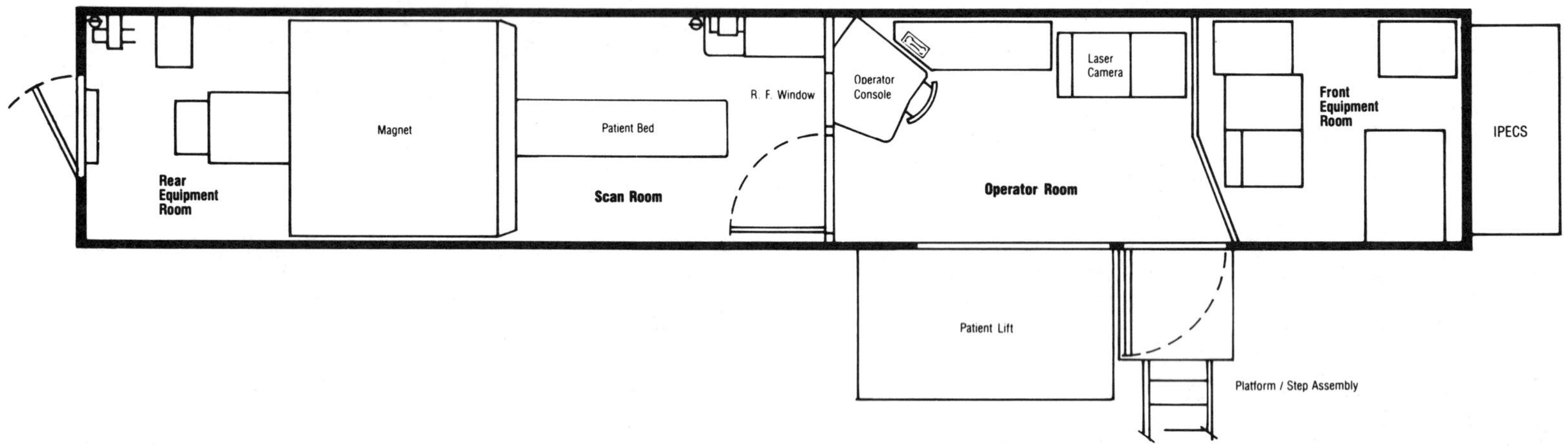

Additional Features

- Master Status Control Panel
- Operator's Viewing Window
- Telephone System with Modem Port
- RFI tested and approved
- Smoke Alarms
- Fire Extinguishers
- Interior Lighting with adjustable intensity
- Emergency Lighting
- Phase Monitor
- Film Illuminator
- Coil Storage Cabinet in Scan Room
- On-Board Storage
- Water Tank Assy. for Humidifier

Available Options

- Built in Oxygen/Suction System
- Patient Lock-Box
- Patient Entertainment System
- Sink w/Hot & Cold Water
- Code Blue Option
- Roadside Emergency Escape Hatch
- Automatic Fire Suppression System
- Non-Magnetic Patient Gurney
- 50Hz Power

Specifications

Overall Length: 48 ft.
Overall Width: 8 ft.
Overall Height: 13 ft. 6 in.
Power Requirements: 480v, 3 Phase @ 150 amp service
On-Board Generator for Environmental Systems
Generator Fuel Tank Capacity: 50 Gallons
Hydraulic Patient Lift Capacity: 1000 lbs.
Personnel Door Width: 44 in.
Patient Lift Entry Width: 75 in.
A/C-Heating Capacity: Accommodates Signa Advantage system heat load and ensures patient comfort.
Meets applicable section of the following codes: UBC, SBCC1, BOCA, NFPA70, NFPA101, NEC
Full 1 Year Service Warranty: Extended warranty/maintenance packages available.
5 Year R.F.I. Warranty

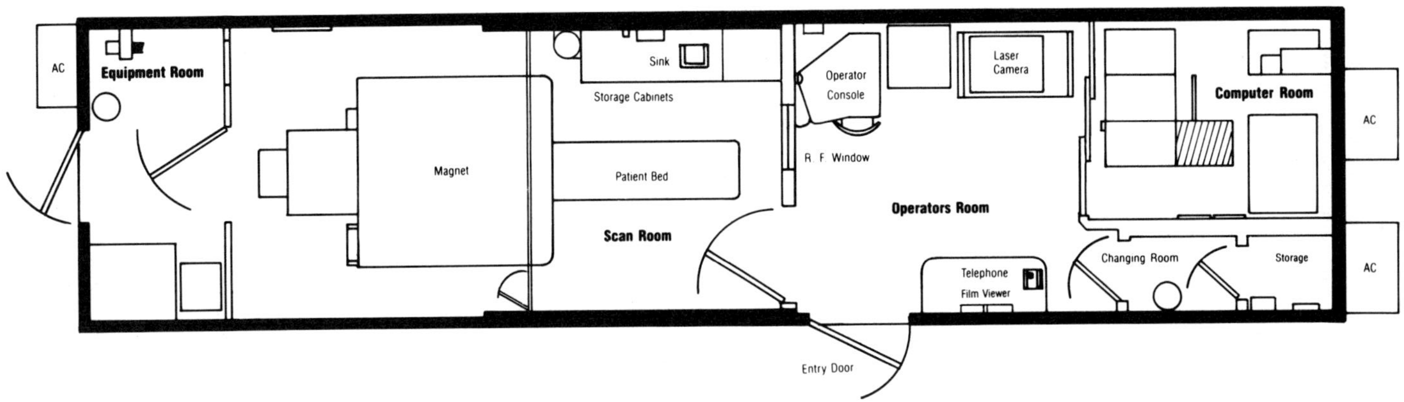

Additional Features

- Master Status Control Panel
- Operator's Viewing Window
- 2 Line Telephone System
- RFI tested and approved
- Built-in Magnetic Shielding
- Smoke Alarms
- Fire Extinguishers
- Interior Lighting with adjustable intensity
- Emergency Lighting
- Phase Monitor
- Film Illuminator
- I.V. Track
- Coil Storage Cabinet
- On-Board Storage
- Patient Change Area

Available Options

- Automatic Fire Suppression System
- Built in Oxygen/Suction System
- Additional Work Surface Area
- Patient Lock-box
- Patient Entertainment System
- "Code Blue" Button
- Sink w/Hot & Cold Water
- Water Tank Assy. for Humidifier
- 15 KVA Transformer (Requires 150 amp Serv.)

Specifications

Overall Length: 50 ft.
Overall Width: 12 ft.
Overall Height: 10 ft. 9 in.
Total Weight: 83,000 lbs., incl. .5T Signa System
74.800 lbs. incl. 1.0T or 1.5T with Active Shield
Power: 480v, 3 Phase/220 1 phase @ 100 amp service
or 415-380v/240-220v, 150 amp service, 50 hz system for overseas units
Personnel Door Width: 48 in.
Service Door Width: 44 in.
A/C-Heating Capacity: Accommodates
Signa Advantage system heat load and
ensures patient comfort.
Meets the following codes:
UBC, SBCC1, BOCA, NEC
Full 1 Year Service Warranty: Extended
warranty/maintenance packages available.
5 Year R.F.I. Warranty

Courtesy of Ellis & Watts, Batavia, Ohio. Used with permission.

electronically overlaid with mechanical drawings showing the location of air-supply registers and return-air grilles and electrical drawings showing light fixtures and ceiling-mounted power-supply connections. This technique not only aids in the coordination of the various building trades, it also reduces the need for multiple background drawings.

For large hospitals and medical centers, computer-generated construction drawings can assist the owner in keeping track of real estate and other physical assets. Some computer-aided facility management (CAFM) packages include interactive databases that convert floor plans into inventories of space and equipment. Many identify departmental boundaries and compare the facility-related operating expenses of a department against its operating budget.

The growing use of computers as design, production, and management tools will continue to expand and refine the practice of health care architecture, thus enabling the design profession to contribute to the needs of a rapidly changing medical profession. The ability of computers to communicate ideas between the two professions is a powerful one.

The Challenge

Resources are shrinking. Requirements are expanding. Designing and building an imaging facility was never easy; now it is even more difficult. Addressing economic, technological, and patient mandates is not enough; today, the architecture of imaging facilities must satisfy these needs with a solution that is both innovative and affordable. The challenge is greater and the risks are higher than they were in the past.

In spite of, or perhaps because of, a more difficult challenge, today's imaging centers and hospital departments are more dynamic and patient oriented than ever before. Successful imaging architecture blends dynamic space and form with logical planning and construction. If the design team does not understand imaging functions or equipment, it is all too likely that design efforts will either ignore, or become overpowered by, technical and functional constraints. On the other hand, if the nature of imaging is understood, design opportunities will be recognized and form and function will enhance one another.

Successful imaging facilities are those that address at least four major challenges. These are:

1. *Improve the medical experience.* Simply stated, this means designing for people, their emotions, and how they function. Improving the medical experience will benefit patients, staff, referring physicians, owners, and visitors.
2. *Anticipate change and integrate flexibility with design.* Build into every design the ability to change, both internally and externally. Although the nature of future changes may be unknown, the fact that change will occur is a given. It is both possible and necessary to provide flexibility today to accommodate tomorrow's changing needs.
3. *Maintain quality with less expense.* Incorporate cost-effective imaging systems, plan spaces for efficient staff functioning, and specify appropriate materials and building components.
4. *As imaging becomes more decentralized, avoid unnecessary duplication of equipment and facilities and ensure that information transfer between remote sites is integral.* Many hospital imaging functions are becoming decentralized and distributed throughout the campus. As health care providers continue to form service networks, distant sites become functionally linked to each other. In either case, do not duplicate facilities or equipment if it is not cost-effective in the long run. Plan now for future application of all aspects of electronic information management as a means of linking remote sites.

References

1. Eisenberg, R. L. *Radiology: An Illustrated History.* St. Louis: Mosby-Year Book, 1992, pp. 51–52.

2. Eisenberg, pp. 68–69.

3. Howell, J. D. Diagnostic technologies: X-rays, electrocardiograms, and CAT scans. *Southern California Law Review* 65(1):534, Nov. 1991.

4. Eisenberg, p. 67.

5. Howell, p. 536.

6. Howell, p. 532.

7. Swett, H. A. Computers: power tool for imaging diagnosis. *Diagnostic Imaging,* June 1992, pp. 97–109.

8. Swett.

9. Egerter, D. E. Tool of the future: ultrasound stethoscope. *Diagnostic Imaging,* Jan. 1991 (supple.), p. A64.

10. Lathrop, J. P., Krauss, K. P., and Shows, G. P. Operational restructuring: a recipe for success. *Healthcare Viewpoint,* 1988, p. 3.

11. Lathrop and others, pp. 3–6.

12. Freiherr, G. Policies seek to avert future shock. *Diagnostic Imaging,* Jan. 1991, p. A69.

13. Freiherr.

14. Dakins, D. A. Tour of RSNA program identifies top attractions. *Diagnostic Imaging* 3(11):A30, Nov. 1991.

15. Bushong, S. C. *Radiologic Science for Technologists: Physics, Biology, and Protection.* 5th ed. St. Louis: Mosby-Year Book, 1993, p. 9.

16. Sochurek, H. *Medicine's New Vision.* Easton, PA: Mack Publishing, 1988.

17. VandenBrink, J. Network solutions to radiology problems. *Diagnostic Imaging* 17(supple.)(4):8, Apr. 1995.

Part 2

Development of an Imaging Facility

It is not enough to take steps which may some day lead to a goal; each step must be itself a goal and a step likewise.

Goethe

Chapter 3

Organization of an Imaging Project

Of all building types, health care facilities are perhaps the most complex, and among the various types of health care facilities, imaging facilities are perhaps the most challenging to design. To successfully meet that challenge, the planning team must be well organized and aware of the forces, both internal and external, that influence project development.

The architecture of imaging facilities encompasses such a vast range of facilities and spaces that it is not possible to exhaustively reference all the conceivable requirements for every imaging project. For example, the organizational needs of an internal remodel that replaces a single radiography room will differ from those of a new building containing comprehensive, state-of-the-art diagnostic and treatment systems. Similarly, the needs of a major renovation project will differ from those of a small, newly constructed imaging center. It is the very nature of these differences that makes development of any imaging facility so challenging.

This chapter describes some of the activities that must take place prior to designing and planning an imaging facility and explains how the facility owner or administrator can best prepare for the often difficult decisions that will need to be made. It also discusses how to build a foundation for a well-organized design and management process by covering planning stages and project team selection. Although this chapter is written primarily for individuals with little or no previous experience with imaging facility development and construction, experienced owners and architects also will find its content useful as a review or checklist.

Strategic Planning and Master Planning

The ability of the project team to make astute decisions depends, in part, on the degree to which all members of the team are working toward common goals and are familiar with the process of developing an imaging facility. For novices and veterans alike, often the initial steps that set the project in motion are the most important. The temptation to "make a building" before researching the context in which imaging services and the facility itself will operate should be resisted. Much of the groundwork preceding architectural design does not focus directly on a building itself but, rather, on the external forces that either enable or preclude the owner and architect from designing a successful project and managing a successful process. Strategic planning and master planning address these external factors, as well as other important variables in the process.

Strategic planning, an essential prerequisite to site and facility development, is the application of an external and internal analysis of the factors that determine an organization's future. In the context of a provider of imaging services, it is the process by which an organization evaluates its surroundings and sets goals to achieve its objectives for providing imaging services. This, in turn, leads to the creation of a responsive site and facility master plan that will guide the continued growth and development of real estate and facilities, as necessary, to achieve these goals.

Although development of a single imaging project may not in and of itself require a comprehensive strategic or master plan, reference to existing strategic and site/facility master plans serves as valuable guidance to any development project. If a strategic plan is not in place, one probably should be initiated whether or not immediate facility development is anticipated.

The strategic plan sets forth objectives for future growth of the organization and defines tactics necessary to achieve the goals of the operation. Without a common strategy, it is doubtful that project team members are working toward a common goal; and without defined tactics, it is doubtful that they are working together at all.

In contrast to a strategic plan, a *master plan* provides the framework for growth by (1) mapping the conditions of existing property and structures, (2) identifying opportunities and obstacles to future development, and (3) charting the application of resources to effect sequential development consistent with the strategic plan's intentions. Both strategic plans and site and facility master plans specify various periods of time within which primary goals are targeted.

For imaging facilities, a *technology plan,* which defines strategies for implementing new medical technologies, should be a part of the strategic plan. The technology plan describes a rational basis for technology assessment and acquisition and thus provides an alternative to decision making that is driven solely by departmental politics.

The components of strategic planning and master planning set the stage for purposeful design. Each step in this predesign process has particular objectives. The steps are:

1. Establish goals and evaluation criteria
2. Perform market analyses and feasibility studies
3. Perform site and facility evaluation studies
4. Develop a working budget
5. Develop a project schedule
6. Develop functional and space programs
7. Align scope, budget, and schedule
8. Prepare site and facility concept plans

A brief discussion of these key predesign activities follows.

Step 1. Establish Goals and Evaluation Criteria

To achieve architecture that is both aesthetic and functional, high-quality design requires that the goals of a project be well defined and clearly stated. Clearly stated goals will in turn help align the expectations of each member of the project team. Examples of project goals include:

- Strategic:
  - To provide the best imaging services in the region
- Economic:
  - To provide a physical environment that will maximize staffing efficiency
  - To improve physical accessibility and allow for patient convenience by eliminating "operational bottlenecks," thus reducing waiting time
  - To avoid unnecessary duplication of equipment
- Political:
  - To make imaging services accessible to patients residing in outlying areas of the region
  - To provide convenience for referring physicians and affiliated provider organizations
- Medical:
  - To reduce the incidence of lost films
  - To improve cardiac imaging capabilities

- Temporal:
  - To allow for incremental growth and modification over time without disrupting existing services
- Physical:
  - To integrate building systems that will accommodate continuous change
  - To separate inpatient and outpatient zones and circulation routes
  - To create a physical image that reflects state-of-the-art medical technology without losing sight of personal interaction between patients and health care providers

Project goals also should be stated in terms of measurable evaluation criteria. This will help project team members recognize whether they are drifting away from the goals and objectives with which they began. The importance of clearly stating both project goals and evaluation criteria prior to commencing facility design cannot be overemphasized. Evaluation criteria to consider include:

- Strategic:
  - Is the solution consistent with the core goals of the strategic plan?
  - Does the solution give the organization a strategic advantage?
- Economic:
  - Is the solution economically feasible and fiscally responsive?
  - Does it make good business sense? Is it consistent with the demands of the marketplace?
- Political:
  - Does the solution serve the community well?
  - How does it affect, and how is it affected by, competitors?
- Medical:
  - Does the solution enable high-quality health care to be provided?
  - Are the medical needs of the community met? Is the solution consistent with the institution's goals for focusing on certain medical programs?
- Temporal:
  - Can the solution be implemented in such a manner as to maximize its impact?
  - Does it provide for phased implementation?
  - Does it provide flexibility for adapting to an unknown future?
- Physical:
  - Is the solution durable?
  - Does it enhance the organization's image?

Step 2. Perform Market Analyses and Feasibility Studies

A market analysis should be considered an integral component of strategic planning. However, it is unlikely that a strategic plan is so current or so specifically targeted to imaging services that it may serve as an accurate guide to the feasibility of a new or newly expanded service. Implementation of new services represents such a significant expenditure of resources that analysis of the current and anticipated market conditions is essential.

A market analysis should identify the anticipated demand for services and calculate the potential return on investment (ROI). It also should consider the likely introduction of similar services by other nearby institutions. In this way, it offers a conceptual framework for determining the viability of new services and programs.

The market analysis should be as realistic as possible. Therefore, the opportunities for a new or expanded market should not be exaggerated. Conversely, overly conservative estimates of demand for imaging services may lead to an undersized facility or less-efficient use of staff and equipment. A balanced and realistic view of external conditions will result in the greatest ROIs. A qualified strategic planning analyst, who can bring an objective vision to the planning team, should be considered.

Upon completion of a general market analysis that supports the viability of new imaging services, a more detailed feasibility study should be conducted to further assess viability of the specific imaging project that is anticipated. This feasibility study should include realistic estimates of facility size, construction costs, equipment costs, additional project costs, and anticipated operational costs. (See chapter 4, "Management of the Process.")

Preliminary estimates for building size can be calculated using generic guidelines, but these figures should be refined later (based on more accurate data) if they are to be used for anything other than feasibility studies. Similarly, preliminary unit construction costs (dollars per gross square foot of construction) can be obtained from a cost estimator, an architect, or a building contractor, provided these individuals are familiar with current projects that are similar in both scope and location.

Construction costs vary considerably by region and building type and will vary further depending on the bidding climate. For example, the cost of building an imaging facility as part of a hospital will differ from that of an imaging suite located within a medical office building. Similarly, the cost of a magnetic resonance imaging (MRI) suite will be greater than that of a basic radiographic facility. An escalation cost factor also must be considered.

The cost of equipment will vary considerably depending on its capabilities, the vendor, and, most important, the purchaser's ability to negotiate a good price. In some cases, existing equipment may be able to be reused. For the purposes of the feasibility study, the cost of equipment for a recent comparable project should suffice, provided a healthy contingency is added and the equipment budget is refined once additional details become known. The cost of equipment can easily exceed construction costs, and equipment maintenance contracts—paid over the useful life of the equipment—can exceed the purchase price of equipment.

If the project involves a freestanding building on a new site, the feasibility study should consider the need for delivery of electrical, gas, water, and sewer services to the building. The study also may consider an evaluation of the geotechnical aspects of the site to determine any unusual subsurface conditions that might affect construction and thus construction costs.

If installation of the imaging project is to occur within an existing structure, the feasibility study should consider the capacity of the existing structure to support the anticipated increase in equipment load and demand for utility services. A renovation project may not allow for planning that is as efficient as it would be in new construction, due to physical constraints inherent in the existing structure. As a result, the renovated project may require more space, be less efficient for staff, and compromise future flexibility, and its configuration may be limited by a restrictive infrastructure. (See chapter 17, "Renovation versus New Construction.") It should be kept in mind that the cost of renovation is not necessarily less expensive than the cost of new construction.

Step 3. Perform Site and Facility Evaluation Studies

If an existing site is inadequate for the proposed program or if no site is presently owned by those individuals proposing the new facility, a new site may need to be selected. Whatever site is proposed (new or existing), it will need to be analyzed to determine how well it will accommodate the needs of the new facility.

Site selection and site analysis are integral components of the market analysis and feasibility studies. As such, site data must be integrated back into the assumptions made in the preceding steps. The site selection and analysis will generate financial data, such as the purchase price of the preferred site and the cost of improvements required after purchase. Site evaluation and selection criteria include:[1]

- Proximity to patients and other providers
- Major road access
- Accessibility by public transportation
- Direct-site access
- Size and usable area

- Site configuration and orientation
- Zoning restrictions
- Legal and physical restrictions
- Environmental impact

(A detailed description of the site selection and site analysis processes is included in chapter 9, "Site Design.")

If an existing facility is to be renovated or added to, it should be evaluated to determine how well it can accommodate its new function. Facility evaluation criteria include:

- Present age and remaining useful life expectancy
- Compliance with current codes
- Structural capacity
- Capacity of, and ease of adding to, the existing electrical and mechanical systems
- Presence of toxic or hazardous materials
- Size, shape, and configuration (for example, does the location of structural columns allow an efficient configuration of imaging rooms and adjacent support spaces?)
- Interior and exterior appearance of existing facility

Step 4. Develop a Working Budget

The process of developing a working budget is cyclical, not linear. As the project progresses and more detailed data about the project's scope and complexity become available, the budget should be reevaluated and confirmed. (See chapter 4, "Management of the Process," for a discussion of types of costs and cost considerations at each phase of a project.)

During these iterative examinations, however, the magnitude of the budget should remain more or less stable. If cost estimates conflict with the budget, the scope of the project might need to be modified at the outset to conform to the limitations of available capital. If the budget is arbitrarily changed in the middle of design, the programming, planning, and design processes will need to be revisited. For these reasons, the initial preparation of a working budget should be as comprehensive as possible.

Although the owner is chiefly responsible for developing and preparing the project's capital budget, it is the architect and cost consultants who are responsible for verifying that the budget is appropriate for the scope and quality of intended work. If the two are in conflict, they must be brought into alignment before detailed programming or design activities begin. Additional consultants often provide an estimate of both fixed and movable equipment costs.

It is very important that both the owner and the architect consider the capital budget in tandem with the operating budget for the facility. In some cases, the operating budget may eventually exceed the total cost of building an entire facility.

> While work on development of the capital budget is in progress, the owner should see to it that an operating budget is also prepared. The correlation between the two budgets will be apparent when it is time to decide whether it is better policy, on the one hand, to increase an expense classification in the capital budget with resulting decrease in expense in the operating budget or, on the other hand, to hold the line in the capital budget and take care of the offsetting effect in the future operating budget. Similarly, consideration should be given to whether it is wise to plan in the capital budget for such eventualities as future installation of special equipment or for [increased electrical, heating or air conditioning capacities] to meet foreseeable needs in the future.
>
> Both the owner and the architect should realize that, in many instances, an increase in the original capital investment to pay for good construction and high-quality materials will decrease the future cost of repairs and maintenance. Use of inferior construction and cheap materials to save capital dollars and to reduce the [initial cost of the facility] may add many dollars to the annual operating budget. A system known as life-cycle costing . . . attempts to evaluate capital costs and lifetime maintenance costs. The purpose

is to determine whether an item that is more expensive initially is or is not more economical in the long run because it has lower maintenance costs.[2]

An owner's construction contingency should appear as a line item in the budget. This contingency, often 10 percent of the estimated construction cost for new construction and up to 20 percent for renovation, is provided to account for unknown conditions that might arise during construction. It is not intended to be used by the owner to increase project scope. If it is, it will have been spent before construction begins and will not be available when needed.

A design contingency should be included in addition to the owner's construction contingency. The purpose of the design contingency is to account for the absence (at this early stage) of detailed drawings that describe how design concepts will be implemented. Prior to beginning schematic design, the design contingency might be equal to 10 percent of the estimated construction cost for new construction and 15 percent for renovation. Later, it might be reduced to 2 to 3 percent of the new construction cost and 7 to 8 percent of the renovated construction cost by the time the project is bid. The design contingency is not intended to be used by the owner to increase project scope.

Contingency figures should be neither too lean nor too fat. An inflated estimate of cost might seem to limit the exposure to risk by guaranteeing that the construction project will be achieved within the assumed budget. However, the true risk of this is unnecessarily limiting the amount of program area by being too conservative in developing the project budget. Should construction bids or cost estimates reveal that more program area is possible within the original budget, the additional program area will be designed at a premium price and with considerable compromise.

Step 5. Develop a Project Schedule

The schedule is a road map that highlights milestones critical to the project's development. (See chapter 4, "Management of the Process," for information and details on how long each phase of the process typically takes.) The schedule should be neither so loose that it has little meaning nor so rigid that it cannot accommodate important developments that will arise during the course of design and construction. Like the budget, the project schedule will require occasional adjustments.

Budget and schedule are intimately related. As the magnitude of one increases, in most cases so does the magnitude of the other. Both owners and architects should be careful not to squeeze either the budget or the schedule so tightly that it will have a negative impact on the quality of the project.

For imaging projects that require careful coordination of many diverse disciplines (architects and planners, equipment installation experts, radiologists, technologists, and administrators), the project schedule is as much a tool for communication as it is a calendar. It describes the work for which team members are responsible and the time by which the results of their work must be made available, so that other team members can accomplish their tasks.

A number of key questions should be asked prior to establishing the initial project schedule. These include:[3]

- When must the project be occupied? Is this tied to a critical date?
- Is it possible or desirable to occupy the project in stages?
- How long should it take to construct the project? Can site preparation or other work begin before design is complete? Can or should the entire project be fast-tracked?
- How long will preconstruction activities (design, planning, and so on) take? When can design work begin, and how complete will it be before construction begins? Are there other activities (environmental impact studies, regulatory agency reviews, public approval of financing, for example) that, if delayed, will extend the project schedule?
- When will the debt and equity capital for the project be available?
- What regulatory and financial reviews are required? Who will perform them, what information will be needed, and how long will they take?

If financial and regulatory agency approvals are needed, they need to be incorporated into scheduling plans:

> Financial and regulatory approvals usually involve go/no-go decisions, so they almost always lie on the critical path. For complex projects requiring many interconnected approvals . . . the architect providing project scheduling services may need to map out a "decision schedule" as well as a design and construction [or project] schedule.[4]

Figure 3-1 provides an example of a decision schedule and figure 3-2 provides a sample project schedule.

The project schedule will be determined, in part, by the selected method of project delivery, for example, design-award bid, fast-track, or design/build. The project duration will in turn influence the level of compensation the architect will seek. For example, a very short duration may require that the architect employ additional staff or pay overtime premiums. However, a prolonged schedule might require that the architect attend to the project for a longer duration than might otherwise be necessary. If the schedule (from the time of its inception) is either unusually long or unusually short, there should be good justification for this. If the architect feels that the schedule, relative to the project scope, is inappropriate, this should be brought to the owner's attention as soon as possible.

Step 6. Develop Functional and Space Programs

Functional and space programming provide a road map for facility planning and design. The functional program identifies past and present workload and operational characteristics and translates them into a model for future operations. For areas undergoing significant

Figure 3-1. A Decision Schedule

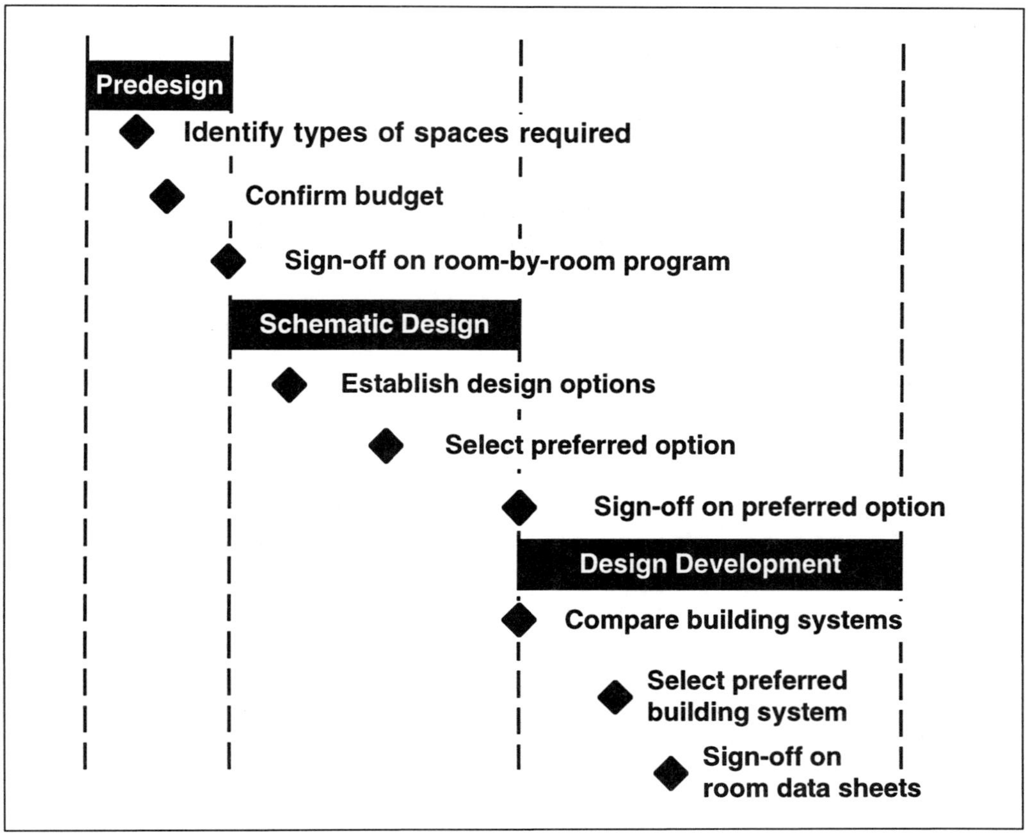

Figure 3-2. A Project Schedule

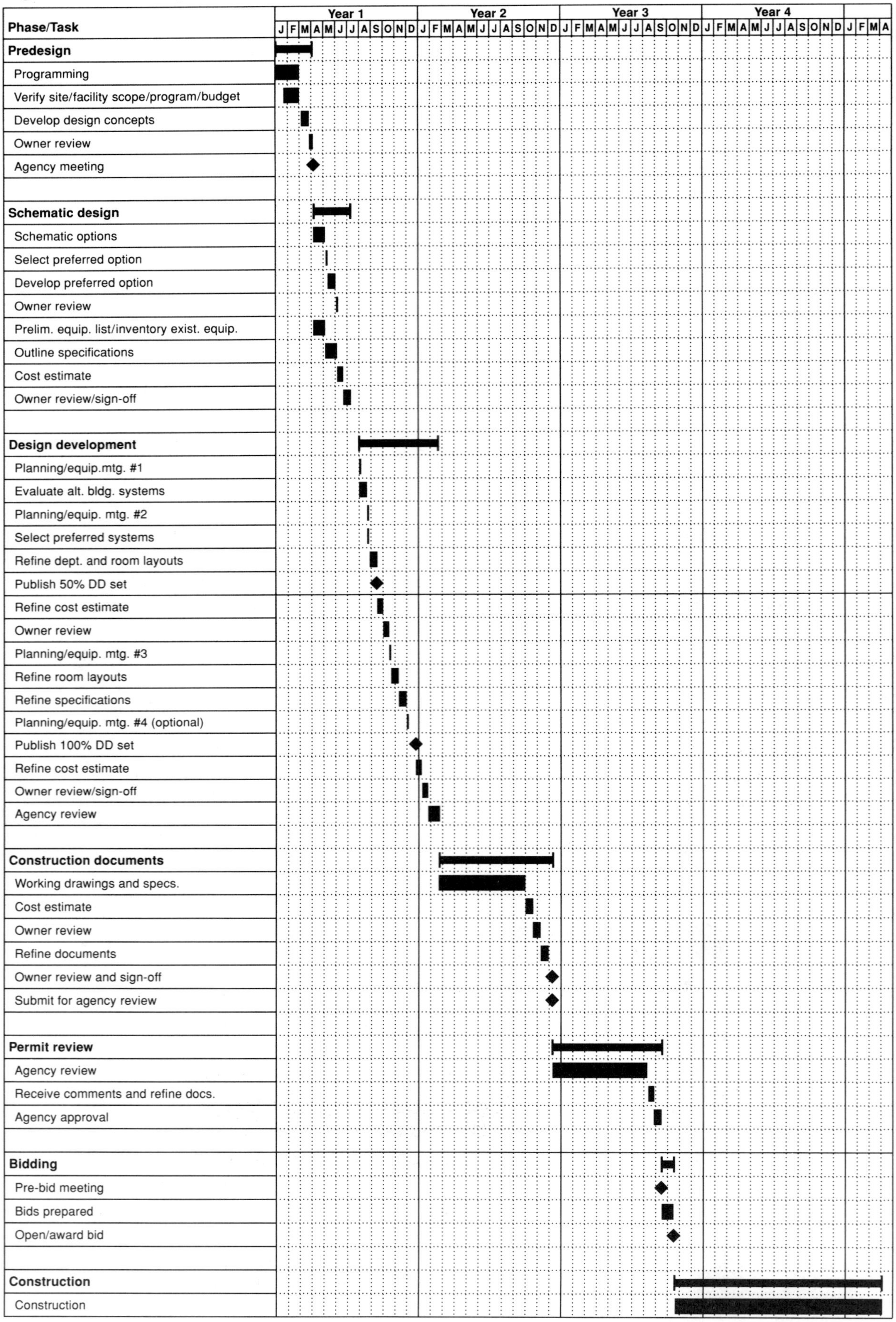

reengineering, however, past operational characteristics may have little relevance to future approaches. Space programming translates the functional program into spatial data: size, quantity, quality, and space adjacencies. A detailed space program identifies each assigned space to be provided in the facility (public areas, patient areas, and staff areas) along with multipliers to account for unassigned circulation space and rooms to house mechanical equipment. (See chapter 12, "Space Requirements.")

> The functional program defines the project in terms of purpose, scope, functions and facility requirements. Based on the assessment of community needs and individual programs for services, it sets forth the needs to be fulfilled, the specific services to be provided, the staffing patterns, and the proposed operational policies and procedures. Anticipated utilization factors, service loads, and facility elements are estimated in order to complete the functional data.
>
> The functional program ultimately becomes the statement of the building requirements that the architect must solve. Unless the functional program is worked out in advance, the architect will be required to make many assumptions and suppositions. Therefore, to avoid future major changes, the closest possible cooperation between the [functional programmer, the owner] and the architect is required in developing the functional program. [Note: In many cases, programming services are provided by the architect.]
>
> The architect should not be expected to decide [which] services [will] be provided in the [imaging facility] or its methods of operation; such decisions are normally outside [the architect's] particular competence and responsibility, although he [or she] may well assist in reaching conclusions on these matters. Although there should be allowance for flexibility and professional judgment in the design of the facilities, every functional consideration affecting the architectural [space] program should be resolved and clearly stated in advance of the design phases.[5]

A room-by-room space program is a description of the individual spaces that constitute the entire imaging service. A well-written program is more than a list of rooms; it serves as an accurate model of the imaging facility. As such, it makes it possible to visualize the operation of the completed project. For example, adjacencies of one room to another present a logical progression of imaging service delivery. The space program for renovating an existing facility should consider the utilization of existing services and spaces and should address the implications of reusing existing construction. However, such reuse might introduce inherent inefficiencies into the space program.

Development of the functional and space programs should not be rushed. These are important tools, and they provide an essential step between feasibility and design. The very process of programming will encourage the project team to reflect on important design and functional aspects that may not have been considered otherwise. It is easier and far less costly to make revisions to the building program than to effect the same changes while the building is under construction. The entire planning team should review and formally approve the space and functional programs before advancing to any subsequent design phase.

Functional and space programs should be comprehensive. They should consider and represent the flow of people, material, and equipment through the facility. The programs serve as a checklist and provide data useful in confirming preliminary budget estimates.

The space programs should address physical planning concepts in the abstract. Where examples of physical relationships are necessary to illustrate a desired concept, they should be diagrammatic. In this way, they will not preclude subsequent design solutions.

Space and functional programming activities might include tours of other facilities that contain types of equipment and services comparable to those being planned. Such facility tours also are useful during schematic design.

Finally, the functional and space programs should reiterate the project goals and objectives set forth in the strategic plan. The project criteria should clearly describe scope, purpose, quality, schedule, and budget. (See the appendix at the end of this chapter.)

Step 7. Align Scope, Budget, and Schedule

Once the project scope, budget, and schedule are identified, these three variables should be compared to verify that they are in balance with one another. The verification process will likely require that one or all three need to be refined. Now, rather than later, is the time to ensure alignment.

It usually is a good idea for each variable to be formally approved in writing. Later, a description of project scope, budget, and schedule will be incorporated into the agreement for design and planning services between the owner and the architect, where they will become terms of the contract.

Formal written approval does not imply that no further changes will be made. However, it does suggest that if one variable changes, all three are likely to change respectively. By documenting the starting point at which all three were in balance, it is easier to monitor when and by what level of magnitude deviation occurs. It also helps identify whether budgetary deviations are due to any changes in scope.

Step 8. Prepare Site and Facility Concept Plans

Once scope, budget, and schedule are aligned, concept plans should be developed. The purpose of concept planning is to determine and test options available for initial and future growth on the site or within the confines of existing construction. Concept plans should include options for:

- Site circulation, including that of patients, staff, and services
- Parking
- Circulation within the building(s), specifically the flow of people, equipment, supplies, and waste
- Land acquisition
- Building massing and configuration

A concept diagram is shown in figure 3-3.

Alternative concept plans should be examined and evaluated. One preferred option should then be developed in greater detail, and one or two alternate versions of the preferred concept plan may be warranted. Concept planning should conclude with a written evaluation of both the preliminary and preferred concepts, including the strengths and weaknesses of each and their associated implementation costs.

Project Team Selection

As soon as the risks of moving forward with the project have been evaluated, the owner should assess the capabilities potentially available in-house. Does the organization include individuals experienced with managing design and construction projects of this type? What is the cost of dedicating most of their time to the project and having others take over the remainder of their responsibilities? If sufficient experience does not exist internally, perhaps a project management or construction management consultant should be considered.

> Construction–project management involves the concept of a single focal point of responsibility for the planning, coordination and direction of all phases of design, procurement and construction of a health care building project.
>
> The scope of work includes complete responsibility for the coordination and direction of the work of all of the architects, engineers, vendors/suppliers, consultants and contractors who may participate in the building project.
>
> Construction management, on the other hand, refers to the construction mode—when someone representing the owner controls the construction work, which (usually) is bid upon and constructed by different contractors.

> Generally, the same control also can be exerted by . . . a general contractor. The traditional definition of construction management covers the group or segment of management activities that are above and beyond any normal architectural and engineering services; those activities may be carried out during the predesign, design, and construction phases, during which the construction manager who's responsible for the project retains control over quality-, schedule-, and cost-related considerations.[6]

Except in the case of small projects developed by large institutions with in-house architects and engineers, a team of architectural and engineering consultants probably will be hired to design the project and assist in administering the contract documents during construction. If programming and master planning services are to be provided by the design architect, the architectural team should be selected soon after the preliminary budget and schedule have been established. (Programming is a preliminary stage that involves research to determine the true nature of the project and future needs, and is discussed in chapter 4, "Management of the Process.") The selected architect can help verify that the budget and schedule are in balance with project scope.

Figure 3-3. Example of a Concept Diagram

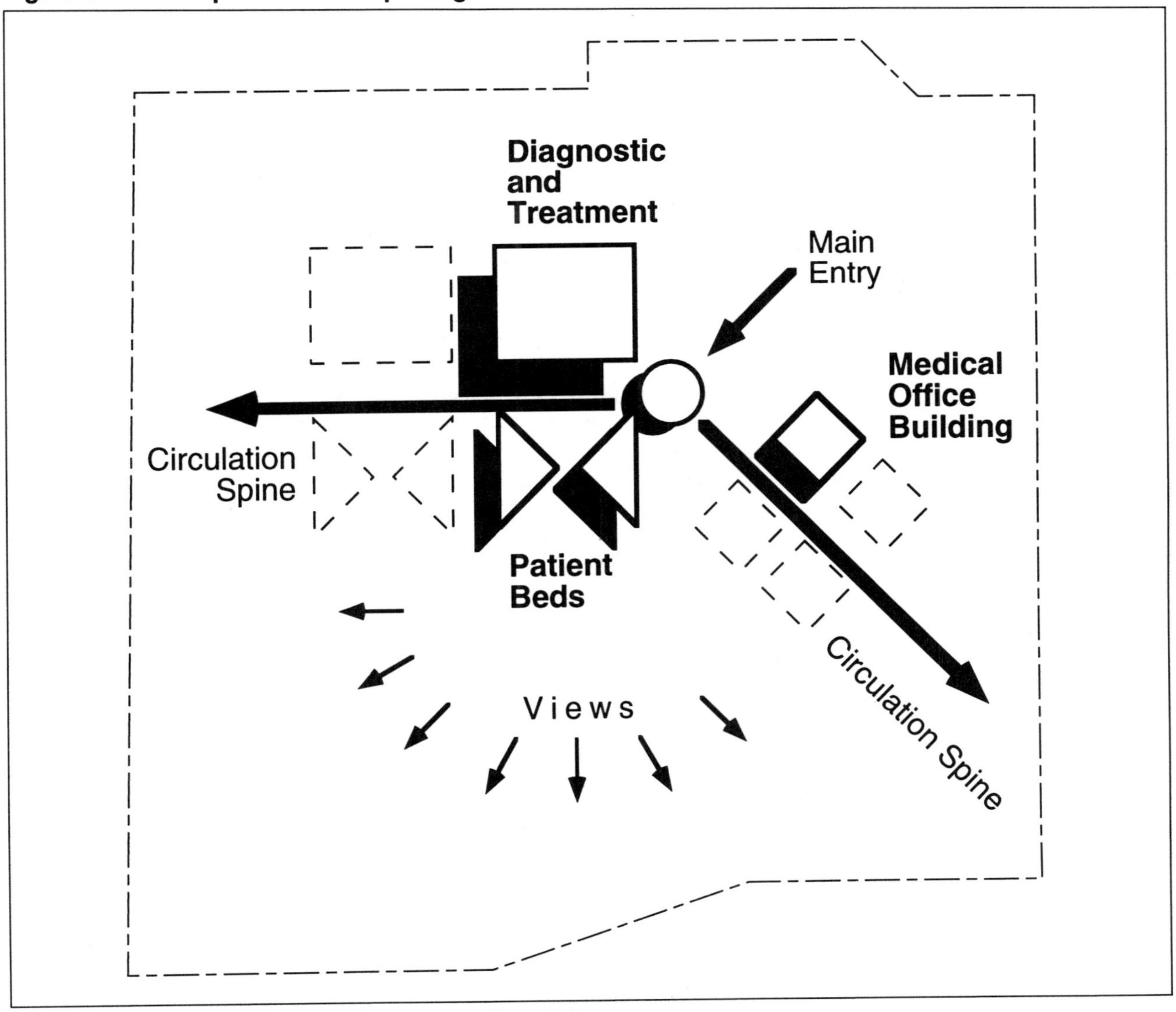

Courtesy of Stone Marraccini Patterson, San Francisco. Used with permission.

However, if programming and/or master planning services are to be provided by someone other than the design architect, two selection processes will occur: one for programming and master planning consultants after establishment of a preliminary budget and schedule; and one for the architectural design consultant after functional and space programming is complete. In this case, both consultant teams can help verify that schedule and budget are in balance with project scope.

Selecting the appropriate architectural team is an important and often difficult decision. An experienced team is needed to successfully complete the project. Thus, it is essential to select consultants who understand the special nature of imaging facilities in general, as well as the unique requirements of the specific project to be developed.

The architectural selection process consists of four basic steps. These are:[7]

1. *To define goals and criteria for the selection process.* These will be used in selecting consultants and identifying who will be involved in the selection process, who will be involved in the project management process, and what the reporting and communications structure will be.
2. *To prequalify potential architectural candidates.* Experience can be demonstrated through a proven track record for similar projects. Recent experience with comparable projects in the same regulatory jurisdiction is important. Out-of-town consultants may be unfamiliar with local and state regulatory agencies and their policies. However, in the case of designing for new imaging technologies that exist in few other places, the preferred architectural team may bring together an out-of-town specialist with a competent local firm for a combination of design expertise and knowledge of local codes and regulations.

   Checking references is essential. Both recent clients and contractors who have built projects designed by the architect should be contacted. Critical reviews should be clarified before making a final judgment. Touring similar facilities designed by the architect is an excellent opportunity to evaluate the architect's abilities and to visualize what a new facility can be like.
3. *To develop a "short list" of candidates.* A short list serves to narrow down the number of prequalified architectural consultants to the 5 or 6 most qualified teams. A longer list of candidates (10 or more) makes the selection process more difficult and indicates to the architects that there may not be a clear decision-making process in place.

   More than just finding the most qualified health care architectural team, the short list should focus specifically on finding the most qualified team for the particular project under consideration. Depending on the particular needs of the imaging facility, the two criteria may be different. The ability to develop the best short list will be predicated, in part, on how well the specific needs of the project are defined.
4. *To conduct the interview.* The interview should be conducted by a small group consisting of people from the organization who will be directly involved in the project from planning through construction. Each individual should be familiar with the written proposals and come prepared to participate fully in a dialogue with the architects as they present their ideas and their firms' qualifications.[8]

Other helpful guidelines concerning the interview include the following:[9]

- An agenda should be set and the candidates should be told in advance what is expected of them.
- If possible, interviews should not all be compressed into one day. A sufficient amount of time should be allowed for the information to sink in.
- No architect should be asked to criticize another; nothing significant will be learned by doing this.
- Interviews should be as informal as possible. Participants will learn more from the interviews and the interviews will be more enjoyable.
- Candidates should be told when a decision will be made, and whatever timetable is given should be adhered to.

Selecting an architect means selecting a team, including various consultants who will work with the architect. (See chapter 4, "Management of the Process.") The key individuals who will work with the owner on a day-to-day basis sometimes are more critical to the project's success than is the firm itself. Consider the following:

- A specific individual (usually the project manager) should be appointed to serve as the primary contact for the design team.
- The principal-in-charge has overall responsibility for the project. He or she should be someone who can dedicate sufficient time to the project.
- It should be determined whether the team members at the interview will be the same individuals who will serve on the project team.

Selection of a good project manager also is a key issue. Often, the skills of a good project manager are different from those of a good designer. Although the project manager should have a keen sense of design and the project designer should also be a good manager, it is likely that the most qualified individual in one area might not be as strong in the other. The abilities of both the project manager and the project designer are key to the success of the project.

The *project manager* is the focus and catalyst of the architectural process. He or she will maintain the most direct relationship with the owner. Characteristics of a good project manager include experience in all areas of professional architectural practice and specific experience with imaging facilities, the ability to efficiently use the resources of his or her firm, strategic thinking, the ability to detect problems before they develop, and good communication skills.

The *project designer* should be both visionary and realistic. He or she will give the project form and personality. The project designer must have the ability to both communicate design concepts and generate strong design solutions. On the other hand, if the owner and the designer have vastly different design philosophies with little or no common ground, this can have a detrimental effect on the entire design process. When examples of projects are presented during an interview, it is important to verify whether they were designed by the designer who will be assigned to the project in question or by other members of the firm.

Aside from experience and qualifications, a successful architectural project relies heavily on interpersonal chemistry. The owner needs to feel comfortable with the team members, because their daily working relationship will continue for years. Some important considerations include:

- How well the members of the architectural team appear to work with each other and with their own consultants
- How long the key members have been with the firm
- The extent to which the proposed project team members have previously worked together as a team
- The owner's intuition, based on the team's interview presentation

References

1. Lifton, J., and Hardy, O. B. *Site Selection for Health Care Facilities.* Chicago: American Hospital Publishing, 1982 [out of print].
2. Rea, J., Frommelt, J. J., and MacCoun, M. D. *Building a Hospital: A Primer for Administrators.* Chicago: American Hospital Publishing, 1978 [out of print], pp. 31–33.
3. Haviland, D. *The Architect's Handbook of Professional Practice. Volume 2: The Project.* Washington, DC: American Institute of Architects, 1987, p. 16.
4. Haviland, pp. 16–17.
5. Rea and others, pp. 21–22.

6. Hammelman, D. J. Project management vs. construction management. *Health Facilities Management* 5(7):22, July 1992.

7. Flaws, J. A. Which architect should you pick? *Health Facilities Management* 5(7):34–40, July 1992.

8. Flaws, p. 40.

9. Flaws.

Appendix. Example of a Functional and Space Program for Diagnostic Imaging

I. Existing Conditions
  A. Current and future programs
    1. Components of diagnostic imaging in this evaluation include inpatient imaging, MRI, and special procedures.
    2. All inpatient and outpatient angiographic, interventional fluoroscopic, and CT-guided biopsy procedures are performed in this area of service.
    3. All inpatient CTs and all inpatient and outpatient neuroradiology and head and neck CT scans are performed in this area of service.
  B. Current facilities
    1. The existing facility is approximately 15,000 DGSF.
    2. Archive records and files are stored in approximately 3,000 NSF of space in a remote area.
    3. The existing facility includes 1 MRI, 2 CTs, 3 general radiographic, 1 chest, 1 mammography/breast biopsy, 2 interventional fluoroscopy, and 3 angiographic special procedures.
  C. Facility deficiencies
    1. Traffic flow and circulation through the service is restricted, resulting in cross-traffic between staff, inpatients, and outpatients.
    2. Many of the inpatient holding areas are crowded, limit supervision, and have inadequate space for family and relatives to stay with patients.
    3. Most procedure rooms are undersized for current practices.

II. Planning Assumptions
  A. Operational policies and procedures
    1. MRI is to be located between the inpatient and outpatient areas. One MRI will be provided, initially, as part of the inpatient area. An adjacent area will be shelled for a future unit to be installed as part of the outpatient zone.
    2. All special procedures work for inpatients and outpatients will be located in the proposed facility. It is assumed that at least 40 percent of the special procedures work will be done on an outpatient basis. The staging and observation of postprocedure outpatients will occur in the adjacent day surgery area.
    3. Facility planning is to anticipate the eventual integration of electronic image management and communications systems, with digital image transmission links between the diagnostic imaging service, operating rooms, pathology, emergency, and the nursing units. The primary space implications for this goal is a plan for installation of conduit and eventual wiring, workstations, and image storage equipment.
  B. Staffing and scheduling
    1. Existing/projected staff by shift:

Position	Day	Evening	Night
Faculty, administration, research	4	0	0
Residents/students	4	0	0
Technologists/nursing	12–14	0	0
Clerical	4	0	0
Other	6–7	0	0
Total:	30–33	0	0

  C. Workload
    1. Historical data show inpatient procedures peaking in fiscal year 1993 at 35,225 examinations. The ratio of inpatient examinations to admissions has declined from 2.2 exams per admission in 1990 to 1.76 in 1993.
    2. Ultrasound and other procedures provided outside the main inpatient department accounted for 2,486 examinations in 1993. Workload within the inpatient service included 3,245 CT examinations, 1,463 angiographic procedures, 3,156 radiographic exams, 8,026 chest exams, 1,104 fluoroscopic examinations, and 489 MRI studies.
    3. Outpatient examinations provided in the department during 1993 included 2,204 MRI exams, 1,643 outpatient CT exams, and 734 angiographic procedures.
    4. A one-month sample of patient records during September 1993 reported that 506 of the 3,408 examinations performed in the department were performed in the evening or on the weekend. This represents approximately 15 percent of the total workload for that period.
    5. Special studies are currently under way to provide additional data regarding average procedure time and equipment utilization rates.

III. Planning Guidelines
   A. Desired relationships
      1. Access from the intensive care unit (ICU) and surgery is necessary for the provision of imaging to these patients.
   B. Design considerations
      1. Provide for future flexibility by providing some shelled space for future use and allowing for future external expansion.
      2. Consider universal room design for basic procedure rooms.
      3. Plan for decentralized image processing.
   C. Special and technical equipment
      1. MRI equipment, magnetic shielding, radio-frequency shielding
      2. CT units
      3. Special angiographic rooms
      4. Interventional fluoroscopy
      5. Standard radiographic and radiographic/fluoroscopic rooms
      6. Image-processing systems to be determined
   D. Support systems considerations
      1. Instruments for special procedures and invasive fluoroscopy will be provided in central processing. Movement of clean and soiled material between the service and central processing should be considered in the planning of the service.
   E. Building systems considerations
      1. Shielding for all radiographic, CT, and MRI equipment must be incorporated into the design of the building. The effect of imaging equipment on adjacent areas—and the effect of adjacent areas on imaging equipment—must be evaluated during design.
      2. MRI, CT, angiography, and interventional imaging rooms should be equipped with built-in suction, compressed air, oxygen, and gas-scavenging systems.

IV. Room-By-Room Space Listing

Area/Room	NSF[a]/Unit	Unit	Total NSF	Comments
MRI				
Scan room	300	2	600	
Control	130	2	260	
Computer room	200	1	200	
Laser imaging	100	1	100	
Patient valuables	60	1	60	
Archival storage	90	1	90	
Patient holding	80	6	480	
Patient toilets	50	4	200	
Interpretation/consult	0	0	0	See specific procedures
Subtotal:			1,990	
Special Procedures				
Angiography	480	3	1,440	
Interventional/ fluoroscopy	480	2	960	Includes control
Control (angio)	120	3	360	Adjacent to angio
Storage/supply	180	3	540	
Patient holding/prep	100	3	300	
Postprocedure observation	0	0	0	In day surgery area
Interpretation	240	1	240	
Clean/soiled utility	80	2	160	
Patient toilet	50	2	100	
Tray makeup	100	1	100	
Darkroom	100	1	100	
Light room	40	1	40	
Subtotal:			4,340	
Radiographic/fluoroscopic				
Fluoroscopy	320	2	960	Includes control
Cytology	0	0	0	In fine-needle area
Radiography	280	3	840	
Control	40	3	120	
Patient toilets	50	3	150	
Barium prep area	80	1	80	
Patient prep area	80	2	160	
Darkroom	100	1	40	
Light room	40	1	40	
Subtotal:			2,390	

(Continued on next page)

Area/Room	NSF[a]/Unit	Unit	Total NSF	Comments
Patient Support				
Outpatient waiting	20	40	800	Near day surgery
Reception				
Public toilets	80	2	160	
Patient gowning area	240	2	480	Includes linen supply area
Gowned waiting	20	30	600	
Patient toilets	50	2	100	
Soiled utility/trash	80	1	80	
Inpatient holding	80	4	320	
Dressing, standard	16	10	160	
Dressing, handicapped	35	3	105	
Subtotal:			2,805	
Staff Support				
Office, asst. chief	100	2	200	
Technical work area	1,200	1	1,200	
Office, radiologists	120	4	480	
Secretarial/transcription	85	1	85	
Viewing room	360	1	360	
Film sorting QA	180	1	180	
Film file holding	360	1	360	
Conference/education	240	1	240	
Physician viewing room	240	1	240	
Lockers/lounge	180	2	260	
Staff toilets	60	4	240	
Storage	360	1	360	
Subtotal:			4,205	
Total NSF:			15,730	
Net to department grossing factor:			1.5	
Total NSF × Departmental gross square feet =			23,595	

[a]NSF stands for net square feet.

Chapter 4

Management of the Process

Experience, knowledge, and creativity are requisite ingredients for innovative design. Unfortunately, these qualities alone will not bring success to most imaging projects. Too many things will go wrong without continuous leadership and coordination. In an aerospace program, for example, the world's best engineers cannot keep a space shuttle in orbit without an expert manager to direct the knowledge path of each rocket scientist while the shuttle is being designed, constructed, and operated. Similarly, imaging projects cannot be kept on track without experienced managers.

Some imaging facilities require technical specialists as part of the team, along with medical planners, structural engineers, and interior designers. But, regardless of team composition, a manager is always at the helm. Both the architect and the owner should assign a full-time manager with specific responsibilities to the project, and together these two managers will lead the project team. (See table 4-1.)

The project manager's job is to construct a road map and make sure that everyone follows it. Managing an imaging project may involve tasks that are more complex than those required for other projects. Specific project manager tasks include establishing goals, scheduling, budgeting, and directing in such a way that the design team can obtain consensus on critical issues. For example, radiologists will likely want to defer equipment selections until the latest date possible to ensure that the equipment is state-of-the-art (or at least the most current model available), but the manager representing the owner must make sure that such decisions are made in a timely manner and that there is a mechanism in place to accommodate changes to those decisions when they become necessary.

For the architect, management includes coordinating engineering, equipment, and other consultants as well as maintaining the project budget and schedule. For the owner, management includes coordinating the needs of administration, medical staff, support staff, patient advocates, and consultants as well as managing budget and schedule. Imaging equipment selections can be particularly complicated because they must be made earlier than most other medical equipment selections. This is because imaging equipment has such a profound influence on facility layout and the detailed design of mechanical, electrical, and structural systems. Also, the lead time in obtaining detailed, site-specific information about imaging equipment is likely to be longer than with other equipment. Even short delays in equipment selection can produce long delays in facility design and construction.

Sometimes it is not apparent just how many steps in the design and planning process are contingent on detailed, site-specific equipment data. For example, design of some radiography or fluoroscopy procedure rooms must remain generic until the control console, image intensifier, table, and various accessories are specified. Although a generic or universal layout (as described in chapter 13, "Room Design") might be acceptable for simple basic procedure rooms, delaying the specific layout of special procedures rooms is likely to affect the entire project schedule because long lead items will arrive late, requiring some of the construction trades to perform their work out of sequence. In many states, the regulatory review required to obtain a building permit also would need to be deferred until adequate equipment information is available. This can have a considerable impact on the construction schedule.

In the case of magnetic resonance imaging (MRI), substituting one equipment model for another could require replanning several rooms and modifying the structural, mechanical, and electrical systems. Postponing equipment selections may delay the preparation of contract documents, which in turn will delay construction.

This chapter provides a working knowledge of the key factors that contribute to the management of a successful project. The first part covers roles and responsibilities of the various project team members, alignment of expectations among project team members, and communications factors. The rest of the chapter briefly describes each project phase, budget implications, and scheduling considerations.

The Project Team: Roles and Responsibilities

Successful architecture is borne out of collaboration. It requires a team of skilled professionals who are willing and able to work together interactively. In essence, the team is made up of the owner, the architect, and the contractor, with the architect and contractor responsible to the owner.

For small projects, the team might be limited to an administrator, a radiologist, a technologist, a physicist, an architect, engineers, and equipment vendors. For large projects, it should include most of the individuals listed in table 4-1. The first step in a successful collaboration is to define each team member's responsibilities.

Table 4-1. The Project Team (Design and Planning Phases)

Owner	Architect/Engineers/ Other Consultants	Contractor[a]
• Project manager	• Principal	• Construction manager (optional)
• Radiology administrator	• Project manager	• General contractor (optional)
• Radiologist	• Project architect	• Cost estimators (optional)
• Chief technologist	• Designer	• Others (optional)
• Radiation physicist	• Interior designer	
• Facility operations and maintenance representative	• Medical planner	
• Others	• Programmer	
• Equipment planner[b]	• Technical coordinator	
• Equipment vendors[c]	• Mechanical engineer	
• Radiologic nurse	• Electrical engineer	
	• Structural engineer	
	• Cost estimator	
	• Equipment planner[b]	
	• Others	

Notes:

a. The contractor or construction manager's involvement during design and planning phases is considered optional (but desirable) in this table because the work during these phases can be performed without their involvement. If a contractor or construction manager is involved at this time, it usually is to assist with recommendations regarding constructability, to provide a second cost estimate, or to help with complex issues of phasing or subdividing the project into separate bid packages.

b. Equipment planners sometimes are consultants to the architect and sometimes consultants to the owner.

c. Equipment vendors may not actually be consultants. Often their services are tied to product sales. Nonetheless, their input can be helpful. Information from vendors is necessary in order for the architect to perform design and planning services, but the architect has no contractual relationship with the vendors. Therefore, all vendor-furnished information should come to the architect via the owner.

The Owner's Responsibilities and Consultants

The owner's key management responsibilities include stating the goals of the project and obtaining consensus from a diverse group of facility users. Radiologists, technologists, nurses, radiology administrators, hospital administrators, and maintenance personnel all may have differing opinions on particular issues. In addition, the owner may seek the advice of consultants in the areas of finance, equipment procurement, radiation protection, and staffing. Effective leadership suggests a process through which all key personnel are involved in executive decision-making and brainstorming activities; in smaller work sessions, individual spokespersons are selected to represent each group.

Additional owner responsibilities include establishing a strategic plan, a project budget, and schedule parameters, as well as providing information about existing site and facility conditions. Specific owner responsibilities are defined in article 2 of AIA (American Institute of Architects) document B141: Standard Form of Agreement between Owner and Architect.

Within any facility, a variety of groups will overlap in their use of various spaces, circulation routes, equipment, and functions. The owner should assist the architect in identifying all user groups potentially affected by planning and design decisions. User group input should be sought during the early phases of the process, such as programming, schematic design, and design development (all described later in this chapter). The architect's ability to understand the nuances of the medical imaging process is critical at this phase.

The Architect's Responsibilities and Consultants

The architect provides design and management leadership for the project team, collects information from the various user groups, and coordinates the input of the many consultants needed for a complex imaging facility. This planning is done by a multidisciplinary team led by the project manager. Civil and structural engineers, landscape architects, mechanical and electrical engineers, specialized health care planning consultants, interior architects and designers, and cost consultants all play a role in facility design. The architect must coordinate the documents of these disciplines with the architectural documents.

Although information from equipment vendors needs to be provided for the architect's use, vendors should not be considered the architect's consultants. Their primary relationship is with the owner. Thus, ultimate responsibility for providing critical equipment-related information to the architect rests with the owner. In addition, the architect usually is not involved in owner–vendor negotiations for purchasing imaging equipment. Although some architectural firms have in-house equipment planning specialists, most firms obtain the services of outside consultants. In either case, medical equipment planning services do not necessarily include equipment acquisition or procurement. Generally, equipment planning services are considered to be additional services, as defined in AIA document B141. (See chapter 5, "Equipment Planning.")

The architect's own staff brings to the team a diverse set of skills and abilities. Planning, design, management, and technical expertise, as mentioned earlier, are not always of equal strength in any one individual. A principal-in-charge has overall responsibility for the project. The project manager has management expertise and day-to-day contact with the owner. Technical expertise usually is supervised by the project architect and technical coordinator and together they coordinate the preparation of construction documents and establish standards for drawings and specifications. Project designers and planners give form to the building and work closely with the project architect to address the owner's design and planning-related needs and goals. (The architect's responsibilities are defined in article 1 of AIA document B141: Standard Form of Agreement between Owner and Architect.)

Alignment of Expectations

The planning and design of an imaging facility is an iterative, or repetitive, process. Many different techniques and management styles are employed. Because numerous individuals are involved in a facility's planning, design, and construction, an enormous amount of information must be collected and verified. In addition, each health care institution varies in its philosophy, practice, and methods.

Another factor that makes the process challenging is that technology continues to develop, growing increasingly more complex and demanding in terms of design requirements for the accommodation of new equipment and processes. Thus, there is little opportunity to create comprehensive "standards" for imaging facilities that can be reused on different projects. For this reason, it is necessary that the architectural team and the departmental users share their cumulative knowledge, experience, and thoughts about the facility before the project is under way.

Also, the owner, the architect, and the contractor need to agree on the specific roles each party will play throughout the course of project development in order to establish a clear path for decision making. Project goals and parameters—such as types of service that will be accommodated, space allocations for each service, type of project delivery anticipated, and a detailed description of the project budget indicating the relative proportion of funds allocated to each department or building component—should be determined as early as possible, so that there will be no "surprises" at the conclusion of individual design phases.

Before work can begin, the owner and the architect must define the project scope so that both parties agree on the services each is responsible for providing. These should be spelled out for each phase of work and integrated into the project schedule. In addition, each party's services should be clearly defined in the owner–architect agreement. This agreement should clarify what services the architect is to provide and what services are not identified as basic services. (See AIA document B141 for a description of both basic and additional services. Note that the AIA documents can be modified for each specific project.) For example, a renovation project should begin with a detailed assessment of existing building and site conditions. If no accurate "existing conditions" drawings exist, an on-site survey should be performed. However, it should not be assumed that this survey is part of the architect's basic services unless it is specifically stated in the owner–architect agreement. Similarly, the kinds of information that must be provided by the owner and his or her consultants also should be defined before the project begins.

The architect is responsible for meeting the stated budget, but this can occur only if budget and project scope are appropriately matched. At the end of each phase of work, three things must be in balance: cost, quality, and quantity. Two can be fixed, but one must remain flexible in order to make up for extra demands from the fixed elements. If these factors are aligned during the initial (programming) phase, they should not drift apart in successive phases. However, if an imbalance develops, the next phase of work should not begin until the discrepancy is corrected.

To a certain extent, it might be possible to reduce quality in some areas, but only minimal savings will be seen before it becomes so inferior in the long run that it no longer is either desirable or economical. If a serious deviation among cost, quality, and quantity arises, either the budget will need to be increased or the project scope decreased. If the latter alternative occurs well into design, any construction cost savings will be negated by the increased cost of completing the project.

Communication

Clear communication is key to the successful management of the design and construction processes. The more complex the facility, the more important the clarity of communication. The architect plays a primary role in integrating the knowledge and input of the many individuals involved. The owner's project manager, as a spokesperson for the various facility user groups, must be forthcoming with concerns and questions as soon as they arise, so that all the necessary information will be at hand as early in the process as possible. The contractor should keep the architect informed (via the owner) of any potential conflicts that arise during the course of construction. No one involved in the process can afford to "wait and see" if a problem will work itself out later on.

Sometimes the information presented by the architect is not conveyed in a manner that is clearly understood by either user group members or administrators. Although an architect looking at an X ray of a fractured wrist probably can recognize the individual fingers and bones of the hand, he or she is unlikely to comprehend the severity of the fracture or its treatment implications. However, this is understandable because most architects are not trained in reading X rays! By the same token, the often-overlooked converse is that most radiologists, technologists, and administrators are not trained in reading architectural drawings. The architect must be aware that what seems clear and self-evident might have very little meaning for the audience to whom it is being presented. Whenever possible, graphics should be presented using a language common to both the facility users and the architect.

Language, whether written or spoken, often is confusing. Jargon and acronyms may convey confusing or double meanings that we sometimes are aware of. With technical subjects such as architecture or radiology, a term that is universally understood within one profession may be unknown or take on an entirely different meaning in another. For example, most architects understand the acronym *CAD* to stand for *computer-aided design* or *computer-aided drafting.* But for many medical professionals, the term may signify *coronary artery disease* or possibly *computer-assisted diagnosis.* Similarly, a subspecialty of radiology—*interventional radiology*—has a precise medical definition. However, the types of rooms used for interventional procedures vary from fairly basic to highly sophisticated spaces. Therefore, it cannot be assumed that one vision of an interventional room is the same for everyone.

Vague terms such as *square footage* or *dollars per square foot* often are thrown about without precise clarification. For example, if a hospital wants to expand its existing radiology department by 800 square feet into adjacent space that was just vacated, how much new space is required? The question cannot be answered without more information. If the estimate of 800 square feet for required expansion space was arrived at by taking into account net program area plus corridors, wall thickness, and mechanical chases, an 800-square-foot area of vacated space probably is sufficient. However, if the 800-square-foot expansion represents only the net area required, a net-to-gross multiplier (of approximately 1.5 to 1.6) needs to be factored in. Now approximately 1,200 to 1,280 departmental gross square feet (DGSF) are needed.

As another example, if an entire building, such as a freestanding imaging center, contains 8,000 square feet of net program area, the overall building size is estimated by factoring in another multiplier (a department gross-to-building gross multiplier) of approximately 1.3 to 1.35. Therefore, 8,000 net square feet (NSF) of program area requires approximately 15,600 to 17,280 ($8{,}000 \times 1.5 \times 1.3 = 15{,}600$; $8{,}000 \times 1.6 \times 1.35 = 17{,}280$) building gross square feet (BGSF). (Figure 4-1, on p. 53, shows the relationship between BGSF, NSF, and DGSF.) As a general rule of thumb, the overall amount of BGSF will be approximately double the NSF.

The problem becomes more complicated when discussing cost. Unit costs, such as $200 per square foot, generally refer to the construction cost per BGSF. However, if the cost of building an imaging department is compared to that of building an administration department, these comparative unit costs might refer to departmental area (DGSF), assuming that the building shell and service core are already built. Interior "tenant improvement" costs are significantly lower than the cost of an entire building enclosure. As a general rule, the type of area measurement (NSF, DGSF, or BGSF) being discussed should always be defined; it is important to not simply refer to square feet or dollars per square foot.

With that in mind, assume that a 25,000-BGSF freestanding facility requires a budget of approximately $5 million, which both the architect and the owner agree is appropriate for the imaging facility. A problem arises when the owner refers to a $5 million *project budget* and the architect refers to a $5 million *construction budget.* Although they may think they are in agreement, in the architect's mind the project budget (which includes the cost of financing, the cost of land, professional fees, and so on) may be 60 percent (or more) higher than the construction budget, for a total budget of $8 million. To avoid confusion, it should be stated that the 25,000-BGSF facility costs about $200 per BGSF to build excluding project costs and therefore requires a construction budget of $5 million. It should further be stated that this figure excludes the cost of major medical equipment and furniture.

Project Phases

Whether the end product is a renovated department in an existing hospital or an entire, new, freestanding building, the design and planning process parallels that of diagnosing and treating a patient. (See figure 4-2.) In both cases, the early stages provide the most opportunity for determining future needs and developing a course of action that will yield an optimal outcome. As the plan progresses, opportunities to rechart the course become limited and costly, in human as well as economic terms.

Of course, new information will come to light and problems may occur during the course of the building process, just as may happen during the treatment process. Thus, it is important that the project team establish a means for incorporating new information and remedying problems as soon as they occur.

One solution is to involve the key decision makers early in the project. In this way, individual team members do not bring "new ideas" to the table halfway through the process, causing costly repetition of previous efforts. Another technique is to structure the process so that global issues are addressed initially and details are discussed during those subsequent project phases that are most appropriate for detailed issues. In this way, fundamental decisions will not be overlooked due to the team becoming sidetracked by specific issues less critical to that stage of the project.

Finally, a policy requiring user groups and administration to formally sign off at the conclusion of each phase, prior to commencing the next, will help the process move forward. The sign-off process is not intended to hold individuals responsible for the conclusions arrived at during each phase but, rather, to document consensus on critical issues and to provide a baseline from which subsequent changes can be measured. In addition, a formal sign-off process provides clear documentation summarizing each of the project's phases.

Although the terms *planning for change* and *changing the plans* sound similar, each one's meaning implies a world of difference. The former should be an integral component of any project that is undertaken. (A variety of methods for designing flexibility into the project are discussed in chapter 8, "Design Concepts.") Although it may not be possible to predict exactly how imaging facilities will need to change in the future, it *is* known that they are going to change. Conversely, changing the plans at an inappropriate time can trigger critical events that will cost money, delay schedules, and sacrifice both functionality and appearance.

Opportunities for change become increasingly limited and costly as the project progresses. Conversely, early project phases provide opportunities for considering various alternatives. Sometimes this period of exploration is not used as effectively as it could be, which, unfortunately, may result in unnecessary last-minute changes.

Understanding the kinds of decisions that need to be made in each project phase helps reduce the frequency and magnitude of unnecessary changes. A brief description of project phases follows.

Feasibility Study

The basic questions asked in a feasibility study for building an imaging facility are not unlike those asked by an individual in deciding whether to seek medical care. The first issues to be examined are:

- What is the need for taking action?
- What are the consequences of doing nothing versus taking action?
- Can I afford (physically and financially) to take action?
- Can I afford not to?

The feasibility study is simply a commitment to examine the go–no-go decision more closely. It is an effort to gain more knowledge of the situation but not yet a commitment to design or construct a building. Usually it is money well spent, even if the resulting conclusion is "no go."

Figure 4-1. Defining Units of Area

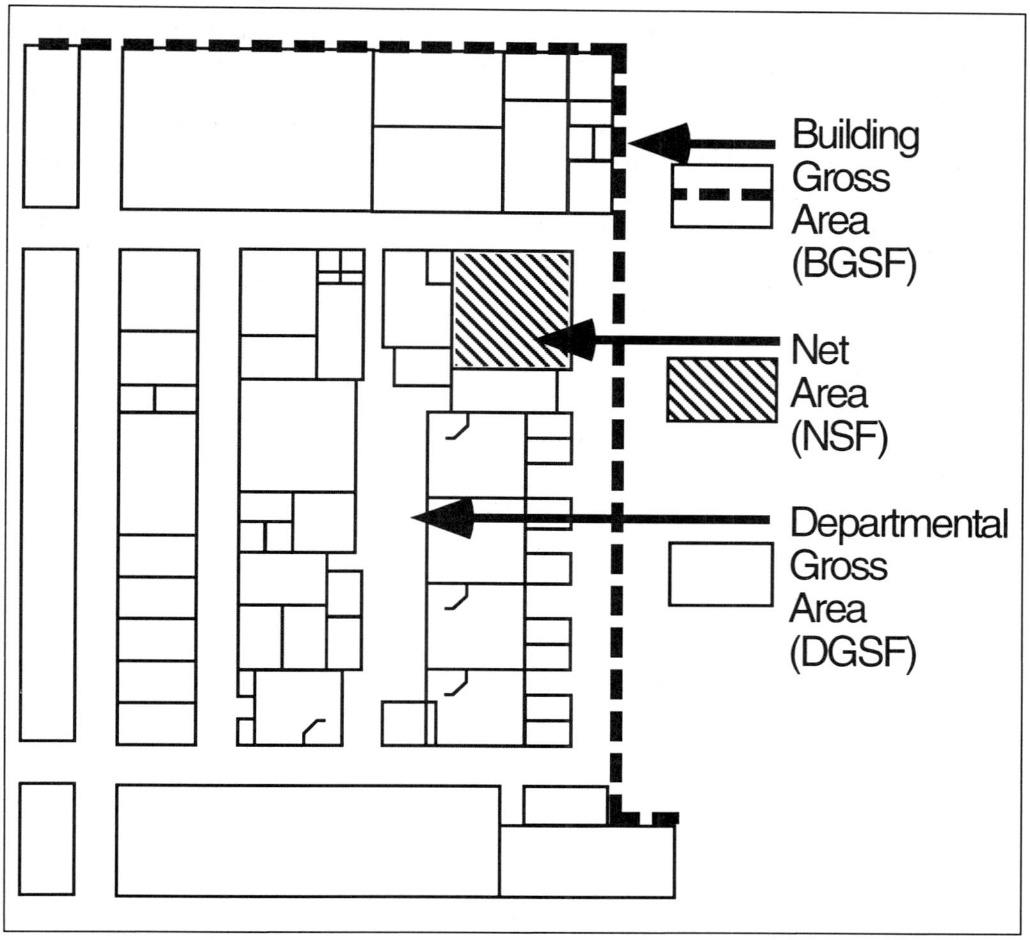

Figure 4-2. The Architectural Process in Medical Terms

Project Phases	
Program	History and Diagnosis
Design	Treatment Plan
Document	Medical Report
Construct	Treatment

Programming

The programming phase for an imaging facility is similar to recording a patient's history. This is the point at which the true nature of the project is identified as carefully as possible and a plan developed for addressing additional needs that may emerge in the future. Program information is typically obtained through a series of meetings or interviews with various users of the facility. (The programming process is discussed in more detail in chapter 12, "Space Requirements.")

The programming phase concludes with a "diagnosis" in the form of a functional and space program or report describing proposed space allocations, adjacencies, and environmental features that should be considered for future as well as present conditions. (See the appendix at the end of chapter 3, "Organization of an Imaging Project," for an example of such a program.)

Appropriate issues to be addressed during programming include:

- Flow of patients, staff, visitors, and equipment
- Space requirements of each room
- Adjacencies of one functional area to another
- Staffing projections
- Workload projections
- Operational issues
- Quality of the built environment
- Relative cost of construction
- Projections for future expansion

This is the time to identify rooms that might be used initially for one function and then converted to another at a later date. For example, a clerical work area might be transformed into a computer workstation, once electronic image management is fully embraced. Knowing that the function may be changed in the future can influence the amount of space allocated for that function.

There is no substitute for comprehensive functional and space programming. Time spent developing a thorough program is likely to save time and money that otherwise would be required if the program were to need modification after design had begun. The final program should be carefully reviewed and signed by both the medical staff and the administration prior to beginning design. Written sign-off is suggested.

Schematic Design

Schematic design is the first of two design phases. For the imaging facility, this phase is similar to the development of a course of treatment that typically follows diagnosis of a patient. The required adjacencies and circulation patterns, which were identified and tested during programming, should remain intact as the written program report is translated into three dimensions. During this period of synthesis and testing, additional information emerges that will refine the previously developed program. During schematic design the facility begins to take on a personality.

Alternative plans are now developed and alternative future outcomes are considered. This is the time to explore a variety of forms within which the functional and space program can be realized. Throughout schematic design there is constant interaction among designers, planners, engineers, and facility users. Additional work sessions (similar to, but more detailed than, the programming phase interviews) reveal more data regarding equipment preferences and how the facility will be used. The architectural team needs to take great care in communicating abstract design concepts using language and graphics that are clearly understandable to individuals who may have no previous experience "reading" architectural drawings or models.

Suddenly, the words and numbers used in the programming phase to describe individual spaces become more visually understandable. As the plans take form, the project seems to become more real. Sometimes, as the design becomes more tangible, there also is a desire to reconsider earlier fundamental decisions. Strong leadership, coming from both facility users and design consultants, is needed to prevent the process from becoming sidetracked.

The first stages of schematic design might begin with a series of block or single-line diagrams. (See figures 4-3 and 4-4.) These are generalized sketches that test the space program to verify whether all the rooms and departments can be arranged to provide both the required functional adjacencies and a reasonable aesthetic form.

Circulation and flow patterns are essential elements of the block and single-line diagrams. How these patterns will change when new technologies are employed is a consideration that should be addressed during this early design phase. It is much easier to make changes on drawings or the computer than it is to move concrete and steel; once construction begins, changes will be more costly and difficult. Flexibility designed into the plan initially will allow an effective and affordable response to future change; unplanned, forced changes usually result in functional compromise. The operational costs of a facility design that does not adequately support required functions can exceed the associated cost of construction.

By the end of schematic design, a preferred plan should be selected from among the various alternatives. Schematic design concludes with a series of somewhat developed, but still generalized drawings and study models that depict the size, configuration, and arrangement of each space or room. (See figure 4-5.) For imaging facilities major medical equipment has a significant influence on room size, configuration, and arrangement. Therefore, preliminary equipment selections for fixed imaging and other fixed equipment should be made

Figure 4-3. Example of a Block Diagram

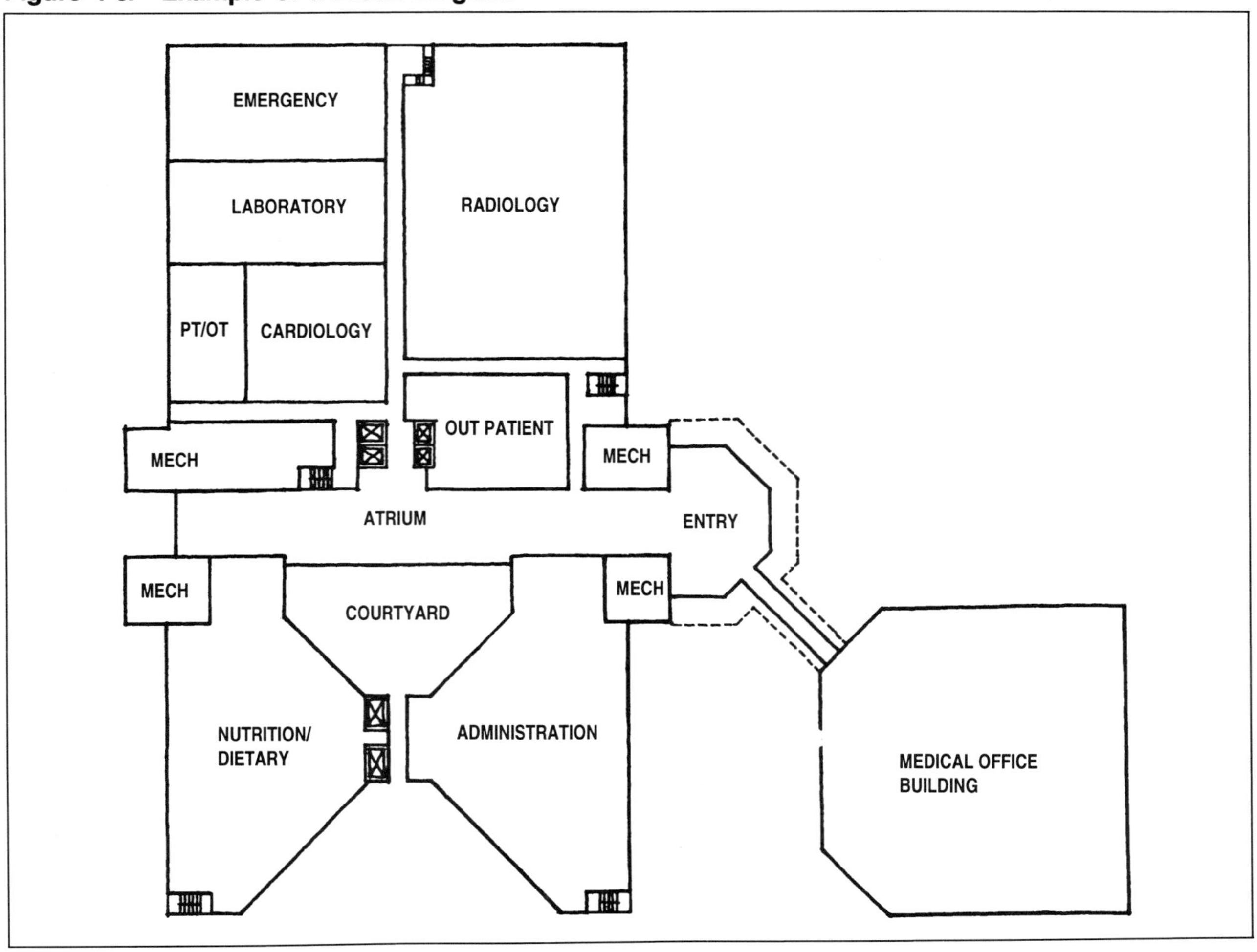

Courtesy of Stone Marraccini Patterson, San Francisco. Used with permission.

at this time, if at all possible. Each room should be identified with a name and room number; this provides a framework from which the equipment planner can develop an equipment list or database.

Design Development

Design development, the second and final design phase, includes a detailed revisit of the preferred schematic design and serves as an examination to both verify the previous "diagnosis" and build on it in detail. This is the time to evaluate finishes and materials, refine equipment requirements, examine furniture arrangements, and finalize the needs of the electrical, mechanical, security, and communications systems. This also is the time to finalize detailed

Figure 4-4. Example of a Single-Line Schematic Departmental Layout

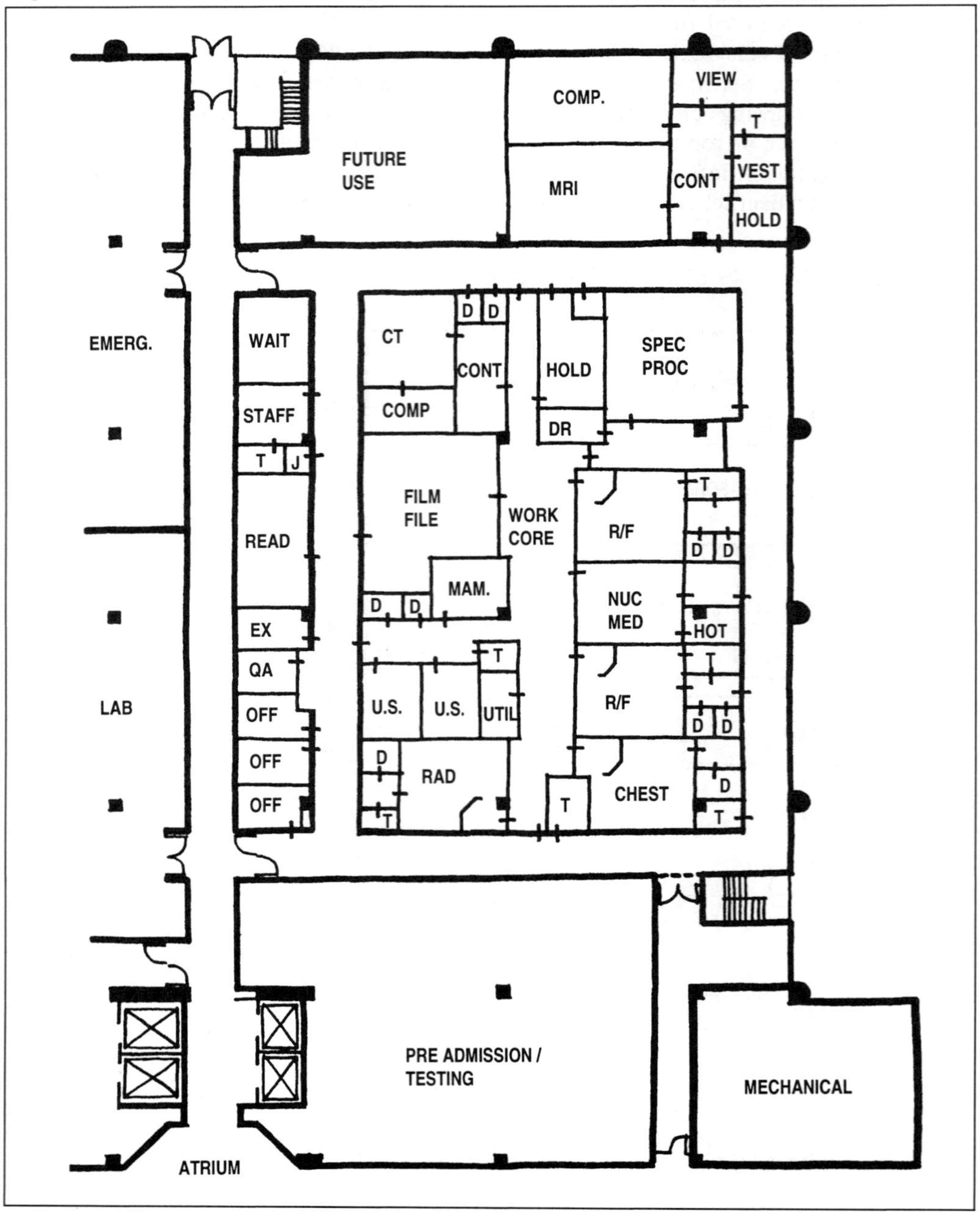

Courtesy of Stone Marraccini Patterson, San Francisco. Used with permission.

Figure 4-5. Example of a Schematic Design Partial Plan

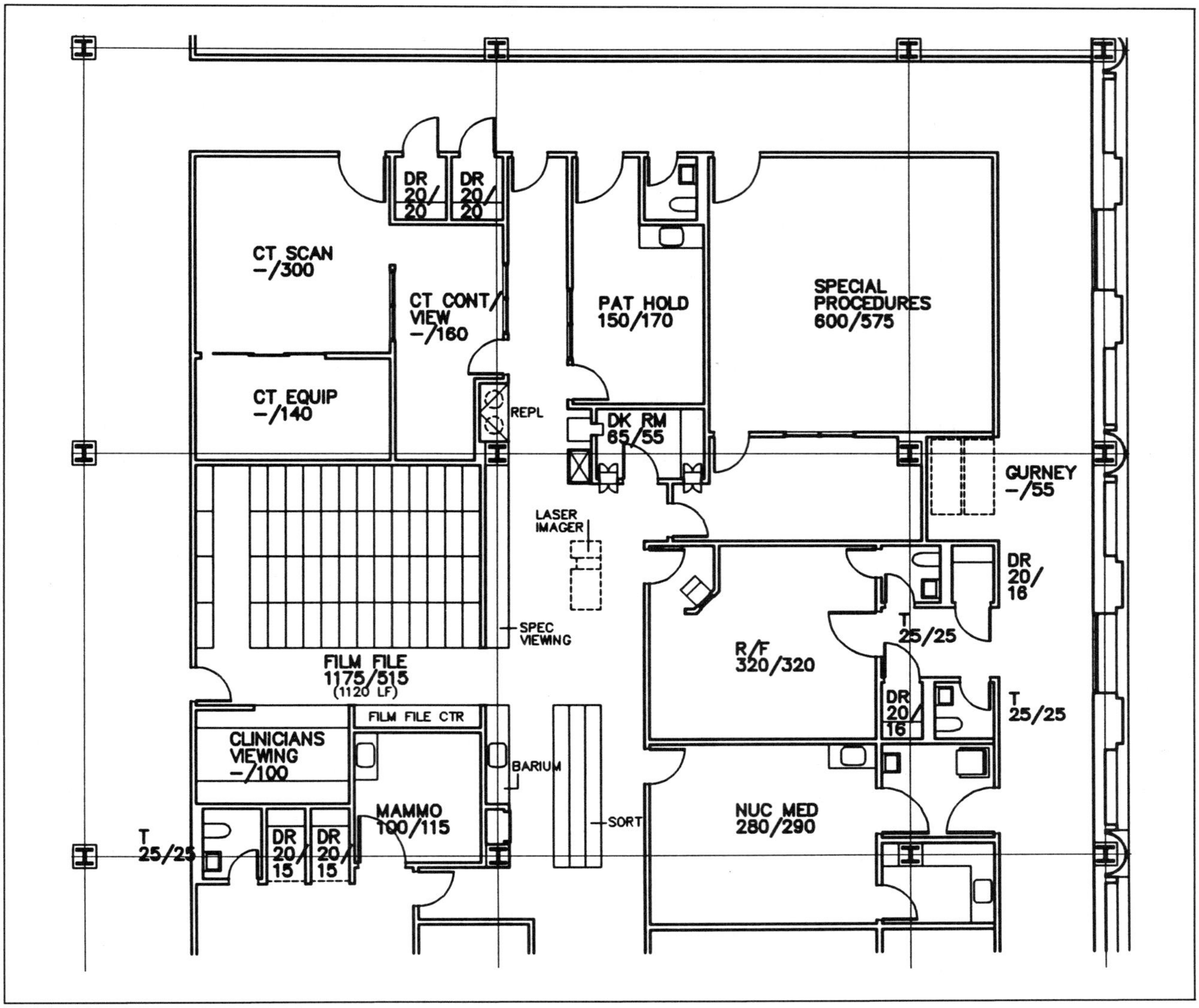

Courtesy of Stone Marraccini Patterson, San Francisco. Used with permission.

information about group 2 equipment. (See chapter 5, "Equipment Planning," for a description of the type of information to be collected.)

Circulation patterns and required adjacencies for staff, patients, materials, and information are now fixed. Design development is not the time to be adding new rooms to the program or relocating rooms, just as a physician would not want to rediagnose a patient well after a treatment plan for an initial diagnosis had been developed. Design development is the time to develop the internal and external facility design in detail.

Ideally, all design decisions should be made before the contract document phase begins. This means the design development phase theoretically provides the last opportunity for design changes.

One useful technique employed during design development work sessions is to fill out a series of data sheets, one for each room. A data sheet lists specific requirements such as floor, wall, and ceiling finishes. Sometimes electrical, ventilation, plumbing, and communications requirements; equipment requirements; furnishings; and so on are combined with architectural room data. Often they are documented separately by each specialty consultant.

Special attention must be given to coordinating architectural, engineering, equipment, and interior design information to prevent information from being overlooked or documented twice. Additional coordination is needed to ensure that accurate and current data find their way from the design development documents to the contract documents. Because there is so much detailed information in the equipment list, it usually is advantageous to keep this document separate from, but coordinated with, the room data sheets.

For rooms where architectural, engineering, and equipment requirements are highly interrelated, equipment, architectural, engineering, and interior design user group meetings might occur together. Although this requires more time of the consultants and makes the user group meetings very long, it can eliminate coordination problems later on.

The information contained in the room data sheets will later be incorporated into the contract documents, drawings, and specifications. For this reason, it is necessary to ascertain which items are to be furnished and installed by the contractor and identify them separately from those items for which the owner is responsible. Contractor items are described in detail in the contract documents and owner items are not (although they sometimes are identified on the drawings and referred to as "owner furnished–owner installed," or OF–OI, in the specifications). Because owner-furnished equipment is not a contractor responsibility, it usually is not described in detail in the contract documents. However, utility lines, piping, and couplings—which provide power, water, and so on to the owner-furnished equipment—are contractor responsibilities. Therefore, they must be clearly documented in the contract documents.

Although the equipment-related information is not provided to the contractor until the bidding phase and is not incorporated into the final documents in detail until the contract documents phase, everything related to the equipment must be analyzed and coordinated during the design development phase. This is no small task! Equipment selections for imaging facilities have a tremendous impact on both the *design* and *construction* processes.

Contract Documents

Just as the programming, schematic design, and design development phases document communication between owner and architect, the purpose of the contract documents phase is to provide information to the contractor. In a sense, contract documents (which include construction drawings, specifications, and other exhibits) report in detail the proposed "treatment plan" for building the facility. However, they describe the desired results or outcome; they do not dictate construction methods.

During the contract documents phase, drawings and specifications that convey the physical requirements of the facility to the contractor are prepared. (See figure 4-6.) These documents should provide enough detailed and coordinated information for the contractor(s) to develop a comprehensive bid or negotiated fee. Otherwise, areas in which the documents are vague provide the contractor with opportunities to ask for additional funds, or change orders, during construction.

Regulatory Agency Review

Depending on the project's scope and the jurisdiction in which the project resides, the duration of regulatory agency review(s) may be as short as a few weeks or as long as more than a year. An estimate of the review period should be factored into the project schedule.

The type of review process required may be determined by both the project's occupancy classification and its location. For example, in some locales hospital imaging projects are reviewed by the state, whereas nonhospital outpatient facilities are reviewed by the local reviewing agency. Some projects may be reviewed by multiple agencies. In addition to the building permit review, some projects also will require neighborhood approvals, an environmental impact report (EIR), licensing, and other formal regulatory reviews.

Bidding and Negotiation

The bidding or negotiation phase is determined by the project delivery method selected by the owner. Examples include the traditional design–bid–build method or a number of approaches

Figure 4-6. Example of a Construction Drawing Partial Plan

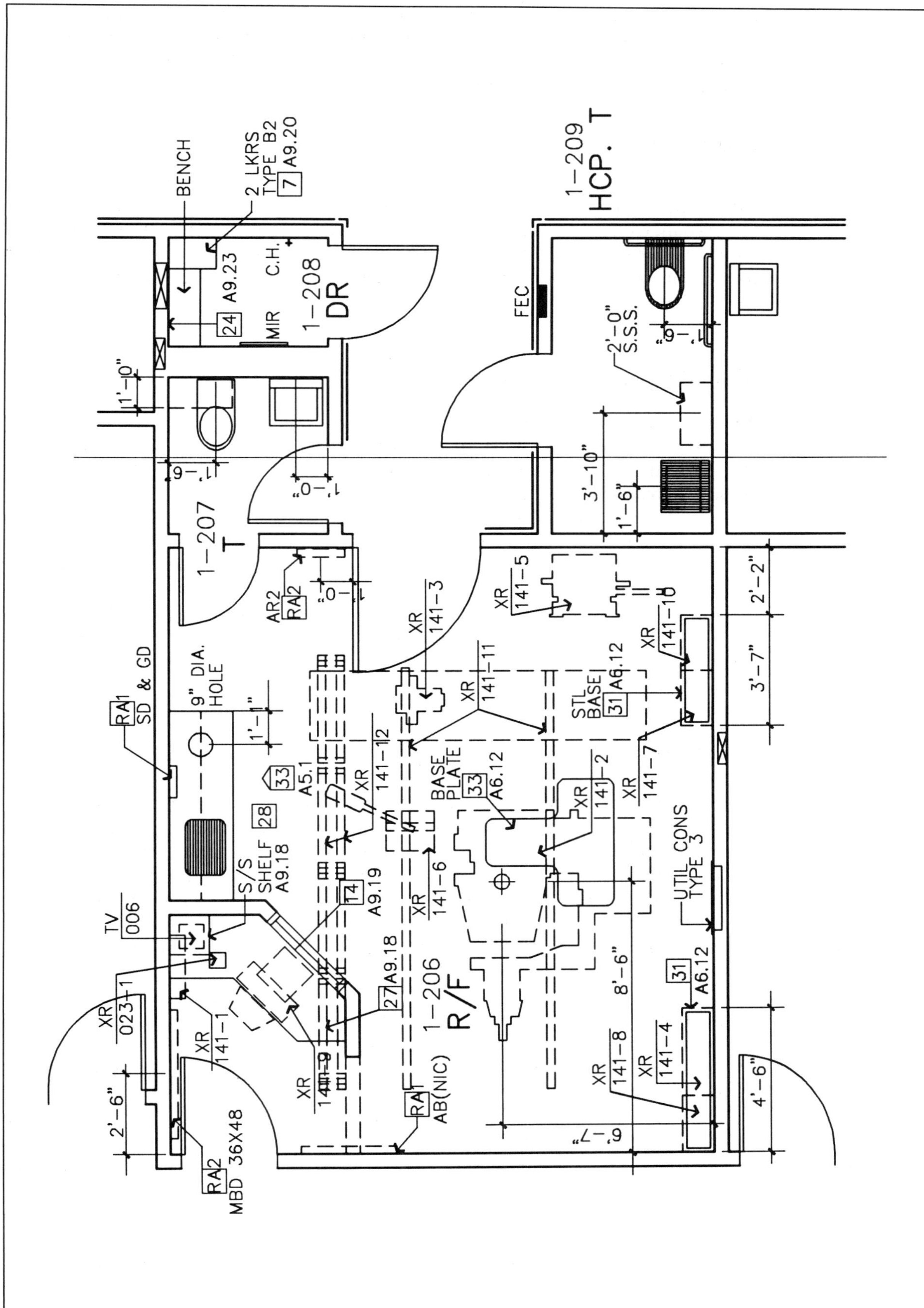

Courtesy of Stone Marraccini Patterson, San Francisco. Used with permission.

in which a contractor, who is selected prior to completion of design, will negotiate a construction fee instead of competitively bidding the project. The approach to project delivery should be selected at the beginning of the project, as it will influence both the project schedule and the method in which documents are prepared.

Construction

The architect's role during the construction process usually is limited to "administering" the contract documents. This means that he or she will clarify—via the owner—questions initiated by the contractor. Additional architect responsibilities include verifying payment requests and visiting the site as specified in the owner-architect agreement. The architect has no direct contractual arrangement with the contractor; therefore, the architect has no authority to "supervise" the contractor.

The Project Schedule

The *project schedule* is simply a tool that charts the various activities of the project, relative to time and each other. In addition to being a project management tool, the schedule is a communication tool: It identifies who is responsible for each activity and what will be affected as each activity is carried out or delayed.

Usually, there will be one or two "key drivers" of the schedule. For example, the cost of money (compound interest) may be a key driver. As the schedule lengthens, the finance charges for funding the project increase. If the project is funded by publicly approved bonds, the conditions of funding may require that a substantial portion of the funds be spent by some predetermined date. Possibly, the project is one of a series of projects—all of which are tied to a master schedule—that makes space available for one project when another is completed.

Tasks—the basic element of any schedule—include all activities that must be completed throughout the duration of a project. For each of the project phases described earlier, a series of tasks can be identified. Each task will have a relationship to others. Some tasks must precede others, some will succeed others, others may occur simultaneously, and still others will be independent.

All tasks have a duration. For example, if an equipment vendor requires six weeks to prepare technical equipment drawings, equipment selection will precede technical drawing preparation, which in turn will precede contract documentation of that equipment. Thus, the task of preparing the technical equipment drawings by the vendor has a duration of six weeks. The schedule tracks the various interdependent relationships among tasks and adjusts all related activities when the duration of one task is changed.

Milestones are interim deadlines that are either self-imposed or stipulated beyond the control of the project team. *Self-imposed milestones* include planned presentations to executive committees; *external milestones* include deadlines for filing an application for public funding.

Each activity implies resources or staffing to get the job done. For some activities, such as preparation of construction details, adding staff may decrease the task duration. For activities that depend on the completion of related activities, additional staff resources might not reduce the task duration.

Because the schedule tracks temporal relationships among tasks, it will be adjusted continuously. *Critical path activities* involve sequences of events that will have a negative impact on milestones if their duration "slips" too far; *noncritical path activities* may slip without having major negative impact on the overall schedule.

The appropriate duration for each project phase depends on the project's scale and complexity. For a moderate-size, newly constructed hospital imaging department, an approximate duration for each phase is shown in figure 4-7. Obviously, numerous variables, such as decision-making structure, regulatory review requirements, and the sophistication of equipment, will influence the duration of each project phase.

The schedule can be presented in a variety of forms, including Gantt or bar chart, PERT (program evaluation and review technique), and critical path chart. A Gantt view (named for its inventor) displays the name of each activity with a corresponding time line representing the task's duration and location within the schedule. (See figure 4-8.) A PERT view displays each task as a box with lines representing the type of relationship (predecessor, successor, and so on) connecting the task to other tasks. (See figure 4-9.)

Project Budgets

The project budget is likely to go through many phases during the life of the project. It should include a design contingency to accommodate minor changes that might occur during the design phases.

A preliminary budget must be established during feasibility planning and before any design decisions can be made. This budget serves as a yardstick by which existing funds

Figure 4-7. Approximate Duration of Project Phases for a Newly Constructed Hospital Imaging Department

Programming phase	2 months
Schematic design phase	4 months
Design development phase	6 months
Contract documents phase	9 months
Permit review phase	10 months (duration varies with regulatory review process)
Bidding/negotiation phase	2 months
Construction phase	18 months
Subtotal:	51 months = 4 years, 3 months

Figure 4-8. Project Schedule: Gantt View

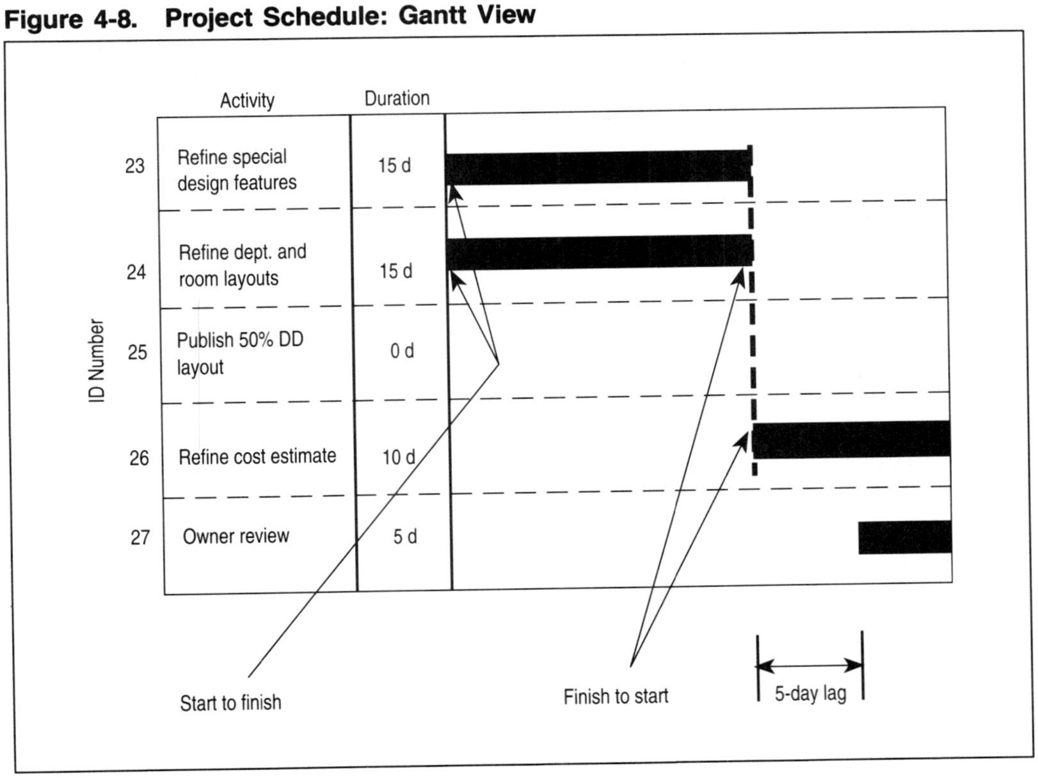

Figure 4-9. Project Schedule: PERT View

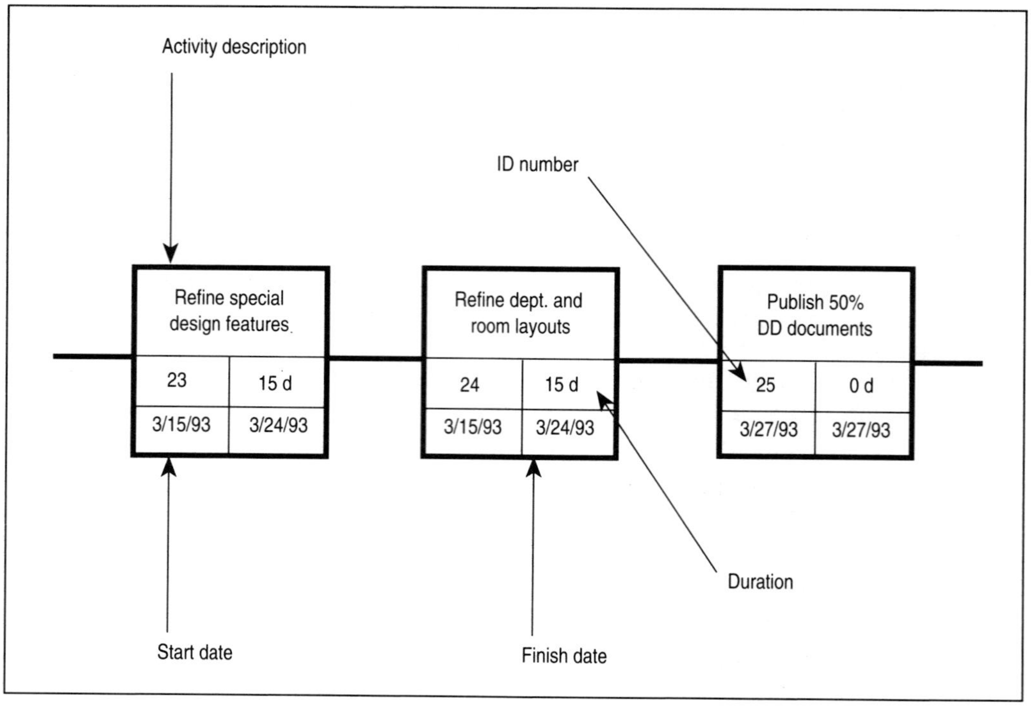

can be measured against required capital. It also establishes cost parameters within which both owner and architect must be able to work. If either party doubts the appropriateness of these limits, his or her concerns should be addressed as soon as possible.

Elements of Project Cost

Construction costs are only a part of overall project costs. The cost of land, as well as financing, operating expenses, and maintenance expenses also must be considered.

The budget estimate form identifies the major elements of project cost. (See figure 4-10, pp. 64–65.) These elements are organized into three distinct categories:

- Direct construction costs
- Indirect construction costs
- Project development costs

Direct Construction Costs

Direct costs include:

- *Building:* Including the costs of structural components, walls, floors, partitions and finishes, and their associated labor costs.
- *Site development:* Including site improvement costs, such as grading, excavation, backfill, and the installation of utilities throughout the site.
- *Landscaping:* Including types and arrangements of foliage, walkways, benches, and so on.
- *Fixed nonmedical equipment and systems:* Including permanent building-related equipment (but not medical equipment). Confusion between fixed and movable equipment can lead to misinterpretation of project cost estimates. For example, built-in paging systems are fixed equipment, whereas desk telephones are movable equipment. The cost of fixed equipment (usually referred to as *group 1 equipment*) is generally carried

as part of the construction budget, whereas the cost of movable equipment (usually referred to as *group 2 equipment*) is generally carried as part of the equipment budget. (See chapter 5, "Equipment Planning," for further discussion of this subject.)

- *Utilities:* Systems and equipment (including electrical; plumbing; heating, ventilating, and air-conditioning (HVAC); and fire protection systems), either inside the building or extending (usually 5 feet or less) just beyond its external limits.

Indirect Construction Costs

Indirect costs include:

- *Site acquisition:* Including the purchase price of land and associated expenses, such as the cost of mitigating environmental hazards associated with the site.
- *Contractor's profit and overhead*
- *Escalation*
- *Furnishings*
- *Movable equipment and other non-building-related equipment:* Referring to equipment that is not considered to be a part of the building construction. Although usually fixed, imaging equipment often is budgeted with movable equipment. (See chapter 5, "Equipment Planning.")
- *Allowances and contingencies:* Referring to a predetermined amount, usually a percentage of direct construction costs, set aside for unforeseen conditions, such as undesirable subsurface site characteristics, or for anticipated but fluctuating costs that might increase by the time the project is bid.
- *Miscellaneous:* Including artwork, signage, and so on.

Project Development Costs

Project development costs include:

- *Professional fees:* Architect and consultant fees.
- *Site survey*
- *Insurance*
- *Attorney and accountant fees*
- *Postconstruction leasing and advertising (if applicable)*
- *Financing:* Including interim construction financing, as well as long-term financing expenses.
- *Permit fees:* The costs of regulatory reviews, building permits, and so on.
- *Taxes*
- *Miscellaneous development*

Some items, such as landscaping, may be controlled by the project team; others, such as prevailing interest rates, are beyond the team's control.

Development of Construction Cost Estimates

Cost estimates become more complex as the project progresses and more information becomes available. Broad-brush estimates are adequate at preliminary stages, but later phases should include estimates with enough detail to enable the project team to compare the value of alternative designs.

Construction cost estimates used for feasibility studies are commonly determined by multiplying an appropriate unit cost by the estimated gross building area or volume. During programming, expensive specialty areas can be distinguished from less-expensive general use areas. For example, a special procedures imaging room might cost $250 per DGSF (plus the cost of equipment) as compared to a storage area that might cost $65 per DGSF. This classification of cost relative to the type of space provides greater accuracy in the estimate.

Figure 4-10. Budget Estimate Form

Project name	______	Building gross square feet	______
Location	______	Net square feet	______
	______	Net/gross ratio	______
	______	Total project cost/ square foot	______
Owner	______	Direct construction cost/ square foot	______
Job number	______	Site area square feet	______

Direct construction costs

Building cost (gross area × unit cost/square foot)	______
Site development	______
Landscaping	______
Fixed equipment	______
Utilities	
Heating/ventilating/air conditioning	______
Plumbing, fire protection	______
Electrical systems	______
Subtotal	______

Indirect construction costs

Site acquisition	______
Contractor's profit and overhead	______
Furnishings	______
Allowances and contingencies	______
Miscellaneous (describe)	
______	______
______	______
______	______
Subtotal	______

Figure 4-10. (Continued)

Project development costs

Professional fees

Architectural	______
Consultant (______)	______
Consultant (______)	______
Consultant (______)	______
Site survey	______
Insurance	______
Legal	______
Accounting	______
Financing	______
Interim	______
Long-term	______
Permit fees	______
Taxes	______
Miscellaneous (describe)	
______	
______	
______	______
Subtotal	______
Total project cost	______

Notes: ______

______

______

Source: Rostenberg, B. Design Planning for Freestanding Ambulatory Care Facilities. Chicago, American Hospital Publishing, 1986 [out of print], pp. 29–30.

At the completion of each design phase, either a statement of probable construction cost (a cost estimate) should be developed or a previous one revised. The type of estimate prepared at each phase might be as follows.

Conceptual Cost Model (Programming Phase)

A conceptual cost model can be assembled at the programming phase. Based on the program documents and an understanding of the intended quality of construction, the conceptual cost model assumes a unit rate ($/SF) of construction cost for each major component of the facility. For example, *high-tech spaces,* such as procedure rooms and film-processing areas, would be assigned one unit rate and *general use areas,* such as offices and storage areas, would be assigned a different unit rate. An allowance for furniture, fixtures, and equipment also should be assigned. If possible, the equipment allowance should be based on a preliminary list of proposed medical equipment rather than an average $/SF rate. The conceptual cost model probably will be prepared by the architect's cost-estimating consultant using equipment costs provided by the equipment planning consultant.

Outline Subsystems Estimate (Schematic Design Phase)

Alternative layouts need to be compared during the schematic design phase (development of conceptual or schematic drawings). Options for major elements of each building subsystem (structure, HVAC, and so on) should be briefly examined and tentative selections made. For example, a steel structural frame may be more expensive than concrete, but also may provide flexibility in its ability to accommodate future changes. Selection of building subsystems also will be influenced by materials availability, applicable building codes, regional conditions (such as seismic activity), and prevailing wage rates. A typical outline subsystems estimate includes an estimate for each of the project's major subsystems.

Expanded Subsystems Estimate (Design Development Phase)

As more detailed information becomes available, tentative selections made can be tested during the schematic design phase. An expanded subsystems estimate compares alternative building components and assemblies (for example, precast concrete versus aluminum wall panels) by assigning unit costs per square foot of area or other unit of measure. The outline estimate developed during schematic design can be expanded to permit comparisons of alternative subsystems or entire building systems.

The expanded subsystems estimate is detailed enough to provide reasonably accurate predictions, and yet design options are still flexible during the design development phase. If estimated construction costs exceed those anticipated in the project budget, this can be resolved by substituting more cost-effective building components rather than redefining the entire project scope.

Unit Rate Estimate (Construction Documents Phase)

While the final details for construction are being assembled into the contract document package, the project team needs to be aware of the cost ramifications that will result. Previously developed subsystems estimates now can be analyzed in even greater detail. The unit rate estimate incorporates costs of the individual elements that make up each subsystem. For example, the construction cost of basement walls may include concrete, formwork, waterproofing, and damp-proofing.

Material quantities multiplied by the respective unit costs plus the cost of labor yields the total direct cost of construction. Indirect costs, such as contractor's profit and overhead, also must be included to make this figure meaningful. Additional items include cost escalation contingencies and allowances for the requirements specified in the general conditions of the construction contract. Sometimes a detailed cost estimate is provided when the contract documents are 50 and 90 percent complete.

Chapter 5

Equipment Planning

Equipment planning is an essential and often complex process integral to the development of any imaging facility. Coordination of architectural and equipment planning activities becomes complex, in part, because the imaging facility is affected by medical equipment more directly than are other types of health care facilities. Most imaging equipment has unique requirements for structural, electrical, mechanical, and communications systems.

Most imaging projects warrant the involvement of an equipment planner. Some architectural firms specializing in the design of health care facilities offer equipment planning capabilities from within their own organizations; others look to equipment planning consultants for this service. In some instances, the owner may want to contract with the equipment planner directly as an "owner's consultant." Any of these arrangements is acceptable, provided the equipment planner is knowledgeable about equipment currently available, trends in medical imaging, and the specific needs of the owner. Ideally, the architect, the engineers, and the equipment planner would have some previous experience working together on medical imaging projects.

It is important to note that although equipment vendors provide information to the architect that is necessary for design and planning, their role is different from that of equipment planners. The equipment vendors' planning information generally is provided in support of their primary goal, which is to sell equipment. Their planning information usually is specific to their own line of equipment. In contrast, equipment planning consultants do not necessarily recommend one brand of equipment over another, although they might assist owners in selecting equipment by helping them understand differences among available brands.

This chapter discusses the scope of equipment planning services and responsibilities. It also describes approaches to equipment classification and how to establish an equipment budget.

Scope of Equipment Planning Services

The responsibilities of the equipment planner can be limited or quite broad. Basic equipment planning services might include:

- Assisting the owner in making equipment selections
- Establishing and tracking the equipment budget
- Compiling an "equipment book" including manufacturer's installation data and "cut sheets" (equipment specifications) and obtaining other relevant data from equipment vendors
- Developing room-by-room equipment lists indicating the general location of equipment
- Obtaining from the vendor and forwarding to the architect (via the owner) installation data necessary to develop architectural and engineering components of the building

- Organizing and directing equipment user group meetings in which the specific equipment needs of facility users are identified

Additional services, which may be beyond the scope of basic equipment planning services, may include:

- *Assisting the owner in procuring and installing equipment and negotiating a purchase agreement with the vendor:* Although the equipment planner can be helpful in this area, many health care providers are affiliated with some type of bulk purchasing service and can negotiate competitive prices themselves. The difference between an aggressively negotiated price and list price is considerable. Negotiated pricing also should include extended service contracts, which in themselves can eventually add up to a considerable sum.

  Unless procurement and price negotiating are part of the equipment planner's services, the architect and equipment planner's work should be clearly separated from the owner's equipment negotiating process. If the architect, equipment planner, and facility users need to meet with equipment vendors in order to clarify the equipment's space or utility requirements, that team should make it clear to the vendor that the meeting is solely for planning purposes and that similar meetings are being held with other vendors. If the vendor assumes that the owner has already "selected" his or her brand of equipment, the owner's negotiating edge may be compromised.
- *Additional user group equipment meetings:* Departmental user group meetings consist of a series of long, intense, interactive work sessions. Ideally, every piece of fixed and movable equipment, except those items for which the architect or interior designer is responsible, is identified, discussed, and documented.

  In order for these meetings to be conducted in a time-efficient manner, by the time of the first equipment meeting, each department user group should have a general idea about the equipment it is considering to purchase or reuse. In this way, the equipment planner can be an additional resource in describing some of the specific attributes and requirements of each unit, rather than having to begin with more basic issues. Equipment vendors probably will be the most qualified to describe the specific characteristics of their line of equipment. However, in most cases, the equipment planner brings a more objective viewpoint.

  Departmental user groups must be aware of the budget within which they may select their equipment. Although the equipment planner, with the architect, may be developing and tracking the equipment budget, the allocation of funds among various departments must be determined by the owner. Developing "wish lists" instead of reasonable equipment selections that fit within the limitations of the budget can destroy the intention of the user group meetings, initiating redesign and causing additional work and schedule delays.
- *Coordinating tours to visit facilities where similar equipment is in operation and presentations by equipment vendors:* One good way to learn more about the equipment that currently is in use is to visit similar facilities that have recently opened. In most cases, the department staff are more than happy to share their opinions and observations. When conducting such a tour, it is best to select a facility that is similar in scope to the one being designed. Additionally, the facility selected should be one that has been operational long enough for the staff to develop more than just first impressions, but not one that is so old that the equipment does not compare with what currently is on the market. It is important to keep in mind that facility design and construction takes a few years at best; therefore, even a brand-new facility may contain equipment that already is a few years old. Equipment vendors also may organize tours—of their own showrooms and of current facilities showcasing their equipment—as part of their sales efforts. Such tours can be both educational and economical. However, again, vendor-organized tours tend to be less objective than those organized by the architect or equipment planner.

Trade shows are another good source for learning about current equipment as well as staffing, management, and business issues relating to the operation of imaging facilities. Each year, the Radiological Society of North America (RSNA) holds the world's largest gathering of medical personnel and equipment. The conference, which usually occurs in Chicago during the week after Thanksgiving, includes the largest display of medical imaging equipment assembled under one roof. Many equipment vendors "unveil" their latest technological developments at the RSNA.

Equipment Classifications

The way that equipment is classified often determines whether its cost will be associated with the building construction budget or a separate equipment budget. Although equipment usually is divided into fixed, major movable, and minor movable categories, no single universally accepted rule for specific equipment classification exists. As a result, equipment classifications often cause confusion regarding both budgetary issues and procurement and installation responsibilities.

Of all equipment types, medical imaging equipment (and some physiological monitoring equipment) seems to cause the most confusion. This is because imaging equipment usually is fixed or physically attached to the building, and fixed equipment usually is furnished and installed by the contractor. However, imaging equipment generally is furnished by the owner and installed by the equipment vendor.

Equipment traditionally has been grouped into three classifications: group 1, fixed equipment (this group is further divided into fixed plant and fixed nonplant equipment); group 2, major movable equipment; and group 3, minor movable equipment.[1] (See table 5-1.) *Group 1, fixed nonplant equipment* includes equipment that is permanently attached to the physical structure or utility services of the building, but is not necessary for the building services to

Table 5-1. Equipment Classifications

Group 1, Fixed Equipment	Group 2, Major Movable Equipment	Group 3, Minor Movable Equipment
• Permanent connection	• Plug-in connection	• No physical connection
• Usually part of construction budget	• Usually part of equipment budget	• Usually part of owner's operational budget
• Usually furnished and installed by contractor	• Usually not furnished or installed by contractor	• Usually does not require installation
• Usually specified in the contract documents	• Usually referenced in the contract documents (contractor may be responsible for necessary utilities and anchorage, but not the equipment itself)	• Usually not specified or referenced in the contract documents, because it has no impact on the facility
	Exceptions included in group 2:	
	• Fixed medical imaging equipment	
	• Fixed physiological monitoring equipment	
Examples:	Examples:	Examples:
• Fume hoods	• Movable ultrasound units	• Surgical instruments
• Sterilizers	• Exam tables	• IV stands
• Medical gas headwalls	• Fixed imaging and physiological monitoring equipment	• Pots and pans
		• Kitchen flatware

operate. (An example of fixed nonplant equipment is a medical gas headwall unit.) Fixed plant equipment also is physically attached but includes equipment integral to building services, such as boilers, chillers, and air handlers. The two types of equipment are very different.

Group 1 equipment generally requires physical modification to the building or its utility systems in order for it to be installed, removed, or replaced. As a result, it usually is indicated on the architectural and engineering documents as being a part of the facility, and its cost is therefore considered part of direct construction costs. The following list clarifies the types of equipment:

- *Group 1, fixed plant equipment:* Examples include boilers, chillers, air handlers, energy management systems, and conveying systems such as elevators and lifts.
- *Group 1, fixed medical equipment:* Examples include fume hoods, sterilizers, hydrotherapy tanks, medical gas headwalls, and power columns. Although medical imaging equipment usually has the characteristics of fixed medical equipment, it usually is classified as group 2 equipment. This places its cost in the equipment budget and not the construction budget.
- *Group 1, fixed nonmedical/nonplant equipment:* Examples include walk-in refrigerators, kitchen cooking equipment, laundry equipment, built-in casework, and conveyors such as dietary tray return systems. Dietary equipment usually is the responsibility of a food service consultant, not the medical equipment planner. Similarly, most other group 1, fixed nonmedical/nonplant equipment is coordinated by someone other than the medical equipment consultant.

Architectural and engineering documents should "reference" owner-furnished–owner-installed (OF–OI) equipment that requires electrical, mechanical, and structural components, because these utility components are furnished and installed by the contractor as part of the construction contract. One way to reference OF–OI equipment is to indicate its outline on the construction drawings and to identify it as OF/OI in the specifications. (See figure 4-6 [p. 59] in chapter 4, "Management of the Process.") In this way, the contractor provides the physical environment that must adhere to unique requirements determined by the equipment vendor, whereas the vendor—not the contractor—is responsible for the equipment itself.

The contract documents also should include a detailed equipment schedule, often included as part of the specifications. For each piece of equipment, the schedule identifies (1) an equipment number; (2) an equipment description; (3) whether the contractor or owner is responsible for its purchase and installation; (4) equipment width, depth, and height; (5) weight; (6) heat output; (7) mounting details; and (8) room location number. (See table 5-2.)

Group 2, major movable equipment includes medical equipment that may have architectural or engineering impact, although it customarily is moved from place to place without disrupting the physical components of the facility. Equipment having the following qualities may be considered to have architectural or engineering impact:

- Power voltage in excess of 120 volts (alternating current)
- Power draw greater than 2 amperes
- Requires a dedicated electrical circuit
- Requires emergency power
- Size, weight, or configuration that may affect room design, dimensions, or casework

Most movable equipment rolls on wheels, and if it requires electromechanical services, the connection is made with a simple plug-in receptacle. As noted above, fixed imaging equipment is an exception to the rule, as it usually is classified as group 2 equipment even though it is fixed.

Some types of medical furniture and furnishings may be considered group 2 equipment if they require electricity or otherwise affect facility design. If the cost of medical furniture is to be carried in the equipment budget, a clear distinction between medical and nonmedical furniture must be made so that it is neither counted twice nor unintentionally omitted.

Table 5-2. Example of a Partial Equipment Schedule for MRI

Number	Description	Responsibility	Width (in.)	Depth (in.)	Height (in.)	Weight (lbs.)	BTU/HR	Mounting Detail	Room Number
XR1	Control desk	OF–OI	48.25	30.25	27.50	126	NA	W-14	1-153
XR2	Image monitor	OF–OI	21.25	17.50	18.25	44	273	C-23	1-153
XR3	Patient monitor	OF–OI	17.50	16.25	14.75	33	171	C-23	1-153
XR4	Patient couch	OF–OI	117.25	26.75	35.25	770	1,023	F-07	1-153
XR5	Electronics cabinet	OF–OI	19.25	15.75	18.75	220	685	W-12	1-153
(Continues . . .)									

Often the budget is divided into two distinct categories: one for medical equipment and one for furniture, fittings, and nonmedical equipment (FF&E). Care must be taken to carefully define each category and to identify who is responsible for inclusion of each item in the contract documents and the budget. For example, office furnishings usually are the responsibility of the interior designer whereas medical furnishings may be the responsibility of the equipment planner. Thus, a table lamp and secretarial desk are listed in the furniture budget whereas an exam light and an exam table are listed in the equipment budget.

Casework can be another source of confusion. Built-in casework (which can be either custom-built or premanufactured and purchased) is considered part of the facility, rather than equipment. The architect is responsible for documenting and budgeting built-in casework. However, premanufactured exam room casework, which is not physically attached to the facility, may be considered medical equipment and, thus, may be the responsibility of the equipment planner. Premanufactured office-type casework, which is not physically attached to the facility, is considered furniture and is the responsibility of the interior designer.

It is important that items whose classification is unclear be identified and identified only once. Problems occur when these items are either double-counted or missed entirely. The following list clarifies group 2 equipment:

- *Group 2, medical equipment:* Examples include movable ultrasound and electrocardiography machines, patient beds, exam tables, medication carts, movable monitors, and sometimes fixed imaging and physiological monitoring equipment.
- *Group 2, nonmedical equipment:* Examples include tables, chairs, desks, and miscellaneous furnishings. The cost of these items is more appropriately listed in the furniture budget than in the equipment budget. However, it is a good idea to verify which equipment items (such as an MRI operator's console) routinely come with matching furniture (such as an operator's chair). The cost of furniture that is part of a medical equipment purchase is usually listed in the equipment budget.

Group 3: minor movable equipment consists of miscellaneous equipment and instruments that have no physical connection to the physical plant and are small enough that they have little or no effect on facility design. Minor movable equipment often is purchased by the owner and does not appear in either the construction or the equipment budget, and includes the following:

- *Group 3, minor movable equipment:* Examples include surgical instruments, pots and pans, and kitchen flatware.

A system of classifying equipment is found in *Guidelines for Construction and Equipment of Hospital and Medical Facilities.* Currently, this document is written by a special task force of the American Institute of Architects/Academy on Architecture for Health (AIA/AAH), with assistance from the U.S. Department of Health and Human Services (DHHS). It is a revision of a series of periodically updated documents that began in 1947 as part of the implementation regulations for the Hill–Burton program, and serves as an aid in the design and construction of hospital and medical facilities. Revisions to the document reflect dramatic changes to health facility planning that have occurred in subsequent years. In addition, the document is referenced by the DHHS and sometimes is referenced by certain state licensing agencies.

Chapter 4 of this document refers to equipment. The nomenclature for equipment classifications is slightly different from that described above, although the intent is similar. Excerpts from the *Guidelines* document are included in appendix C at the back of this book.

Establishment of an Equipment Budget

One of the first tasks in any project is to establish a preliminary budget. (See chapter 4, "Management of the Process.") As the project moves forward and more specific information regarding both the building and its contents becomes known, the accuracy and level of specificity of the budget increases. Individual components of the construction budget include both an equipment budget and a furnishings budget. Regardless of the nomenclature used for classifying equipment, every effort should be made during early phases of the project to establish which types of equipment are in each of the budget components and how many dollars are assigned to each component.

During the feasibility study phase, the project budget often is estimated by taking an overview of all the activities and services associated with the project. The largest single component of the project budget usually is the cost of facility construction; its magnitude is estimated by multiplying an average cost per square foot by an anticipated size (in terms of building gross area). Often equipment and furniture budgets are estimated in this phase by either a percent of construction cost or an allotment of dollars per square foot. An assignment of $10 to $15 per DGSF may be appropriate for furniture at this early stage. However, a percent of construction for the equipment budget (sometimes a figure equal to 30 to 40 percent of the construction budget is used to determine the budget for groups 1 and 2 medical equipment) can be misleading unless a distinction is made between a project with a lot of expensive major technical equipment and one with relatively little.

A better approach is to itemize—to the degree possible—the quantity, type, and unit cost of group 1 and 2 medical equipment and add a reasonable contingency factor. If the institution has purchased imaging equipment in the past, an anticipated discount can be used, based on past experience. Fixed plant equipment is already factored into the construction budget.

During the programming phase, every room in the proposed facility is identified. This allows confirmation and/or adjustment of the previous equipment and furnishings budget. For most imaging exam rooms, the type of equipment (for example, basic radiography versus digital fluoroscopy) is identified. Although specific make and model numbers are still unknown, a fairly accurate budgetary range can be established. However, if additional exam rooms are added (or perhaps deleted) after programming is completed, both design efforts and budgetary efforts may have to be repeated.

The schematic design phase is the time when room adjacencies are established and the building begins to take on its form. For most health care projects, equipment selections are far from being made during this phase. However, imaging projects pose a notable exception. Because the specific requirements of major fixed imaging equipment have such a dramatic impact on facility design and documentation, preliminary selection for imaging equipment should be made during the schematic design phase.

Once the equipment is identified, it usually takes a minimum of six to eight weeks for the equipment vendor to develop technical drawings for the architect and engineers to use. These technical drawings are essential for the architect and engineers to have before design phase services are completed.

The suggestion that preliminary selections for imaging equipment be made during schematic design will cause understandable resistance from the radiology staff. The mere thought of being asked to identify such equipment some three to four years before the building is ready for occupancy will not be readily accepted. The intent here is not to order equipment this far in advance, but rather to obtain necessary information required for facility design. This is one of the most difficult predicaments inherent in the architecture of imaging facilities.

On the one hand, facility users may want to postpone equipment selections until the latest date imaginable to ensure the latest technology available. However, delaying equipment selections delays development of significant aspects of design and engineering. On the other hand, detailed information, which varies from one equipment unit to another, is needed early in the design and planning process.

Although no perfect solution to this situation exists, the following approach helps minimize potential problems. During schematic design, the radiology staff should be asked what specific equipment they would select if the facility were to open tomorrow. In this way, equipment identification decisions are not simply delayed, they are made on a preliminary basis using the limited information available. However, architectural and engineering design can proceed on the basis of the identified equipment selections. If equipment selections change as the design continues to be developed, the owner may need to absorb the cost of any major architectural or engineering changes that might result.

An alternative is to defer further design of portions of the project until equipment in those areas is selected. However, this approach can lead to substantial delays for the entire project. In either case, the architect may want to advise the owner to establish a special construction contingency reserved for redesign required by last-minute changes in equipment selections.

A concept called *universal room design* can help accommodate various types of basic imaging equipment and, thus, allow for some equipment decisions to be deferred. (Universal room design is discussed in chapter 8, "Design Concepts.")

Reference

1. Pulaski, J. P. Equipment planning and coordination: a different point of view. A presentation for the New York City AIA Health Facilities Committee, Sept. 25, 1991.

Part 3

Imaging Techniques

A disease known is half cured.

Thomas Fuller
Gnomologia
1732

Chapter 6

Imaging Modalities

Imaging is essential to modern medicine. Angiography and ultrasound can demonstrate blood flow and visualize the inside of the heart without major surgery. Epilepsy and migraine headaches are understood better because metabolic changes can be detected through nuclear medicine and biomagnetics.

However, every imaging technique has both advantages and disadvantages for the radiologist and the patient. Some potentially lifesaving techniques show precise anatomic detail; others show images that are less precise physically but reveal exquisite metabolic function. Some procedures have dangerous side effects. Most are expensive, and some are very expensive.

Because the technology of imaging changes so rapidly, it is challenging to describe each modality in a way that is both meaningful and enduring. Because the technology is complex, architects and planners may not be aware of the subtle differences among similar imaging procedures or consider the particular functional, human, and technical requirements for each modality.

This chapter provides the background necessary to understand these imaging modalities. It briefly describes some of the methods available for seeing inside the human body and explains how they are used. The descriptions focus on the principles behind each modality, especially those aspects that will endure the myriad changes each surviving technique will undergo in the ensuing decades. Because the technology is undergoing constant refinement, it often is difficult to obtain current, accurate data necessary for designing the architecture of imaging facilities. Thus, readers will need to supplement each section of this chapter with site- and equipment-specific data available from equipment vendors. (Readers are also directed to chapter 13, "Room Design," for additional planning criteria and the functional, human, and technical issues to be considered when planning for the modalities described in the current chapter.)

Basic Radiography and Fluoroscopy

X rays have the ability to ionize substances as they pass through them, thus changing previously neutral particles to charged particles called *ions*. Radiography and fluoroscopy identify parts of the human body that are capable of blocking or absorbing ionizing radiation.

Basic *radiography* records anatomic structure as a stationary photographic image on X-ray-sensitive film sandwiched between X-ray-photon-excitable phosphorus. This is known as *film-screen radiography*. *Fluoroscopy* records a moving image that is viewed on a television-like monitor. (See figure 6-1.) In either approach, a shadow is created when X rays passing through the patient are differentially absorbed by tissues. Due to its high calcium content, bone absorbs, rather than transmits, most of the X rays that strike it.

Figure 6-1. Basic Fluoroscopy Setup

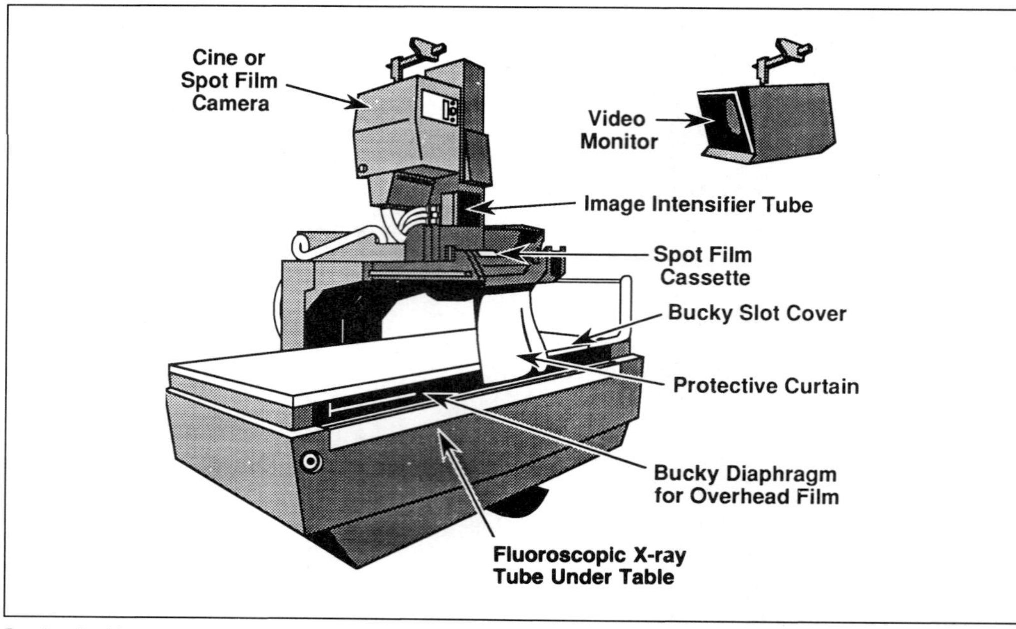

Reprinted, with permission, from Bushong, S. C. *Radiologic Science for Technologists: Physics, Biology, and Protection.* 5th ed. St. Louis: Mosby-Year Book, 1993, p. 353.

Although the lack of X-ray-absorbing elements in muscles, blood vessels, and organs renders soft tissue less visible than skeletal structure, radiographic imaging can be adapted to view such soft tissue. To accomplish this, an X-ray-absorbing contrast agent, such as a barium- or iodine-laden compound, is either ingested or injected to help visualize the area in question.

Radiographic procedures using contrast agents include:

- *Arteriograms:* For visualizing arteries
- *Arthrograms:* For viewing cartilage, ligaments, and tendons of a joint
- *Cholecystograms:* For examining the gallbladder
- *Intravenous pyelograms (IVPs):* For seeing inside the kidney, ureters, bladder, and urethra
- *Myelograms:* For viewing the spinal cord and nerves

Some contrast agents occasionally can cause unpleasant side effects. At many institutions, nonionic or low-osmolality contrast agents (LOCAs) are preferred agents for some basic and special radiographic and fluoroscopic procedures. They also are used for some contrast-enhanced computed tomography (CT) procedures. Although advocates of these agents claim they are safer and less likely to cause systemic reactions than high-osmolality contrast agents (HOCAs), LOCAs are extremely expensive. Emergency resuscitation equipment and capabilities should be readily available wherever any contrast agents are used.

In spite of the numerous specialized radiographic procedures available today, basic radiography at its relative low cost remains the workhorse of the radiology department. Simple chest X rays still constitute much of the radiologist's workload. (Figure 6-2 shows an automated dedicated chest unit.)

Mammography

Radiographic techniques such as mammography are of particular importance for their value in early cancer detection. (Figure 6-3 shows a mammography unit.) Traditional mammography

Figure 6-2. Dedicated Chest Unit

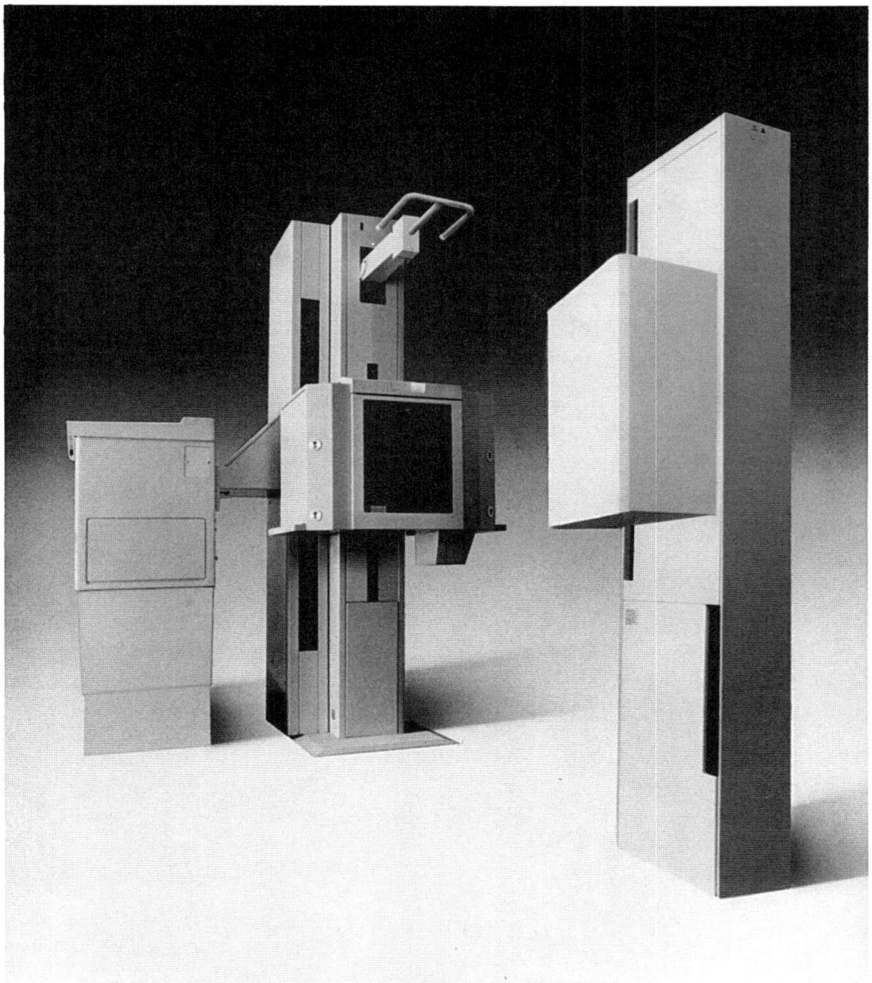

Courtesy of Picker International, Cleveland, Ohio. Used with permission.

employs low-level radiation to identify tumoral calcifications and to characterize palpable lumps and unpalpable cysts or lumps in breast tissue. Once a growth is detected, further investigation may be necessary to determine whether it is malignant. About 80 percent of breast cancer patients who are treated following early detection remain free of cancer for at least five years.

Breast lesion biopsy can provide definitive histologic diagnosis of suspect breast lesions. "The need for breast biopsy will likely rise dramatically in the coming years as more women undergo screening mammography and they and their physicians seek definitive diagnoses of lesions."[1] Three types of biopsy procedures are common: surgical excisional biopsy, fine-needle aspiration biopsy (FNAB), and needle-core biopsy. Fine-needle aspiration, needle-core biopsy, and lumpectomy developed in recent years primarily as alternatives to the trauma and expense of radical surgical procedures. Each procedure may use either mammography or ultrasound as a means of guidance for localizing lesions that require biopsy.

To detect nonpalpable breast lesions, most percutaneous breast biopsies use some form of mammographic guidance. Although orthogonal mammography has been used traditionally, lately attention has turned to stereotactic mammography as a means of targeting mammographically suspect lesions, because stereotactic techniques allow for theoretic pinpoint accuracy.[2]

Adapted standard mammography machines or dedicated stereotactic units are used for this purpose. The principle is the same for both units: the x-ray tube swings 15° off center in opposite directions, allowing for the stereo image acquisition. [See figure 6-4.] The position of the lesion in each view, compared with standard reference points, allows for the calculation of the coordinates describing the lesion's location within the breast.

The adapted standard mammography stereotactic units use an add-on device that attaches to the conventional mammography machine. These units generally require the patient to stand or sit as she would normally be positioned for a mammogram. This can be awkward and uncomfortable, as the patient must turn her head 90° and hold it back away from the x-ray tube while it is in position for the stereo views. The biopsy procedure takes place literally right under her nose with the needle in full view.

The drawbacks of the adapted standard mammography units are largely eliminated [with dedicated stereotactic mammography units, which position the patient prone on the unit's table]. The x-ray tube, compression plate, and stereo and biopsy apparatus are all located beneath the table, out of sight of the patient and free of encumbrances.[3]

Figure 6-3. Mammography Unit

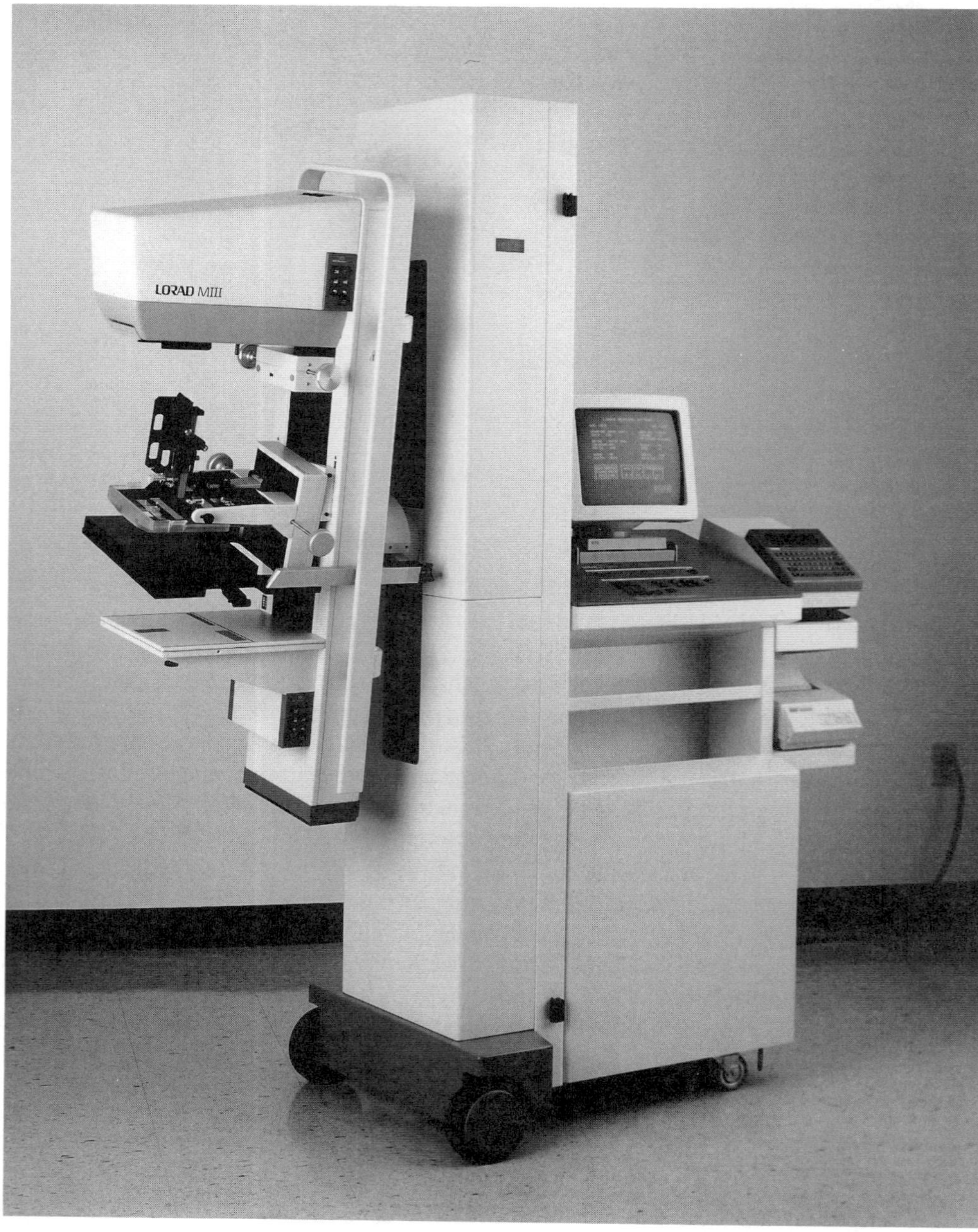

Courtesy of Lorad Corporation, Danbury, Connecticut. Used with permission.

Figure 6-4. Stereotactic Mammography Concept

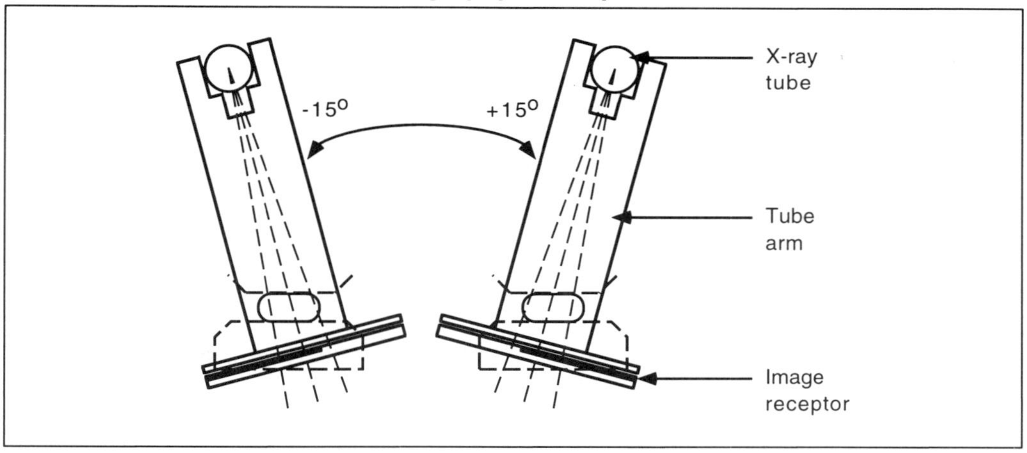

The space requirements for mammography units on which the patient is positioned in the prone position (as shown in figure 6-5) generally are greater than the space requirements for those units where the patient sits or stands upright. Also, additional space will be needed for ancillary biopsy-related instruments in any mammography room where biopsies are performed.

Recently, magnetic resonance imaging (MRI) has been used for breast imaging in non-clinical applications. (MRI is discussed later in this chapter.) Dedicated MR mammographic systems are under development.

Special Radiography/Fluoroscopy Procedures

Special radiography/fluoroscopy (R/F) procedures include a number of techniques that employ radiographic or fluoroscopic imaging equipment for guidance during complex exploratory and interventional procedures. Such procedures may require special computerized equipment, may combine diagnostic and interventional techniques, and may require the involvement of many specialists to attend to the patient simultaneously. The room in which special procedures take place usually is larger than a basic procedure room. The exact size of a special procedure room will depend on the array of equipment used and/or its intended use. (See chapter 12, "Space Requirements.")

Interventional techniques now involve specialists in cardiovascular interventional radiology, neuroradiology, and cardiology. These procedures are often highly tailored because of the diagnostic information previously derived on that patient from other imaging modalities, such as CT, MRI, or diagnostic ultrasound. In new installations, equipment usually is capable of computer-based digital image acquisition rather than primarily film-based acquisition. Fluoroscopy affords immediate internal visualization of structures that require highlighting with contrast material.

Interventional Radiology

Interventional radiology bridges the indistinct boundary between surgery and imaging. (See figure 6-6, p. 83.) With this family of techniques, fluoroscopic views of blood passage through vessels enable real-time monitoring and intervention through essentially painless catheter operations within the circulatory system.

> One of the most promising areas of medical imaging is the field of interventional radiology. . . . Viewing the human circulatory system as interconnected roadways or a vast river complex with countless tributaries, the radiologist has devised methods of entering and traveling within the system to reach almost every internal recess of the body. The utilization of these arterial passageways is at the heart of interventional radiology.[4]

Figure 6-5. Stereotactic Mammography Unit on Which Patient Is Positioned in the Prone Position

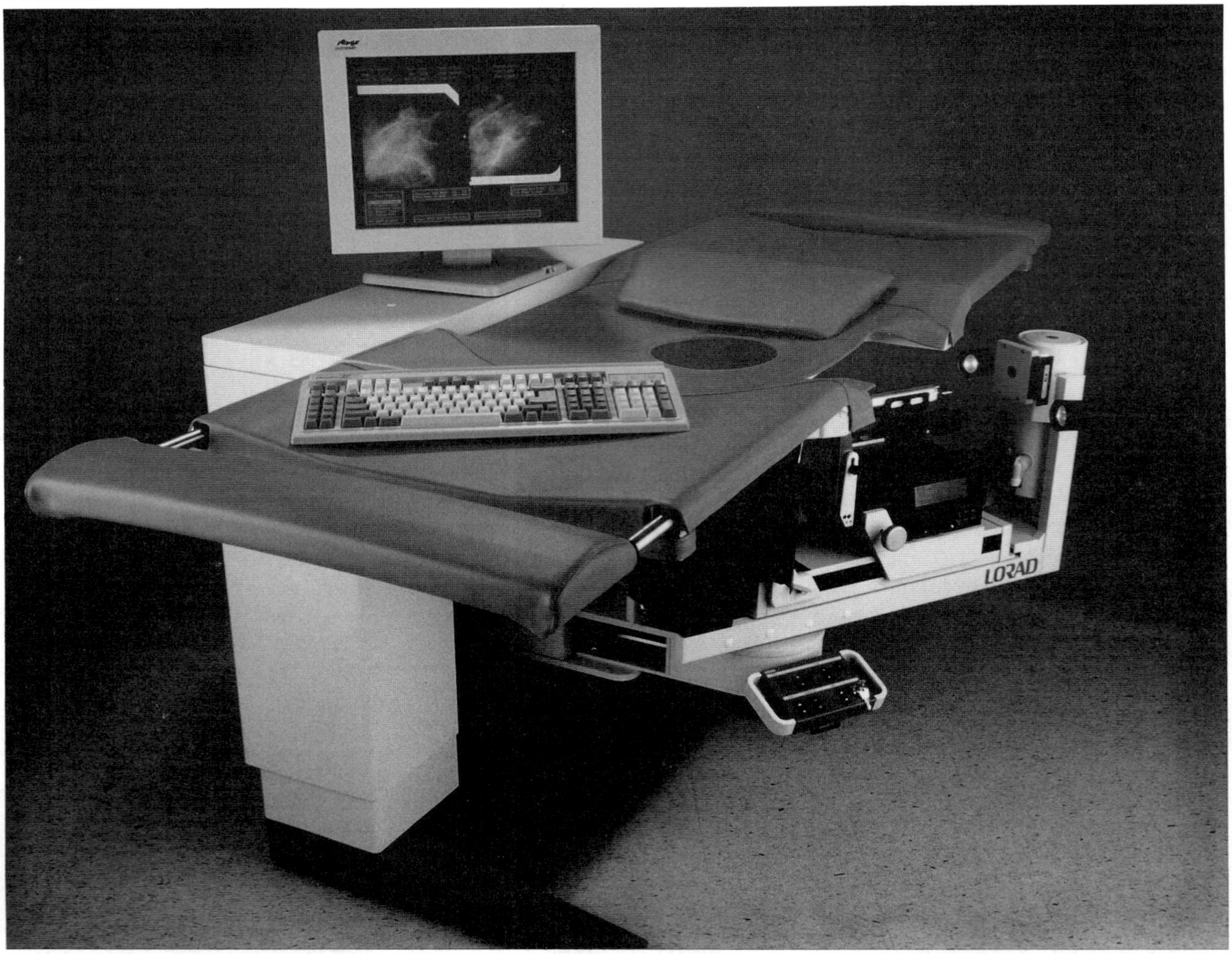

Courtesy of Lorad Corporation, Danbury, Connecticut. Used with permission.

Cardiac Catheterization

Cardiac catheterization is a special interventional procedure involving the insertion of catheters into an artery or a vein as an access point for eventual entry into the heart. Once it reaches the inner chambers of the heart, the catheter is used as a conduit for ancillary devices that obtain pressure readings, collect blood samples, and inject contrast material to improve visibility of the heart's chambers and the arteries serving the heart. This information is then used to help ascertain the heart's pumping capacity or to diagnose constricted coronary vessels, partial or total blockage of the coronary arteries, defects in the walls separating the chambers, or damaged heart valves. Cardiac catheterization often serves as a final diagnostic step for determining whether a patient should undergo heart surgery.

Cardiac catheterization has grown tremendously as both a diagnostic and therapeutic procedure. For example, the number of these procedures has increased from 500,000 performed in 1976 to 995,000 performed in 1990. In the past 10 to 12 years, many other procedures have been used by cardiologists to treat patients suffering from coronary artery disease, congestive heart failure, valve disease, arrhythmias, and congenital defects. One common popular procedure is percutaneous transluminal coronary angioplasty (PTCA), which uses a balloon to open plaque-filled arteries.[5]

Some believe that the rising number of therapeutic procedures may contribute to a greater need for cardiac catheterization systems. Therapeutic procedures take two to three times longer than diagnostic procedures, a factor that also fuels this need. Smaller, suburban hospital cath labs typically handle diagnostic studies and then refer patients who need therapeutic procedures to larger hospitals with surgical backups.[6]

Following is a description of what equipment is needed for a cardiac cath lab and how a cardiac catheterization procedure works:

> A basic cardiac cath lab suite is comprised of a high-quality fluoroscopic system with a floor or ceiling mounted C-arm and/or U-arm, a programmable film changer, a high-power X-ray generator, an X-ray tube with high heat capacity and a variable focal spot, a TV camera cine camera and/or digital angiographic system, an exam table, a special collimator with compensation filters to smooth out the different densities of the chest and a power or hand injector for the contrast [material].
>
> To evaluate the cine images gathered, a cine processor, cine projector, video tape machine and player, or a combination of these are needed. Digital images are read on a video or computer screen.

Figure 6-6. Interventional Radiography

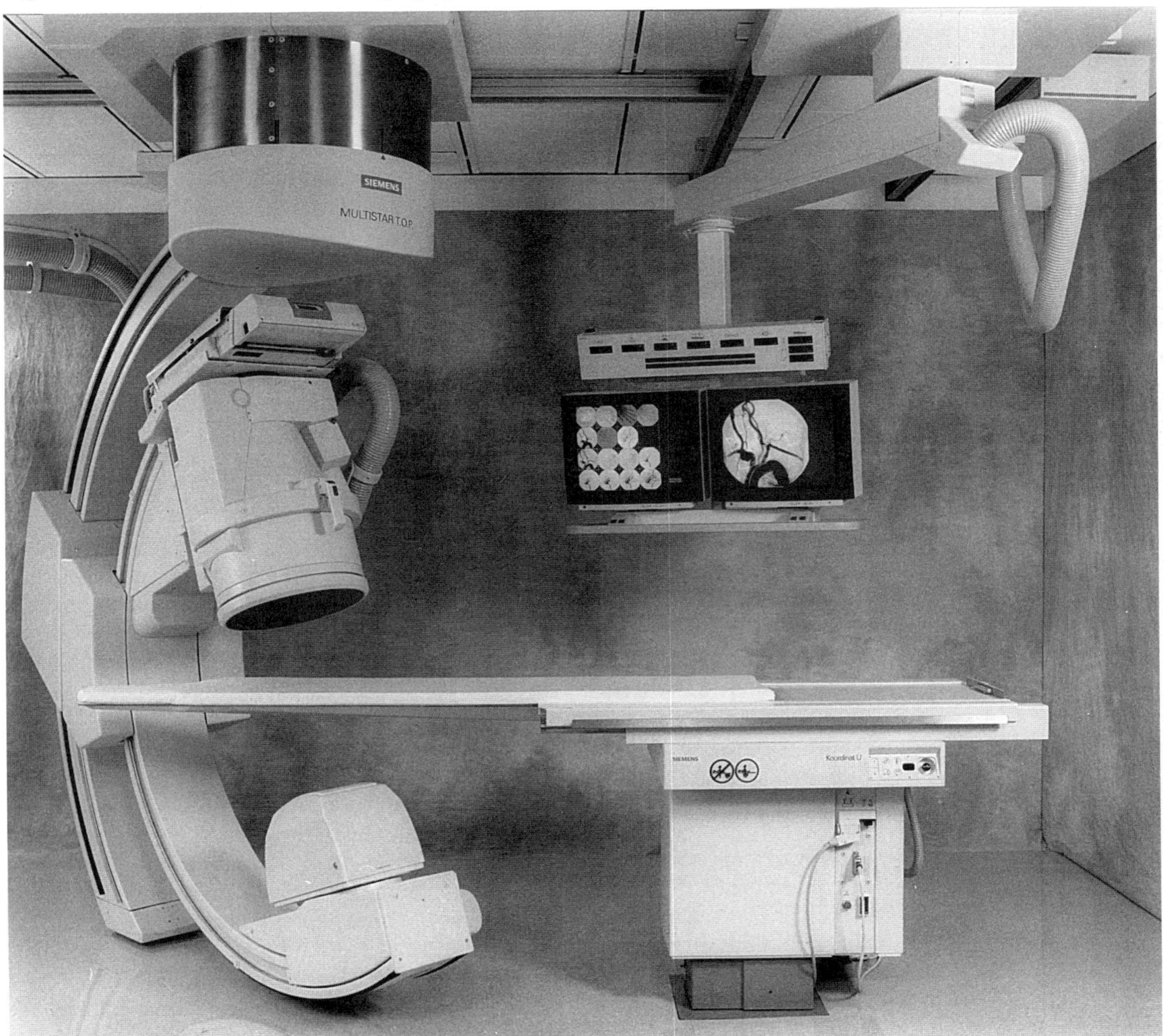

Courtesy of Siemens Medical Systems, Inc., Iselin, New Jersey. Used with permission.

During a cardiac catheterization procedure, a catheter is inserted [into the] patient's brachial or femoral artery. A thin wire is advanced through the artery, into the aorta, and on to the heart to act as a guide for the catheter insertion. This occurs under the watchful eye of a fluoroscopy system. When the wire is withdrawn, the catheter remains and is used to inject contrast agents into the coronary arteries or heart, facilitating X-rays of anatomy and blood flow. Being opaque to X-rays, a contrast agent allows tissue to show as shades of gray. This enables physicians to map blockages in arteries. Without an agent, hard and soft tissue differentiation would be impossible via X-ray.

A run, in which the injector pushes contrast through the veins while the cine camera or digital system and X-ray system monitor its path, lasts between 5 and 13 seconds, during which the patient must hold his or her breath. In a full exam, which can take from 10 minutes to 5 hours, there are about five to ten runs, often using different sizes and shapes of catheters in different areas of the heart, depending on the problem area.

The configuration of devices that takes these X-ray images is known as a cardiac catheterization radiographic/fluoroscopic unit. This unit can have a cine camera or 35mm high-speed camera, which takes 30 or 60 frames per second, or digital image acquisition system. With cine film, X-rays are read following the catheterization to determine the extent of cardiac problems and the percent of arterial blockage, or stenosis. Of late, however, the industry has been moving away from 35mm cine film in favor of digital-based systems, [which were first introduced around 1983–1984].[7]

Digital film is becoming the preferred method of image acquisition because of its lower cost, accuracy, clarity, and ability to give more real-time measurements, although cine film is still used. Some predict that in four to five years cine film will be the exception in new purchases.[8]

On average, hospitals spend about $50–$60 on cine film for each patient. . . . Using digital film, five to six patient studies cost [about] $35. Digital's faster acquisition and diagnosis, and its immediate playback capabilities also allow higher throughput for the lab. Digital [acquisition] eliminates the need to process film, reducing its accompanying product, chemical and employee costs as well as storage and retrieval problems. . . .

As cath labs gradually move toward digital acquisition, other changes are occurring in the lab, driven by physician demands for access to smaller vessels and hospitals' needs to cut costs. To reduce costs, speed is important to perform more procedures in less time but with more accuracy. . . .[9]

Because catheterization poses some risks, it usually is performed only on patients who are considered to be good (safe) candidates for surgery. Usually the patient has already undergone an echocardiogram and a treadmill stress test. Although diagnostic cardiac catheterization initially was exclusively an inpatient procedure, it now is routinely performed on an outpatient basis as well.

Several diagnostic catheterization studies are described below:

Pressure readings from the various chambers of the heart are transmitted from the tip of the catheter to a monitor in the catheterization lab. Differences in the pressure from one side of a heart valve to the other can help diagnose a scarred or narrow valve. Pressure readings also help assess the heart's overall ability to pump blood.

The catheter is also used to take *blood samples* from the various chambers of the heart which are then analyzed for oxygen content. This can help detect leaks or defects in the wall that separates the heart chambers. For instance, if the blood that fills the right atrium has an oxygen content of 70 percent but the blood in the right ventricle has an oxygen content of 90 percent, it means that the oxygen high blood must have leaked into the right ventricle from the left ventricle. These measurements can identify defects, and to some extent the percentages can be used to calculate the size of the defect and whether it needs surgical repair.

> *Coronary angiography* is probably the most common reason cardiac catheterization is ordered. The catheter is inserted into an artery and guided up to the aorta, the [major] blood vessel that receives all the heart's freshly oxygenated blood before it goes to the body. From the aorta, the catheter is guided to the openings of the coronary arteries and dye is injected. The coronary arteries are the arteries that supply the heart muscle itself with the blood it needs to live. Any blockage or narrowing should show up very clearly on the x-rays taken right after the dye injection. If there is severe blockage of these arteries, surgery may be considered.
>
> [During] *left heart angiography,* the catheter may be withdrawn from the coronary arteries and threaded through the left atrium into the left ventricle where a large amount of [contrast material] is injected and more x-ray [motion studies are conducted]. These x-rays, or ventriculograms help the cardiologist detect abnormal motion characteristic of [a] weakened or scarred muscle wall. By carefully examining how much dye is pumped out of the ventricle during successive heart beats the ejection fraction can be calculated. This is the percentage of the blood that is pumped out of the left ventricle with each heart beat. In a normal heart, about 60 percent of the ventricular blood is pumped out. In a diseased failing heart, 30 percent or less may be pumped. The ejection fraction is a critical . . . determination of which patients will be able to survive surgery.
>
> [During] *pulmonary angiography,* a catheter is inserted in a vein and guided through the right side of the heart until it reaches the pulmonary arteries, the blood vessels that carry blood to the lungs. [Contrast material] is injected and x-rays [are] taken that reveal the structure of—and any abnormalities in—the arteries that supply the lungs. [Pulmonary angiography is] most often used to detect a pulmonary embolism (blood clot), a potentially very dangerous condition where part of a lung is deprived of blood and oxygen. This in turn puts a great strain on the left side of the heart. Diagnosis of pulmonary embolism is one . . . instance in which cardiac catheterization may be done on an emergency basis.[10]

Cardiac catheterization is not limited to diagnostic procedures. Treatments such as temporary pacemaker insertion and permanent pacemaker implantation cause the cath lab to behave more like an operating suite compared to many other imaging rooms. As a result, when a cardiac cath lab is planned, there often is a political "discussion" as to whether the lab is to be part of the imaging department, the cardiology department, or perhaps the surgery department. Any number of issues may be involved in making this decision. For example:

- What mix of patients will be treated in the cath lab?
- What mix of procedures will be performed in the cath lab?
- Is more than one large procedure room capable of invasive angiography? If so, will the other room(s) be reserved exclusively for noncoronary patients?
- Will the ICU department be using the cath lab for catheter insertions?
- Is the cath lab intended to be used exclusively for diagnosis? For research? For both?
- Where is space available?
- Do the prevailing regulatory agencies require proximity to a surgical program?
- How extensive is the current heart program? Does one exist?
- Who is funding the project?
- Who will staff the cath lab?

Various arrangements have been tried over the years. Following is a brief look at the cath lab's evolution:

> Historically, the cardiac catheterization laboratory began as a subdivision of cardiology, utilizing fluoroscopy to implement physiological studies. With the advent of contrast radiography and advanced roentgen diagnostic methodology and equipment, radiology departments assumed a vested interest, particularly where case loads were low, facilities shared, and the equipment [was] in the precincts of radiology. Facilities vary widely in situation and structure—ranging from fully equipped units, in and staffed by Cardiology,

with their own laboratory, developing, viewing, and storage areas, to units in Radiology, run by radiologists. Concentration, however, in one discipline or another is not a guarantee of excellence in either. Of the two extremes, the cardiology facility is more likely to include a greater variety of physiologic and electrophysiologic studies, and the radiology facility to stress anatomic aspects. Many grades of compromise and cooperation have evolved with the laboratory physically in one bailiwick or another.[11]

Digital Radiography/Fluoroscopy

Although much of basic radiography is still film-based, there is a growing trend toward digital or computed R/F. This is especially true where special examination procedures are involved. True digital R/F systems afford flexibility through enhanced speed, broader dynamic range, and high probability that each exposure will be accomplished. (See figure 6-7.) The incidence of repeat examinations in intensive care units, pediatrics, emergency departments, and operating rooms is decreased by using digital R/F.

Figure 6-7. Digital Radiography

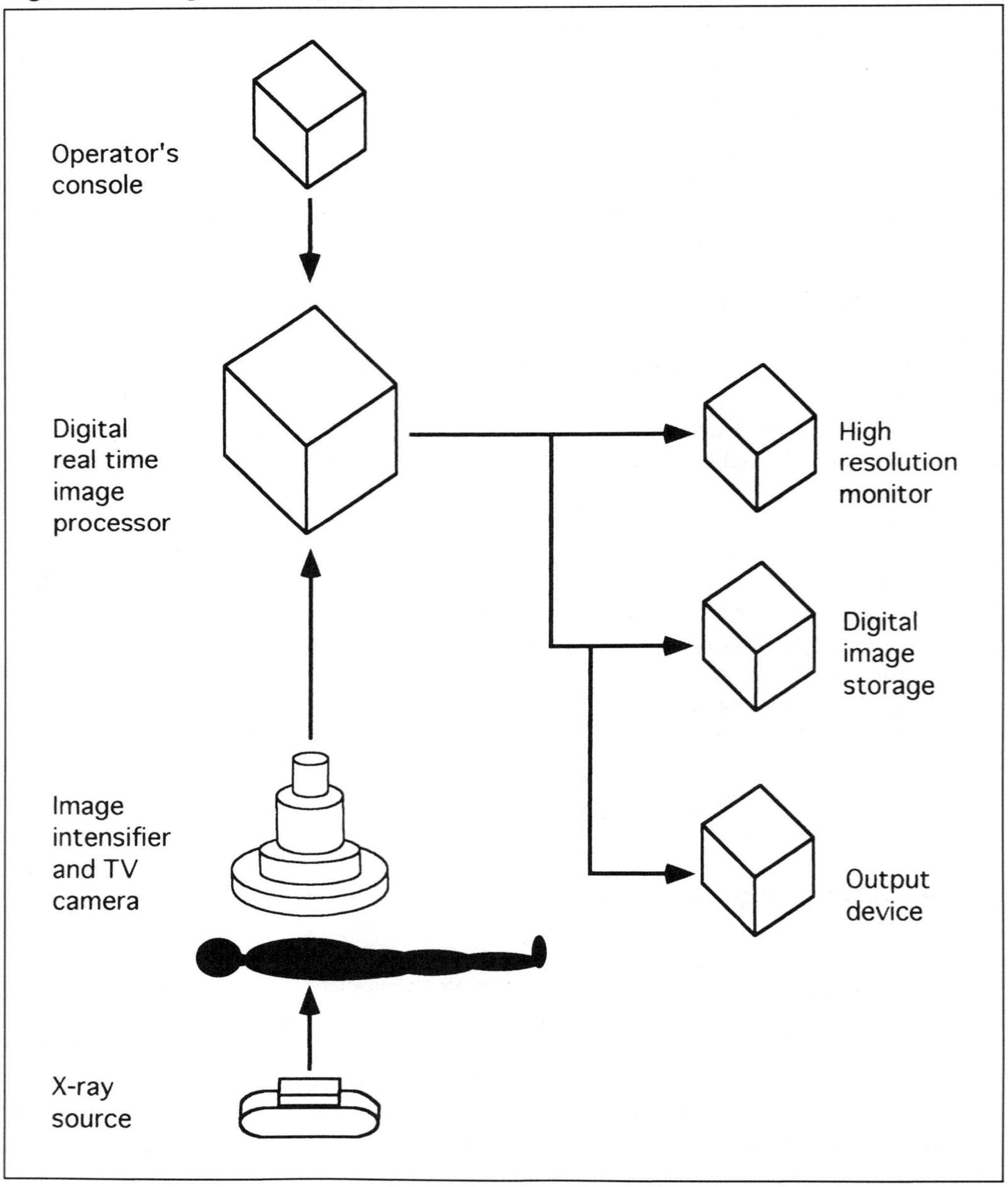

In digital radiography the variations of signal produced by the x-rays passing through the patient are translated into digital information by a converter. The numbers, like the signal, vary according to light and dark areas of the picture formed by the x-rays. A series of coded numbers assigned to a picture area is converted into pixels or picture units. Each pixel varies in brightness. When reassembled by a computer, they form a whole image not unlike that of a radiograph. Picture units vary in size and govern the sharpness and definition of the final image.[12]

Digital techniques have many advantages over conventional processes. These advantages extend to patients as well as to radiologists and referring physicians. Digital video fluoroscopy—the automated replacement of the conventional film-screen cassette and photostat procedures used in traditional fluoroscopy—is a faster, better method of X-ray imaging than conventional methods. Advantages include the ability to enhance images, enhance edges for better viewing and diagnoses, manage files better, create cine loops (like little movies), and go to film if desirable.[13] In addition:

> The latter capability—choosing whether or not to go to film—is particularly advantageous. Whereas traditional x-ray techniques require processing each image—and quite a few are shot, just to be sure the doctor gets what he or she wants—digital fluoroscopy allows doctors to print only those shots they deem useful or appropriate. This has cut film costs and processing times in half in some places.
>
> Speed and efficiency are also associated with digital fluoroscopy, engendering patient appreciation with the technology. Imagine you're on the table being x-rayed. While you're still on the table, the film has to be processed and checked by the radiologist to make sure there is no need for a retake. Thanks to automation, the image can be acquired and viewed immediately on a high-resolution monitor. Also, with mechanical equipment, if the film jams you lose the images and they have to be reshot. This is not pleasant for patients on two levels. First, no one wants more radiation exposure than is absolutely necessary. Second, it adds time and contributes to aggravation. On the other hand, a film jam presents only a minor inconvenience when going to hard copy from digital data. With digital data, you can recreate the image from the original information [without having to reexamine the patient].[14]

Another process that also results in digital image transmission involves nondigital film originals scanned into a digitizer. Computed data can then be printed (on paper or film) via a laser printer, viewed simultaneously by many people via a computer monitor (CRT), or transmitted via a cable or network. Once hard copy is transformed into digital data, the image can be integrated into a computer-based image management system. Duplicates also may be printed. Each duplicate is derived from the same digital data, and so each image is like an original. This feature eliminates the need to lend (and sometimes lose) original films. (See chapter 7, "Image Management and Film Processing.") However, image quality depends on the quality of both the original film-based image and the data transfer chain.

Although basic digital R/F has not yet overwhelmed the marketplace (price and operational difficulties in the transition from an analog to a digital system have limited its implementation), momentum is building. Offsetting the additional cost of computed (compared to film-screen) radiography are a number of benefits.

First, servicing digital systems actually can be simpler and less expensive in the long run. Many computer-based systems have self-correcting software for common problems. In addition, remote diagnostics—the ability to identify equipment problems without being on-site—will become more comprehensive in the near future.

Second, digital systems allow for radiation dose reduction as compared to analog units. This is due, in part, to the fact that phosphor screens used with some forms of digital radiography require less radiation to expose the latent image. Also, the X-ray beam is more finely collimated or narrowed with digital radiography as compared to traditional techniques. Collimation reduces scatter radiation.

Finally, according to some manufacturers' claims, computed radiography promises easier upgrading capabilities because improvements can be added by replacing software, not hardware.[15] However, such claims may need to be closely examined. Due to rapid technological improvements, upgrading often involves hardware as well as software and can be quite costly.

For some modalities, however, digital acquisition currently does not provide the contrast or density of film-screen radiography. Radiographic spatial resolution is measured in line pairs per millimeter (lp/mm). A higher number of line pairs per millimeter indicates better resolution. A typical chest film has 5 lp/mm; a mammogram has 15–18 lp/mm. Digitized film until recently contained only about 2.5 lp/mm; so did digitally acquired computed radiography.

However, the overall improvements in contrast resolution in nearly all modalities (except mammography) can compensate for and even overcome reduced spatial resolution. With recent breakthroughs, digital systems may soon match the image quality of film. Researchers have been working with charge-coupled devices (CCDs) that offer better spatial resolution than film—between 14.3 and 16.6 lp/mm, although the CCD device is limited by its small diameter (55 mm).[16]

Even though chest films and bone X rays constitute the majority of a radiologist's practice today, these modalities may be superseded in the near future. To meet the increasing demands of medical technology, more radiologists are looking to computed radiography systems.[17] This will also change how these images are viewed on computer monitors, with multiple windowing (zooming in or out) possibilities. According to one futurist's predictions:

> Digital systems will provide the missing link needed to complete implementation of picture archiving and communication systems. Presently, digital systems [including CT, MR, and so on] constitute 20 percent to 30 percent of imaging procedures performed in a modern hospital. But it is predicted that by the year 2000, about half of large teaching hospitals will be performing digital radiography of the chest and by 2020 all imaging procedures in advanced hospitals will be digital.[18]

High-speed (broad-bandwidth) networks and increased options for low-cost image archiving are accelerating this change. Therefore:

> Digital imaging is inevitable, even in the most basic of radiology modalities. As hospitals continue to come under pressure to reduce even more costs, the savings which digital radiography can bring combined with the evolution of the technology will offset the radiologist's resistance and other pressures resisting the trend.[19]

Digital Subtraction Angiography

Special digital image acquisition and manipulation techniques, such as digital subtraction angiography (DSA), provide an enhanced view of the vascular system. To understand DSA, it is useful to review how vascular fluoroscopy techniques work.

Vascular fluoroscopy includes a series of techniques for viewing the human circulatory system in real time. For example, angiography looks at blood flow as indicated by the passage of X-ray-opaque contrast agents through arteries and veins and detects blockage from narrowed or otherwise compromised blood vessels.

Digital subtraction was first introduced clinically in the 1970s in the form of DSA. However, the principles behind digital subtraction date back to analog film techniques reported in the 1930s but not widely used until the 1960s. At that time, enhanced contrast studies were conducted manually by applying photographic subtraction techniques to radiography.[20]

DSA can further manipulate the angiographic image. First, a preliminary image is recorded and stored in a computer. Then, contrast material is injected into the vessel. This enhances the blood vessel and its branches. The computer then electronically "subtracts" the unobscured preliminary (unenhanced) image from each of the spatially enhanced vessels. This results in a masking of nonessential background information (such as the skull in cerebral angiography); an unobscured, precise view of the vessel remains. In this way, delicate coronary arteries, for example, become visible without heart tissue in the background obscuring the image. Smaller vessels may be magnified many times or enhanced with gray scale or occasionally with color for a better view. Most modern systems provide real-time imaging, which enables the viewer to observe vascular movement at the time it occurs. Therefore, the imaging can be curtailed when the desired information has been derived.

Radiographic Tomography

The term *tomography* refers to a variety of methods of viewing thin "slices" of anatomical or functional data and can be misleading if not used carefully. The confusion arises when various tomographic methods, each of which can be extremely different from one another, are thought of as being similar. For example, positron emission tomography (PET) and single-photon emission computed tomography (SPECT) are nuclear medicine techniques and are significantly different from computed tomography (CT) and linear tomography (one type of geometric tomography), which are radiographic techniques. The tomographic procedures listed in this section are limited to radiographic procedures. Other tomographic techniques are listed under their appropriate imaging modality headings.

Conventional X-ray images superimpose multiple anatomical structures—one on top of the other—often causing the area of interest to be blocked by less-pertinent information. Tomography separates thin "slices" of anatomical information by enhancing the contrast of a selected two-dimensional plane while blurring the structures in front of and behind the plane of interest. With geometric tomography, both the X-ray source (imaging tube) and the receptor (film or electronic sensor) move in a coordinated manner, causing only a thin slice of information to appear in focus. (See figure 6-8.) The resulting tomogram contains more usable or discernible information about the area under investigation than a conventional X-ray image can provide.

Figure 6-8. Principles of Tomography

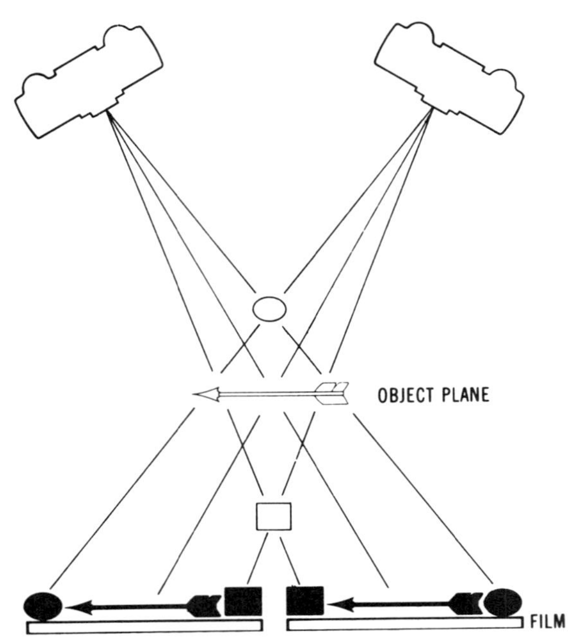

Reprinted, with permission, from Bushong, S. C. *Radiologic Science for Technologists: Physics, Biology, and Protection.* 5th ed. St. Louis: Mosby-Year Book, 1993, p. 327.

Geometric Tomography

The most basic geometric tomographic examination involves a linear movement (linear tomography) in which both the imaging tube and the film travel in parallel planes. Other forms of geometric tomography are multidirectional and are produced when the imaging tube and film are synchronized to move in a circular, elliptical, trispiral, or other geometry. The tube moves forward while the film receptor moves in the opposite direction. (See figure 6-9.) Simple linear tomography often can be performed by adding a tomographic armature to conventional radiographic equipment.[21] The simplest arrangement is to use a nontilting table with a four-way floating top.

Linear tomographic capabilities often are provided in basic radiographic rooms where intravenous pyelograms (IVPs) are performed. However, newer procedures, such as CT and ultrasound, provide higher contrast resolution and a less-invasive alternative to IVPs.

Computed Tomography

With computed tomography (CT), a rapidly rotating X-ray source generates digital data, which are electronically recorded as a collection of points, stored, and then reassembled into narrow slices. CT is useful in its ability to exquisitely discriminate density differences, both in high-contrast objects (such as bone) and in lower-contrast objects (such as soft-tissue structures and organs).[22]

CT requires special equipment that rotates the imaging tube around the patient's head or body, creating multiple X-ray slices. (See figure 6-10.) With CT, radiation is received by electronic sensors instead of film; X-ray signals are transmitted to a computer, processed, and then displayed as an image. Multiple slices from one examination can be further processed by the computer to form a single three-dimensional representation. CT scans identify detailed information, precluding the need for exploratory surgery.

CT was invented by G. N. Hounsfield, a senior research scientist at EMI Limited in Middlesex, England, and announced publicly in 1972. Although he called it *computerized axial*

Figure 6-9. Linear Tomography

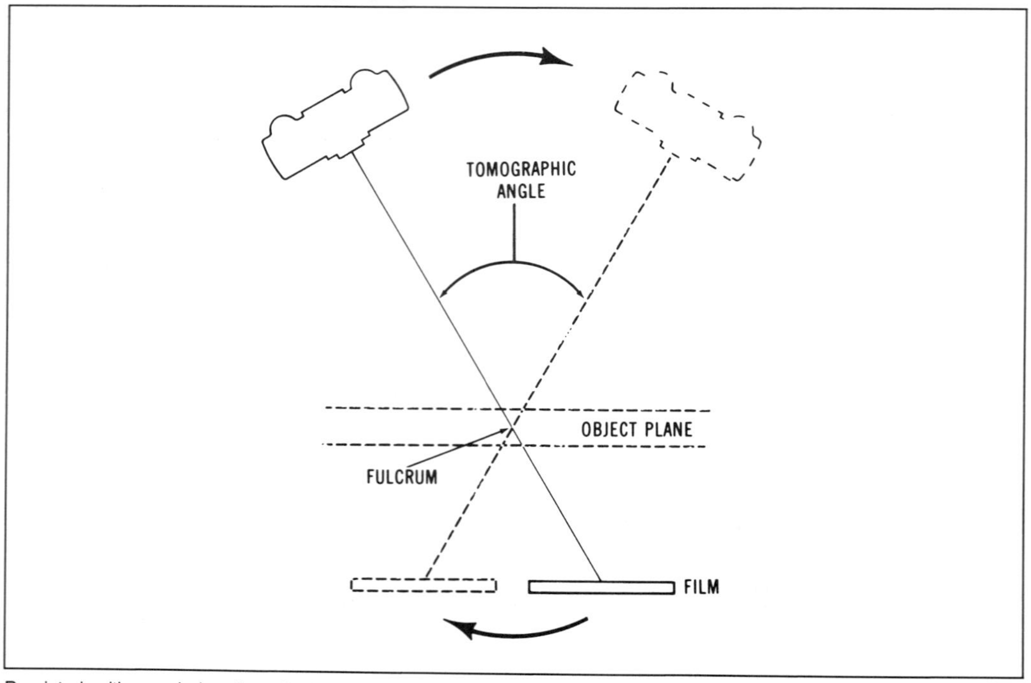

Reprinted, with permission, from Bushong, S. C. *Radiologic Science for Technologists: Physics, Biology, and Protection.* 5th ed. St. Louis: Mosby-Year Book, 1993, p. 328.

transverse scanning, the modality now is commonly known as computed tomography because it no longer is limited to axial projection.

> The basic concept was quite simple: a thin cross section of the head, a tomographic slice, was examined from multiple angles with a pencil-like x-ray beam. The transmitted radiation was counted by a scintillation detector, fed into a computer for analysis by a mathematical algorithm, and reconstructed as a tomographic image. The image had a remarkable characteristic, one never before seen in an x-ray image: it demonstrated a radiographic difference in the various soft tissues; blood clots, gray matter, white matter, cerebrospinal fluid, tumors, and cerebral edema all appeared as separate entities.

Figure 6-10. Computed Tomography

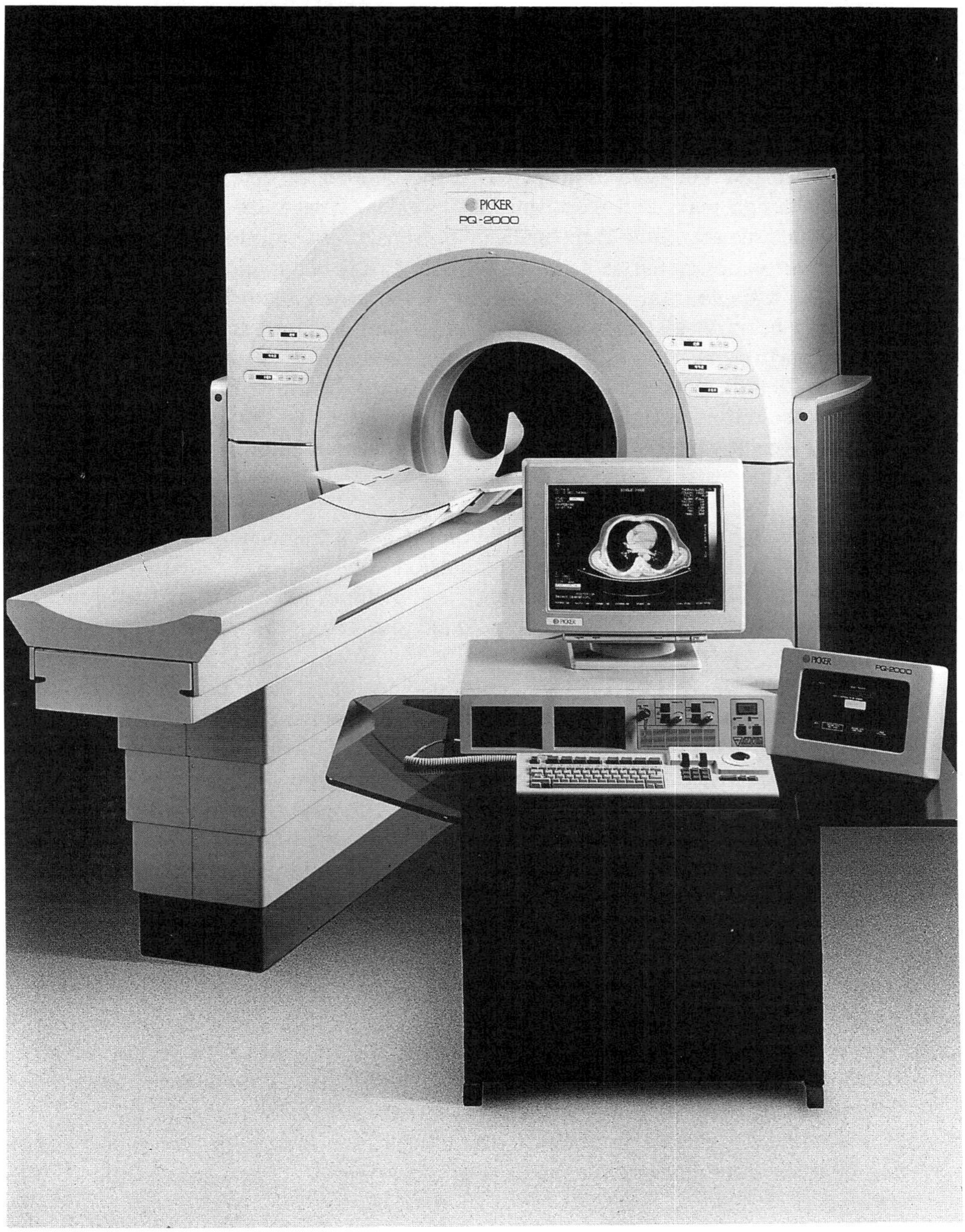

Courtesy of Picker International, Cleveland, Ohio. Used with permission.

> The basic principle behind CT is that the internal structure of an object can be reconstructed from multiple projections of the object. Projections [of an object] can be obtained by passing an x-ray beam through [the object] and measuring the transmitted radiation.[23]

Since the 1972 announcement of Hounsfield's scanner, a number of improvements and variations on the image acquisition techniques of CT have developed. For example, the speed (image reconstruction time), size, cost, and environmental requirements of CT scanners have changed significantly.

> Although it is somewhat misleading, the term "generation" is used to describe the various design types. [When applied to CT scanners,] *generation* does not refer to the state of product development but, rather, to the geometry of the movement of the x-ray tube-detector system [the number of photomultiplier detectors and as a result image reconstruction speed.] First-generation scanners consisted of an x-ray tube producing a finely collimated pencil beam of x-rays and a single sodium iodide photomultiplier detector mounted on a scanning gantry into which the patient's head or body was placed. . . . [The first commercial scanner required more than 5 minutes to complete a scan.]
>
> To reduce the scan time, the second-generation design replaced the pencil beam x-ray with a narrow fan beam and increased the number of detectors. . . . The second-generation design permitted scan times as short as 10 seconds. . . .
>
> To reduce the scan time even further, . . . translational motion was eliminated. The third-generation design uses a wide fan (40°–55°) x-ray beam and a large detector array mounted on a single rotating gantry. In this design, the patient is totally encompassed in the x-ray beam at all times. . . . Scan times [are] as short as two seconds. . . .
>
> The fourth-generation design removes the detectors from the rotating gantry and distributes them in fixed locations around the gantry opening. In this design, . . . only the x-ray tube moves during data collection, rotating inside the circle of detectors. . . . The lighter weight gantry and simpler cabling arrangement allow this scanner to produce scans in the one second range. . . .[24]

Additional techniques that have improved on the initial CT technology include slip-ring technology, spiral or helical scanning, twin-beam CT, double-helix scanning, and electron beam tomography (EBT). Slip-ring technology is sometimes referred to as fifth-generation CT. Electron beam tomography is sometimes referred to as sixth-generation CT. (It is described in a separate section of this chapter.)

Slip-ring design replaces the internal gantry cable with an electrical connection, resulting in continuous gantry rotation rather than having to change direction during each rotation. This, in turn, enables a much shorter scan duration. Slip-ring gantry rotation, coupled with the continuous movement of a patient through the gantry, results in helical or spiral imaging. "The result is [volumetric image] acquisition. There is no interscan delay and whole volumes of information can be obtained in as little as one breath-hold of the patient. With its increased speed and volumetric capabilities, [spiral/helical] imaging [has revolutionized] the way CT is performed. The conventional step-wise slice-by-slice scanning technique will be reserved for patients who can't hold their breath. All other patients will be examined by helical CT."[25]

A twin-beam scanner divides the X-ray beam into two separate beams that simultaneously strike the detector alongside one another. Thus, they collect twice the information per scan. Helical scanning, using a twin-beam CT scanner, covers twice the region of interest per scan and is called double-helix scanning. With double-helix scanning, the entire length of the lungs can be imaged with a single series of scans.[26]

A CT scanner consists of three basic components: the gantry, the computer, and the operating console. Each component, in turn, is composed of several subsystems:

> The gantry assembly includes the x-ray tube, the detector array, the high-voltage generator, the patient support and positioning couch, and the mechanical support for each.

These subsystems receive electronic commands from the operating console and transmit data to the computer for image production and analysis.

The computer is a unique subsystem of the CT scanner. CT scanning would not be possible were it not for the high-speed digital computer.

Many CT scanners are equipped with two . . . consoles, one for the technologist to operate the unit and one for the physician to view the scan image and manipulate its contrast, size and general visual appearance. The operator's console contains meters and controls for selecting proper radiographic technique factors, for proper mechanical movement of the gantry and patient couch, and for computer commands allowing image reconstruction and transfer. The physician's . . . console accepts the reconstructed image from the operator's console and displays it for viewing and diagnosis.[27]

The physician's console has not been broadly used because most interpretation to date has been from filmed images, not VDT analysis. However, this is likely to change with the broader distribution of electronic PACS workstations.

Not too long ago, all CT computers required a special controlled environment that restricted temperature and humidity. Although some units still require a specially controlled environment, many models now have less-restrictive temperature and humidity specifications. Also, many of these new units are smaller than in the past.

Electron Beam Tomography

Electron beam tomography, sometimes referred to as ultrafast computed tomography (UFCT), is newer than conventional CT. One difference between the two is that EBT relies on an electron beam gun instead of an X-ray tube to create X rays. Radiation is generated as a beam of electrons strikes a fixed tungsten ring. The X rays are reflected by the fixed ring and then pass through the patient and onto a fixed detector ring. In contrast to the moving gantry of traditional CT, the fixed EBT rings enable extremely short (50-millisecond) imaging time and eliminate table motion. (See figure 6-11.)

Figure 6-11. Electron Beam Tomography

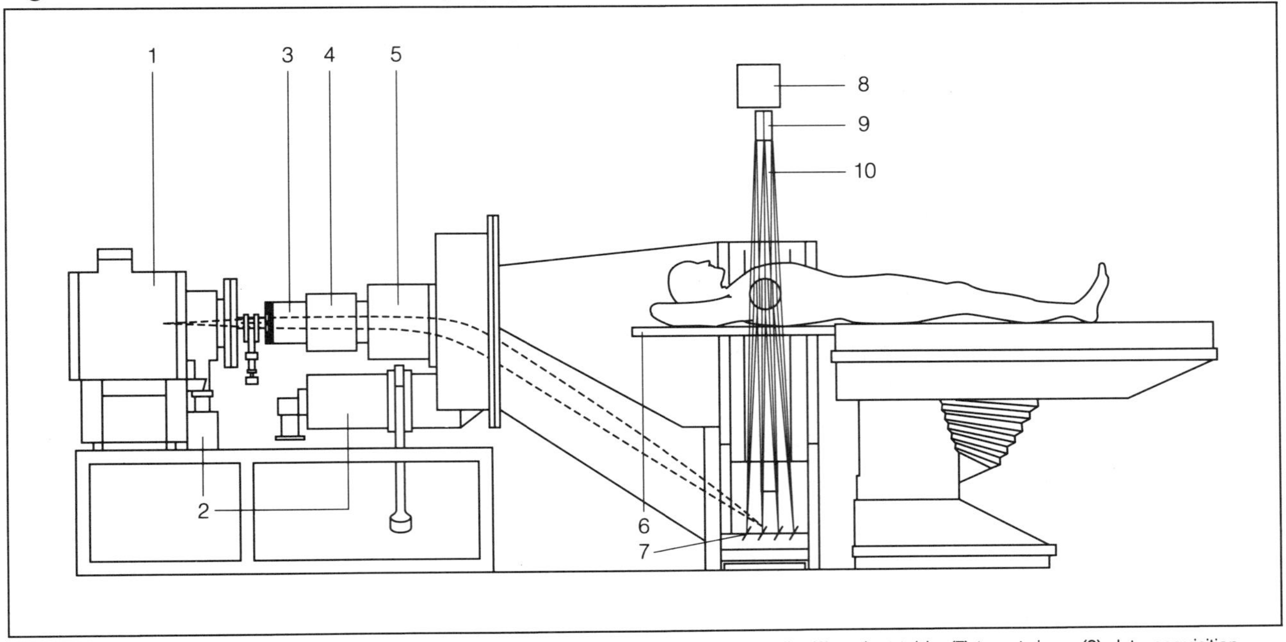

Note: (1) electron gun, (2) vacuum pumps, (3) electron beam, (4) focus coils, (5) deflection coils, (6) patient table, (7) target rings, (8) data acquisition system, (9) detector rings, (10) X-ray beams.

Courtesy of Siemens Medical Systems, Inc., Iselin, New Jersey. Used with permission.

First-generation EBT (originally known as cine CT) was developed specifically for cardiac imaging. Whereas most early images lacked the resolution of conventional CT, this rapid and motion-free technique was innovative in its ability to capture the motion of a beating heart and provide cross-sectional images unattainable from almost any other imaging technique.[28]

Current EBT combines high resolution with its remarkable speed, which results in high patient throughput as well as exquisite imaging. No longer limited to cardiology, applications include airway studies, chest and abdominal imaging, and central nervous system scanning. Because of its tremendous speed, EBT is well suited to pediatric, geriatric, and trauma patients who cannot hold still or should not be moved. Cardiac imaging remains a primary market for EBT, especially applications for noninvasive arterial plaque calcification identification and screening.

Electron beam tomography is expensive compared to conventional CT. EBT instrumentation generally is larger and siting requirements, such as sensitivity to electromagnetic fields, often are more complex. In addition, the electron beam gun assembly usually requires a room separate from the scanning room. (See figure 6-12.) Although many hospitals have "fast CT" units, relatively few currently have EBT.

Figure 6-12. EBT System Layout Guidelines

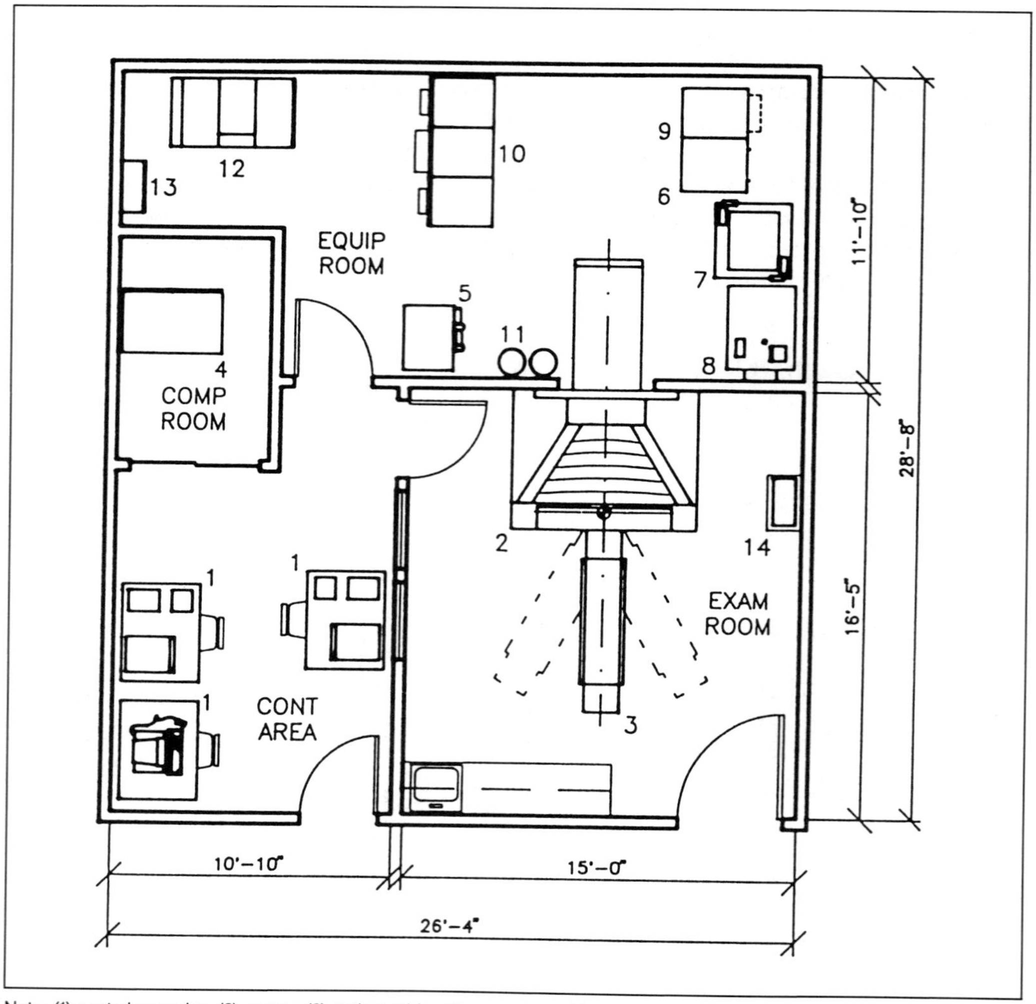

Note: (1) control consoles, (2) gantry, (3) patient table, (4) computer cabinets, (5) chiller unit, (6) HV controller, (7) HV post-regulator, (8) HV raw DC tank, (9) vacuum interlock control, (10) electronic cabinets, (11) nitrogen gas tanks, (12) exide UPS/DPS systems, (13) LEA surge suppressor, (14) EKG unit on shelf.

Courtesy of Siemens Medical Systems, Inc., Iselin, New Jersey. Used with permission.

Ultrasound

One of the dangers of radiographic imaging is the damaging effect of repeated exposure to ionizing radiation. This can be particularly harmful to the developing fetus. Ultrasound, a safer alternative for fetal imaging, has revolutionized the practice of obstetrics over the past 30 years and is leading the way for the development of fetal medicine as a new subspecialty.[29] Ultrasound also is used for many applications unrelated to fetal imaging. For example:

> New applications being developed for computed sonography, more commonly known as ultrasound, are yielding diagnostic information previously unavailable and even are beginning to replace more expensive diagnostic tests in some cases. . . .
>
> Radiologists, cardiologists, obstetricians and gynecologists seem to continuously find new uses for the technology. But the expansion is also setting up turf battles for ultrasound testing among various specialists and between hospitals and non-hospital settings. [Vascular surgeons and neurologists are also competing with radiologists for the use of "vascular evaluation laboratories" in which ultrasound is used.]
>
> Advances in technology are making ultrasound the tool of choice for initial screenings of many problems, in some cases eliminating the need for more sophisticated and expensive tests, such as an MRI scan.[30]

Ultrasound, or sonography, is based on the principles of sonar and records size and shape by tracking reflected sound waves. For example, during abdominal ultrasound, a hand-held transducer emits regular pulses of high-frequency sound and translates the received "echo" into electrical signals. Because tissue density affects sound reflectivity, the returned sound wave's amplitude helps identify tissue type.

Although ultrasound is unable to view bones or gas-filled cavities such as the lungs or intestines and although sonograms do not record size and shape in great detail, ultrasound provides a unique ability to reveal cysts, tumors, and abscesses. Abdominal ultrasound is commonly used to evaluate the kidneys, liver, spleen, lymph nodes, and pancreas and is replacing the cholecystogram as the procedure of choice for examining the gallbladder for stones and thickening of the wall.[31]

Doppler ultrasound records blood flow within the arteries and veins. Abnormal blood flow can indicate clots, blockages, or narrowing of blood vessels. Color Doppler uses color images to depict direction and velocity of blood flow. Three-dimensional ultrasound promises improved volumetric images of the heart, blood vessels, and fetus. Echocardiography enables internal study of the heart.[32]

Pelvic or transvaginal ultrasound is used to visualize the bladder and female reproductive organs. Transrectal ultrasound is used to detect prostate cancer and cancer of the rectum. Both transvaginal and transrectal ultrasound use a small probe in which the transducer is located.[33]

Transcranial Doppler (TCD) directs ultrasonic waves through the skull as a means of assessing intracranial blood flow. This information is used to detect cerebrovascular disease, such as malformation and narrowing of intercranial blood vessels. TCD also is useful for presurgical and postsurgical evaluation of neurosurgical patients and shows promise in identifying the basis of some types of migraine headaches.[34]

The increasing miniaturization of transducers will further extend expertise with ultrasound. One interesting new application is transesophageal echocardiography (TEE):

> Miniature transducers are catheter-mounted and threaded down the esophagus to image the heart from inside. The information gained helps cardiologists make better diagnoses and allows anesthesiologists to monitor the cardiac wall. Surgeons can use TEE with 2-D and Doppler during surgery to obtain information about the patient's heart after performing a procedure.[35]

TEE also is used for esophagogastropic staging of esophageal cancer.

Another new application is intravascular ultrasound (IVUS), which will greatly influence monitoring of interventional procedures:

> IVUS can image all three layers of the vessel wall, and thus may provide a more accurate measure of disease extent. This in turn may aid interventionalists in determining therapeutic end points. In some cases that involve plaque removal within the blood vessel, intravascular ultrasound showed more plaque remaining when angiography suggested that all had been removed.
>
> While interventional radiologists are the most experienced with IVUS, its benefits are not limited to the vascular system. [Intraluminal] catheter-mounted probes are being used in a growing number of applications from assessment of the ureter to the pancreatic duct. Intraluminal ultrasound is going to add a whole new area of clinical capability that wasn't available without the miniaturization.[36]

Miniature transducers and probes are leading to the increased internal use of ultrasound, particularly in the operating room. Ultrasound is used to guide physicians performing procedures such as brain surgery in a way similar to the way a tugboat guides large ships through shallow or unknown waters. (See chapter 14, "Imaging outside the Radiology Department.")

Magnetic Resonance

This discussion of magnetic resonance describes the principles of magnetic resonance imaging and the basic components of MRI systems. Classifications of magnets by type and field strength are also discussed, as are recent developments in magnetic resonance angiography (MRA), magnetic resonance spectroscopy (MRS), and magnetic resonance mammography (MRM). (Readers should also see chapter 15, "Physical Properties Influencing Design," for additional information on designing the physical environment for MRI.)

Magnetic Resonance Imaging

Magnetic resonance imaging uses magnetic and especially radio-frequency (RF) pulses, instead of ionizing radiation, to demonstrate normal versus abnormal anatomy. MRI techniques also have been developed for viewing physiology. Although the principles behind MRI have been used by chemists for half a century, its clinical applications have existed for less than half that time. (See figure 6-13.)

The physical phenomenon of magnetic resonance was first characterized in independent experiments by American scientists Felix Bloch and Edward Purcell in 1946. In 1971, Damadian used MRI to demonstrate differences in the behavior of water in malignant and benign tissues, and he suggested that MRI possessed "many of the desirable features of an external probe for the detection of internal cancer." In the same year, Lauterbur produced the first two-dimensional MRI image, a cross-sectional portrait of two tubes of water. The potential utility of this technique to medical imaging was obvious, and soon afterward multiple researchers began development of clinical MRI systems, including the first human whole-body MRI scan in 1977. Improvements in the scanning process and image quality continue today.[37]

The following explains MRI and its components:

> [MRI] proton imaging noninvasively produces a representation of internal body structures and organs, without exposure to ionizing radiation (x-rays) or conventional radiologic contrast agents. Proton imaging is founded upon a basic physical principle: the nuclei of certain atoms possess an intrinsic angular momentum, or "spin." Because nuclei carry an electrical charge, those that spin generate tiny magnetic fields. These magnetic fields can be brought into alignment by the imposition of a forceful external magnetic field. The addition of radio frequency (RF) energy, at a specific frequency characteristic of the type of nucleus and the strength of the imposed magnetic field, perturbs the alignment of the tiny nuclear magnetic fields. When the RF energy is removed, "relaxation" of the nuclei to their initial state of alignment results in the release of a radio frequency

Figure 6-13. Principles of MRI

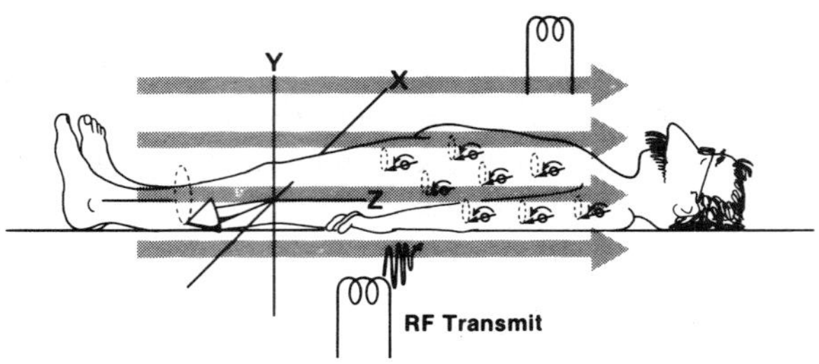

Nuclei will absorb RF energy and flip when the RF is transmitted at the Larmor frequency.

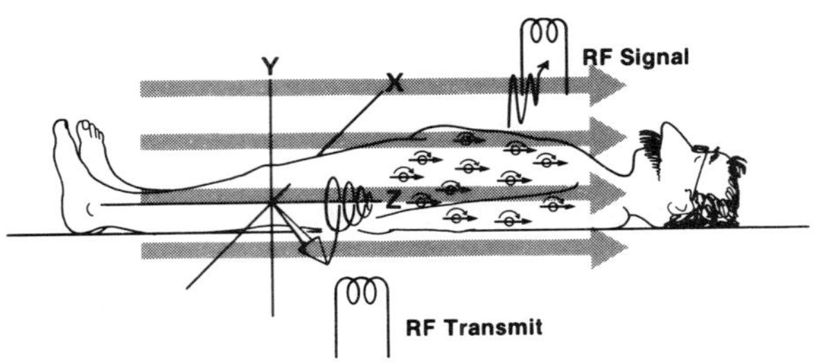

Relaxation occurs when the nuclei return to their normal state of equilibrium after the RF is turned off.

Reprinted, with permission, from Bushong, S. C. *Radiologic Science for Technologists: Physics, Biology, and Protection.* 5th ed. St. Louis: Mosby-Year Book, 1993, p. 456.

signal which can be detected by an RF receiver. The measured signal is a function of a number of factors, including the density of the relevant nuclei in the tissues and two "relaxation time" parameters, T1 and T2, which are affected by the physiochemical environment of the nuclei being examined. Using this signal information, mathematical algorithms reconstruct an image of the anatomy being examined. Current MRI focuses upon hydrogen, an element with a single proton in its nucleus. Hydrogen is particularly amenable to imaging in biologic systems because it is ubiquitous in organic compounds and of course in water.

Thus, four major components are essential to MRI technology:

1. *Magnet.* The magnet must be both powerful and large enough to completely encircle the structure to be imaged. The absolute strength required of the magnet is a point of considerable contention among various investigators and manufacturers.
2. *Radio frequency source.* The RF source must be able to provide sufficient energy to deflect the atomic magnetic fields from their parallel orientation.
3. *Radio frequency receiver.* The RF receiver must be able to detect the energy released during proton relaxation.
4. *Computer and display system.* A computer with a large storage capacity and sophisticated array processor must receive the data and format it into a pictorial display.

These four components of MRI machinery present important implications for both costs and location of this technology. [Special considerations for designing MRI enclosures, such as the influence of magnetic and radio-frequency fields, are discussed in more detail in chapter 15, "Physical Properties Influencing Design."]

Note: MRI is sometimes referred to as Nuclear Magnetic Resonance (NMR) because its imaging principles are based on the behavior of the nucleus of organic elements. The term *nuclear,* however, carries a negative connotation for some people. As a result, the term *NMR* has been almost completely replaced by MRI. Some observers have suggested that "turf battles" between radiologists and nuclear medicine specialists have provided additional impetus for this name change.[38]

MRI has a special ability to view soft tissue and to select areas for visualization that are hidden by dense bone. These areas often are inaccessible by radiographic procedures. Also, a magnetic resonance image has better contrast and provides more biochemical information, for most tissues, than a computed tomogram.[39]

Spatial information about the region of the body being imaged is obtained in MRI by slightly altering the uniformity of the magnet's field. Gradient coils temporarily alter the field in a predetermined fashion, allowing the computer to calculate the precise location of each radio signal's source. The radio signal source location corresponds to the condition of the patient's anatomy or physiology. This signal source mapping is used to form the magnetic resonance image.

To improve the quality of MR body imaging, magnetic contrast agents (magnetopharmaceuticals) are sometimes used. Much research on these agents is being conducted, particularly on newer ones that can target specific tissues or biological reactions.

Magnet Classifications and Principles

Magnets are classified by both field strength and type. Three magnet types are common: resistive, superconductive, and permanent. Neither resistive nor permanent magnets have as great a field strength as superconductors. Field strength quantifies the magnetic field force generated by the magnet and is indirectly related to magnet type. It is measured in tesla (abbreviated T). A 1.0-T magnet has a field strength approximately 20,000 times stronger than the earth's average magnetic force.

Resistive magnets require strong electric currents and dissipate a large amount of heat. To compensate for this, a water-cooling system is integrated into the magnet's coils. Resistive magnets usually do not require external magnetic shielding and, therefore, can be sited within small spaces.

Superconductive magnets are made of special metal alloys that have no electrical resistance at very cold (cryogenic) temperatures. (See figure 6-14.) Superconductors consume less power and expel less heat than resistive magnets, but require a thermoslike container, or dewar, to maintain an internal temperature near absolute zero (−460°F). A sudden loss of cryogen creates a potentially dangerous overheating condition known as a quench. However, quenches are rare; when they do occur, they are more likely during maintenance than during an exam. Superconductive systems require active or passive magnetic shielding or a substantial amount of space.

Permanent magnets can be constructed of materials, such as ceramics, that are easily magnetized. (See figure 6-15, p. 100.) Because the magnetic field of a permanent magnet is not electrically generated, no heat is produced. Permanent magnets may reduce both initial and operating costs significantly for MRI but, because of their weight, are limited to the lower-field-strength category. Like resistive magnets, permanent magnets tend to be inherently self-shielded. Therefore, external magnetic shielding is usually not necessary. For low-field systems, permanent magnets have become more popular than resistive magnets.

Magnets tend to be classified in one of four field-strength categories: ultralow field, mid-field, high field, and very high field. The lower-field-strength magnets have more limitations in image quality than do their stronger counterparts. However, the stronger magnets have more limitations in siting because of the area needed to control the force field and because of their weight. Following is a brief description of the characteristics of the four types of magnets:

- Ultralow-field magnets have a field strength of about 0.06 to 0.4 T. Sometimes this category is further divided into ultralow field (0.06–0.1 T) and low field (0.2–0.4 T). Ultralow-field systems tend to use permanent magnets; some of them are of an open design, which has the advantage of causing very little claustrophobia in patients. Low-field systems typically use permanent or resistive magnets. (See figure 6-16, p. 101.)
- Midfield magnets are approximately 0.5 to 1.0 T. These systems use superconductive magnets. Recently, midfield magnets have become popular as a direct result of cost-containment pressures combined with new technology that makes quality imaging from non-high-field magnets possible. The procedure room for some midfield magnets may be about the size of a traditional R/F room. Additional space for control and computer equipment may be necessary. Active shielding may allow the magnet to be placed directly within the imaging department. (See figure 6-17, p. 102.)
- High-field magnets are approximately 1.5 to 2.0 T and use superconductive systems. Typically, they have been the most popular size of magnets. Some vendors suggest that 1.5 T is the minimum field strength appropriate for magnetic resonance spectroscopy. However, this claim does not seem to be confirmed statistically. In general, a high-field magnet will provide a clearer image than will a lower-strength magnet. Active shielding now allows the fringe field of many high-field magnets to be contained within the MR examination room. (See figure 6-18, p. 102.)
- Very high-field magnets are above 2.0 T and use superconductive systems. The Food and Drug Administration (FDA) currently approves the clinical use for humans of magnets up to a field strength of 2.0 T. However, there are a number of test sites in which 4.0-T and stronger magnets are being used for research purposes. The tests are performed on volunteers. Some adverse effects, including headaches and blurred vision, have been reported by control operators, but not by patients.

Although MR performance initially came to be associated with increases in field strength, recent developments have significantly improved the performance of both high-field and

Figure 6-14. A Superconductive Magnet

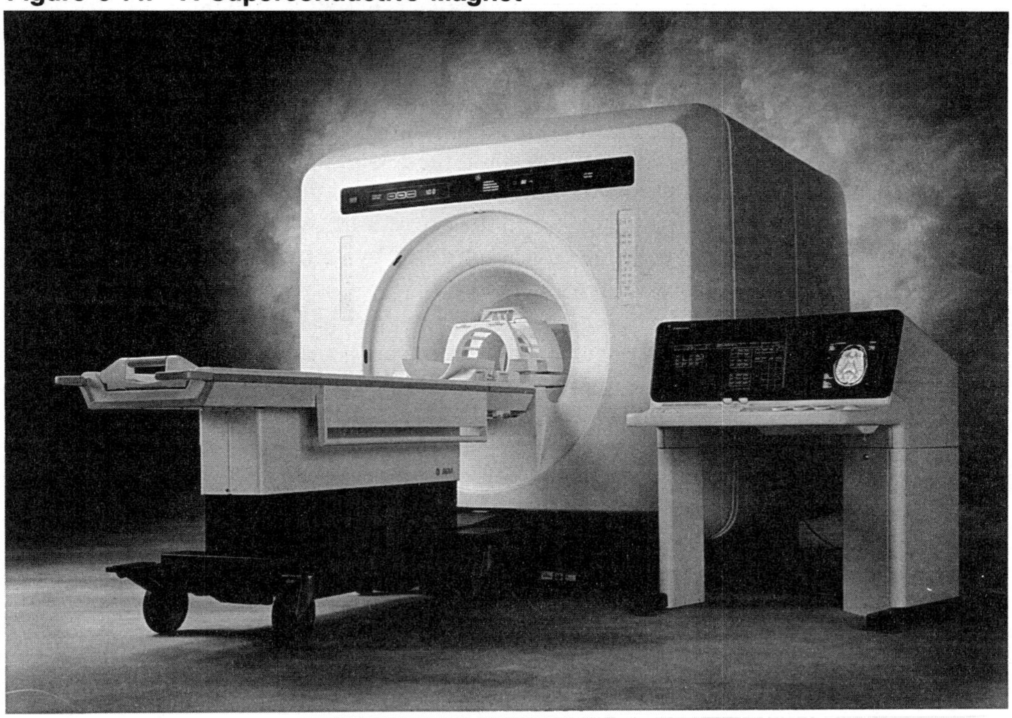

Courtesy of General Electric Company.

Figure 6-15. A Permanent Magnet

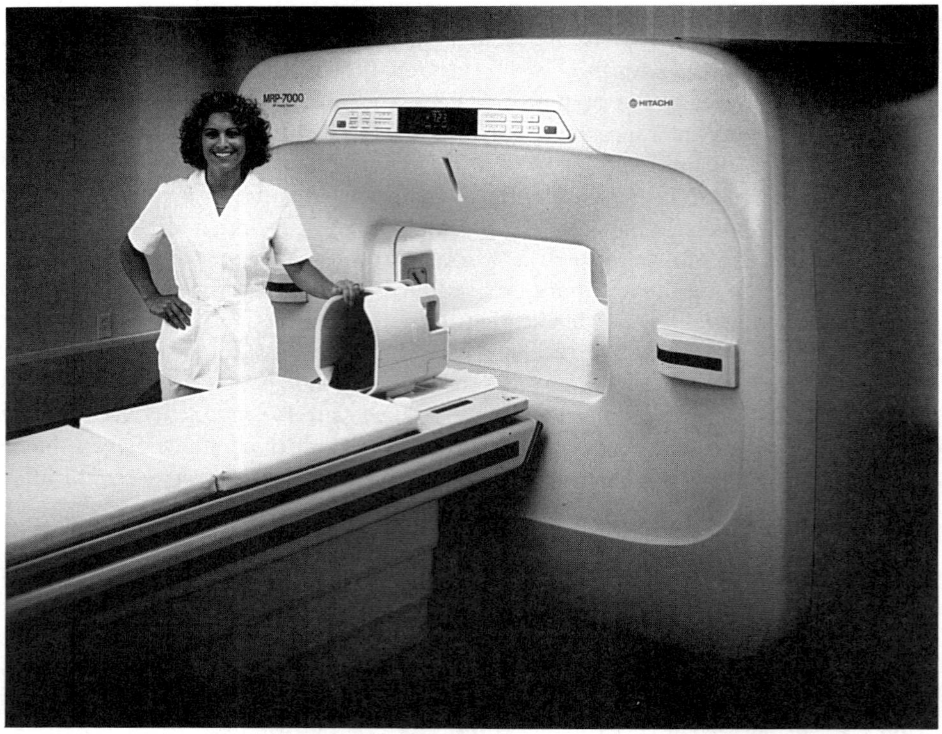

Courtesy of Hitachi Medical Systems America, Inc., Twinsburg, Ohio. Used with permission.

low-field systems. In addition, many of the siting issues for both systems have been simplified in recent years. For example:

> Improvements have come in all of the technologies that go into making an MR image. Over the last 15 years we have learned to manipulate contrast, to reduce artifacts, to extract more and more S/N (signal to noise) from the machine, and to increase throughput by speeding up every aspect of the system operation. Contrary to predictions and fears from people unfamiliar with the technology, superconducting magnet quenches were rare, and the magnets were designed so as to withstand them with no damage. Helium consumption was steadily reduced by the improvements in cryostat design and the use of active cooling systems. Eddy currents induced in the cryostat by switching of the gradient field are the bane of imaging: these are now controlled by actively shielded gradient coils. The cost of magnets has steadily decreased.
>
> In the area of low cost magnets, resistive technology has been superseded by permanent magnet technology. In permanent magnets, second generation designs eliminate eddy currents at the magnet itself, obviating the need for actively shielded gradient coils. Field inhomogeneity and instability problems in these magnets have been corrected by software solutions. Open design permits increased access to the patient and reduces claustrophobia and discomfort. Fluorographic imaging modes open the door to MR-guided interventional procedures.
>
> As technological solutions solve the technological limitation of permanent magnets, we can exploit their unique advantages: low cost, easy siting, trouble-free operation and open architecture.[40]

Magnetic Resonance Angiography

Magnetic resonance angiography (MRA) is a relatively new entrant competing with catheterized computed angiography, ultrasound, and most recently CT angiography as an alternative to invasive vascular imaging. Although not yet clinically competitive with the other techniques, MRA is expected to gain importance in the very near future. Enabled by fast MR image acquisition, MRA may bring the ability to perform functional imaging to magnetic resonance and even outperform PET in that respect. In particular, it may provide new information in assessing regional vascular blood flow to help define how the brain functions. Further:

> This non-invasive technique—made possible by a software enhancement to [some] MR equipment—scans coronary and cerebral blood vessels to look for blockages and/or malformations that cause diseases of the heart and brain.
>
> The traditional method for vascular exploration is x-ray angiography, a radiographic technique involving the introduction of a contrast [material] into the patient's arteries and the use of a long, fine catheter that is passed, under x-ray control, through a peripheral blood vessel into the chambers of the heart or brain. Still the leading method for looking at coronary arteries, x-rays have the advantage over MR in that they are of much higher frequency and, if the [contrast material] provides the proper contrast, can create a much sharper picture. The inherent problems with x-ray angiography, however, include the associated pain, the exposure to radiation, the possibility of the catheter causing an occlusion by dislodging excess arterial plaque, and possible [iodine-related] kidney dysfunction—risks not associated with its non-invasive, radiation-free MR counterpart.

Figure 6-16. Ultralow-Field-Strength Magnet

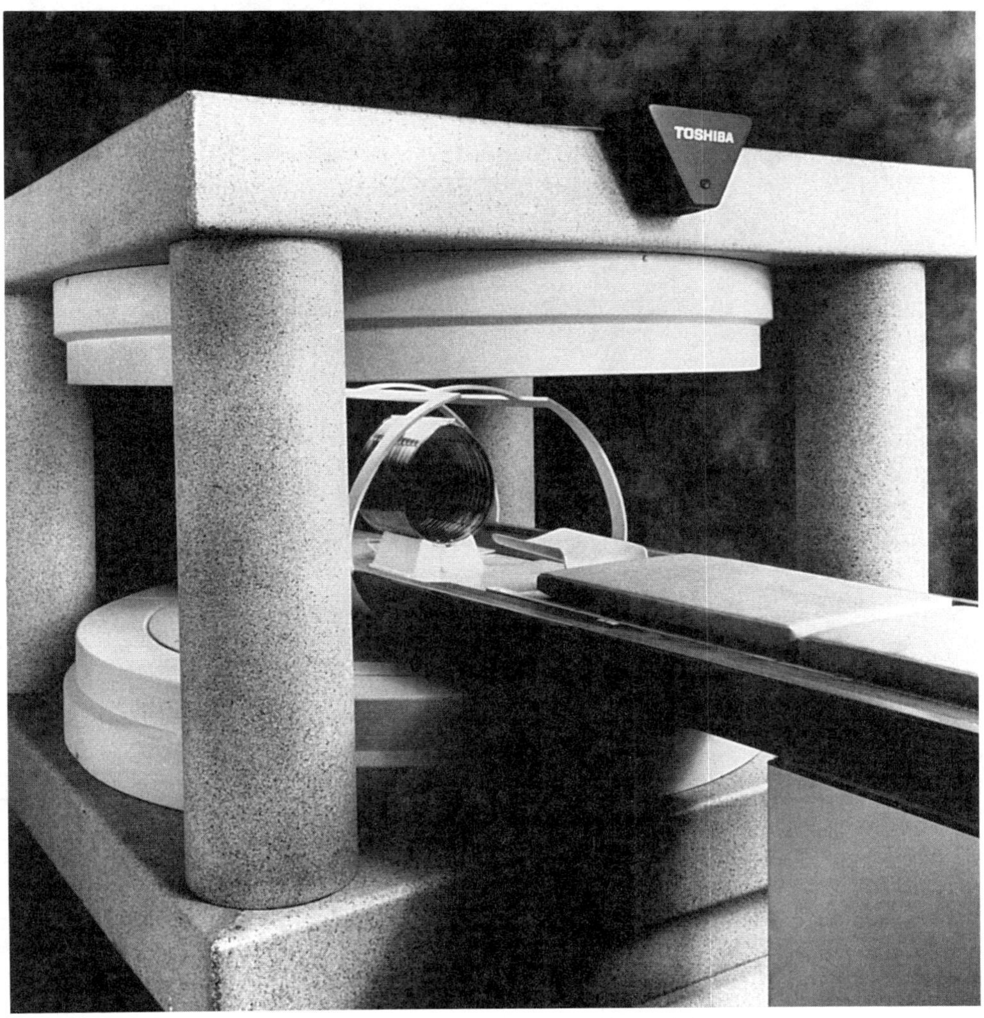

Courtesy of Toshiba America Medical Systems, Tustin, California. Used with permission.

Figure 6-17. Midfield-Strength Magnet

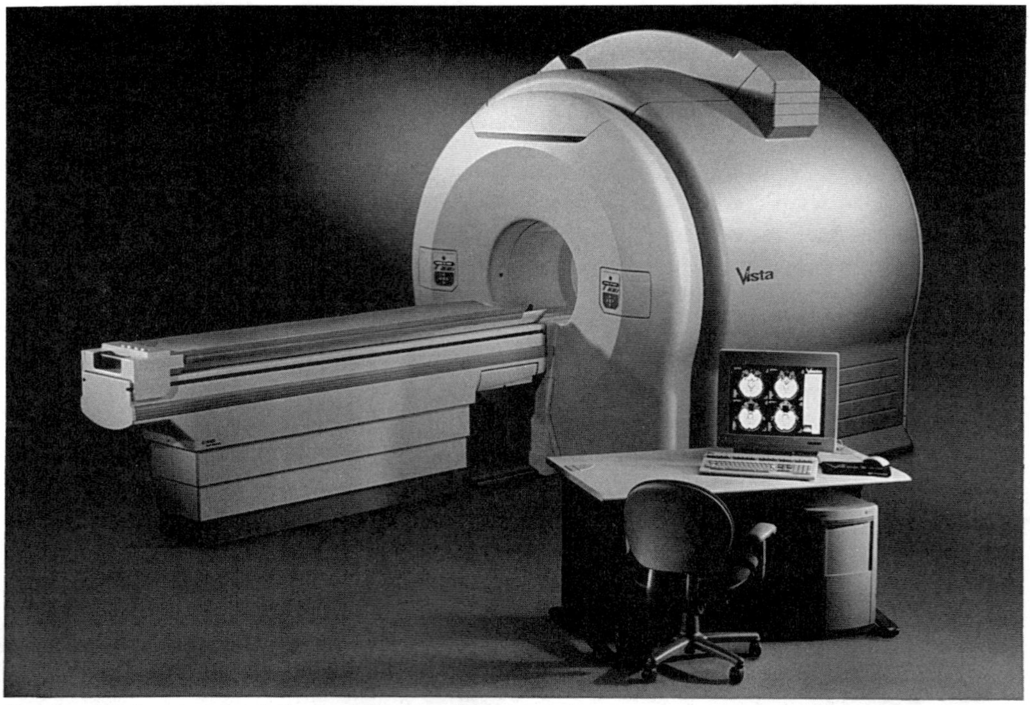

Courtesy of Picker International, Cleveland, Ohio. Used with permission.

Figure 6-18. High-Field-Strength Magnet

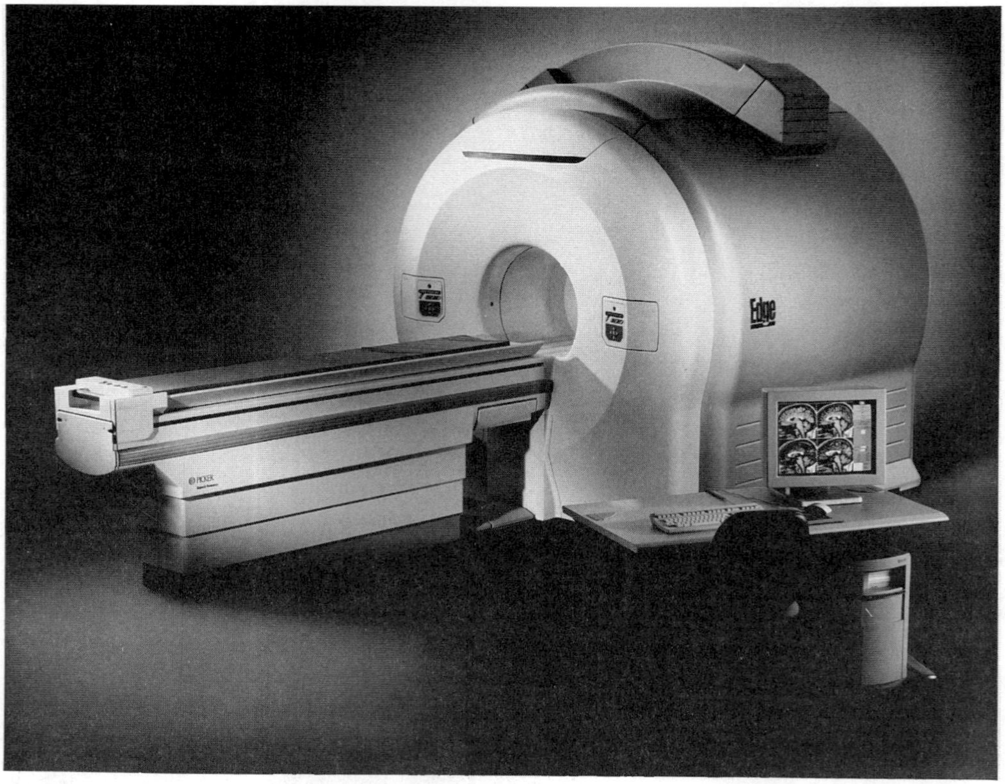

Courtesy of Picker International, Cleveland, Ohio. Used with permission.

> [The use of cardiac catheterization, compared to MRA, can be more risky. For example, insertion of a catheter could rupture an aneurysm, if one is present.] The MR technique [may be] considered more appropriate for diagnosing congenital heart problems in infants, as opposed to exposing newborns to the potential dangers associated with introducing a catheter and [contrast material] into their small vessels.[41]

Compared to diagnostic catheter angiography, MRA could become faster and less expensive (although presently it also is less accurate). One reason that MRA could cost less than conventional angiography is the way it images blood flow. Whereas diagnostic angiography relies on contrast agents, MRA uses pulse sequences inherent in the magnetic resonance process to optimize blood flow. Once the technology is improved, in addition to being less expensive and faster, MRA could become a safer noninvasive alternative to diagnostic angiography. Currently, MRA is applicable to imaging the carotid arteries and is used primarily for brain and renal studies. It is also being extended to the study of peripheral vascular disease.

> Clinical use of MRA is primarily in studies of the head and neck. MRA can provide significant information to complement the traditional brain scan without significantly prolonging the examination time. This combined study provides a noninvasive alternative for patients with suspected cerebrovascular disease. MRA is a useful adjunct, but not yet [competitive] with conventional arteriography.
>
> MRA techniques for the extremities and whole body are also being investigated, particularly measurements of flow velocities. . . . It is difficult to get consistent image quality, especially in the abdomen and chest, where respiratory motion is a problem. Evaluation of renal artery stenosis is considered an area with significant clinical potential.[42]

Magnetic Resonance Spectroscopy

Magnetic resonance spectroscopy, formerly known as nuclear magnetic resonance (NMR) spectroscopy, is a noninvasive method of studying metabolic activity. Tissue chemistry is obtained by MRS, and parallel, spatial information is obtained by MRI. MRS can be carried out on extracts of cells or tissues, body fluids, cell cultures, isolated tissues, animals, and humans. This technique is used increasingly in research laboratories.[43]

The earliest studies of magnetic resonance initially focused on MR spectroscopy. MRI later evolved from the refinement of these basic nonimaging principles of physics and chemistry. As early as the 1940s, scientists were studying the effect of magnetic fields on various materials. In particular, they were interested in how the nuclei of these materials behaved. "MR spectroscopy [has been widely used] in chemistry to obtain detailed information about complex molecules and in physics to study molecular motion. As it became apparent that MR techniques were sensitive to the dynamics of chemical changes, various investigators became increasingly interested in making measurements in living tissues."[44]

MRS requires a magnet with relatively high field strength. Following is a description of the possible field strengths for this technique:

> A 1.5-tesla machine is generally [considered to be] the minimum size used for this technique, [but this is not universally agreed upon]. Although equipment vendors have developed magnets as large as 4-tesla for research since the early 1980s, only recently have such large instruments been installed [for research use] in clinical sites.
>
> The major advantage of 4-tesla MRI is the increase in signal produced by the higher magnetic field. This translates into better signal-to-noise, which can be used to improve spatial resolution or decrease scan time. It also affords better sensitivity for spectroscopy, where voxel size and the time required to obtain various spectra have been limited by signal-to-noise.
>
> Indeed, MR spectroscopy remains the focus of 4-tesla research. The S/N [signal-to-noise] advantage means better separation of chemicals in the spectral domain. This, in turn, will allow researchers to identify compounds with greater accuracy and specificity.

> Researchers hope that high-field MR will propel spectroscopy into an in-vivo diagnostic tool.
>
> In addition to spectroscopic applications, super high-strength magnets provide anatomical images with extraordinary resolution. The 4-tesla magnet enables imaging of the brain and heart with unbelievable clarity. Four tesla should also allow breakthroughs in functional MR imaging and functional brain mapping.
>
> Super high-strength magnets pose questions of safety. FDA guidelines currently limit routine exposure of humans to a field strength of 2-tesla or less. Investigation of potential side-effects will increase before higher field strength magnets become more common.[45]

A homogeneous magnetic field is even more critical in MRS than it is in MRI; therefore, siting the magnet in an environment free of objects that might require shimming is that much more important. MRS still requires further development before it proves its clinical efficacy.

Magnetic Resonance Mammography

Magnetic resonance imaging has been used recently (in nonclinical applications) for breast imaging; the technique is called magnetic resonance mammography (MRM). A specially designed transmit–receive coil is placed over the breast to reduce artifact from other body parts. At present, opinions are divided on how valuable breast MRI will be as an alternative to other mammographic techniques.

> The application of breast MRI can be separated into three major groups: (1) those [examinations] that require improved specificity, (2) those that require increased sensitivity, and (3) those that are used for silicone detection. The techniques and expenses vary dramatically depending upon the clinical approach.
>
> One clinical role for MRI would be that of specificity of breast imaging. . . . MRI has been proposed as a method for reducing the number of biopsies resulting from false positive imaging examinations. The major competition for the specificity model of MRI utilization is the needle. In centers where needle biopsies have been established, MRI is unlikely to provide any advantage in the evaluation of lesions found by conventional breast imaging.[46]

Biomagnetics

Biomagnetics is an emerging imaging technology that is still experimental and awaits clinical usage. Unlike MRI, which views physical anatomy and obtains spectroscopic data, biomagnetic techniques map electrical activity and convert the data into a three-dimensional image.

Magnetic Source Imaging, or Superconductive Quantum Interference Device

A new noninvasive technology, magnetic source imaging (MSI), provides a unique view of the brain, heart, and neuromuscular system. Because MSI uses small superconductive quantum interference devices, the technique also is referred to as SQUID. MSI may become useful in detecting and treating stroke, epilepsy, and cardiac arrhythmias by providing information that cannot be detected by anatomical analysis alone. Following is a description of how MSI works and what it can be used for:

> Biomagnetic fields arise from the flow of electrical currents in neurons and muscle fibers. The biomagnetometer is an instrument that measures these small biomagnetic fields. The result of the measurement, namely the localization and strength of the bioelectric currents, is called magnetic source imaging. MSI is a noninvasive way to measure the electrical activity in the body, especially in the brain. Until the development of magnetic source imaging, the most common way to noninvasively measure the brain's electrical

activity was through the EEG, which involves attaching electrodes to the scalp. Because the skull distorts the pattern of electrical activity detected on the scalp, the usefulness of EEG measurements is limited for certain applications unless the electrodes are surgically implanted directly into the brain itself—an unpleasant, risky and expensive technique. MSI, on the other hand, requires no surgery, and the signals detected are unaffected by the skull.

By accurately locating the origin of specific electrical activities and tracing the evolution of activity as it progresses through the brain, researchers have already mapped the abnormal tissues responsible for focal epileptic seizures and have pinpointed the precise locations where normal neurological functions are performed. In addition to epilepsy, clinical applications include: (1) presurgical location of essential functional brain tissue, (2) brain regions damaged by localization of stroke, especially when CT and MRI images of these regions appear normal, and (3) ways to detect abnormalities that may be associated with the early onset of Alzheimer's.[47]

MSI scans sometimes are performed in conjunction with MRI to determine the exact location of electrical activity while converting it into a three-dimensional representation.[48] In addition:

> The promise of the magnetic source imaging technique lies in its ability to localize specific regions that are not identifiable through traditional imaging methods. Various conditions, such as brain tumors, strokes, ischemia attacks (warning episodes of stroke), and epilepsy, cause electrical changes in the brain's circuitry.
>
> A limited number of biomagnetometers are currently installed in test sites worldwide. The technology is still pending FDA approval in the United States.
>
> The use of the biomagnetometer is twofold. First, it isolates epileptic foci (the precise points from which epileptic seizures are generated). [Second, it is used] to map areas of cortical function, such as sight and hearing, in relation to diseased areas as a means for guiding surgeons away from these regions during brain surgery.[49]

The equipment used for MSI consists of tiny magnetometers that measure the minute biomagnetic fields of electrical energy flowing throughout the entire human nervous system. Small superconductive rings image this electrical flow.[50] The instrumentation must be sensitive enough to detect the slight magnetic fields in the human body without being disturbed by stronger magnetic forces in the environment. External magnetic "noise" is found in electric motors, automobiles, electric power lines, and even the earth's inherent magnetic field. Another source of noise is the human heart itself. The heart's magnetic field is 100 times greater than that which must be detected by the SQUID interface. In contrast, the earth's magnetic field is over one billion times as strong as "SQUID noise."[51]

The biomagnetometer employs superconducting wire, which has no electrical resistance, in order to discriminate subtle electromagnetic signals from external noise. Also:

> Superconductors have an essential role in obtaining the sensitivity required of the biomagnetometer. The low-temperature environment required to maintain their superconducting state is provided by bathing them in a reservoir of liquid helium. The superconducting circuitry and the helium bath are contained in a thermally insulated vessel or dewar.[52]

The MSI apparatus must be contained within a specially shielded room that reduces ambient noise. In some ways, the room is conceptually similar to an MRI enclosure and is designed to keep out magnetic and radio-frequency noise. However, the MSI biomagnetometer is more sensitive than MRI equipment.

> The walls of the shielded room are made from Mumutel®, an alloy of magnetic materials which has a magnetic permeability of 80,000 (compared to a permeability of 1 for air

and all other nonmagnetic materials). Magnetic fields originating from outside the enclosure take the easier path through the highly permeable wall material and are thereby diverted around and away from the biomagnetometer sensor (and the patient).

Another means of magnetic noise control is provided by incorporating into the biomagnetometer sensor a set of magnetic noise detectors whose coils are positioned too far away from the head to detect signals originating from the brain, but they do pick up background noise common to all the magnetic detectors. The background noise measured by the noise detectors can be subtracted out of all the signal detector outputs during the data-processing stage so that only the signals from the brain are left.[53]

Nuclear Medicine

Unlike radiography, which transmits radiation in the form of X rays from an external source through the human body, nuclear medicine views bones, organs, and physiological function by making them an internal source of low-level radiation over a short time interval. Nuclear medicine uses a gamma-emitting radioisotope alone (such as thallium) or one bonded chemically with a relatively simple carrier molecule (such as various technetium complexes, which are called radiopharmaceuticals) to target a particular organ or area. Later, a scanning camera, or gamma camera, records high concentrations of the radioisotopes or radiopharmaceuticals as "hot" spots and low concentrations as "cold" spots. Figure 6-19 illustrates the basic principles. The resultant record, called a scintigram, distinguishes the condition of different types of tissue, bones, and organs. New radiopharmaceuticals are continually being developed, each with a special affinity that directs it toward a particular organ, muscle, or area of physiological function.

Figure 6-19. Principles of Nuclear Medicine

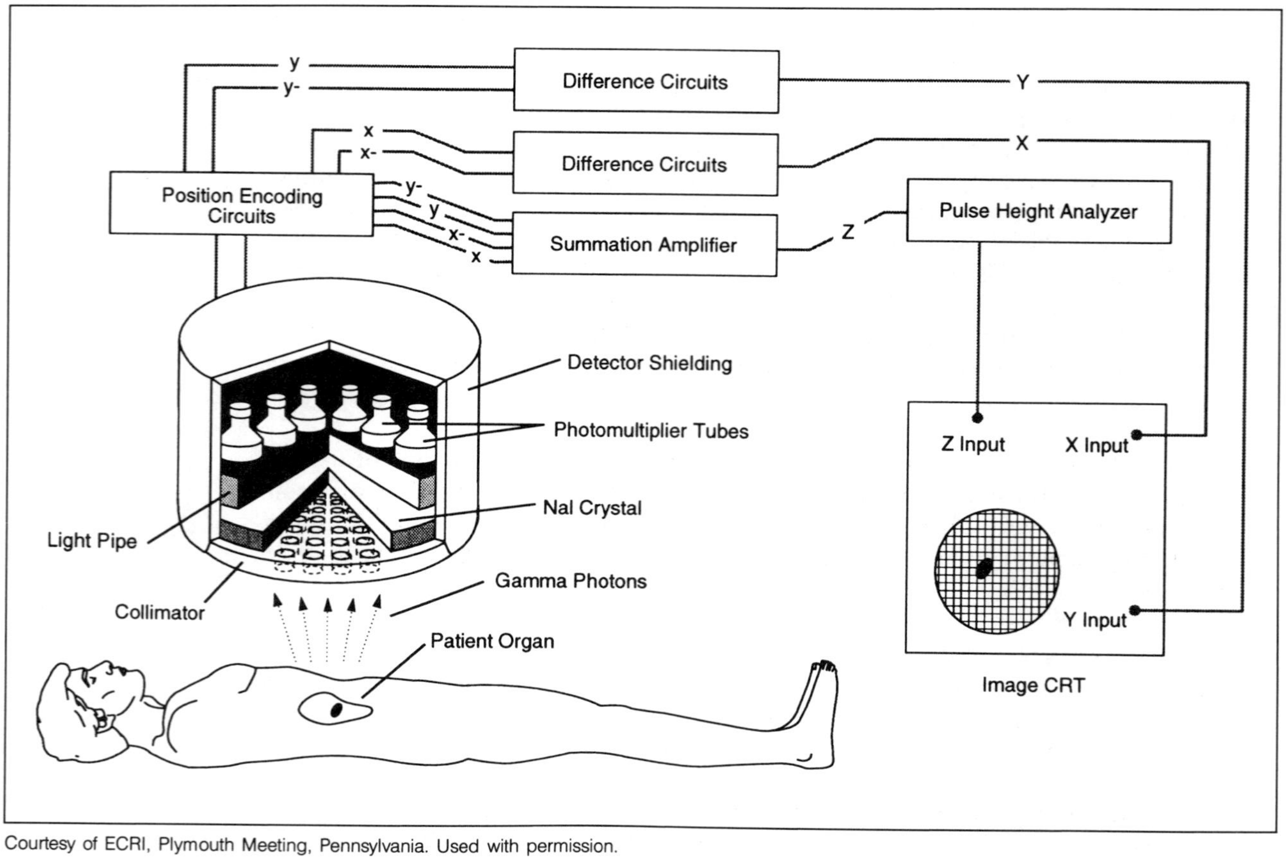

Courtesy of ECRI, Plymouth Meeting, Pennsylvania. Used with permission.

The gamma camera is composed of several elements:

> The gamma camera detects and counts photons emanating from a target organ and maps individual scintillation events in a spatial configuration that creates an image of the organ. A gamma camera system is composed of a collimator, a thallium-activated sodium diode (NaI[TI]) crystal detector, photomultiplier tubes (PMTs), electronic circuitry to determine the location and magnitude of scintillation events, a cathode-ray tube (CRT), and an operator console. A computer is usually incorporated into the system, as well.[54]

Although nuclear medicine lacks the ability to record an image of anatomy with high spatial resolution, it is particularly useful in observing physiology and metabolic activity. As a result, nuclear medicine is helpful in detecting certain tumors, infections, blood clots, cysts, abscesses, and areas of ischemia due to circulatory insufficiency long before they would appear on an X-ray image. In some cases, nuclear medicine scintigrams are "superimposed" on CT or MRI images to provide both metabolic and anatomic information.

> Nuclear medicine continues to be a vital part of diagnostic radiology. Its ability to provide functional information cannot be matched by even the most sophisticated anatomic imaging modalities. Advances in instrumentation, coupled with new radiotracers for both positron emission tomography and single-photon emission computed tomography, will establish [nuclear medicine] as a major force in this decade.[55]

The most common applications of nuclear medicine are bone scans (of the entire skeletal system or of isolated areas), electrocardiographic multiple-gated acquisition (MUGA) imaging (a procedure that traces red blood cells to study the heart's chambers and their muscular activity), thallium scans (a study of blood flow and oxygen uptake in the heart muscles to detect heart disease), perfusion scans (to detect blood clots in the lung's blood supply), and ventilation scans (to monitor the flow of oxygen within the lungs when pneumonia, asthma, bronchitis, emphysema, or lung cancer is suspected).[56] Other common procedures include thyroid uptake scintillation and gas uptake studies. In addition, many nuclear medicine departments also are involved in patient treatment as well as diagnoses.

Single-Photon Emission Computed Tomography

Single-photon emission computed tomography (SPECT), a specialized form of nuclear medicine, is performed on a gamma camera fitted with special computer capabilities. (See figure 6-20.) The technique traces "tagged" radioisotopes to monitor blood flow to the brain and the heart. SPECT, which sometimes is compared to positron emission tomography (described in the following section), does not provide the same image quality as the more expensive PET. In addition, the physical principles of SPECT and PET are quite different. SPECT also uses radiopharmaceuticals with much longer half-lives (days or weeks instead of minutes) that can be produced without a cyclotron. As a result, both equipment and labor costs are substantially less than for PET.

Although PET is more versatile in its ability to view metabolic function, SPECT is a reliable, objective, and low-cost test for confirming certain mental disorders. "SPECT may be the most significant procedure to detect physical evidence of Alzheimer's disease, schizophrenia, and other dementias."[57]

First-generation SPECT equipment consisted of one gamma camera for image acquisition. Later developments incorporated multiple acquisition heads—two, three, and even four cameras. This provides two distinct benefits. First, it reduces procedure time, increasing patient throughput capabilities. Second, the configuration of the multiple-camera assemblies reduces the distance between the scanner and the area being scanned. This results in improved image clarity. Some manufacturers offer SPECT cameras that incorporate slip-ring technology, which was first employed in computed tomography. This further improves image acquisition speed. Most new models of gamma cameras are capable of performing SPECT studies.

Figure 6-20. Single-Photon Emission Computed Tomography (SPECT)

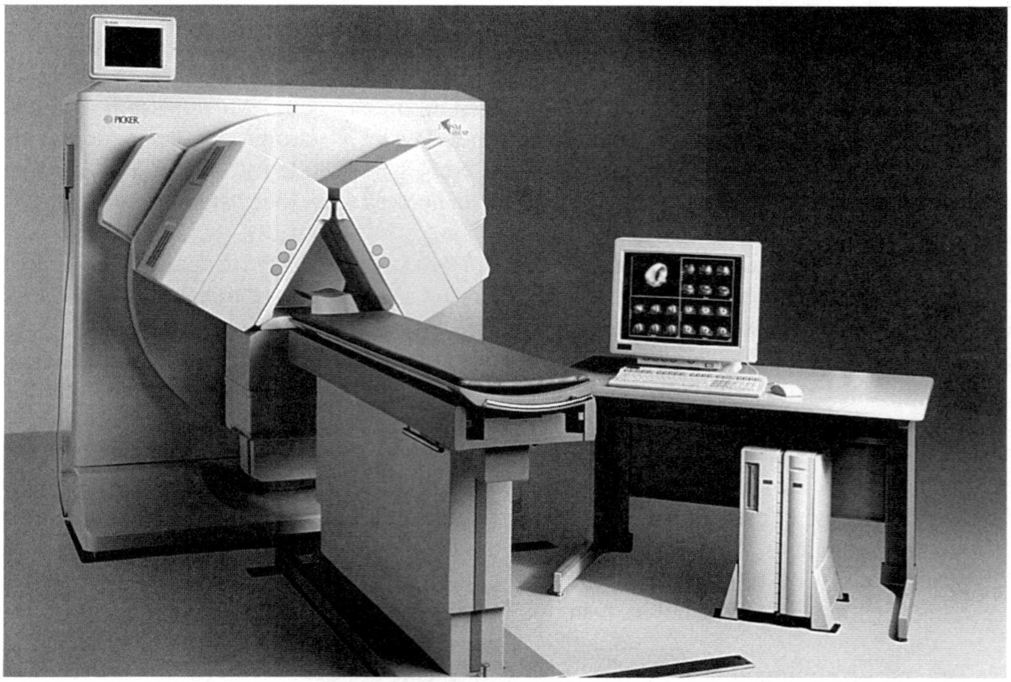

Courtesy of Picker International, Cleveland, Ohio. Used with permission.

Positron Emission Tomography

Positron emission tomography is a specialized form of nuclear medicine. Following is an explanation of how the process works:

> During a PET scan, the patient is [first given a radioisotope dose either by inhalation or by injection], and [later positioned within] an opening in a circular frame [that looks somewhat like a CT gantry]. The frame houses detectors that acquire data for image reconstruction. The data results from the body's interaction with relatively short-lived radioisotopes which provide information about the patient's metabolism. Magnetic resonance imaging (MRI), CT and PET scanners are [somewhat] similar in appearance.[58]

PET uses radioisotopes called positron emitters, which in most cases are manufactured on-site due to their ultrashort half-lives. The PET radiopharmaceutical, consisting of an organic chemical such as sugar or a fatty acid that has been labeled or "tagged" with such a positron-emitting radioisotope, is administered to the patient by injection or inhalation.

This radiopharmaceutical, or radiotracer, then travels to the brain, heart, or other area by participating in the body's chemical and metabolic processes. The principle underlying the use of radiotracers is that they take part in the metabolic process without affecting it; thus, the PET tracer distributes throughout the body according to these processes. The PET scanner records the distribution of the radiotracer in the area of interest by measuring the location of the radiation resulting from the decay of the positron-emitting radioisotope. A PET radioisotope decays by emitting a positron, or a positive electron. This positron travels a few millimeters before it loses its kinetic energy and encounters a regular, or negative, electron. The two then combine, or undergo mutual annihilation, to yield a pair of annihilation photons that are emitted in opposite directions from the event. The fact that each decay event yields two photons that can be detected simultaneously means that these events can be located with precision.

PET, a relatively new imaging technique that is complementary with MRI and CT, is a valuable form of imaging used to study the heart, brain, and other major organs. It also is useful in oncology studies. Some of PET's uniqueness comes from the radiotracer's ability to cross the blood–brain barrier that keeps many chemicals away from the brain. Once across the barrier, determining the distribution of the labeled tracer enables clinicians to observe changes in blood flow, blood volume, and oxygen utilization, and even to monitor thought processes by measuring glucose metabolism.

Figure 6-21 shows additional clinical uses for PET, which were detailed in the following study:

> In 1991, the AHA [American Hospital Association] conducted an extensive survey of medical experts to estimate the extent to which PET is likely to be used in patients with specific clinical conditions. . . . The results of the medical expert survey provide data on the frequency with which PET may be used for these clinical conditions now and in the future.[59]

Assisted by PET, researchers are learning to map the brain and identify which areas are responsible for specific thought activities, epilepsy, and certain types of mental illness. PET also helps distinguish healthy tissue from diseased. Tumors that otherwise would be inaccessible now can be identified, as can areas damaged by stroke or blood clot.

In studies of the heart, PET identifies normal or abnormal blood flow to the cardiac muscles. PET's ability to record metabolic process offers hope of uncovering early disease indicators that appear before anatomic damage has occurred.

Offsetting PET's capabilities is its high cost and the question of whether the cost can be justified by its impact on clinical outcomes. First, for a self-contained PET imaging center, two complex and expensive pieces of equipment are required: the PET scanner and, located adjacent to the scanner, a particle accelerator (such as a cyclotron) to produce the short-lived positron-emitting radioisotopes. Second, a small, highly skilled, and therefore costly staff

Figure 6-21. Use of PET for Clinical Conditions

Cardiology Indications for PET
(Top Five Predicted by Medical Specialists)

Cardiologists	*Nuclear Medicine Physicians*
1. Nonischemic cardiomyopathies	1. Heart transplant
2. Combined heart-lung transplant	2. Cardiac catheter with angioplasty
3. Cardiac catheterization with angioplasty	3. Cardiac bypass graft
4. Cardiac bypass graft	4. Combined heart-lung transplant
5. Fibrinolytic therapy	5. Chronic ischemic heart disease

Neurology/Psychiatry Indications for PET
(Top Five Predicted by Medical Specialists)

Neurologists/Psychiatrists	*Nuclear Medicine Physicians*
1. Hydrocephalus	1. Refractory seizures
2. Cerebral degeneration	2. Stroke
3. Refractory seizures	3. Schizophrenia
4. Dementia	4. Alzheimer's disease
5. Friedrich's disease	5. Depression

Oncology
(Top Five Oncology Indications for PET)

1. Primary brain tumors
2. Primary colon tumors
3. Metastatic brain tumors
4. Primary breast tumors
5. Primary pancreas tumors

Adapted, with permission, from Hoppszallern, S., and Handmaker, H. The future of clinical PET. *Administrative Radiology,* Nov. 1991, pp. 69–72.

must be recruited to produce the PET radiopharmaceuticals and carry out these specialized tasks and procedures. An alternative to having an on-site cyclotron is to rely on a regional distribution center for the longer-lived PET radiotracers. In this way, several scanners may be served by a single cyclotron.

Ongoing research is aimed at developing less-expensive options for clinical PET applications. One alternative is the use of generator-produced radioactive tracers. Cardiogen-82 (a solution of the positron emitter rubidium-82, which is used for diagnosing heart disease) is an example of a noncyclotron PET radiopharmaceutical that is obtained from a commercially available generator. Cardiogen-82 was the first PET imaging agent approved for use by the Federal Drug Administration (FDA). Another alternative is the development of less-expensive accelerators. A small electrostatic linear accelerator, which is less complicated and potentially less expensive to buy and operate than a cyclotron, is under development.[60]

Less-expensive, next-generation PET cyclotrons also are being developed to reduce costs. Several manufacturers offer compact surface-shielded cyclotrons that eliminate the need for a large and expensive vault to shield the machine. These surface shields move on tracks that permit safe operation in a hospital or clinical environment and that allow access for maintenance of the unit.

Compact cyclotrons are low-energy units, typically 11 megaelectron volts (MeV), which is the minimum required to produce the PET radioisotopes. There is a direct relationship between cyclotron size and its energy magnitude. Small cyclotrons are low-energy units, which means a surface shield is economically and technically feasible. Larger, higher-energy machines require massive shielding; a practical, movable surface shield for such a machine presently is not feasible.

Of all imaging modalities available today, PET perhaps is the most technically complex because it involves the daily production and quality control of short-lived radiopharmaceuticals in addition to the operational requirements of the scanner. Therefore:

> As an institution ponders its commitment to establish a PET program, it is vital that its leadership appreciate this tremendous complexity. These decision makers need to understand that PET is far more complex than echocardiography, magnetic resonance imaging (MRI), computed tomography (CT), or even single-photon emission computed tomography (SPECT). . . .
>
> It is certainly true that great advances have been made in the development and implementation of automated radiochemical synthesis techniques and modern cyclotron design has dramatically simplified the operation and reliability of these instruments. However, the fact still remains that a clinical PET program requires a highly skilled team of scientists and technologists working in well equipped, specialized laboratories.
>
> A "PET Startup Team" should be assembled to systematically approach the many [operational] issues associated with establishing the program. As a minimum, it is suggested that this team consist of the following individuals:
>
> - A senior physician, such as the director of nuclear medicine.
> - A medical physicist experienced in nuclear medicine physics and instrumentation.
> - A chief technologist or technical director with administrative and fiscal management skills. If at all possible, it would be most advantageous to also enlist the assistance of a radiopharmacist or radiochemist.[61]

Institutions planning to implement a PET program should first identify the intended nature of the program. Will it be limited to research? Will it provide only clinical services? Will it incorporate both?

> The "clinical only" program [should] define its scope in terms of the type of procedures to be offered. A diversified clinical program is one which offers essentially all clinically useful PET procedures, including neurologic, cardiologic, and oncologic. An example of a specialized clinical program would be one which only offers either neurologic or

cardiologic procedures, but not both. Specialized clinical programs must also further define their scope in terms of their radiopharmaceutical requirements. This will dictate which method is most appropriate for obtaining PET agents. The alternatives are:

1. A fully equipped and staffed radiochemistry lab and cyclotron
2. A generator system
3. Unit doses of [^{18}F] fluorodeoxyglucose (FDG) from a regional distribution center

The "clinical and research" program [should] define its scope in terms of the types of clinical procedures to be offered and types of research protocols to be undertaken. A diversified clinical and research program is one which offers essentially all clinical PET procedures and some amount of research in one or more areas of investigation. The research component may be very broad in nature or limited to only one area of investigation, such as PET neurology. An on-site cyclotron and fully equipped radiochemistry lab are usually required. Some special facilities which serve the research aspects of the program may include an animal lab, a binding lab, a fully equipped clinical (blood) lab, and an expanded radiochemistry lab with a designated area for the development of new tracers. Programs which intend to engage in new target development or other cyclotron-related research may opt for a larger cyclotron, in the 16–30 MeV range. These cyclotrons usually require a shielded vault.

It might also be appropriate to plan a specialized clinical and research program. An example of such a program would be one which offered clinical PET cardiologic procedures and pursued research interests in the development of new PET cardiac imaging agents.[62]

Monoclonal Antibodies/Radiolabeled Pharmaceuticals

Monoclonal antibodies (MoAbs) are radiolabeled tracer elements used in nuclear medicine to both detect certain diseases and deliver medication to specific affected sites. Like some radionuclides, MoAbs often have an affinity for certain organs and travel directly to their target site. Some MoAbs piggyback onto white blood cells, enabling quicker and more effective treatment for certain diseases than was previously possible.

Radiolabeled pharmaceuticals, such as MoAbs, are playing an increasingly important role in fighting disease by tracking metabolic activity and by site-specific medication delivery. Through this process, the division between diagnostic and therapeutic imaging continues to shrink. Hopefully, through the use of MoAbs, nuclear medicine will soon be able to simultaneously "detect" and "correct" a variety of illnesses and injuries. New uses of radiolabeled pharmaceuticals are likely to have a significant impact on medical diagnosis and treatment of disease in the near future.

References

1. Parker, S. H., and Jobe, W. E. Large-core breast biopsy offers reliable diagnoses. *Diagnostic Imaging,* Oct. 1990, pp. 90–97.
2. Parker and Jobe.
3. Parker and Jobe.
4. Sochurek, H. *Medicine's New Vision.* Easton, PA: Mark Publishing, 1988, p. 77.
5. Tierney, M. C. Getting to the heart of cath labs. *Second Source Imaging,* Oct. 1992, pp. 56–62.
6. Tierney.
7. Tierney.
8. Tierney.
9. Tierney.

10. Wurman, R. S. *Medical Access.* Los Angeles: Access Publishing, 1984, p. 23.
11. Laufman, H. *Hospital Special-Care Facilities: Planning for User Needs.* New York City: Academic Press, 1981, pp. 467–71.
12. Sochurek, p. 141.
13. Mahoney, D. P. Picture this. *Computer Graphics World,* Sept. 1992, p. 49.
14. Mahoney.
15. Freiherr, G. *Second Source Imaging,* Jan. 1992, pp. 40–42.
16. D'Angincourt, L. Advances push imaging past recognizable limits. *Diagnostic Imaging,* Jan. 1991, pp. A54–A55.
17. D'Angincourt.
18. D'Angincourt.
19. Freiherr, p. 50.
20. Hillman, B. J., Smith, J. R. L., Pond, G. D., Ovitt, T. W., and Capp, M. P. *Current Radiology.* Vol. 4. New York City: John Wiley and Sons, 1983, p. 1.
21. Bushong, S. C. *Radiologic Science for Technologists: Physics, Biology, and Protection.* 5th ed. St. Louis: Mosby-Year Book, 1993, pp. 325–29.
22. Mahoney, p. 44.
23. Bushong, pp. 407–28.
24. ECRI. *Product Comparison System: Scanners, Computed Axial Tomography, Full Body.* Plymouth Meeting, PA: ECRI, May 1989, pp. 1–2.
25. D'Angincourt, p. A34.
26. DeNike, J. Medical Imaging: An Internal SMP Report. San Francisco: unpublished report, Mar. 1992, p. 2.
27. Bushong, pp. 370–75.
28. Brody, W. R. *Clinical Update,* 1989, pp. 3–4.
29. Sochurek, p. 47.
30. Wagner, M. *Modern Healthcare,* Apr. 6, 1992, pp. 26–27.
31. Freiherr, G. A closer look at techniques reshaping brain study. *Healthweek,* Dec. 2, 1991, p. 4.
32. Freiherr, Closer look.
33. Freiherr, Closer look.
34. Freiherr, Closer look.
35. D'Angincourt, p. A54.
36. D'Angincourt, p. A54.
37. Iezzoni, A. I., Grad, K., and Moskowitz, M. A. *MRI: Overview of the Technology and Medical Applications.* Boston: Little, Brown, 1985, pp. 481–97.
38. Iezzoni, Grad, and Moskowitz.
39. Bushong, p. 399.
40. Kaufman, A. *Administrative Radiology,* June 1991, pp. 61–62.
41. Mahoney, pp. 45–46.
42. Hoppszallern, S. Hospital technology scanner; outlook for MRI services. *Hospital Technology Series* 11(13):6–8, July 1992.
43. Gadian, D. G. Abstracts from Neuroimaging Symposium, Antwerp, Belgium, Oct. 8–10, 1990. *Journal of Neuroimaging* 1(4):207, 1991.
44. Bushong, p. 388.
45. D'Angincourt, L. *Diagnostic Imaging,* Dec. 1991, pp. 81–87, 104.
46. Harms, S. Breast MRI: the potentials and dangers: are you informed? *Administrative Radiology,* Nov. 1992, pp. 111–15.

47. Black, W. C. Biomagnetism: magnetic source imaging. *Medical Electronics,* Oct. 1991.

48. American Hospital Association. Technology scanner. *Hospital Technology Series* 9(2):20, Jan. 1990.

49. Mahoney, pp. 49–50.

50. Sochurek, p. 172.

51. Black.

52. Black.

53. Black.

54. ECRI. *Product Comparison System: Cameras, Gamma, Stationary.* Plymouth Meeting, PA: ECRI, Nov. 1992.

55. D'Angincourt, Advances push imaging, p. A40.

56. Sochurek, pp. 67–68.

57. American Hospital Association. Executive Briefing. *Hospital Technology Series* 9(1):1, Jan. 1990.

58. Herman Smith Associates. *Technology Update: PET Scanning Approaches Clinical Reality.* Hinsdale, IL: Herman Smith Associates, Jan. 1988.

59. D'Angincourt, Advances push imaging, pp. A44–A45.

60. D'Angincourt, Advances push imaging.

61. Faulkner, D. B., Kearfott, K. J., and Manning, R. G. Planning a clinical PET center. *Journal of Nuclear Medicine Technology* 19(1):5–19, Mar. 1991.

62. Faulkner and others.

Chapter 7

Image Management and Film Processing

The practice of radiology requires information management. Picture images and text data (patient history, medical identification, insurance coverage, and so on) are merged together, manually or in an automated fashion, and dispersed to various locations for review. The systematic management of radiographic images can be complicated by the number of diverse systems for acquiring, storing, and transporting information. In particular, the use of both film- and computer-based images has resulted in the development of two distinct image management systems — manual and electronic — for many radiology departments and imaging centers.

This chapter discusses types of images, ways they are stored, and how they can be converted from one format to another. It also addresses the management of manual and electronic imaging, concentrating on the planning considerations for tomorrow's image management. (Additional planning information can be found in chapter 13, "Room Design.") A brief discussion of teleradiology is followed by a section describing various aspects of image-processing systems, including ways to organize the system, types of processing for film and electronic images, and methods for recovering the silver used in film processing.

Types of Images

Techniques that enable "imaging in motion" require the storage and display of video, cinematic, or sequential digital images. Video images typically are made for temporary use and visualization on a video monitor; they cannot be easily enhanced or modified. However, video images can be transferred to film via a multiformat camera to provide a permanent record.

Cinematic (cine) images are film images that show temporal studies of anatomic or metabolic information. As is the case with video images, cine images cannot be easily enhanced. Like motion pictures, cine film is viewed by projection. Cine films are used mostly for cardiac catheterization studies; the exam is called *cine fluorography.* Cine film typically comes in 100- and 500-foot rolls, is either 16 or 35 millimeters wide, and requires special processing equipment similar to that used in the motion picture industry.[1]

Cine films should not be confused with roll films 70 to 105 millimeters wide used in spot film cameras. The latter are made from the image intensifier's output and are sometimes called *photospots.* Spot films are produced on conventional film-screen cassettes by direct X-ray exposure.

During a fluoroscopic exam where the image is viewed on a video monitor, spot films enable the radiologist to record an X-ray image for later study without interrupting the exam in progress. The spot film camera is similar to a motion picture camera, except that only one frame is exposed at a time. Because of their large size, spot films do not need to be projected for viewing; they can be viewed directly over a film illuminator. Rolls of spot film usually can be processed with a typical radiographic automatic film processor.[2]

An adjunct to cine fluoroscopy is video tape recording of images. However, the image quality is not as good as the quality of cine film. The typical cardiac catheterization exam uses video to temporarily record the entire procedure. In comparison, cine fluoroscopy is used selectively for a permanent record of the heart's activity. It is this record that is typically used for making a diagnosis.

Electronic image recording provides the opportunity for modifying, manipulating, and enhancing images. Image enhancement, performed on computer workstations, is becoming an increasingly important component of many imaging modalities, such as magnetic resonance imaging (MRI) and computed tomography (CT). For example, gray scale helps discriminate one type of tissue from another. As another example, three-dimensional images can be "constructed" from a series of planar, or two-dimensional, images. Both color and three-dimensional images are of great value in presurgical planning and radiation treatment planning. The development of three-dimensional and color imaging results in extremely large image files.

As shown in figure 7-1, different methods of recording images are common for different imaging modalities. For example, digital recording is inherent in CT and MRI, but new for ultrasound and conventional radiography.

Image Storage and Conversion between Formats

In a manual image management system, film originals are stored in central film files and usually hand carried from one location to another. However, with electronic image management, digitally acquired images (MR, CT, ultrasound, and nuclear medicine, for example) are stored on magnetic or optical media and transmitted electronically for display or manipulation. Most of these modalities commonly print images on film or paper via a laser camera (or a video printer in the case of ultrasound).

Figure 7-1. Methods of Recording Images for Different Imaging Modalities

- *Ultrasound*
  —Video recording is common.
  —Digital recording is new.
- *CT, MRI*
  —Fully digital recording is inherent in those processes.
- *Conventional Radiography*
  —Single sheets of film in cassettes is common.
  —Digital recording is new.
- *Angiography/Special R/F*
  —Radiographic recording on cut film using a rapid film changer is common.
  —Video recording is common for temporary image viewing.
  —Permanent images are acquired using spot sheet film and spot roll film.
  —A spot film device (multiformat imager) is used to record multiple permanent images on a single film.
  —Permanent digital recording is possible, but image quality is inferior to spot film.
- *Cardiac Catheterization*
  —Cine film (cinefluorography) recording is common.
  —Digital recording is possible, but image quality is inferior to cine.
  —Video recording is common for temporary image viewing.
- *Digital R/F*
  —Same as angiography and special R/F above.
- *Nuclear Medicine (Gamma Camera)*
  —Video recording is common for temporary viewing.
  —Permanent images are acquired using digital recording processed into cut film with a laser camera and an automatic film processor.
- *Mammography*
  —Images are recorded on cut film, which requires processing at an extended speed and for a longer period of time. Digital imaging is under development.

The absence of standardized formats among equipment vendors and among imaging modalities limits universal interconnectivity of individual devices within an electronic image management system. However, at present the two systems, manual and electronic, do have some ability to be interconnected. This situation is improving because of the efforts of standards developers such as the American College of Radiology–National Electrical Manufacturers Association (ACR–NEMA) in the United States and the Comite European de Normalisation (CEN) in Europe. In addition, electronic images can be printed on either paper or film. The resulting hard copy can then be stored manually with other film images. Digital to hard-copy conversion usually is performed on a laser imager connected to the digital system. This is often necessary in order to review the image with other health care providers. In some cases, it is a legal requirement.

As another option, hard copy can be converted or scanned into a digital format so that it can be easily transmitted. This requires a scanner or digitizer that transforms the graphic data on the film image into corresponding pixels, or electronic picture elements, which in turn are recognized by the computer.

Manual Image Management

Manual image management systems assume that film hard copy will be hand carried from exam room to processor to viewer to film file. Usually, the file area is centrally located. It should be close to radiologists' offices, referring physicians' viewing areas, film-processing areas, and the film file librarian, if possible. When light-sensitive processing techniques are employed, passboxes can be installed in the walls between procedure rooms and darkrooms to shorten the distance that film must be carried.

Although many imaging modalities are moving away from film-based operations, the ones that remain (basic radiography of the chest and abdomen, for example) still comprise the major workload for most departments. In addition, because new images of a patient are compared to previous ones, manual image management will remain for some time even as electronic systems become more common.

Electronic Image Management

Unlike manual image management, electronic image management systems transmit digital images across electronic networks. For more than a decade, it has been said that computerized image management in the radiology department will change the practice of medical imaging so dramatically that it will be almost unrecognizable. The promises are familiar: "Soon every radiology department will have comprehensive picture archiving and communications capabilities. . . . Film will disappear from medical imaging. . . . Radiologists will diagnose directly from CRT monitors. . . . Image resolution, storage, and retrieval obstacles will be solved in the near future. . . . Every manufacturer of information management equipment will be using universal standards." But the transition to electronic image management has been slow. Ironically, as most imaging modalities rapidly adopt computer enhancements, the electronic management of images falls far behind. The reasons are clear.

Obstacles to Digital Image Management

Early attempts to develop picture archiving and communications systems (PACSs) and image management and communications systems (IMACSs) offered one solution to all the problems of image management: Convert the entire department to a digital system. This solution was risky for department managers and required radiology professionals unaccustomed to computer technology to change the way they worked.

Many radiologists are still uncomfortable with filmless imaging. The resolution of cathode-ray tube (CRT) images for many modalities is still inferior to film radiographs. This difference was particularly obvious when the first digital images were introduced. Although electronic image management eventually can improve operational efficiency, this requires considerable training and modification of old habits. In addition, both manual and electronic systems need to operate in parallel until the latter becomes well established.

Electronic image management systems are expensive and do not directly generate new revenue. In comparison, the purchase of new diagnostic equipment also is costly but can be considered in terms of the additional diagnostic and therapeutic cases it can accommodate; thus, its cost may be easier to justify. Furthermore, the reduced space requirements for digital image storage may be insignificant and are not realized immediately, because both manual and digital image storage will coexist for some time until a comprehensive electronic system is fully operational. Thus, the purchase of electronic image management systems can be difficult to justify; many of their benefits are difficult to quantify in terms of a precise return on capital investments. Other obstacles to the implementation of electronic image management concern legal issues such as requirements for the printed archival of images, inconsistent licensing requirements for practicing medicine electronically across state lines, and ambiguous legal opinions about consistency of diagnosis when one image is viewed on various computer monitors, each with different physical specifications and in different settings.

Advantages of Digital Image Management

Of course, digital image management offers many benefits. The challenge is to ensure that the benefits outweigh the costs.

Digital image management can address the concern that medicine, in general, is becoming increasingly decentralized. Hospitals, outpatient clinics, and physicians' offices comprise a complex continuum of patient care. In the proper format, digital information can be electronically transmitted from one remote site to another more rapidly than hard copy.

Another advantage is that the quality of computed images is rapidly improving. For some modalities it is becoming easier to control than film. In addition, instantaneous review (via monitor) during acquisition reduces the need for repeating patient exams. As a result, utilization of imaging equipment improves when it is not tied up during film processing or for repeat exposures. A reduction in the number of repeat examinations also lowers the radiation exposure of patients.

Additionally, digital images are easy and quick to retrieve. Computer storage is unlikely to result in lost or misplaced film. Duplicate films (prints or transparencies) can be made instead of lending originals.

Digital archiving lends itself to most new imaging modalities. CT, magnetic resonance, and digital angiography depend on manipulation of digital information. Following is an explanation of how digital archiving works and what its advantages are:

> A digital image exists as a matrix of discrete points (pixels). Each pixel has an associated numerical value that represents a gray scale level in the image. The benefits of digital imaging technology include the ability to manipulate an image's numerical values for optimization of image quality, the ability to view the image on a cathode ray tube (CRT) display, and the ability to store and manage the image's numerical values in computer memory.
>
> While the introduction of these digital imaging modalities has revolutionized radiology, analog images—conventional projected radiographs—still account for more than 60 percent of the average radiology department's workload.[3]

Planning for Tomorrow's Image Management

Proactive planning enables future changes to the imaging department that are both cost-effective and functionally beneficial. If the possibility that changes will occur is considered during planning, rather than as an afterthought, facilities sometimes can be designed to accommodate them, thus avoiding the need for expensive alterations. For example, installing a fiber-optic backbone network with only a few partial or component PACS stations initially will accommodate several feature expansion phases if the network is strategically placed. Although the specific needs of future image management systems may be unknown today, some general requirements can be identified. Each component of the image management system might change independently from the others.

The following sections cover some technical considerations regarding image acquisition, processing, storage, and transmission that affect planning for an image management system. One strategy for acceptance of total digital image management includes envisioning a comprehensive system, implementing the system on a limited basis, and evaluating the system within the context of the facility's overall information management system.

Image Acquisition

Digital images are either converted from film or a reusable phosphor plate or acquired through a computed radiography system. Planning for digital image acquisition must consider space and power requirements for either a digital image scanner or conversion to a computed radiography system. In addition, where phosphor plate computed radiography (CR) replaces film-screen radiography, space for other components of the CR system will be needed.

> In order to achieve a digital radiograph with computed radiography, it is necessary to have a means of exposing the phosphor plate, a means of identifying the digital image with patient identification and exam information, a digitizer system for generating the actual image from the phosphor plate, a system for manipulating digital image data to optimize image quality, and a method of displaying the resultant image.[4]

For images that are not digitally acquired, films can be scanned and transferred to digital format, although this is not always cost-effective and image quality is compromised. Following is an explanation of how digital scanning occurs:

> Earlier attempts to acquire digital radiographs included film digitizers, which function by scanning a conventional x-ray film image and recording the amount of light transmitted through the film. Film digitizers are considered an indirect means of acquiring digital images because they depend on a conventional x-ray film image being produced first. The image quality of these systems is therefore limited by the quality of the conventional film image used.[5]

Some departments are converting to computed radiography (where the image is acquired digitally) for chest and orthopedic exams. This alternative may require modification of existing equipment and/or additional new equipment. Therefore, it can be costly, and image display resolution still needs improvement. However, not all computed radiography systems require total retrofitting of existing equipment.

> Computed radiography systems are made possible by the technology of photostimulable luminescence. Reusable photostimulable phosphor plates are used as image receptors to store the x-ray image until it is generated by the computed radiography system.
>
> The first step in producing a computed radiography image is the exposure of the phosphor plate to the patient exam. Most available and proposed computed radiography systems use a cassette similar to a conventional radiography cassette except that the film/screen system has been replaced by the reusable phosphor image plate. The cassette is similar to that used in conventional radiography and this allows implementation without the necessity of retrofitting of x-ray equipment or exam rooms.[6]

Nonetheless, computed radiography systems have implications for facility design. Space considerations as well as patient throughput are affected by these systems.

> Some computed radiography systems employ dedicated tabletop or wall mounted units which contain the entire computed radiography system (phosphor plate and digitizer system) rather than employ cassettes. Although these systems do away with technologists' handling of cassettes, they do require retrofitting of exam rooms or accommodations in plans for new rooms. Wall mounted units are significantly larger than conventional film/screen wall bucky systems. Another disadvantage of dedicated computed radiography units is that the x-ray equipment is unavailable during the phosphor plate digitizing time (approximately forty seconds), and this may limit patient exam throughput.[7]

(See the section entitled Imaging in the Intensive Care Unit in chapter 14, "Imaging outside the Radiology Department.")

Image Processing/Display/Manipulation

The reader/processor, or digitizer, is where the phosphor plate's information is digitized and translated into a recognizable image. In most computed radiography systems, the technologist needs to enter the phosphor image plate into the digitizer system for processing. Some advanced computed radiography systems feature cassette input and output buffers that automatically enter cassettes for processing. Some of these systems also have an emergency exam image input slot that allows the technologist to bypass cassettes waiting in the queue.[8] Following is an explanation of how image processing works:

> Within the digitizer, the image plate is removed from the cassette and is slowly passed in front of a scanning laser beam to liberate its latent image. The latent image is detected and recorded digitally, and the image plate is either erased by exposure to bright light and returned directly to the cassette, or is moved to an internal buffer for future erasure—from which an already erased image plate has been returned to the cassette. The cassette with the erased image plate is then returned to the technologist and is available for reuse.
>
> The final step in the computed radiography imaging chain are the display and archival of the acquired image. A computed radiography image may be displayed for diagnosis on film or on a monitor.
>
> Because of the currently limited resolution and dynamic range of monitor displays, the primary method of displaying the computed radiography image has been by printing the image on film with a laser printer. The laser printer may be either contained within the computed radiography device or exist as an external system to which the computed radiography device is interfaced.[9]

After the film is entirely exposed, it is sent through a conventional chemical processor. The film can then be shown in a view box as a conventional radiography film would be and can be archived in the department's film archive.[10]

Because the chemical processor of the laser printer adds some time to the imaging process, some computed radiography systems include a preview monitor. This is a low-resolution display that shows the image as soon as it is acquired by the digitizer. The technologist can then determine whether a retake is needed due to inadequate patient positioning without having to wait for the final film image. Thus, the monitor allows the technologist to interact with the digitizer and approve or reject the image before printing.[11]

A computer workstation is a critical part of the electronic image management system. It is either located adjacent to or remotely located from the location where the image is first acquired. The computer workstation is where past and present images are compared and medical records can be reviewed. (See figure 7-2.) The workstation should be capable of viewing numerous images simultaneously and accessing data from hospitalwide information bases.[12] Traditionally, many radiologists have been reluctant to diagnose from anything other than hard film because, until recently, CRT images have been vastly inferior to film images. However, improved resolution of monitors is providing a new level of comfort for workstation interpretations.

Figure 7-2. Radiology Computer Workstation

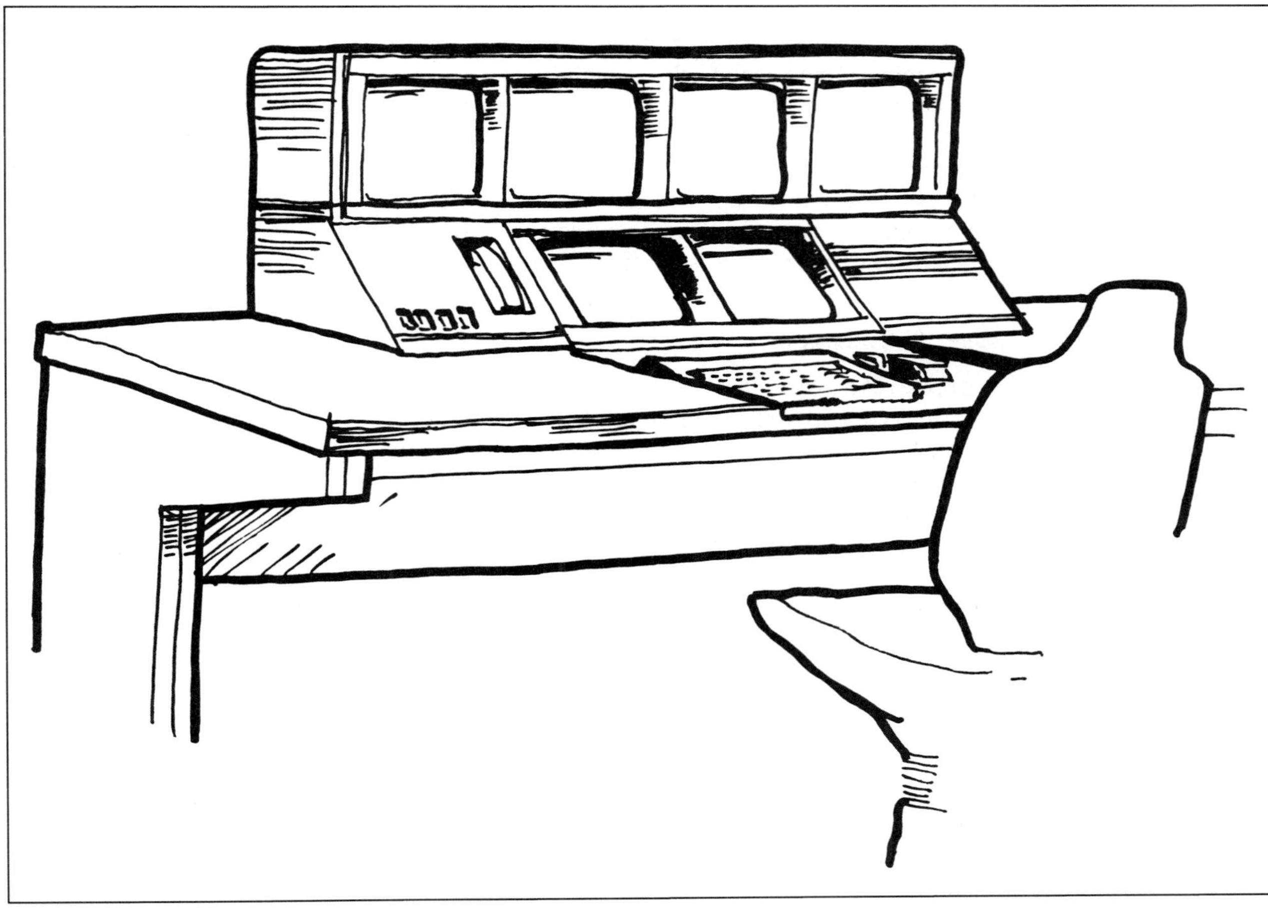

As technology and acceptance of PACS (Picture Archival and Communication Systems) develop, the use of high resolution monitors to display computed radiography images may cause the use of printed films to become obsolete.[13]

If computer workstations will be added in the future, space should be allocated in a location conducive to small group conferences. CRT orientation should be considered relative to what will be viewed. For example, vertical orientation of the monitors is appropriate for chest and abdominal images, and horizontal orientation is best for comparing a series of nuclear medicine studies. Lighting should be indirect, dimmable, and placed to avoid glare on the monitors. (See the section entitled General Considerations for Computer Workstation Environments in chapter 13, "Room Design.")

Image Storage

The enormous amount of data contained in every medical image suggests the need for a higher-capacity storage medium than is typically used in other industries that deal with computed information. Although laser optical disks have greater storage and retrieval capacity than magnetic media, industrywide improvements are necessary before total image management is perfected even on optical disks.[14] Digital tape is replacing many optical disk systems because it provides comparable image storage capacity at significantly lower cost. However, magnetic tape requires a controlled storage environment and must be periodically rewritten when it is used as an archival medium.

Decisions regarding how radiology information will interface with hospitalwide information systems will influence the size and location of storage banks. For example, an integrated hospital information system (HIS) and radiology information system (RIS) could be accessed from a workstation with a single computer terminal but would require a large data archive. In comparison, an HIS that is not integrated with the RIS might require two separate computer terminals and separate data archives.

Technical advancement in storage media is also growing rapidly. For a given size medium, the storage capacity provided by newer recording methods will double about every two to three years. This also means that a given capacity archive will require less space when the storage and hardware are updated. Eventually, digital storage should reduce total storage area requirements, but only after these requirements have increased during the initial period when both electronic and manual storage operate simultaneously.

Image Transmission

Fiber-optic cables carry large amounts of data rapidly to remote locations, but they are more costly than copper wire and have limited turning radii. The tradeoff between copper and optical fiber is one of speed versus cost. Fiber-optic cables can be an order of magnitude faster than copper, but they are less than an order of magnitude more costly. Standard telephone lines also are capable of carrying data but more slowly than a dedicated network. Telephone transmission is acceptable when speed, spatial resolution, a wide gray-scale range, and a large area of interest are unnecessary—for example, when information will not be used to make a primary diagnosis.[15] (See the later section of this chapter on teleradiology.) Microwave transmission, another costly alternative, is effective for sending large amounts of data over great distances. Satellite links that require antennas 2 to 12 feet in diameter are expensive, but they can be cost-effective when large transmission distances are involved.

The key to planning future transmission lines is to identify, early on, what type of data is to be sent, where it will be sent to and from, how frequently it will be sent, and the importance of transmission speed. As a rule, it is best to assume that images will contain increasingly large amounts of data in the future. This is particularly true of three-dimensional images, which now are being used for presurgical studies and radiation treatment planning. In some instances, it may be cost-effective to initially install a fiber-optic backbone network and some empty conduit or cable trays during facility construction and then run additional wires or cable later, when the information system is about to be expanded. When they are sized and located properly, early installation of the conduit or cable trays may eliminate the need for major demolition and renovation when the system needs to grow.

A Strategy for Acceptance of Total Digital Image Management

As partial digital systems prove their value in the radiology department, more comprehensive applications can be adopted. One strategy is to first develop a limited, or partial, image management and communications system (IMACS) linking the radiology department to a selected area, such as the intensive care unit (ICU), where the value of rapid retrieval and transmission of images is apparent. (See the section entitled Imaging in the Intensive Care Unit in chapter 14, "Imaging outside the Radiology Department.") Hard copy from the radiology department can be digitized and sent over dedicated cable to a workstation in the ICU.[16]

Because these areas generally need limited image data, transmission networks can be simple and affordable. Because rapid retrieval and transmission of computed data will directly benefit patient care in these areas, incentives to adapt to a new way of working will be automatic and rewards will be easily recognized. As each increment of electronic image management is gradually tested, accepted, and incorporated into daily routine, another aspect of automation is added to the system.

For this approach to work, however, a comprehensive system must first be envisioned and each component must be based on universal ACR–NEMA design standards, so that future components can be added without compromising overall functionality. Also, implementation of image management systems should be evaluated within the context of the hospital's entire information management system, not merely within the context of the radiology department. That is:

The decision to computerize the functions in a radiology department, or to upgrade a current system, will involve people outside of the department. In all likelihood, the radiology department's system will have to link with other departments. Systems selection should be based on the benefits that will be accrued by the hospital. Key decision makers need to be aware of the hospital's overall strategic plan for information management so that a radiology information system (RIS) makes good operations sense for the organization.

Dr. William R. Brody of the Johns Hopkins University in Baltimore has a list of questions to consider before purchasing a RIS/PACS/IMACS. The questions were based on firsthand experiences in selecting a PACS system.

1. How will scanners be interfaced to the system? Analog interfaces may contribute to degradation of the image.
2. How will images be transferred from the various parts of the RIS/PACS/IMACS? How long will it take to transfer the images from one place to another?
3. How will the images be stored? Can stored images be moved from one workstation to another?
4. Will resolution on screens at PACS workstations be good enough/will the workstations be fast enough?
5. How user friendly will your RIS/PACS/IMACS system be? Will the equipment be compatible with future versions of the computer hardware and software from the same vendor?
6. How secure will your data be? Is there a safeguard against loss of information due to power failures, crashing disks or lightning strikes?
7. How many people will it take to run the system? How much maintenance will be required and how will hardware and software upgrades be handled?
8. Can the system easily be expanded? How many users will the system accommodate at one time and how much image storage will be kept on-line?
9. Will the PACS/IMACS and the RIS interface?[17]

Teleradiology

Teleradiology enables faxlike transmission of medical images between remote sites. The system allows for almost-instantaneous conveyance of images across the country or from an imaging facility to a physician's office or home. In many instances, radiographic and other data can be interpreted by a qualified radiologist who is in a location distant from where the image is being acquired. This is particularly useful for enabling one radiologist to cover several emergency departments during off-hours. (See the section entitled Imaging and Emergency Medicine in chapter 14, "Imaging outside the Radiology Department.") Furthermore, teleradiology provides a convenient method of delivering interpreted images to referring physicians for review and placement in the patient's file.

Pioneered in the late 1950s and 1960s, teleradiology has only recently become popular. Today, it remains largely underutilized, particularly by primary care physicians. Film images can be digitized for transmission; digitally acquired images can be sent directly via electronic networks.[18] Also:

> A large number of telecommunications techniques are available using laser fiberoptic systems, microwave links, or satellite relay networks. The problem with these techniques is the high cost of using them to transmit radiologic images, but their advantage is the high speed with which images can be transmitted. Currently the most economical transmission mode is the standard phone line.
>
> The typical phone-based digital teleradiology (DTR) system uses a standard film illuminator mounted horizontally. A conventional screen–film system that has a medium

> to wide contrast latitude is preferred for the transmission of conventional radiological examinations such as chest, abdomen, and extremities. Most films used in the hard copy formatting of nuclear radiology, ultrasound, computed tomography (CT), and magnetic resonance imaging (MRI) work well on low cost DTR systems. The film to be transmitted is placed on the illuminator, and this image is focused onto the active element of a video camera mounted above the view box. An optical zoom lens . . . is mounted on the front of the video camera. The DTR system usually has a setup mode where the film can be viewed directly on the video screen while the f-stop and zoom of the optical lens are adjusted. The video camera uses charged-couple device (CCD) technology and is linked to a microcomputer by a shielded cable.[19]

One of the potential problems with digital teleradiology is an image with limited contrast resolution, particularly when the quality of the original image is poor. This is true with telephone, fiber-optic, and microwave transmission because the quality of the digitized image can be no better than the quality of the original. For this reason, it is important to immediately examine original films prior to their transmission.[20] If the resolution of the original image is poor, it may need to be reacquired before it can be sent to a remote site. Some teleradiology systems are adequate for reviewing follow-up examinations but are not ideal for primary diagnoses.

Processing Systems

The generation of film-based hard copy requires film processing. Chemical processing involves liquid development, fixing, and washing. Washing requires fresh water. Some paper printers and newer film printers do not require wet chemical processing.

The layout of processing areas within a facility is derived from the type of processing system(s) employed. (See chapter 13, "Room Design.") Ideally, the technologist should not have to travel far or leave the patient to process film. In large departments and imaging centers, a special film-processing technician may be responsible for processing film, whereas radiologic technologists are responsible for attending to the patient and conducting the imaging examination.

Protocol for guarding the environment against contamination from chemicals used in film processing are written by the Environmental Protection Agency (EPA) and must be strictly followed. Special corrosion-resistant piping is required in many places where processing equipment is installed. Federal, state, and local requirements restrict the manner in which chemicals are discharged into the sewage system.

Organization of the Film-Processing System

Three concepts for organizing film processing are common: centralized, clustered, and equipment dedicated. *Centralized* film processing is appropriate for small or medium-size departments. With a centralized configuration, the film-processing and sorting area is circled by examination rooms. Patients enter the exam room from the patient corridor side and staff enter the exam room from the control side, where the processors are located. The distance from exam room to processing area is short when the size of the department or imaging facility is relatively small. Once the facility becomes large enough that this distance increases considerably, a clustered configuration may be more appropriate.

Clustered film processing reduces the technologist's travel distance. With this concept, exam rooms are grouped around decentralized film-processing and sorting areas. The processing equipment within each cluster is appropriate for the needs of the adjacent exam rooms. For example, several radiography/fluoroscopy (R/F) rooms might form one cluster. Mammography and ultrasound rooms might form another cluster. Although a clustered arrangement usually requires more processing equipment than a centralized concept, this added expense could be offset by savings generated by increased patient throughput and overall staffing efficiencies. Also, this type of arrangement provides for backup because alternative processors are available.

Equipment-dedicated processing takes the clustered concept even further. Rooms with very high use (for example, chest rooms) would have their own film processor directly attached to the imaging equipment or at least within the room. Technologist travel time is virtually eliminated, and the patient does not need to wait long while the developed image's quality is reviewed. Both equipment costs and potential staffing efficiencies are greater with equipment-dedicated processing than with either the centralized or clustered arrangement. In general, when an exam room is specially equipped for only one or two procedures, a certain degree of flexibility is given up. However, if the projected workload for those procedures is sufficiently high to suggest minimal vacancy of that room, a dedicated arrangement is worthwhile. (See chapter 13, "Room Design.")

Traditional Light-Sensitive Processing

Traditional light-sensitive processing is still popular for many imaging modalities. For systems other than daylight processing systems (discussed in the next section), this process requires either a lighttight darkroom or a light-sensitive processor directly attached to the imaging instrument. In each case, exposed film is loaded directly into one side of the processor. The film may be delivered one sheet at a time (when individual films are loaded into film cassettes) or in groups (when film magazines are loaded sequentially with multiple films). Film cassettes and magazines may be either hand delivered or loaded automatically via a conveyor or automatic film loader.

Traditional film processing that does not involve a dedicated processor within the exam room requires both a darkroom and a light room. The film processor usually is located in the light room with the feed tray extending into the darkroom by way of a lighttight opening in the wall. Exposed film enters the darkroom via passboxes in the wall and is placed in the feed tray. Each film then passes through a chemical solution in the processor, where the image is developed. (*Note:* Some dry processing techniques exist where neither a darkroom nor wet chemistry is required for image processing.) The exposed image is then conveyed out of the film processor on the light room side, where exposure quality and clarity is reviewed. The film is then sorted for further review and eventual filing.

Light-sensitive processing that occurs in the exam room follows a similar sequence, except the darkroom is replaced by the film processor itself. The exam room should be capable of being completely darkened so that film can be safely removed if the processor fails. A darkroom is still required within the general vicinity for loading film cassettes and magazines, although some manufacturers offer daylight packaging, which allows magazines to be loaded in room light. Air exhaust, water supply, and drainage are required for most processors, regardless of location.

Daylight Systems

Daylight film processing for radiology departments has become popular in the past two decades. Some daylight systems use special film cassettes that allow film to be loaded in the daylight. Others require special filtered daylight, which enables the technician to see but does not expose the film.

Daylight systems provide a number of advantages. First, because a darkroom is not part of the processing sequence, both space and time can be saved. Waiting to enter a controlled darkroom is eliminated, thus increasing film-processing throughput capabilities. Second, daylight systems are easy to locate within or adjacent to the exam room. This reduces not only the technologist's travel distance but also the need for leaving the patient alone. Film quality can be checked quickly, and so the patient does not need to wait and the exam room is not tied up. Daylight systems have been marketed as a space-saving technology. However, the total amount of space required is nearly the same as that required for conventional light-sensitive systems. The amount of darkroom space saved is usually made up by the amount of daylight processing space required. The third advantage is that daylight processing is compatible with many analog and digital image acquisition modalities. Depending on workload and department configuration, a daylight processing area can support radiography, fluoroscopy, computed tomography, magnetic resonance, ultrasound, and nuclear medicine procedures. Newer daylight loading systems further simplify work for the technologist. He or she simply inserts any size daylight cassette into the cassette handler. The handler senses the size of the cassette and the type of film it contains. It then unloads the cassette, passes the exposed film to the processor, and reloads the cassette with unexposed film.

Image Format, Multiformat Cameras, and Laser Cameras

Conventional radiographic images usually are stored on film. Digital CT and MR images usually are stored electronically on magnetic tape, magnetic disk, or optical disk. Electronically stored images sometimes are recorded on multiformat film for future viewing. Electronic-to-film recording is performed by a multiformat camera, which uses a cathode-ray tube and a lens/shutter system to form images on the film. The camera usually generates 8-by-10-inch or 11-by-14-inch films. Multiple images (up to nine on an 8-by-10-inch sheet) are arranged on the film. However, small multiformat images may be too small to display detail at normal viewing distances. The smaller 8-by-10-inch and 11-by-14-inch sizes also do not fill standard 14-by-17-inch viewbox panels, thus allowing light to spill in around the film edges.

Laser cameras also are used to generate hard-copy images from digital data. Compared to the multiformat camera, laser cameras often produce higher-quality images (higher sharpness, density range). High-quality image output requires a wide dynamic range and a high degree of accuracy in transforming digital data. Dynamic range is the density difference between clear film and the blackest film. Accuracy refers to both the number of gray lines within the dynamic range and the spatial resolution of the recorded image. Over the years, laser imaging has become a standard for generating high-quality image output from computer-processed modalities.

Silver Recovery

Silver halide crystals have been used in photographic processing for more than a hundred years. Almost 40 percent of the silver used worldwide in industry is used in conjunction with photography.[21] Although silver is integral to most photographic processes, it is neither consumed nor damaged. Because it is a limited resource—and an expensive one at that—recovering the silver used in film processing is prudent and can be cost-effective. (See figure 7-3.)

Silver remains in various forms, depending on the stage of the developing process. The motivation for silver recovery depends, in part, on the market value of silver at the time. Where the recovery is done is another question.

> Silver to be recovered from the fixer solution is in the form of a soluble thiosulfate complex. The silver to be recovered from unexposed film is in the form of the insoluble silver halide; the silver to be recovered from exposed and processed films is in the form of elemental silver. Recovery processes differ in their complexity depending on the form of the silver to be recovered. Recovering the soluble silver in the fixer solution is relatively simple and practical both within and without the confines of the radiology department. Recovery of the developed silver from the film itself is more complicated and, therefore, impractical for the individual radiologist to consider doing within the premises.[22]

Two recovery methods of soluble silver from the processor solution are common within the radiology department: metallic replacement and electrolysis. Of the two methods, metallic replacement tends to be less expensive, easier to install, and easier to monitor and operate. However, electrolysis yields silver in a purer state. The purer silver requires less processing, can be sold for more money, and costs less to ship. Also, the metallic replacement process forms a silver sludge that can cause blockage in the system if drains are improperly designed and periodic cleaning does not occur.[23]

Figure 7-3. Silver Recovery

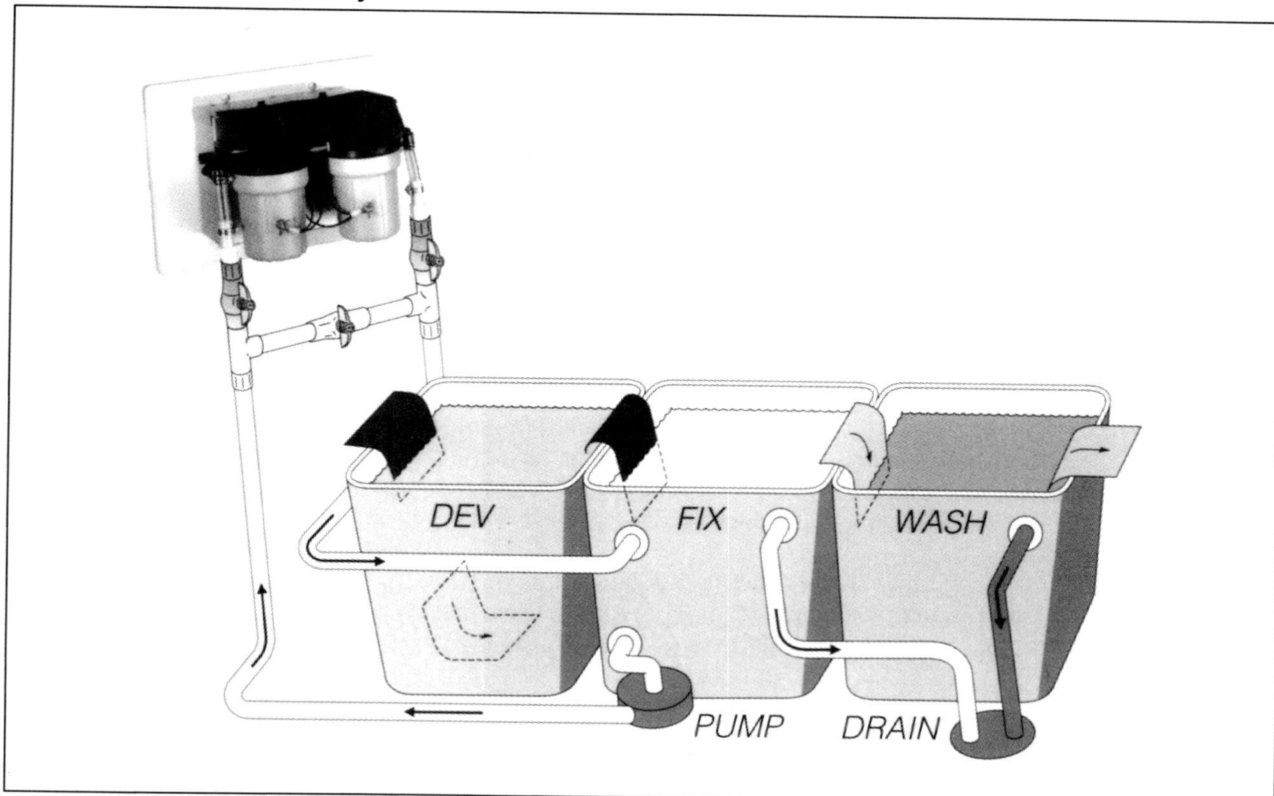

Courtesy of Byers Industries, Inc., Portland, Oregon. Used with permission.

The EPA and local regulations governing the discharge of heavy metals should be reviewed and strictly followed. Regulations specify the maximum allowable concentration of silver that may be discharged. Mechanisms for monitoring the concentrations of silver and other chemicals need to be integrated into the processing system.

> According to the National Association of Photographic Manufacturers (NAPM), pollution prevention will be a dominant concern throughout the 1990s. Hospitals and healthcare providers use silver-based systems and photoprocessing effluents to develop x-ray studies as well as film from other diagnostic imaging procedures. Healthcare providers need to be aware of the laws and regulations in their area and carefully study the alternatives of photoprocessor add-on controls and solution haul-away to be in compliance. While regulations are expected to increase unrecoverable costs to healthcare providers, some approaches are significantly more costly than others and may result in liability problems.[24]

The EPA has mandated new regulations affecting how radiology departments discharge silver into the water supply. A coalition has been formed to study the impact of these regulations.

> The U.S. Environmental Protection Agency (EPA) has enacted regulations that limit the release of silver into the water supply to 5 parts per million (ppm). The EPA's National Toxics Rule, required by the 1987 Clean Water Act amendments, resulted in the EPA's water quality criteria. Implementation of these criteria is now taking place at the state level, and adoption of the criteria is automatic in 22 states. Although most states and municipalities regulate silver based on federal criteria, in some areas the limits may be as low as 1 ppm of silver in the water.
>
> The NAPM and other concerned organizations have formed the Silver Coalition to address the EPA criteria and regulatory controls. Environmental studies indicate that

silver compounds emitted during photoprocessing, unlike the highly toxic free silver ion, are not acutely toxic in the environment and do not pose a chronic health threat. The Silver Coalition has asked that the level of regulatory control be tailored to the degree of risk involved.[25]

Certain waste treatment techniques and equipment can reduce the amount of silver released into the environment or that needs to be hauled away. Following is one example:

> According to medical imaging industry experts and hospital administrators and clinical engineers who have researched the issue, one acceptable method of reducing the silver content of the water involves the use of a recirculation system, also referred to as an electrolytic recirculating unit along with two ion exchange canisters for overflow. The addition of a tank in which wastes from the silver recovery process neutralize each other may produce the desired results. The costs vary with the number of film-processing units (a small hospital may have 3 units and a large hospital 19). Add-on controls must be adjusted for each film-processing unit, based on the volume and type of diagnostic imaging procedure being performed. For example, high-contrast x-ray film uses more silver than ultrasound film.[26]

As another approach to mitigating environmental pollution, some manufacturers are developing radiographic film-processing systems that do not use chemicals. It is anticipated that they will eventually have a significant impact on the industry.

References

1. Bushong, S. C. *Radiologic Science for Technologists: Physics, Biology, and Protection.* 5th ed. St. Louis: Mosby-Year Book, 1993, pp. 199–200.
2. Bushong, pp. 199, 200, 352, 364.
3. Hayden, L., and Nilges, E. Digital radiography with phosphor plates. *Computers in Radiology,* Apr. 1991, p. 44.
4. Hayden and Nilges, p. 45.
5. Hayden and Nilges.
6. Hayden and Nilges.
7. Hayden and Nilges.
8. Hayden and Nilges, pp. 45–46.
9. Hayden and Nilges.
10. Hayden and Nilges.
11. Hayden and Nilges.
12. Hayden and Nilges.
13. Vannier, M. W., Lemke, H. U., and Ruger, W. Workstations speed up soft-copy imaging. *Diagnostic Imaging* 13(11):183–85, Nov. 1991.
14. Drew, P. G. In pursuit of the elusive PACS. *Diagnostic Imaging,* Jan. 1991 (supple.), pp. A9–A11.
15. Drew.
16. Drew.
17. Bouchard, E. A. Radiology's demands give birth to new management technology. *Advance—Administrators in Radiology,* Apr. 1993, pp. 11–12.
18. Newell, J. D. *Digital Imaging in Diagnostic Radiology.* New York City: Chirchill Livingston, 1990, p. 71.
19. Newell, p. 72.
20. Newell, pp. 72–75.

21. Fischer, H. W. *Radiology Departments: Planning, Operation, and Management.* Ann Arbor, MI: Edwards Brothers, 1982, p. 216.
22. Fischer, p. 217.
23. Fischer.
24. Hoppszallern, S. Hospital technology scanner; stringent EPA silver standards increase cost of film processing. *Hospital Technology Series* 11(13):13–14, July 1992.
25. Hoppszallern.
26. Hoppszallern.

Part 4

Design and Planning

It is a bad plan that admits of no modification.

Pubilius Syrus
Moral Saying
1st Century B.C.

Executive Summary of Part 4

As mentioned in the preface, part 4 is the heart of this book. It is in the chapters of this section that imaging facility planning and design concepts are described and discussed in detail.

Chapter 8, "Design Concepts," looks at the four essential elements of good facility design: convenience, image, flexibility, and economy. *Convenience* encompasses those design factors that make the facility accessible and easy to use; *image* refers to the facility's "personality" or identity; *flexibility* concerns the facility's ability to adapt to future change; and *economy* considers expense, in terms of both initial cost and recurring value.

Chapter 9, "Site Design," deals with site selection and analysis. *Site selection* involves three principal considerations: location, accessibility, and development potential. *Site analysis* involves balancing the building program with the choice of site, and occurs initially in the selection process and then in the design process.

Chapter 10, "Work Flow and Circulation," discusses the human and work traffic patterns that must be considered in imaging facility design and layout. This chapter also describes the transport and communications systems required between the imaging area and other health care service areas.

Chapter 11, "Department Location and Configuration," describes the physical layout of the imaging department and its location within the hospital relative to interdepartmental and intradepartmental traffic and work flow. The special considerations of freestanding imaging facilities also are discussed.

Chapter 12, "Space Requirements," introduces a general methodology that can be used to determine the imaging facility's space requirements and identifies the variables that influence facility size. Additionally, this chapter describes how to project the type, size, and number of procedure rooms, as well as their support space.

Chapter 13, "Room Design," provides basic guidelines for planning and designing procedure rooms, image-processing areas, reading rooms, and so on, as well as guidelines for universal room design and rooms in which computer workstations are located. This chapter also includes an appendix that outlines specific guidelines for room design based on the requirements of different imaging modalities.

Chapter 14, "Imaging outside the Radiology Department," discusses the space requirements and design needs of departments such as surgery, emergency medicine, and intensive care that also perform imaging activities and thus require imaging equipment. This chapter also includes a discussion of design considerations for technology docks.

Chapter 15, "Physical Properties Influencing Design," describes the physical properties and characteristics of imaging procedures and equipment that must be considered in the design of imaging areas. These properties include equipment size and weight, radiation protection, and special considerations for MRI installations.

Chapter 16, "Utility Requirements," addresses the requirements of utility systems—electrical, HVAC, and plumbing—that are unique to medical imaging facilities. This chapter also provides a number of references to established codes and standards that commonly apply to these systems.

Chapter 17, "Renovation versus New Construction," explores the issues involved in deciding whether to construct a new imaging facility or to renovate an existing one.

Chapter 8

Design Concepts

A well-planned facility cannot replace good medicine or the efficient management of an imaging department; but, if approached creatively, it can enable radiologists and their staff, administrators, technologists, and other health care providers to perform their jobs to the best of their abilities. A soothing, healing environment comforts fearful patients and reduces their apprehension of the unknown. Such an environment also can help lower the staff's level of stress. A poorly planned facility, on the other hand, can compromise the abilities of all those who use it and can be expensive to staff and operate.

This chapter discusses the four key ingredients of good facility design: convenience, image, flexibility, and economy. Although some of these factors may be more prominent than others in certain projects, all of them must be considered in order for a design to be truly successful.

Convenience

How easy is it for a patient arriving at a facility for the first time to find the front door? (See figure 8-1.) How visible is the facility from a distance? How simple is it to navigate through the site to find a parking space or a drop-off zone? For many patients and visitors, convenience is the most important factor contributing to their impression of service quality, even if the convenience (or inconvenience) they experience is not directly related to the quality of the medical services they receive. For staff and referring physicians, convenience can have direct economic and operational benefits.

Convenience begins beyond the building's boundaries. For example, the building site should be accessible to pedestrians, private automobiles, and public transit. Directional signage should clearly identify site entrances and parking areas. Whether a facility has a single entrance or separate entrances for inpatients and outpatients, ample patient and visitor parking should be located within 300 feet (if possible) of the appropriate entrance and should be clearly identified. Parking designated for disabled persons should be located adjacent to these entrances. Additionally, the paths of travel from the parking areas to the building should be level and protected from adverse weather conditions. To that end, both state and federal requirements for accessible design have become stricter in recent years. The most notable example is the Americans with Disabilities Act (ADA), which was signed into law in 1990 and took effect in January 1992.

Once a patient has found his or her way onto the site and has identified the building's main entrance, graphics and directional signage inside the building should enhance a clear system of circulation. From the moment patients arrive at the site to the time they leave, their path of travel should be obvious to them without their having to ask for directions along the way.

Successful wayfinding experiences, those occasions when everything goes well, are seldom thought about. On the other hand, an unsuccessful wayfinding experience is not soon forgotten and may incur both direct and indirect costs. For people having trouble finding their way, time may be lost or appointments missed. For employees in a particularly confusing building, work time may be lost by frequently giving directions and having to learn new routes.

There are other costs associated with disorientation. There is considerable evidence to support the notion that spatial disorientation is disruptive and causes stress. The amount of stress produced by disorientation depends on the individual's ability to cope with uncertainty and varies with specific situations, such as the need to be on time for an appointment. However, in analyzing the relationship between disorientation and design, it is important to consider that wayfinding problems have their own particular costs in the health care environment. Stress caused by disorientation may result in feelings of helplessness, raised blood pressure, headaches, increased physical exertion, and fatigue.[1]

Architectural form and pattern can aid patients in wayfinding or orienting themselves to their destination. For example, a repeating pattern of columns might identify a major corridor. (See figure 8-2.) The use of special materials at intersecting corridors can direct patients to turn instead of continue ahead. (See figure 8-3, p. 138.) Public circulation can be further directed by patterns created with light fixtures, skylights, or atria. Often a distinct landmark, such as a statue, can help orient patients and visitors. (See figure 8-4, p. 139.)

Figure 8-1. Visibility from a Distance

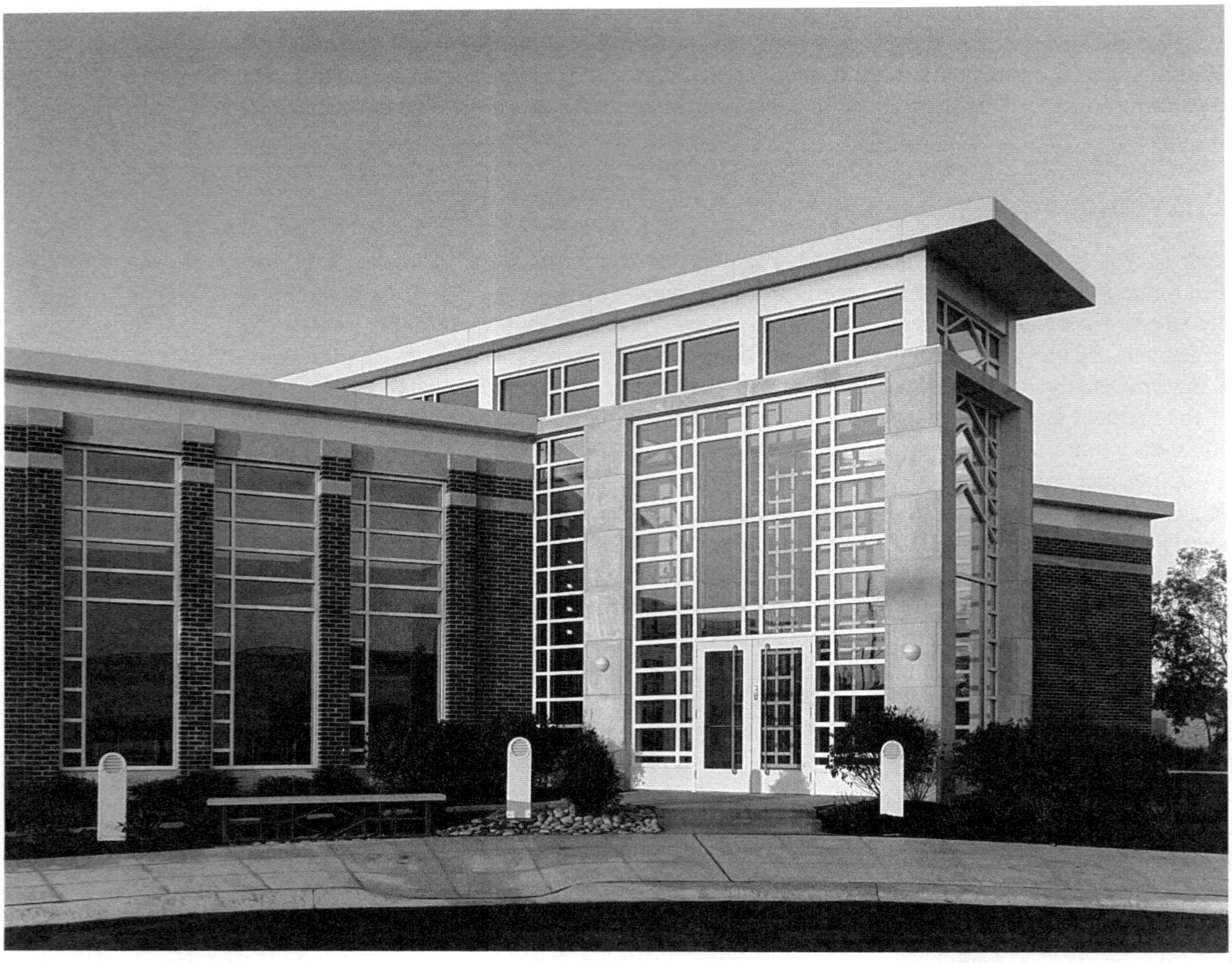

Bridgeview Ambulatory Care Center, Berwyn, Illinois. Architects: Stone Marraccini Patterson. Photo ©Hedrick Blessing (Steve Hall). Courtesy of SMP, San Francisco. Used with permission.

Figure 8-2. Architecture as Directional Device: Repetitive Pattern

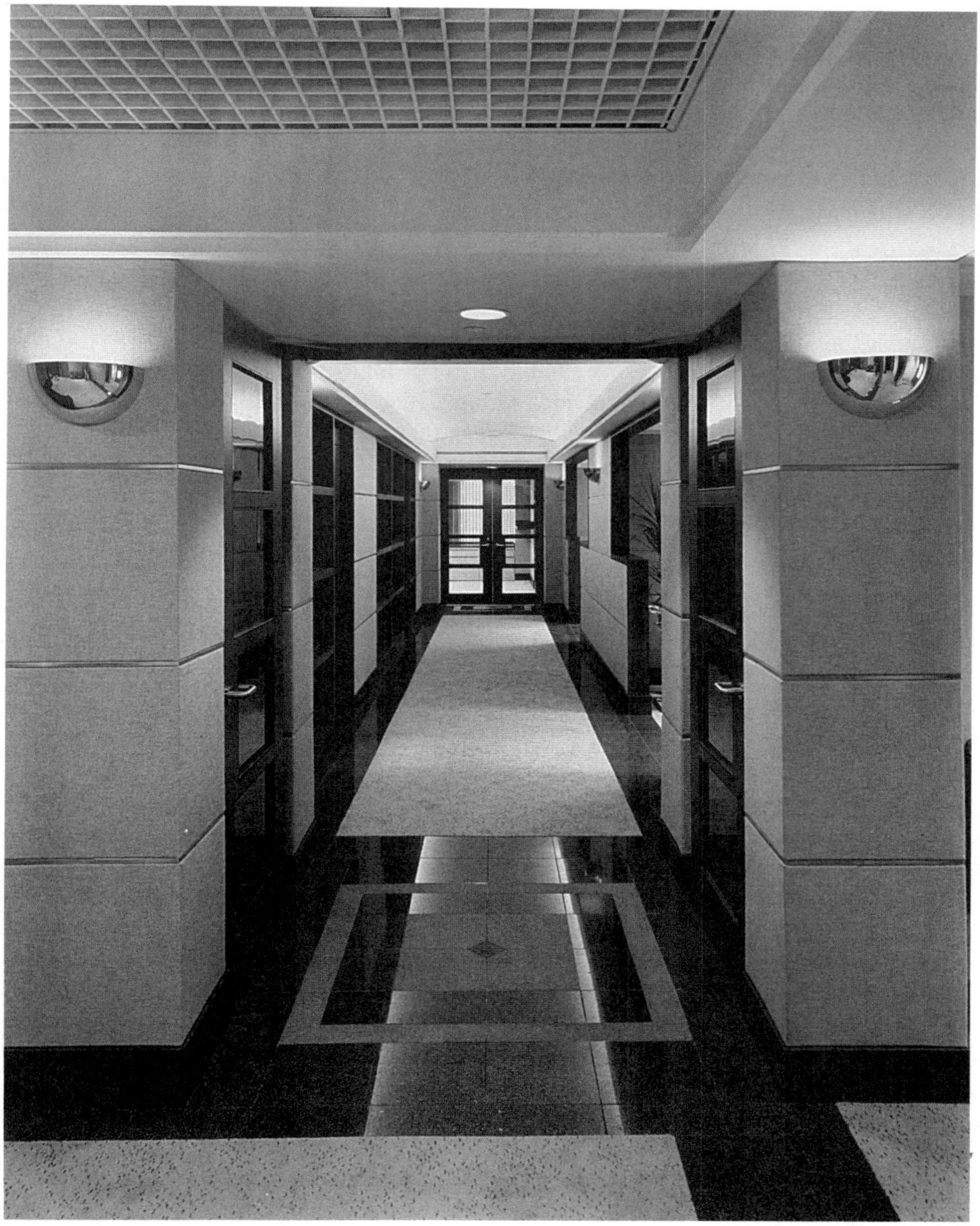

Mallinckrodt administrative offices, St. Louis, Missouri. Architects: Stone Marraccini Patterson. Courtesy of SMP, San Francisco. Used with permission.

A message of patient convenience can be conveyed by the built environment as much as by operational routines (such as extended hours and service-oriented personnel). For example, a reception desk can either be inviting or become a barrier between staff and public. Details such as the relationship of counter height to the receptionist's seating height influence patient and staff communication. A multilevel counter, where staff can talk face-to-face with either seated or standing patients, is convenient. (Low counters to accommodate patients in wheelchairs are now required by code.) An area for confidential discussions about medical procedures, billing status, or other concerns also is convenient.

An imaging facility that offers convenience to staff helps retain and recruit qualified personnel. Staff amenities include short distances for frequently traveled paths, ample natural lighting, and lounges or break rooms where staff members can momentarily leave their highly active work areas. A reading room provided specifically for referring physicians to view films without entering the work area of the imaging department is not only convenient for the physician, but also allows films to be seen without being removed from the department. The reading room is also important where electronic management systems are in place because radiologists and referring physicians may occasionally want to review films together. However, the need to protect against the loss of films is less an issue for departments using image management and communications systems.

Image

Like people, buildings have unique personalities. Each projects a distinct and powerful image. A building's public face serves as its calling card. For many people, a facility's architectural imagery reflects the quality of care provided within. Thus, *architectural packaging,* both interior and exterior, is a powerful tool. A positive image that is clearly visible and skillfully articulated has a profound effect on all who use or pass by the facility.

Image Strategies

The skill with which architectural imagery is articulated is as important as the kind of image conveyed. Various approaches to projecting an image can be successful. They include: softening technology, emphasizing technology, neutralizing technology, incorporating regional imagery, and creating an identity for special groups of patients.

Figure 8-3. Architecture as Directional Device: Corridor Intersection

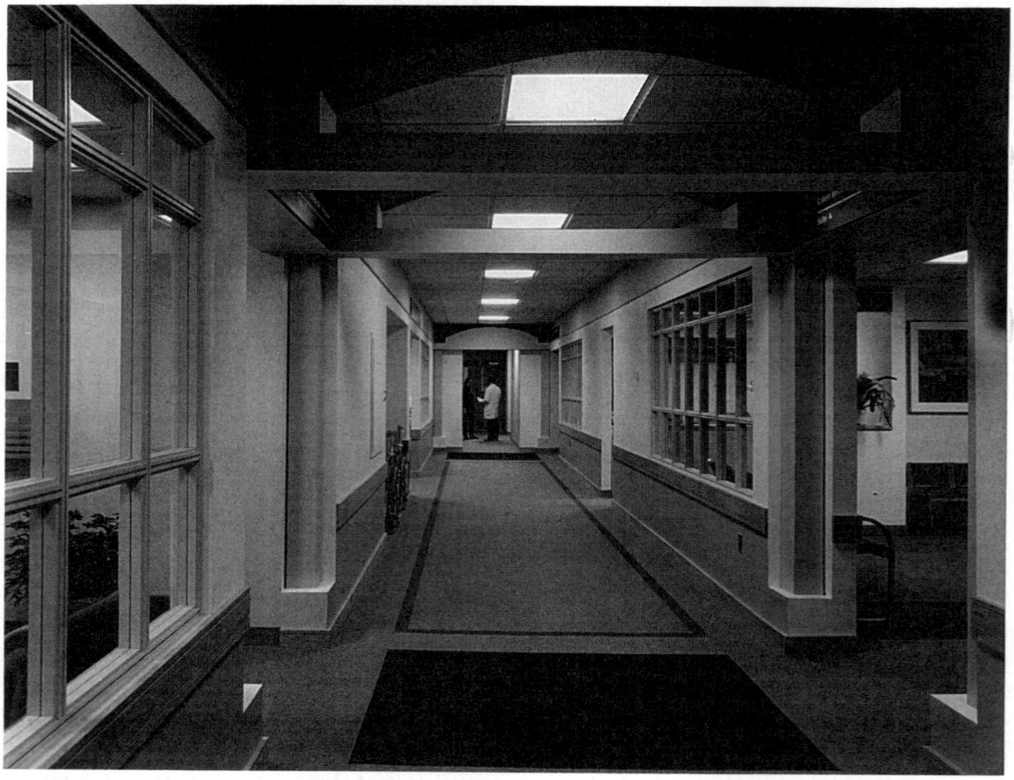

Ambulatory Services Building II, Brigham and Women's Hospital, Boston. ©Steve Rosenthal, 1987. Design by Tsoi/Kobus & Associates and Kaplan/McLaughlin/Diaz, associated architects. Used with permission.

Figure 8-4. Architecture as Directional Device: Landmarks/Atria

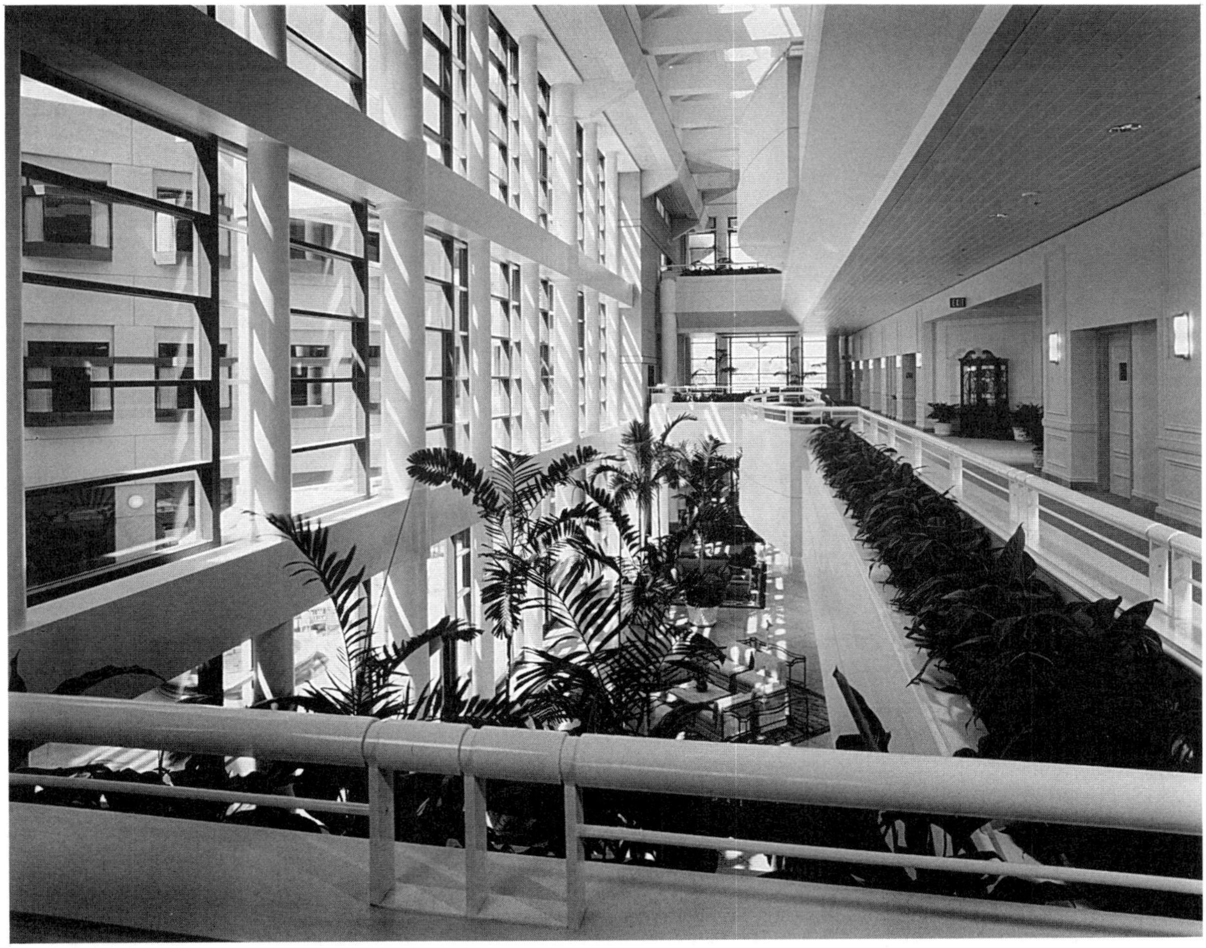

University of California—San Diego. Architects: Stone Marraccini Patterson. ©David Hewitt/Anne Garrison. Used with permission.

Softening Technology

For some patients, the cold, impersonal feeling of medical equipment compounds fears and feelings of helplessness toward the unfamiliar procedures they are about to undergo. Often this sense of alienation can be countered by a less-foreign environment. Familiar objects such as artwork, indirect lighting, quality fabrics and finishes, and even landscaping can help comfort fearful patients. A dedicated space for, and a policy devoted to, patient education also reassures those who are intimidated by the unknown.

Softening technology should begin long before patients come in contact with the "medical machinery." The tone should be set outside the front door and continued through the waiting, reception, and dressing areas. If no attempt has been made to ease patients' fears before they reach the procedure room, the effect will be lost.

Many patients undergoing imaging procedures are conscious and well aware of their surroundings. Patients on gurneys spend much of their time staring at the ceilings of corridors and procedure rooms. Thus, special effort should be made to improve and enhance these often harsh and uninteresting surfaces. (See figure 8-5.)

Acoustic damping of walls and ceilings softens the environment and provides an extra measure of comfort. Proper acoustic design reduces transmission of both airborne noises and those traveling through walls and partitions. Special sound treatment should be provided

Figure 8-5. Imaging Room Ceiling

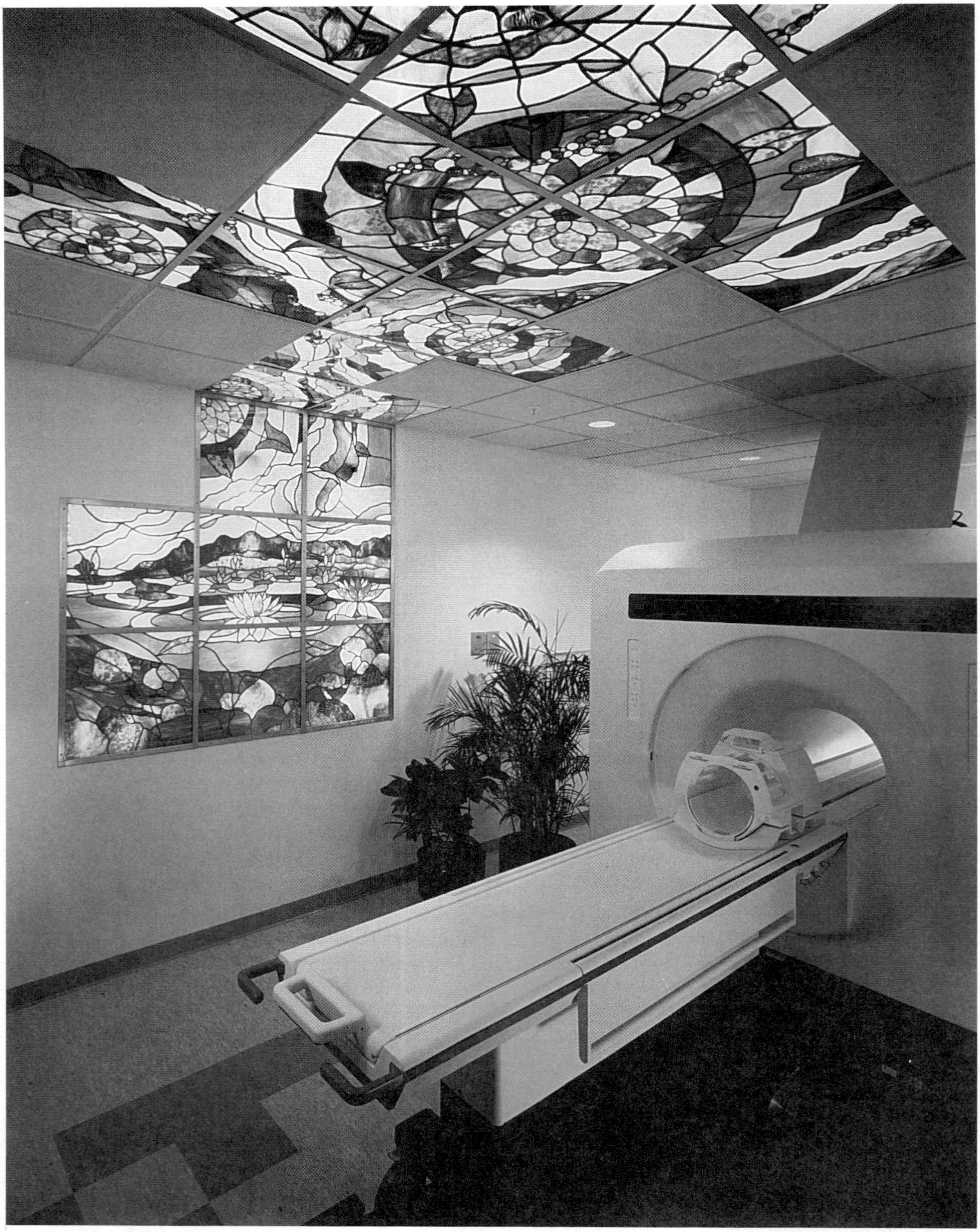

Magnetic resonance imaging room, Tuttleman Center, Graduate Hospital, Philadelphia. Architecture and interior design: Medifac and KPA Design Group. Stained glass: Stigstedt Studio. Photographer: Peter Leach. Used with permission.

in business offices and consultation rooms where conversations must be contained, as well as in excessively noisy procedure rooms.

Some procedures, such as magnetic resonance imaging (MRI), are inherently noisy. A significant number of MRI patients fail to keep their appointments for fear of the noise and the claustrophobia induced by the equipment. Special audio and video systems are available to mask the noise and distract patients from thinking about either the machinery or the medical procedure. In addition, some new magnets (usually low- or ultralow-field magnets) are designed with an open bore to improve access and reduce patient claustrophobia, which is a common problem with this procedure:

> It is a known fact to the experienced user of [MRI] technology that many patients undergo some type of anxiety and fear of the unknown during an MRI procedure; in some cases this will be mild and in others more severe. The very definition of claustrophobia, "the morbid dread of being closed up in a confined space," describes how some patients feel about the procedure.
>
> . . . In [some] reports, as many as twenty percent of individuals attempting an MRI scan could not complete it secondary to claustrophobia. It has been noted that the rate of unfinished scans varies from unit to unit and changes with the experience of the MRI technologist.
>
> The most striking sources of patients' anxiety involve the physical condition and setting of MRI: not being able to move and hearing the unbearable noise. Many patients have already discussed the exam with family and friends; unfortunately, the context is usually negative. Statements like "MRI is the worst experience they've had" [and] "It's like being in a coffin or tomb" are common. [Ironically, compared to other methods of diagnosis and/or treatment, MRI is not painful, just frightening. However, for some people, fear is something that can be mitigated by the surrounding environment and the way care is given by personnel within the environment.][2]

Soft indirect lighting also helps temper the imaging environment. Lighting design is discussed in more detail in chapter 15, "Physical Properties Influencing Design" and in chapter 16, "Utility Requirements."

Emphasizing Technology

In contrast to the strategy of softening technology is the strategy of emphasizing it. Many patients have faith in the marvels of modern medicine. For this reason, a strategy of highlighting the technical components of the physical environment also may be appropriate. In some buildings, the structural system is exposed rather than hidden. This not only creates an opportunity for articulating the architecture, but it also tends to create a feeling of strength and confidence. (See figure 8-6.)

Furnishings, lighting fixtures, and finishes that echo advances in technology may diminish patient fears by reinforcing the quality and capabilities of medical imaging. With this approach, it is important that the human element also be considered. For example, furniture can be arranged to facilitate small group conversations. An image that emphasizes technology might begin on the exterior and then continue through public spaces and private rooms.

Neutralizing Technology

Another alternative is to neutralize technology, in other words, to allow medical equipment to blend into the background. Equipment manufacturers are improving the appearance of their products, which, in turn, enables designers to neutralize the equipment's visual impact.

MRI examination rooms that conceal the magnet from view often tend to neutralize the massive appearance of the machinery. Additionally, careful selection of floor and wall coverings, colors, and lighting can further humanize the imaging environment.

Figure 8-6. Emphasizing Technology

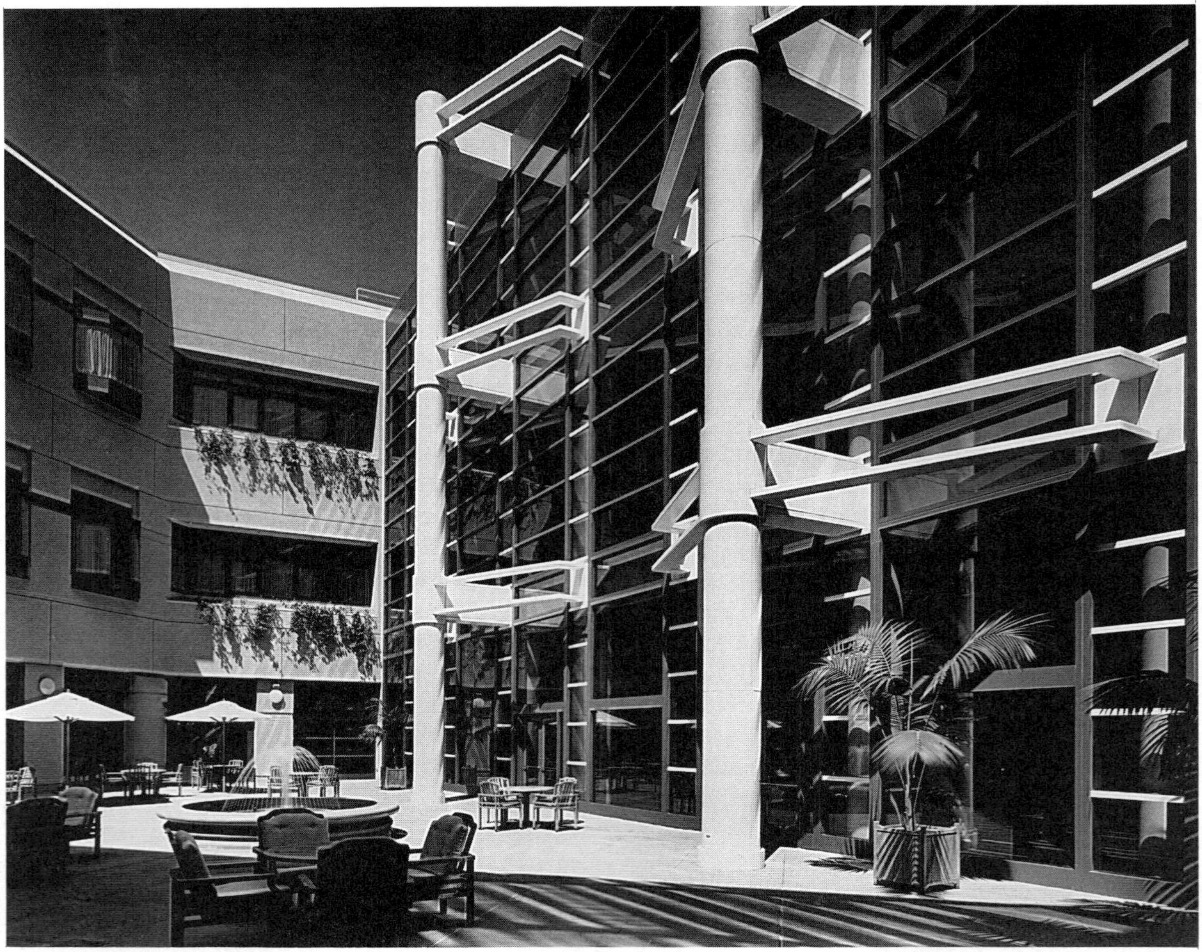

University of California—San Diego. Architects: Stone Marraccini Patterson. ©David Hewitt/Anne Garrison. Used with permission.

Incorporating Regional Imagery

Regardless of whether technology is softened or emphasized, local context can be incorporated into the building's exterior and interior image. Local materials that are indigenous to the region (such as masonry, wood siding, stone, and cement plaster) can be used, perhaps in a more playful way than they have been assembled historically.

Regional imagery can be expressed through form as well. For example, the facade of a large building can be subdivided into smaller elements that echo the forms of adjacent residential structures. (See figure 8-7.) Other references to regional style can be expressed through articulation of window and door openings and roof forms.

Creating an Identity for Special Groups of Patients

Special patient populations provide design opportunities for yet another form of architectural imagery. As the number of diagnostic and therapeutic imaging procedures performed on ambulatory patients increases, many providers elect to differentiate inpatient and outpatient settings. In some cases, one department may have both an inpatient and outpatient zone; in others, there may be two separate imaging facilities or departments.

The distinction between inpatient and outpatient areas can be addressed both architecturally and operationally. Architecturally, each area can be differentiated with special lighting, furnishings, and finishes. Operationally, streamlining outpatient registration paperwork—

perhaps by verifying patients' medical history and insurance coverage prior to the day of treatment—can reduce lengthy waiting periods and thus further strengthen the facility's image. Paperless admitting and registration systems are a common way that imaging and other services are being reengineered to improve work flow and efficiency.

Within the outpatient zone, special populations can be further accommodated. For example, if ultrasound and mammography rooms are clustered together and separated from other traffic, a women's health area with its own entrance can be created within the department. (See figure 8-8, p. 144.) Ideally, this area would be located either toward the front or off to the side of the department so that these patients do not have to travel through the entire facility. Dressing rooms and toilet rooms can be placed within a separate vestibule to maximize privacy. A separate area for patient education also should be considered.

When children make up a significant percentage of the patient workload, a separate children's waiting area is appropriate. (See figure 8-9, p. 145.) This area might have a more playful feeling and be designed in brighter colors than the rest of the department. Furnishings can be kid sized; murals and graphics can be childlike. Special acoustic treatment should contain noise within the immediate area.

> Imagine a radiology department through the eyes of a five-year-old: "Strangers in white clothes come get me and take me into a room and close the door. The rooms have big, scary machines inside. The people in white turn the lights out when we go in. I have

Figure 8-7. Regional Imagery

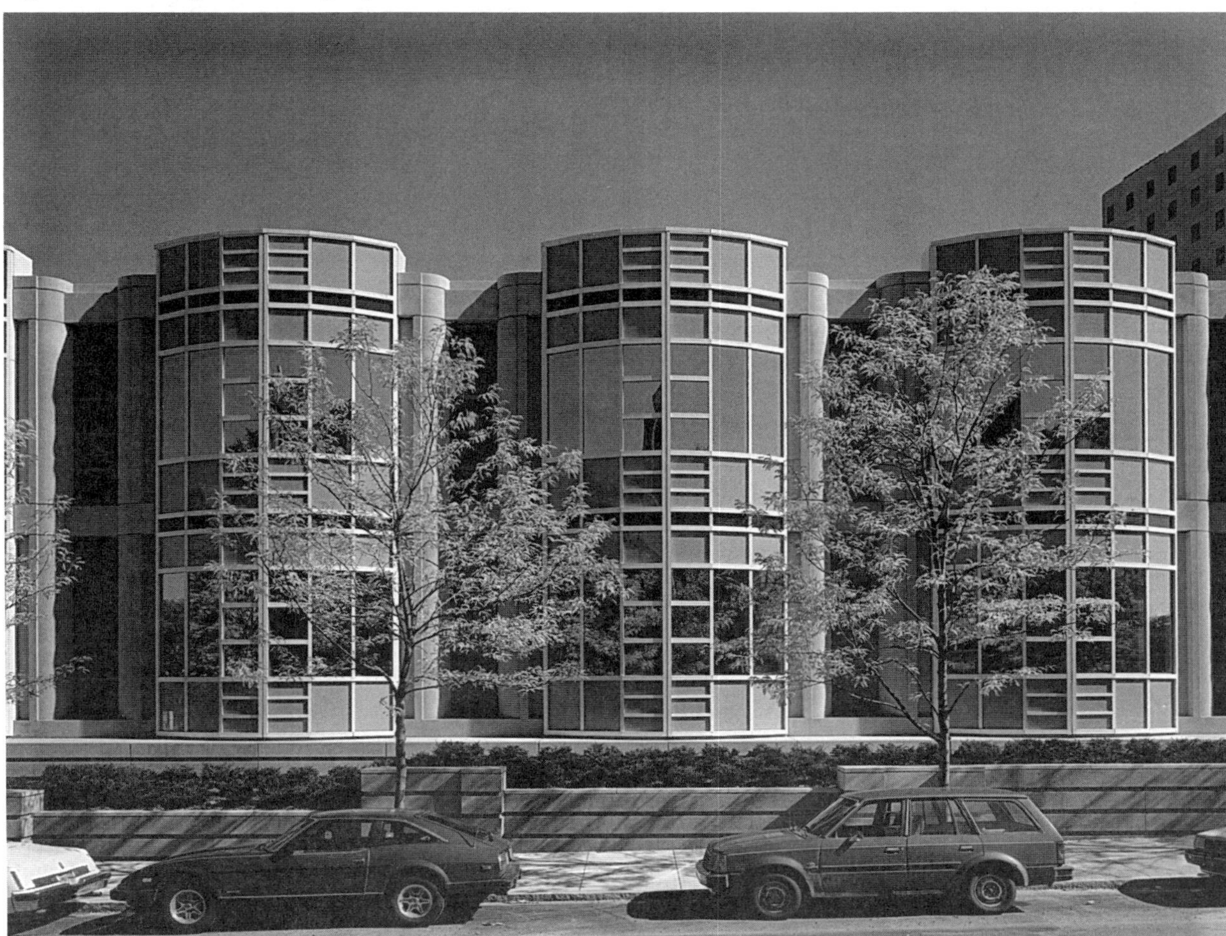

Ambulatory Services Building II, Brigham and Women's Hospital, Boston. ©Steve Rosenthal, 1987. Design by Tsoi/Kobus & Associates and Kaplan/McLaughlin/Diaz, associated architects. Used with permission.

Figure 8-8. Women's Health Screening Area

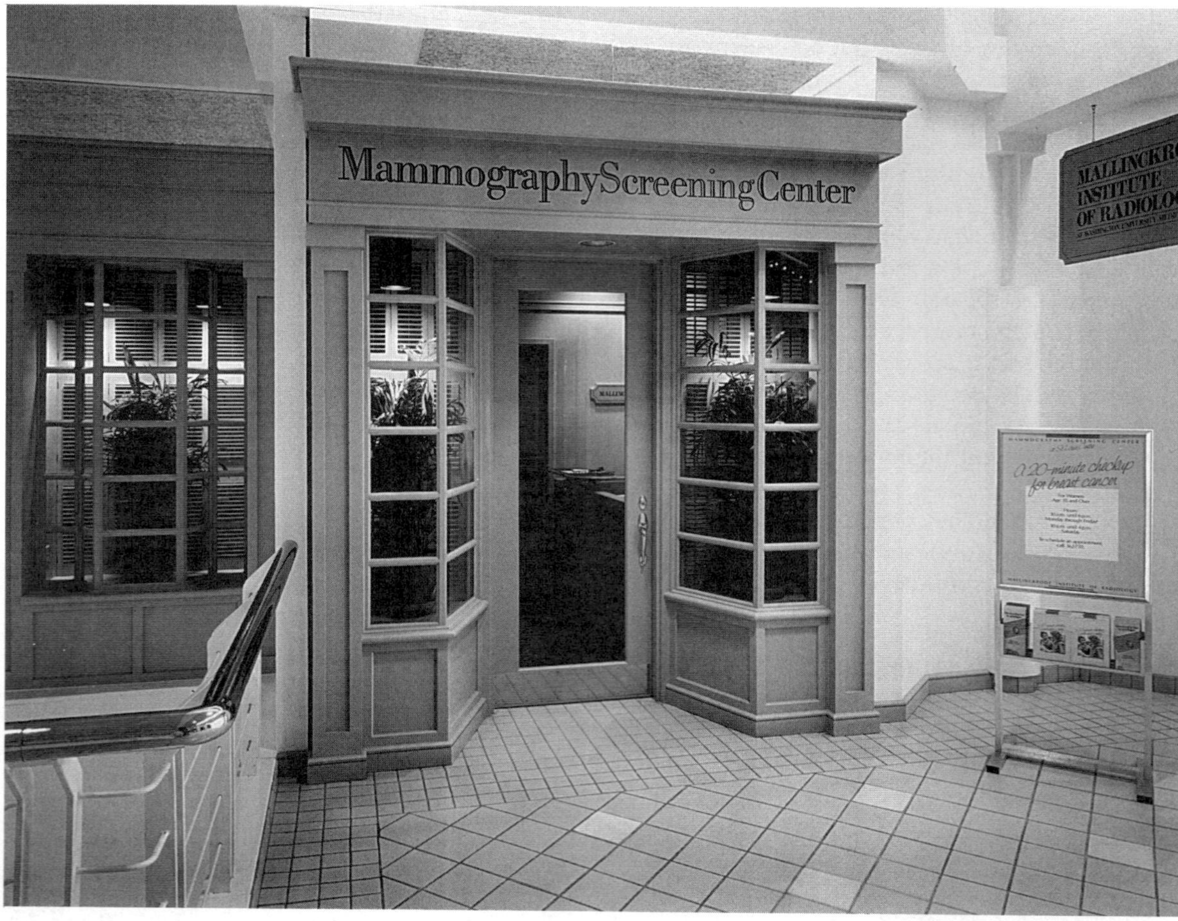

Freestanding Women's Health Center, St. Louis, Missouri. Architects: Stone Marraccini Patterson. Used courtesy of SMP, San Francisco.

> to hold my breath so the man can take my picture. This isn't like mommy's camera. I don't like the dark." To a child, a trip to the radiology department can be a frightening experience. . . .
>
> The physical environment, however, can empower a sensitive care provider to transform a fearful child into a trusting patient. Inside the exam rooms, decorations that are familiar to children may help ease their apprehension. Pictures of animals, cartoon characters or sports teams are excellent examples. Colorful stickers on the X-ray tube and surrounding equipment give children something fun to look at when they lie down on the exam table. Even three-year-old patients can spot whether [or not] a room is designed for children.[3]

In both the women's and the children's areas, recognition of these special patient groups strengthens the facility's image and is usually appreciated by patients.

Flexibility

One of the most challenging aspects of imaging facility design is that of providing flexibility for future changes. During the several years often required for design, documentation, regulatory review, construction, and occupancy of a new facility, both technology and medical practice will have changed considerably. Unfortunately, for this reason it is possible that a new facility could be partially obsolete on opening day if the design does not provide ample flexibility.

Although it is difficult to predict exactly what will change in the near future, it is safe to assume that some change will occur. Imaging facilities can be extremely expensive to modify if flexibility is not integrated into the project from the outset.

Every design solution should enable change to occur in two distinct ways: external expansion and internal conversion. *Expansion* implies both a building that will grow and a site that will accommodate such growth. Structural, mechanical, electrical, and communications systems also must be planned to accommodate such expansion. And in addition to a larger building, the site must be able to expand its parking capabilities and related circulation space. *Conversion* implies a building that will change from within. As with expansion, building systems, department locations, and even room configuration should be planned to maximize flexibility. Both approaches—expansion and conversion—can occur simultaneously. (See figure 8-10.)

In each case, the planning team must first determine which building elements are *fixed,* or *hard,* and which ones are *flexible* or *soft.* (See figure 8-11.) Fixed elements include stairs, elevators, mechanical rooms, and major structural elements. Major nonmovable medical equipment with special structural, electrical, or plumbing connections also is considered fixed. Fixed elements should be arranged so as not to impede future modifications to the facility. In contrast to hard space, offices, lounges, and conference rooms are flexible and can be more easily designed to accommodate future change. Infrastructure systems (electrical, communications, and ventilation systems) must be flexible enough to accommodate change even though many elements of the systems are fixed or permanent.

Figure 8-9. Children's Waiting Area

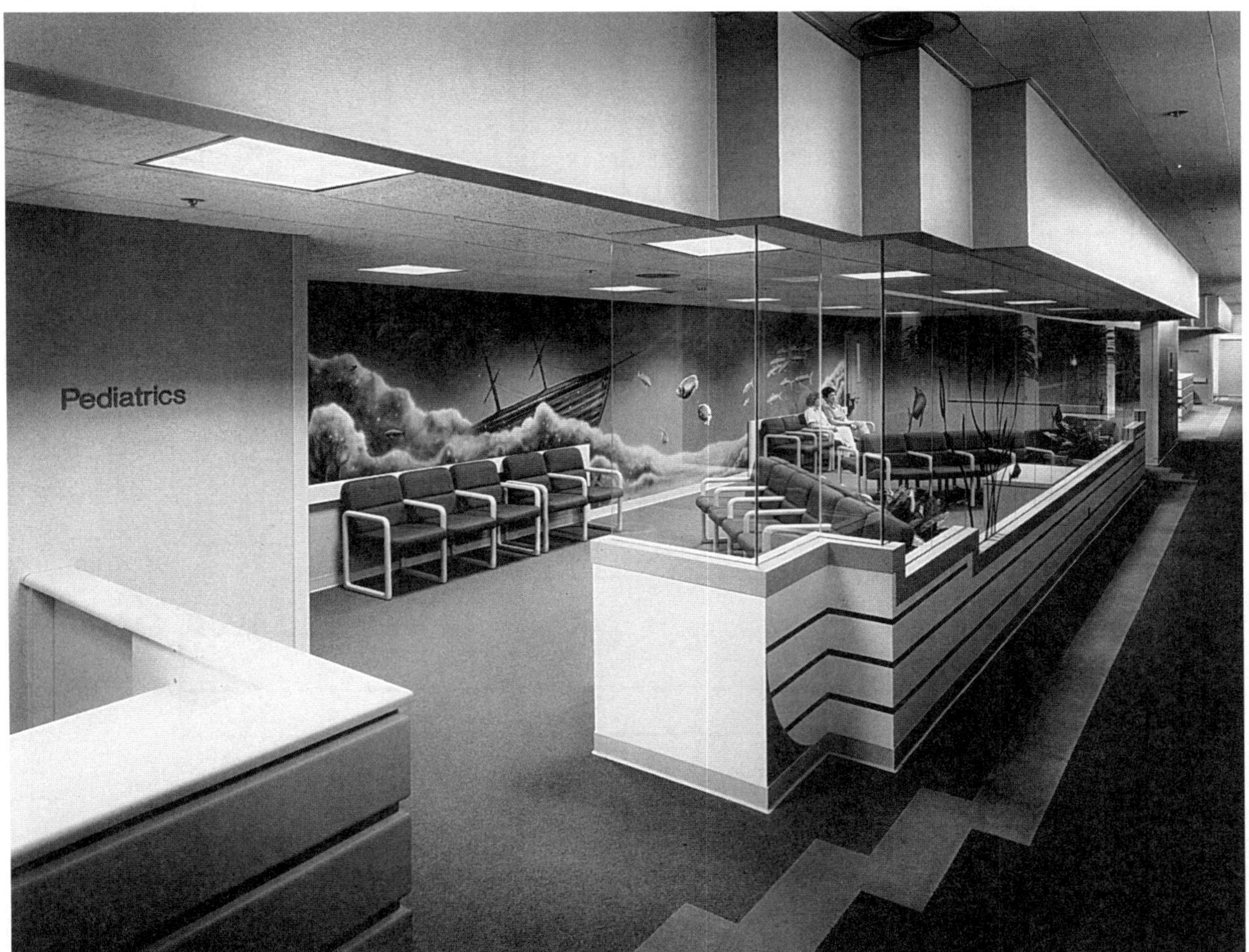

Courtesy of Jain Malkin Inc., La Jolla, California. Photographer: Sandra Williams. Used with permission.

Figure 8-10. Flexibility: Expansion and Conversion

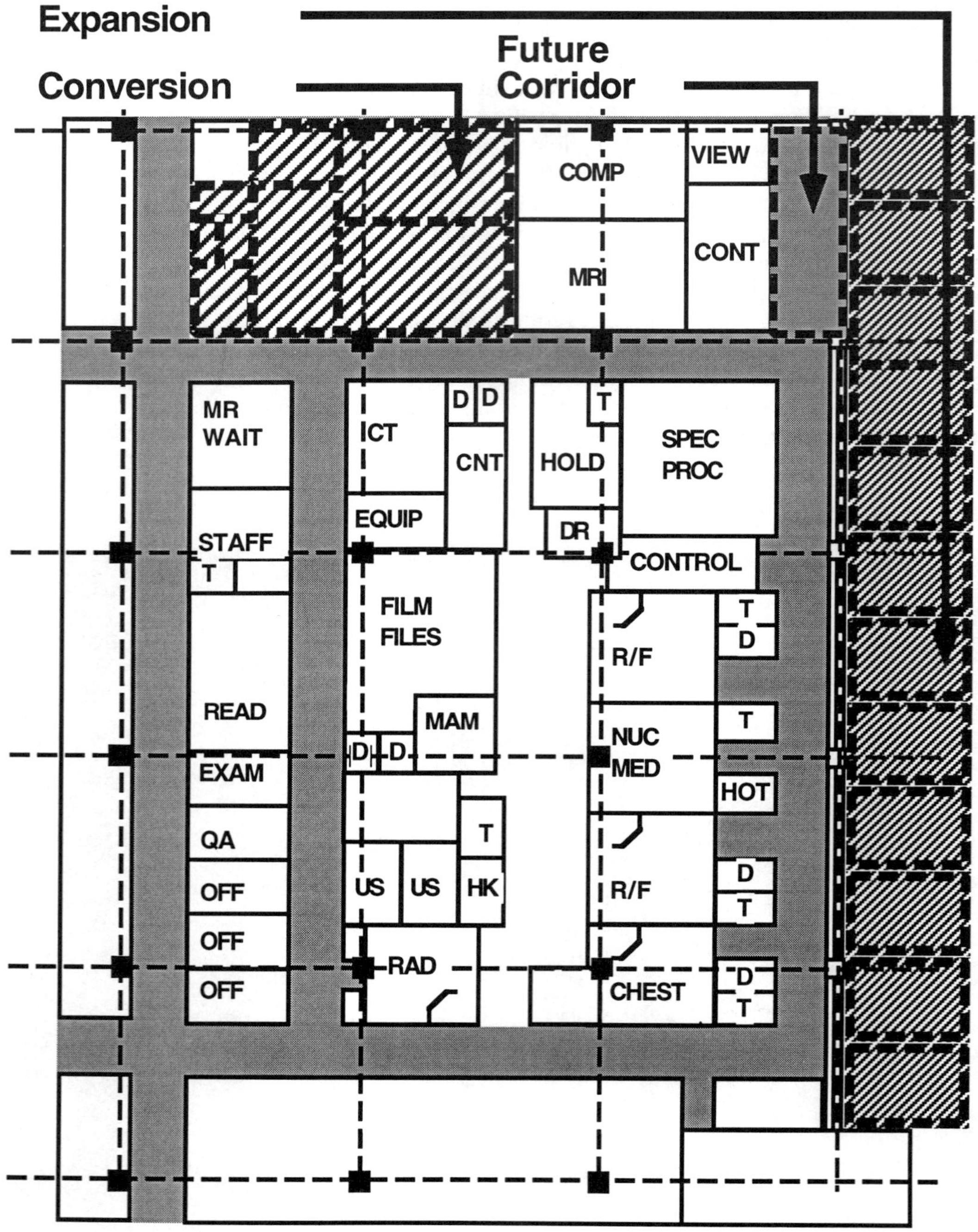

Figure 8-11. Flexibility: Fixed and Flexible Building Elements

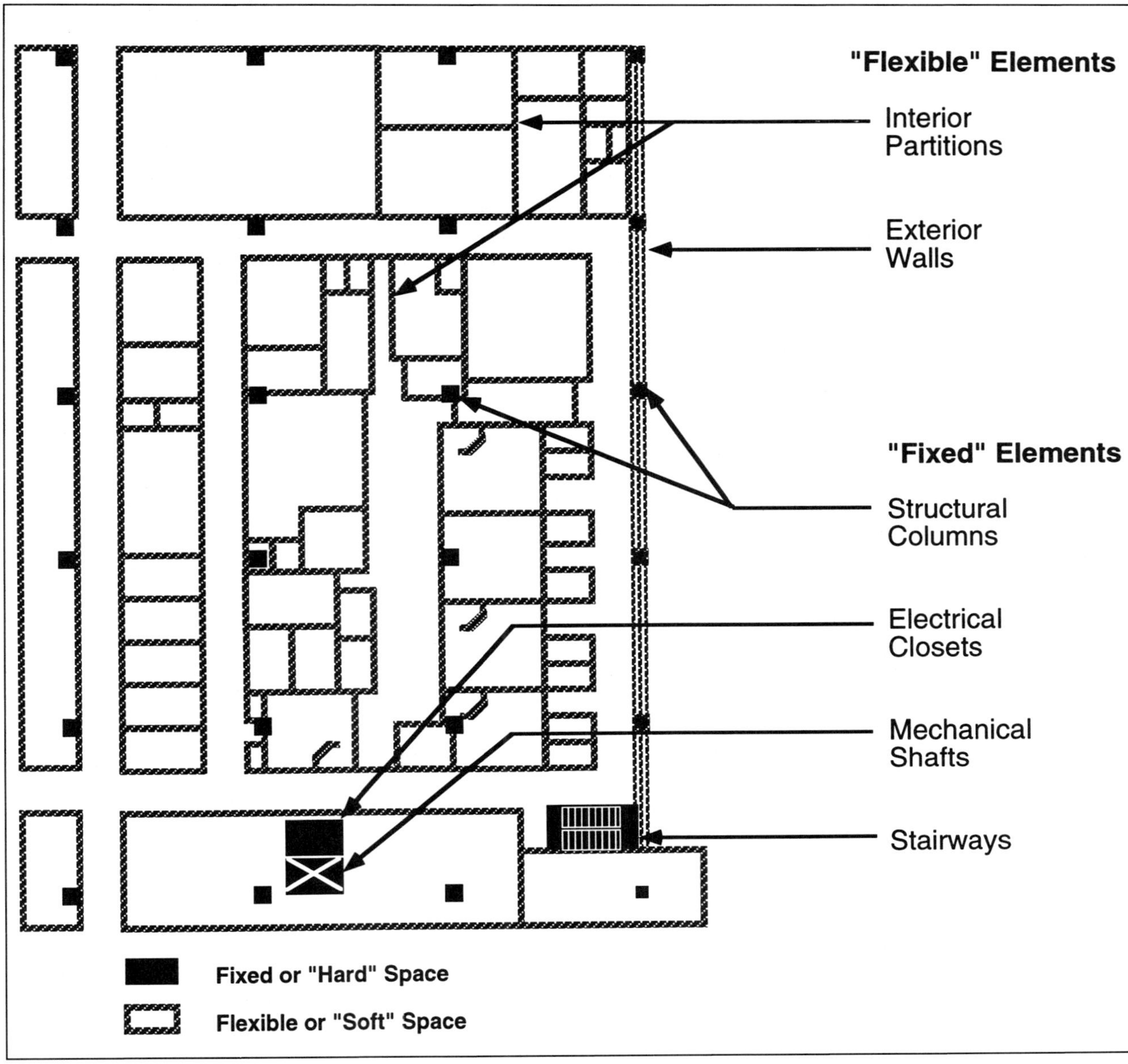

Proactive planning allows future expansion to occur without disrupting existing services. Radiology (and other departments) should be located and designed with a future expansion zone identified at the time the initial construction phase is being planned. Expansion of mechanical and structural systems, as well as extension of exit paths and parking areas, also requires preplanning.

If external expansion opportunities are limited, conversion might be a more appropriate means of accommodating future operational needs. This, too, should be preplanned because conversion requires soft space, such as administrative offices or unfinished shelled spaces, to be modified later to accommodate internal growth.

However, some risk is involved in determining the amount of soft space that must be reserved initially to accommodate future needs. For instance, adequate space must be available to accommodate *functional activity clusters,* or groups of spaces that grow as a functional unit. As an example, the addition of two radiology rooms requires additional dressing areas to be provided and may require additional image processing space. The seating capacity of waiting areas also would need to increase, particularly if the additional procedure rooms are intended for high-volume and short-duration examinations. Converted space that is too small or of the wrong configuration may result in an inefficient use of space. Converted space that is poorly located may result in staffing inefficiencies.

One approach to preplanned conversion involves relocating an entire section of the imaging department when additional space is needed initially. For instance, in some departments, nuclear medicine is combined with radiology. This arrangement can provide expansion opportunities, particularly in small departments. If the two functions are combined initially, it may be feasible to relocate the nuclear medicine component in the future, thus vacating internal space that could be converted for additional radiology functions already within the department boundary.

The Integrated Building System

The integrated building system (IBS) is a specialized planning and construction concept developed to maximize life-cycle, or long-term, flexibility while minimizing both the cost and disruptive nature of equipment and facility changes. Developed initially as part of the Veterans Administration Hospital Building System (VAHBS), the IBS also has been successfully incorporated into many health care facilities that are not part of the VA system. (Note: The Veterans Administration is now known as the Department of Veterans Affairs.)

Objectives of the integrated building system include ease of construction, ease of maintenance, and ease of facility modification. The concept utilizes a series of three-dimensional modules, where each module is organized into three distinct zones: service bay, service zone, functional zone. (See figures 8-12 and 8-13.) Each module is approximately 10,000 departmental gross square feet (DGSF) in size and is self-contained and independent from adjacent modules. The *functional zone* extends from the floor to the ceiling below the interstitial space and is where public circulation and medical treatment occur. The *service zone* is the interstitial space above the functional zone, extending between the ceiling of the functional zone and either the roof or the floor above. This is where mechanical and electrical services are distributed and where maintenance of the utility systems occurs. Each service element—lighting fixtures; power distribution lines; medical gas piping; heating, ventilation, and air-conditioning (HVAC) ductwork; fire protection systems, and so on—has a specific location within the service zone. (See figure 8-14.) The *service bay* is located at the building's perimeter and is as tall as the sum of the functional zones and the service zones together. The service bay houses mechanical and electrical rooms, service shafts, and stairways.

Because the integrated building is divided into modules—each with its own mechanical and electrical system—one module can be modified without disrupting other portions of the building. Changes can be made to building services with little disruption to medical functions, because the functional zone within each module is physically separated from both the service zone and the service bay. Separating functional and service areas provides another important advantage: It allows multiple building trades to work simultaneously. (See figure 8-15, p. 152.) This can shorten the construction schedule, compared to conventional approaches where most building trades work sequentially.

The IBS can provide another measure of flexibility. If each module is designed with long-span structural bays, flexibility in the functional zone will be enhanced because there will be fewer columns to restrict facility layout. The additional depth required for long-span trusses can be incorporated into the interstitial space. Additionally, using the IBS, building components can be mass-produced and repeated from one module to the next, construction schedules are shorter because numerous trades can work simultaneously instead of sequentially (for example, workers can work in the interstitial and functional zones simultaneously), and life-cycle modifications are less expensive.

The fully integrated building system incorporates the following design strategies:[4]

- Service modules range in size from 10,000 to 15,000 DGSF.
- Two-hour-fire-rated walk-on interstitial platforms are located between each service zone and functional zone.

Figure 8-12. Flexibility: Integrated Building System

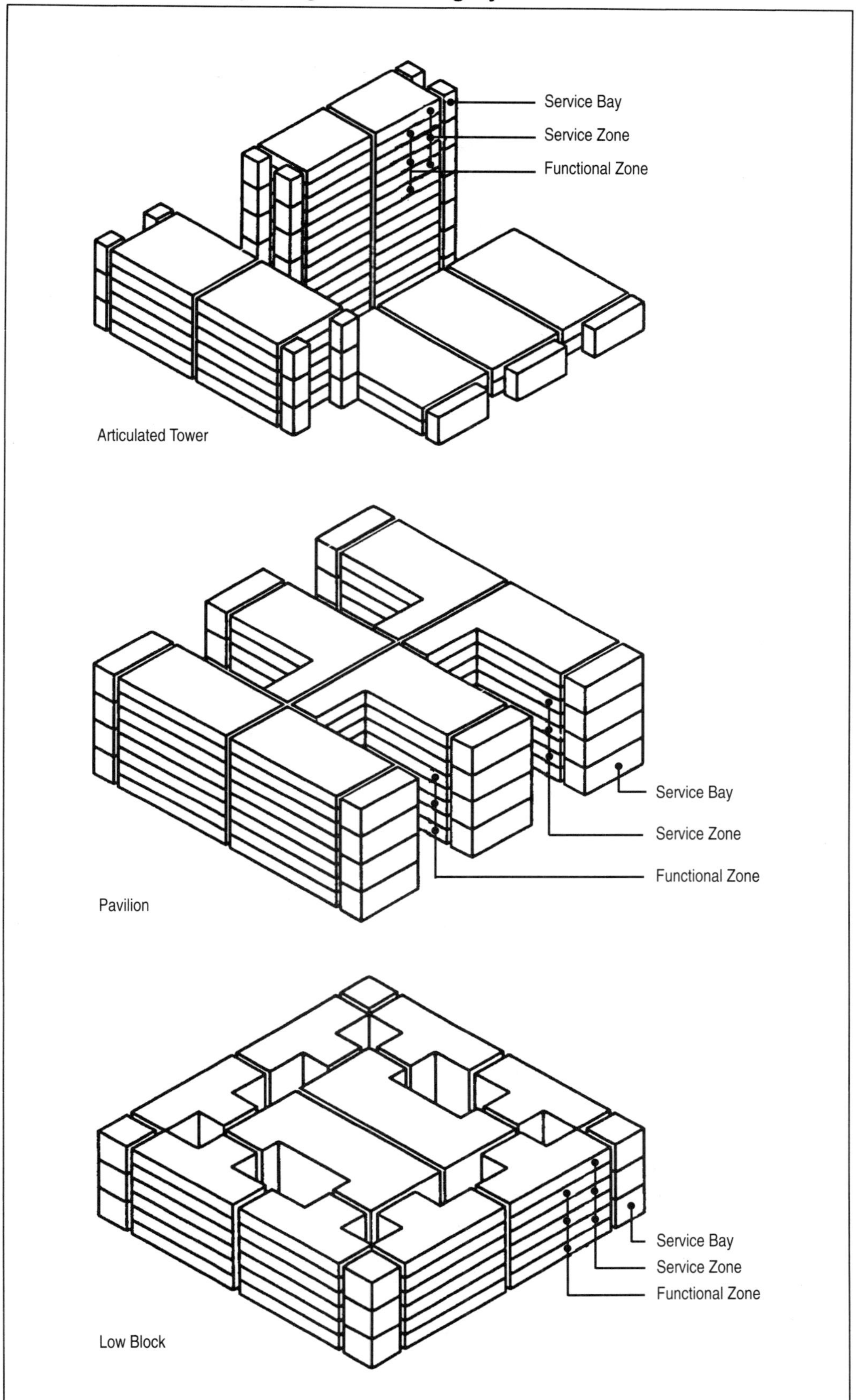

Courtesy of Stone Marraccini Patterson, San Francisco. Used with permission.

Figure 8-13. Section through an IBS Facility

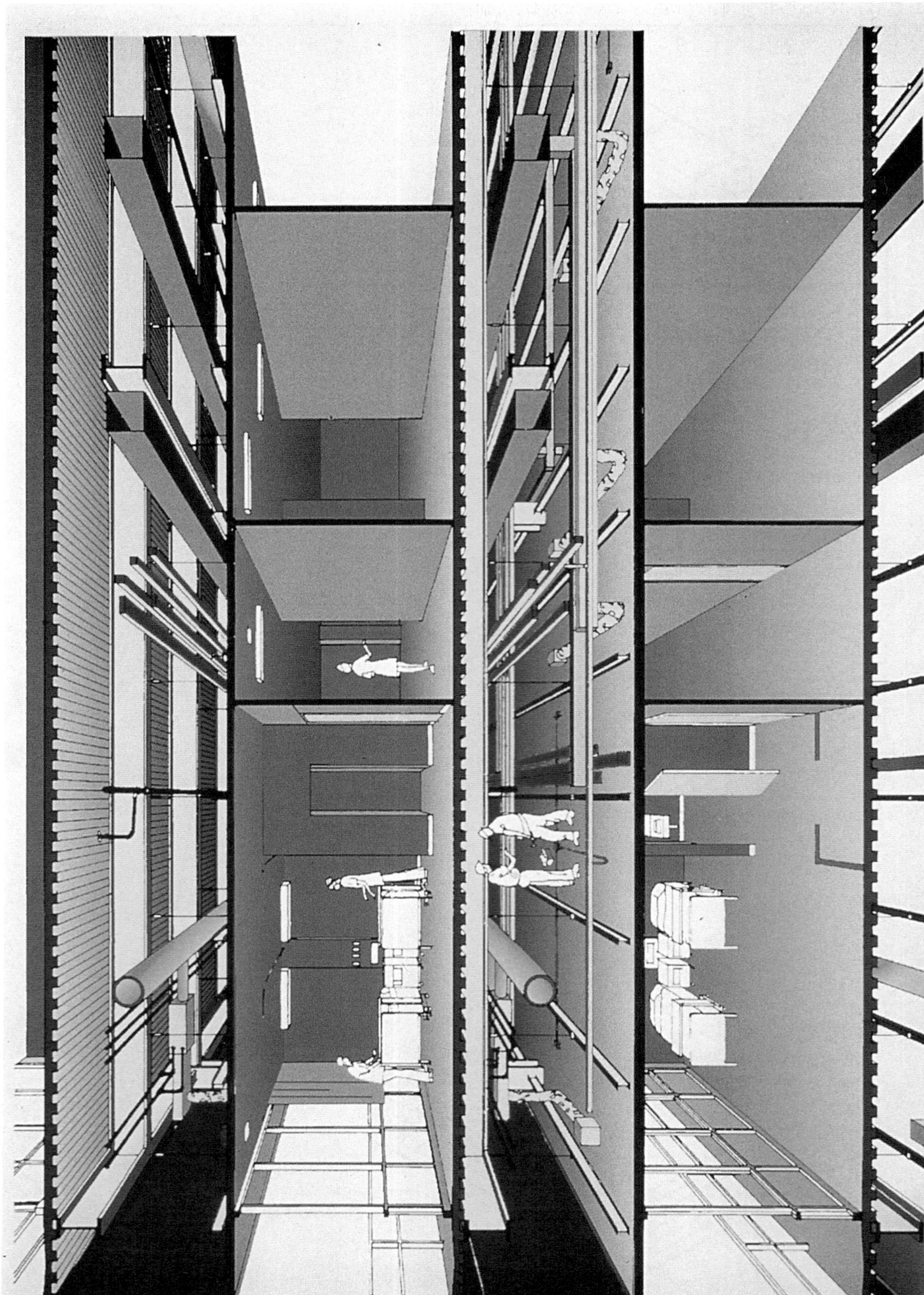

Courtesy of Stone Marraccini Patterson, San Francisco. Used with permission.

Figure 8-14. Section through Interstitial Space Showing Utility Zones

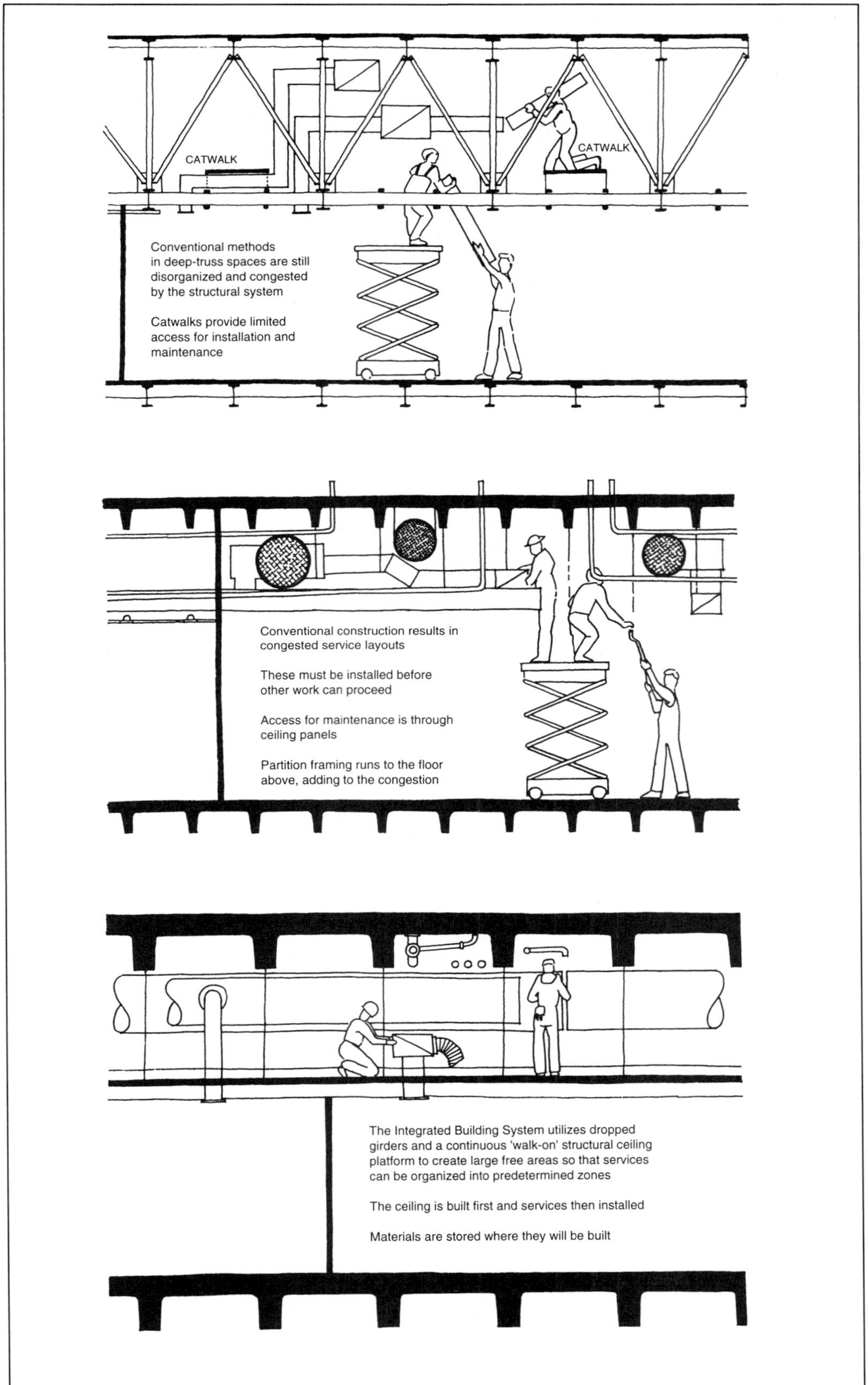

Courtesy of Stone Marraccini Patterson, San Francisco. Used with permission.

Figure 8-15. Sections through Imaging Rooms: Conventional System (top) and Interstitial System (bottom)

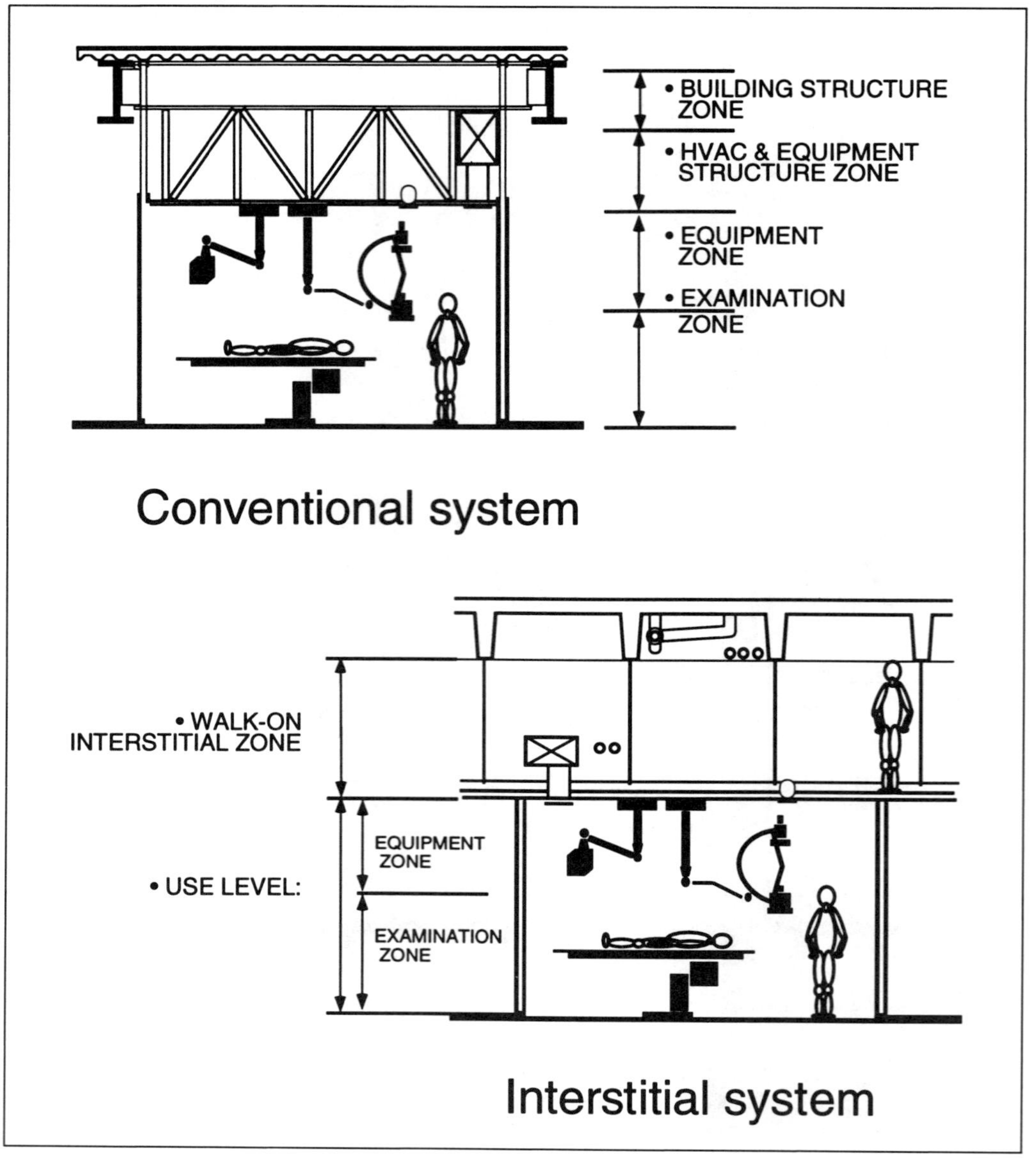

- All building equipment and electrical panels are located in the service bay.
- Access to the service module is from egress stairs.
- Vertical elements such as elevators, stairs, and shafts are located at the boundary of the service modules.
- Required smoke and fire separations are located at service module boundaries.
- All services are fed from the service zone above to the functional zone below (except for gravity-feed systems).
- Repetitive elements are utilized to the extent practical.

In many facilities, a fully integrated building concept is integral to the entire structure. However, alternative hybrid solutions may include interstitial floors without the IBS approach to modular design or interstitial floors only at equipment-intensive locations (such as diagnostic and treatment floors) but not at less-equipment-intensive floors, such as those housing only nursing units. (See figure 8-16.) Hybrid solutions tend to limit the potential for flexibility as compared to the fully integrated building system.

Figure 8-16. Fully Integrated Building System (top), Interstitial System (middle), Hybrid System (bottom)

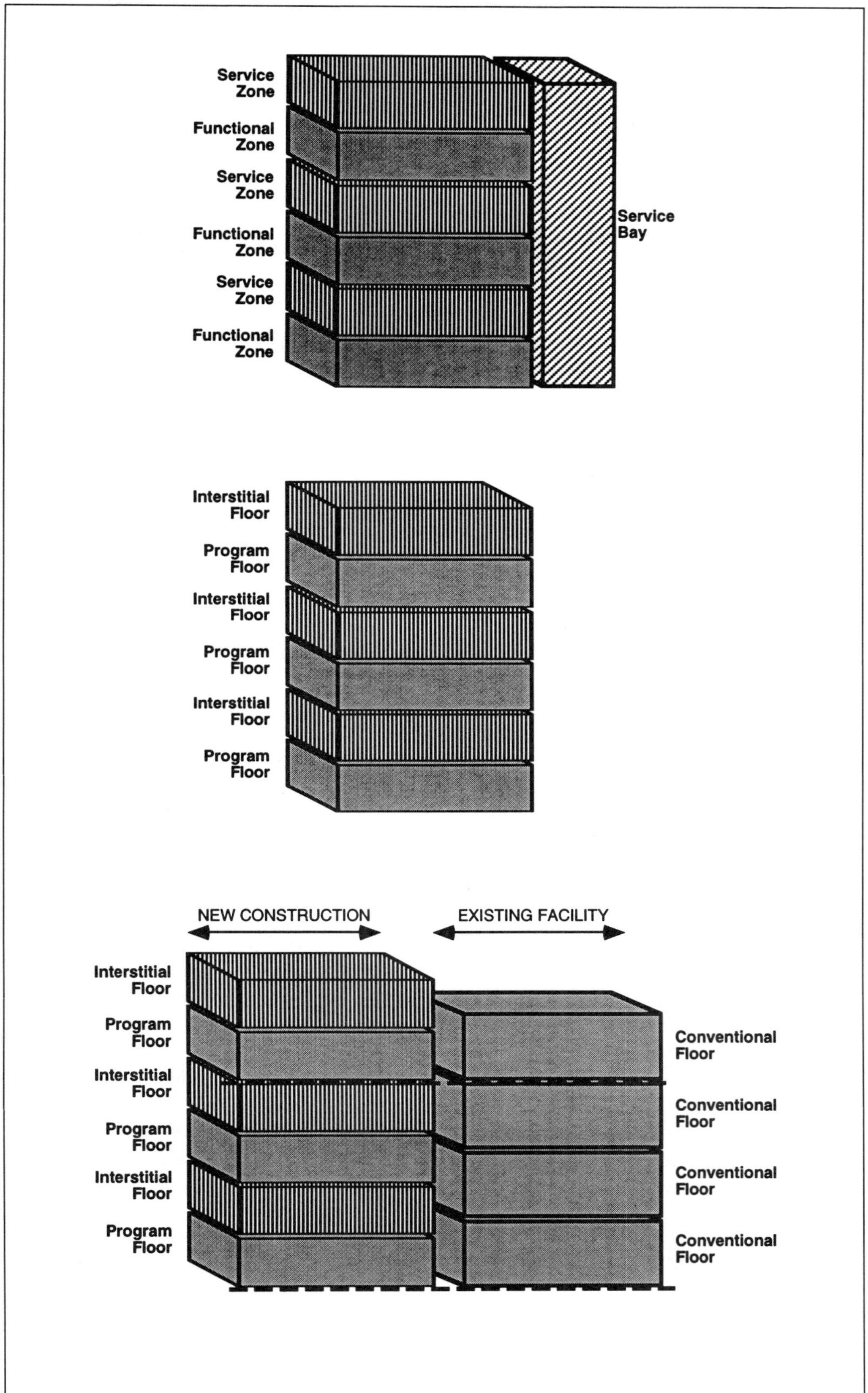

Flexibility for Future Technologies

Preplanning today's buildings to accept tomorrow's technology suggests that department and room design must be flexible enough to accommodate equipment enhancements without necessitating major physical changes to the facility. Three types of technological enhancements are likely: software upgrades, hardware upgrades or replacement, and integration of comprehensive communication systems.

Software Upgrades

Since the advent of computed tomography (CT) following the development of the minicomputer, MRI, some types of ultrasound, and increasingly more general radiography are being digitized. Of those imaging modalities that are still manual and analog, many are becoming more automated. In many instances, software enhancements can extend the usefulness of existing imaging equipment by either increasing its speed or enhancing its diagnostic capabilities. For example, in some instances, enhancements for magnetic resonance angiography (MRA) can add angiographic capability to equipment not initially purchased or designed for that purpose. However, the upgrade may not be as simple to install as some equipment manufacturers claim. In addition, new capabilities often require additional space, for example, for rack cabinets, consoles, and patient holding areas or other support space, as procedural capabilities increase. These extended capabilities may result in additional medical specialties (such as neuroradiology, interventional radiology, and cardiology) using the equipment, thus changing traffic patterns within the department.

> As difficult as it is for manufacturers to design truly upgradable systems and produce coherent upgrades to those systems, that's what hospitals want. By adding features at a relatively low cost, upgrades add to the life span and usefulness of the device while increasing the hospital's ability to survive in the increasingly competitive health care marketplace.
>
> In today's cost conscious budget-slashing atmosphere, it's also much easier to get approval to purchase a few upgrades for the old CT scanner than it is to get the acquisition committee to splurge on a brand new system. Thus, manufacturers who initially underestimated the importance of building upgradable imaging systems are slowly adapting while protesting that their installed devices are, in fact, upgradable.
>
> Like most things that are billed as new and improved, sometimes an upgrade is not really an upgrade. Sometimes it's only half an upgrade, where some of the same components remain but most are new. Sometimes it's not an upgrade at all; it's really a trade-in disguised to look like an upgrade.
>
> A truly upgradable medical device is rare . . . because most upgrades stop short of bringing the original equipment all the way up to the level of the new equipment. Often the original hardware with which the system was built is not sophisticated enough to allow software, network or operating system upgrades to do all the advanced new things that they are capable of doing.
>
> What that means for unwary hospitals is that last year's brand new system may be technically obsolete in one year. If last year's model, now obsolete, can't be upgraded to do the same thing, it leaves them at a competitive disadvantage. Those upgrades that do bring a system up to the same level as a new system generally require more than just an upgrade. Often new hardware or peripherals are needed.[5]

One provision that might simplify accommodation of software upgrades and computerized diagnostic equipment maintenance is the addition of dedicated telephone and modem lines that connect the equipment, via telephone cable, to the equipment vendor. In this way, both computer diagnostics and upgrading of software are accomplished from a remote location. This is becoming common for MRI and CT scanners. Equipment can be monitored periodically, and service engineers can be made aware of inadequate performance before equipment failure or image degradation occurs.

Hardware Upgrades or Replacement

Replacing outdated imaging equipment is more complicated than upgrading software. To simplify this eventuality, *universal room design,* a strategy that results in a generic room layout for certain procedure room types, should be employed where appropriate. (For further discussion, see the section entitled Universal Room Design in chapter 13, "Room Design.") In addition, procedures rooms and computer equipment rooms should be designed in excess of their minimum acceptable dimensions. This "loose-fit" approach provides reserve capacity in terms of space to accommodate both future equipment and still-undeveloped procedures. However, planners should be careful not to provide too much space. A room that is too large for its function is not only unnecessarily expensive, but also may be functionally inefficient if equipment and supplies are not easily within reach when needed.

Electrical and HVAC reserve capacity also is important. However, the mechanical engineer must be careful not to provide so much reserve air-handling capacity that it will become difficult to control humidity. Some consultants suggest providing a minimum of 20 percent reserve capacity for HVAC systems and 50 to 100 percent reserve capacity for electrical systems.

Finally, accommodations for removing or replacing large, heavy equipment (some of which can be broken down into smaller components) need to be considered. The building's structural capacity, as well as doorway and corridor clearances, must be able to accommodate this equipment along an entire route connecting the room where the equipment is housed to the location outside the building where it will be placed onto or removed from a truck or trailer. Potential obstacles along this route should be anticipated and eliminated during detailed planning. For example, if a doorway is too narrow or too low, the door and frame may have to be removed. (It is not uncommon for a door and door frame to have to be removed in order to bring an alternator into a room because the frame is too low.) If corridors are not designed for the weight of the equipment, temporary load-bearing supports may need to be added before the equipment is delivered. Before design solutions are finalized, it is advisable to review maintenance and access requirements with equipment vendors and installers. Each vendor should be walked through building plans and sections in order to identify a preferred access route and verify that each specific piece of equipment can, in fact, be installed or removed.

Comprehensive Communication Systems

The one component of imaging most likely to have the greatest impact on facility design in the future is the refinement of electronic image management and communication systems (IMACSs). IMACSs will affect the architecture of imaging in two distinct ways. First, many traffic and adjacency requirements between those spaces that presently rely on manual transmission of images and written information will disappear, as electronic transmission takes over.

> . . . the impact [of totally digital imaging] on imaging department design could be enormous. Imaging departments of the future will be quite different than they are today. For example, most of the traffic in a film-based imaging department is generated by the movement of images, information, patients, and staff and has traditionally been a major factor influencing the design of imaging departments.
>
> A comparison of routine traffic in a film-based imaging department with [that of] a totally digital department reveals significant changes in traffic patterns. . . . In a totally digital imaging department, digital images replace film and the radiology information system (RIS) replaces much of the paper flow. Images are [permanently] stored on laser disk rather than on film. Cables carry images and data throughout the imaging department and the key locations in the hospital or clinic.[6]

In the future, the physical adjacency of imaging professionals working together will be a less-stringent requirement as comprehensive networks of fiber-optic cable and allied network transmission and receiving stations further link remote sites to others across campus, throughout the community, and even around the world.

Second, space requirements will change. At first, space requirements will increase because space will be needed for both electronic "filmless" and traditional film-based image management systems. This requirement to house both automated and manual information systems will continue until electronic image management becomes more fully integrated into routine health care delivery practice. Once picture archiving and communications systems (PACSs), hospital information systems (HISs), and radiology information systems (RISs) become fully integrated, it is likely that the size of individual "electronic" workstations will be smaller than their "manual" counterparts. (For example, large film alternators will be superseded by small PACS clusters interconnected by various types of networks.) However, it is just as likely that more workstations will be in use by that time, possibly offsetting any overall reduction in the need for space. (For further discussion on designing the physical environment for computer workstations, see the section entitled General Considerations for Computer Workstation Environments in chapter 13, "Room Design.")

Eventually, the amount of space required for storage of hard-copy images may decrease, but this will take some time. The electronic storage of images and information will enable a greater volume of data to be stored in less space, but as most other professions have already experienced, computer-generated information tends to disseminate more printed material rather than less. Additionally, the amount of electronic data that must be stored is increasing at an astronomical rate. This is particularly so for procedures where multiple images compose an examination. For example, CT and MRI may generate hundreds of images of a given anatomical region. How these images will be generated, viewed, and stored in the future is still a challenge, because the standard unit of measure has rapidly evolved from megabytes to gigabytes to terabytes of data.

Although it may be difficult today to anticipate all the forms that an imaging department might take in the future, it is both possible and necessary to plan now for the anticipated integration of electronic information management. The installation of empty conduit or accessible ceiling space throughout imaging areas and at other strategic locations (between the imaging department[s] and other departments, such as intensive care, emergency, medical records, and registration, for example), as well as the provision of communications closets throughout the facility, will allow wires or cable to be installed in the future without demolishing existing walls and ceilings. In addition, locations for future computer-based workstations throughout the facility can be predetermined to ensure that space will be available for that function when needed.

Technology Docks

Another approach to adaptable facility design involves planning for relocatable, mobile, or "plug-in" imaging environments. For example, a technology dock—a simple structure that connects a mobile trailer or building module to the main facility—can be built to facilitate mobile technology that enables multiple users to share expensive equipment for providing special imaging services. The technology dock affords a unique measure of flexibility because it provides a means of housing short-lived technologies, or those in the midst of development, without the same capital investment required of permanent structures. (See the section entitled Technology Docks in chapter 14, "Imaging outside the Radiology Department.")

Economy

The cost of health care is escalating at an astonishing pace. In recent years, construction costs also have been on the rise. At the same time, medical reimbursement rates are shrinking. Among all health care services, imaging involves some of the most expensive construction because of its extensive structural, electrical, and mechanical requirements. With multimillion-dollar imaging equipment, expensive facilities, and diminishing reimbursement, imaging facility design and construction must be efficient as well as functional. Yet, in spite of the expense of equipment, staff labor costs can exceed the value of capital equipment purchases. In fact, facility construction and equipment acquisition costs represent only a small fraction of the cost of health care salaries and operating expenses.

Therefore, the economic value derived from facility design must be measured in two ways simultaneously: the initial cost of space and the recurring value of space. The *initial cost of space* includes the price of construction, furniture, and equipment as well as associated costs for professional fees, land acquisition, and financing. These costs are generated only once, although they may be paid in increments throughout the facility's functional life span.

The *recurring value of space* is measured by the ratio of the value of medical services provided in a space relative to the combined recurring costs for staffing, utilities, and maintenance associated with that space. Maintenance costs include cleaning, repairing, and replacing construction components, finish materials, and equipment.

The initial cost of space is directly influenced by *plan efficiency* as well as the quality of construction components and finish materials. The recurring value of space is influenced by a multitude of variables that affect operations and work flow.

Initial construction cost, which usually is the simplest of the cost indicators to quantify, often is the one most closely analyzed. However, initial construction cost should not be the sole determinant of economy; operational and staffing costs and the ability to provide services efficiently have a greater financial impact than does initial construction cost. For example, an inexpensive heating and air-conditioning system might lower the cost of construction, but that saving could be negligible compared to increased heating and cooling bills or the need to replace the system in the near future. Equipment downtime and the associated lost revenues due to HVAC failure are significant expenses. Poor planning that causes inefficient staffing or an unpleasant working environment also adds a financial burden for the life of the facility.

Plan Efficiency

Facility size directly influences construction cost. The overall building size relative to the number and size of individual rooms programmed into the building indicates how compact the layout is. While floor plans are being developed, a plan efficiency ratio can be easily determined. (See figure 8-17.) The efficiency ratio identifies the amount of net assignable area relative to departmental gross area. *Net assignable area* is equal to the sum of all the functional spaces required to serve the basic program.[7] This includes procedure rooms, dressing rooms, waiting areas, utility rooms, offices, and so on. Excluded from net assignable area are spaces such as departmental corridors, structural columns, walls, and partitions. These spaces usually are considered net unassignable area and are accounted for in the net-to-departmental gross multiplier. Rooms housing equipment required for imaging procedures, such as X-ray transformers and computer rooms, are considered part of net assignable area, whereas rooms housing equipment serving the entire building, such as hospital telecommunication devices, are not considered net assignable area. *Departmental gross area* is equal to the sum of net assignable area and net unassignable area. *Building gross area,* in turn, is equal to departmental gross area plus stairs, elevators, nondepartmental exit corridors, mechanical rooms, electrical closets, shafts, and the thickness of exterior walls. (See figure 4-1 in chapter 4, "Management of the Process.")

Plan efficiency is expressed as a percentage and can be defined as net assignable area divided by departmental gross area. The higher the number, the more efficient the plan is in terms of the amount of usable space it provides relative to the amount of overall space it occupies. Thus, a hospital radiology department that has a plan efficiency of 62 to 67 percent (or greater) is generally considered to have an efficient layout. However, the term *plan efficiency* can be a little misleading, because a plan that is too compact may provide inadequate circulation space or be uncomfortable to work in. Plan efficiency is not necessarily an indicator of flexibility or operational efficiency and thus should not be the sole economic criterion for planning. In fact, a tendency to pack too much functional space into a small, compact area usually will decrease operational efficiency. Another tendency is to program functional spaces, such as imaging procedure rooms, at their minimum—or even below

Figure 8-17. Plan Efficiency (Diagram and Formula)

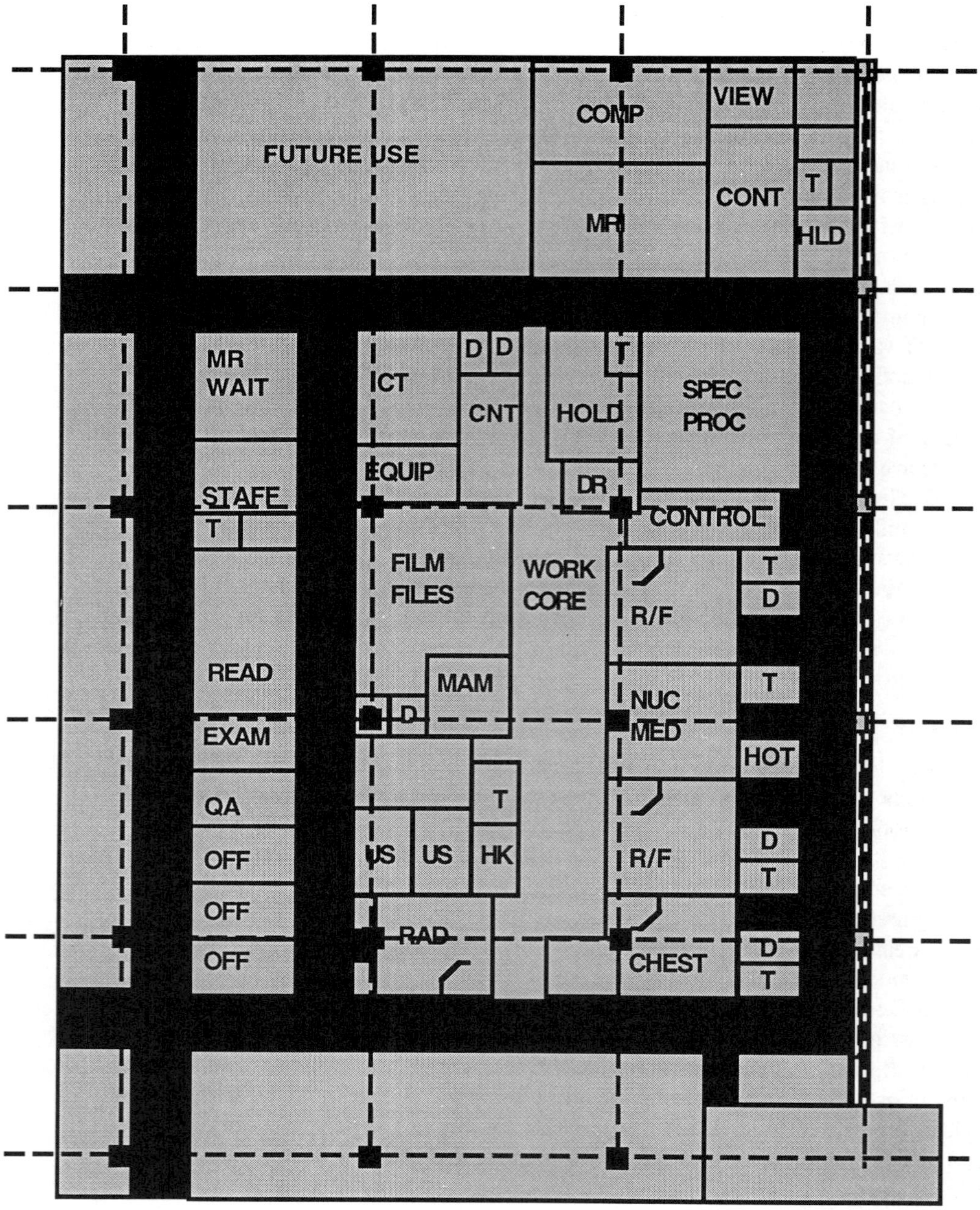

Assigned space

Unassigned space

Plan Efficiency:
= Assigned Space ÷ Total Departmental Area
= 7,282 NSF ÷ 11,060 DGSF
= 66%

Note: Shaded areas represent unassigned space.

minimum—dimensions. This results in a small gross area but can severely limit the types of procedures that may be accommodated in the room. This limitation may be compounded in the future as more complex procedures requiring additional equipment and personnel are performed.

Another way to measure plan efficiency is to analyze the program and plans in terms of their revenue-generating potential. Each room can be classified as either *activity space, support space,* or *administration space.* (See figure 8-18.) The number of activity spaces, such as examination and procedure rooms, is directly related to workload and thus the revenue-generating capacity of the facility. Support and administration space, such as offices, waiting areas, and image-processing areas, contribute indirectly to workload and revenue-generating capacity. (The terms *revenue-generating* and *non-revenue-generating* came into use when the health care payment system was based on fee for service. However, even under capitated arrangements, the number of activity spaces relates to the amount of work that can be performed; therefore, the amount of space is still related to cash flow in capitated systems.)

The proper amount of support and administration space enables each activity space to operate to its maximum potential. For example, if there are not enough dressing rooms for each radiography room, patient throughput will be limited and so will cash flow. However, if too many dressing rooms are constructed, they will not be fully utilized and initial construction costs will be higher than necessary.

By labeling activity space with one color or tone and support and administration space with another, a pattern will emerge indicating both revenue-generating and non-revenue-generating space. This graphic comparison of space allocation illustrates the relative cash flow of a facility as determined by the ratio of revenue-generating spaces versus non-revenue-generating spaces. (See figure 8-19.) However, it should be kept in mind that at many facilities basic imaging procedures represent a high volume of moderate-cost workload, whereas special imaging procedures generate a lower volume, with each procedure involving a significantly higher cost.

It is essential that space programming be complete and the final space program be reviewed, approved, and signed by both administration and all departmental user groups before schematic design begins. If, for some reason, the net assignable area in the program changes during schematic design, the projected departmental gross area should be modified accordingly, because it has significant budget implications. Too often, there is a tendency to add net program area during schematic design without increasing the gross area because there is no contingency in the budget for the additional space. This results in undersized rooms, insufficient support space, and storage areas that are likely to end up being used as offices. Attempts to increase net area without also increasing gross area will result in operational inefficiencies in one form or another. Area increases without corresponding budget increases will similarly create significant obstacles to effectively managing the project.

References

1. Carpman, J. R., Grant, M. A., and Simmons, D. A. *Design That Cares: Planning Health Facilities for Patients and Visitors.* 1st ed. Chicago: American Hospital Publishing, 1986, pp. 58–59. [A second edition of this book was published in 1993.]
2. Depies, M., Balint, S., Guell, M., McGovern, J., and Towle, C. MRI anxiety. *Administrative Radiology,* July 1991, pp. 43–48.
3. Greer, K. A. Pointers to transforming the frightened child into a trusting patient. *Advance for Radiologic Science Professionals* 5:16, Apr. 20, 1992.
4. Stone Marraccini Patterson. Internal report. San Francisco: SMP, 1992.
5. Curran, C. Equipment upgrades: linking old to new. *Second Source Imaging,* Oct. 4, 1992, pp. 37–42.
6. Brovold, R. Bridging the film digital gap. *Administrative Radiology* 7:57–61, Nov. 1991.
7. Pena, W. *Problem Seeking: An Architectural Programming Primer.* Houston: Cahners Books International, 1977, p. 108.

Figure 8-18. Space Types: Activity, Support, and Administration

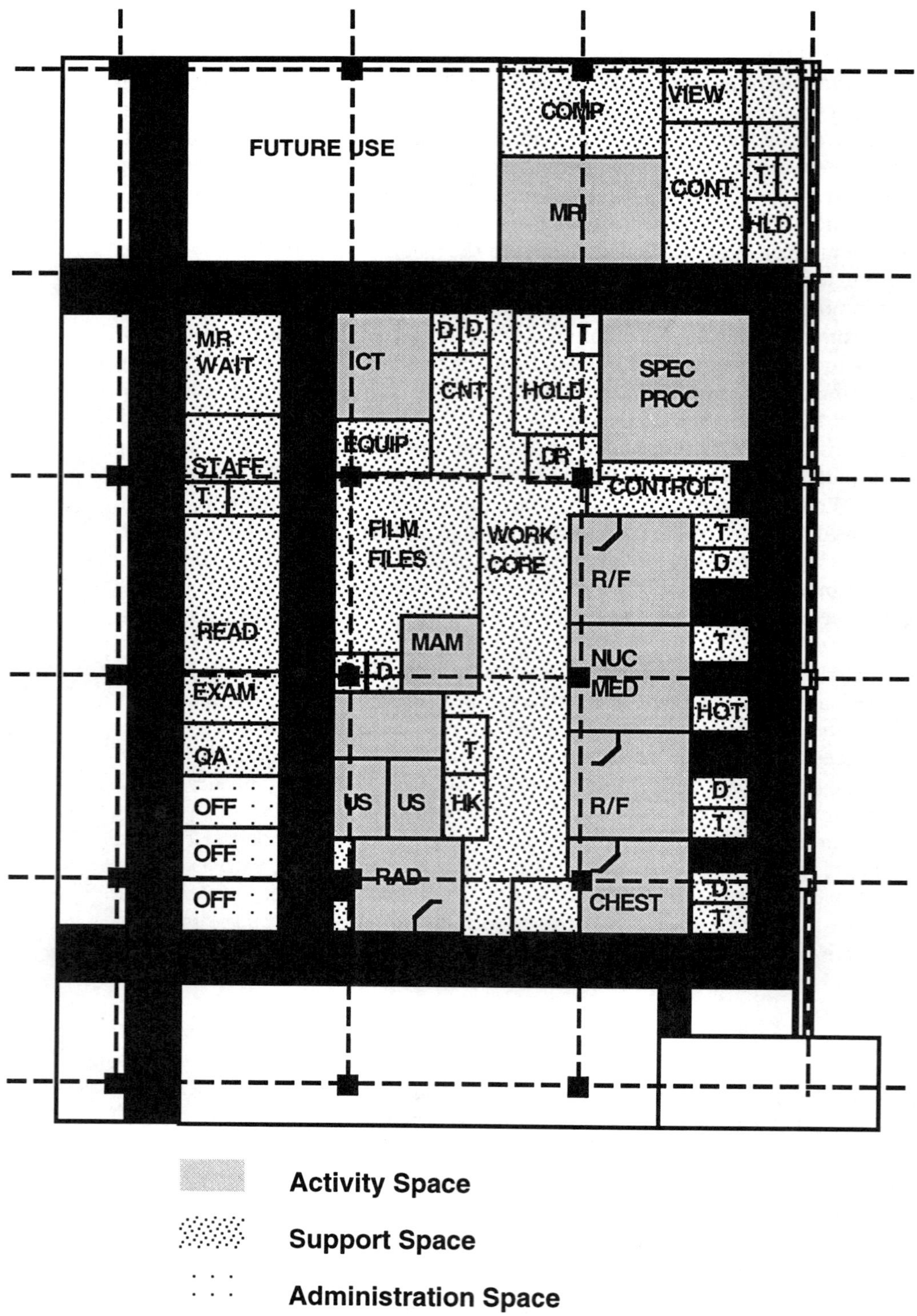

Courtesy of Stone Marraccini Patterson, San Francisco. Used with permission.

Figure 8-19. Graphic Comparison of Space Allocation

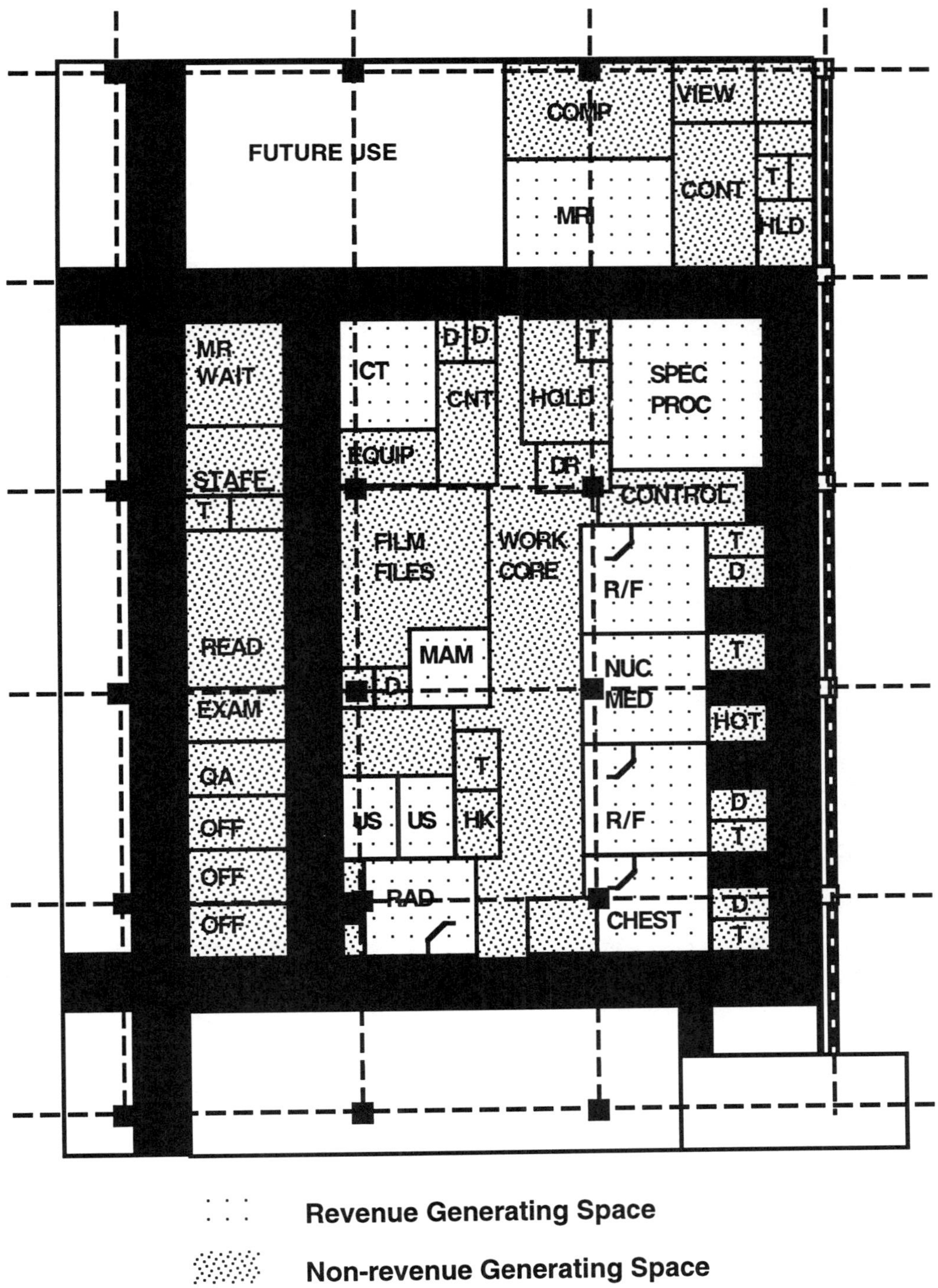

Chapter 9

Site Design

Site design and building design are integrally related. There is no question that inadequate site design can compromise an otherwise successful building. Thus, the optimal size and configuration of structures to be built on the site cannot be determined without first evaluating its characteristics, all of which can affect the project's accessibility, adaptability, and economics. Those characteristics include any legal or physical restrictions that must be taken into account. For example, a sloped site might suggest a service entrance at the lowest floor and a public entrance at the next-higher level, providing grade-level access to both entrances. Additionally, zoning restrictions must be considered. For example, local zoning laws may prohibit a tall building on one site but not on another. Finally, to be successful in the long term, site design should consider both initial and future construction phases.

This chapter discusses two aspects of site design: site selection and site analysis. *Site selection* involves issues such as the location's accessibility; the land's usability and configuration potential; any existing legal, physical, and zoning restrictions; and the possible impact on the environment of the facility and its activities. *Site analysis* begins as part of the site selection process and then is integrated into the initial design process.

Site Selection

A variety of issues should be considered before arriving at final site selection.[1] A comprehensive examination of related concerns is found in the book entitled *Site Selection for Health Care Facilities,* written by Lifton and Hardy.[2]

Because the perfect site may not exist or be available, a few best choices should be identified and compared to one another. In this way, the relative strengths and weaknesses of each can be analyzed and a sensible selection made.

Although certain site-related issues might be more important for one project than for others, the most important issues affecting site selection usually are those relating to location, accessibility, and development potential of the site. The following list includes some of the key issues discussed in *Site Selection for Health Care Facilities.*

Proximity to Patients and Referring Providers

Any service facility should be located near the people who use it. Of course, for certain specialized services, it is likely that some patients will travel some distance for their care and treatment. Because imaging services usually are the result of referrals from primary or other health care providers, the distance between the imaging facility and referring physicians must be considered. Similarly, the location of other facilities providing similar services can have an impact on the success of a new facility.

The first step in assessing a site's location is to project who the potential users of the facility are, where they live and work, who the referring providers are and where they are located, and what the nature of referral patterns is expected to be. The proximity of alternative sites to these potential users and referring providers should then be measured in terms of both mileage and time, taking into account existing roadways and traffic patterns. Projections should be made based on future as well as existing conditions. A site on the outer fringes of a current target area might be in its center in five years if growth trends are in that direction.

Both hospital-based and freestanding imaging centers are likely to be part of a large health care network or managed care consortium. Therefore, medical images and other data will need to be accessed by many health care professionals.

Teleradiology—a method of transmitting images to remote sites—is becoming a viable and important approach to transferring such medical data and picture images between distant sites. Also, as managed care goals for cost containment limit the activities of many medical specialists, teleradiology may provide a cost-effective means for radiologists to extend their expertise to many primary and emergency care providers throughout a given region. (Teleradiology is described further in chapter 7, "Image Management and Film Processing.") Although electronic information management and communications systems utilizing fiber-optic or satellite data networks will be able to link remote sites, it is necessary that each facility utilize compatible software and hardware components.

Major Road Access

A well-designed building is of little use if it is not easily accessible. Even a building that is well located within its projected market area must be easily accessible by private car, on foot, or by mass transit. Furthermore, these routes should be convenient for both staff and patients. A slow and indirect route or one with constant traffic congestion is tedious. "Generally the ideal is for a [facility] to be close enough to a major highway that access to the general area of the site is easy from all directions, yet not so close to the road that noise and congestion result."[3]

Accessibility by Public Transportation

The importance of access by public transportation depends on the general location of the site (urban versus rural) and the degree to which public transportation already exists. If the quality of the existing public transportation network in the region is marginal or if the network is not heavily used, accessibility by public transportation is less important than it would be in an area where people rely more on this type of transportation. In general, however, the more easily individuals can reach the site without assistance or having to drive themselves, the more accessible the facility will be.

In addition to being convenient for patients, public transportation should be considered an amenity for staff. Both existing and future public transportation routes should be examined, and the possibility of requesting that they be altered might be considered for large projects. If the new imaging facility is part of a larger building and is associated with other health care facilities as part of a managed care network, an independent shuttle system may be beneficial if there is enough demand for transportation between remote sites. Such a system could be particularly beneficial for connecting a hospital-sponsored satellite imaging facility with an affiliated hospital.

Direct Access

Depending on the nature of the imaging facility, a variety of transportation routes within the site may be required—for example, emergency, nonemergency, patient, service, and staff. If a technology dock for mobile imaging units is to be provided, additional site circulation routes may be necessary. (See the section entitled Technology Docks in chapter 14, "Imaging outside the Radiology Department.")

All circulation routes should be clearly visible from the street and coordinated so that they do not conflict with one another. It also is important that on-site traffic congestion and peak parking loads be anticipated. Provisions should be made to ensure that these peak loads do not complicate off-site circulation.

A site with streets on many sides will likely enable adequate segregation of traffic, making it easy for special routes, such as those used primarily for patient arrival, to be directed to specific areas on the site without interrupting other routes, such as those reserved for staff circulation. "The ideal situation is to have three sides of a site on existing streets or roads, allowing easy access to the site once vehicles have reached the general area."[4] It should be assumed that many users of the facility are already under stress and do not need the further aggravation of having to decipher a cryptic transportation network.

Size and Usable Area

The actual size of a site is not necessarily an accurate indicator of the amount of area that is usable. In determining the amount of usable land needed, building configuration, parking, and circulation patterns must be considered. Local building codes often require building setbacks and may further restrict the usable area, including parking and circulation layouts.

Consideration also should be given to the need for expansion, as the site might be of adequate size for present needs but not for future growth. "A contingency allowance of 30 percent [for expansion] has been suggested by some authorities, although no data have been collected on whether or not this is an appropriate allowance. Some provision for the future, regardless of whether or not it is arbitrary, is important."[5]

Configuration and Orientation

In addition to size, the geometry and configuration of a parcel of land can determine its relative usable area. For example, a long, narrow parcel might not have the depth required to lay out buildings, parking, and circulation efficiently, whereas a smaller but more regular parcel would. The site configuration should accommodate the greatest amount of design freedom—building configuration, location within the site, circulation, and parking arrangements. Although a square or slightly rectangular geometry is most likely to allow such freedom of design, other configurations can be considered. However, sites with gross irregularities or unusual topography may present unnecessary design constraints.

The following questions pertaining to site geometry should be considered:

- What is the geometry relative to the street frontage? (For example, does the site's long or short dimension face the street?)
- Does it allow for easy access and egress?
- Does it allow for separate public and service access?
- Does it allow for individual parking clusters along the perimeter of the building or for only one central parking lot?
- Can convenient circulation routes be arranged around and through the site without disturbing the building depth and/or configuration?

Zoning

Most municipalities have zoning requirements based on land use. Local codes should be reviewed to see if any restrictions exist. If they do, it sometimes is possible to have land rezoned or to obtain a *conditional use permit,* although this often is a lengthy and costly process.

Some zoning ordinances specify required setbacks and restrict the size, height, and type of building. Most codes specify required parking areas and loading zones, often on the basis of a building's occupancy classification. Before design begins, a thorough investigation and interpretation of applicable codes and ordinances must be completed. The existing zoning of adjacent sites also should be examined. For example, will neighbors be compatible in terms of noise, character, appearance, and traffic?

Legal and Physical Restrictions

Once the site has been evaluated in terms of configuration and orientation, it must be examined more closely to see whether any legal or physical restrictions will adversely affect its development potential. Legal restrictions may be in the form of easements, covenants, trust agreements, or previous subdivision rules. They may restrict the location of construction on the site, the type of use, or the size or height of a building. Easements usually can be identified by contacting the relevant utility company, reviewing the site survey (if one exists), and/or examining the existing title to the property. This is the time to enlist the help of architectural, engineering, and legal consultants.[6]

Restrictions also may be the result of physical conditions. Hills, swamps, and rivers are easily detected, but floodplains, inadequate bearing soil, and contaminated groundwater are less obvious. These conditions all require further professional investigation.

Although it is common for a site to have some restrictions, each restriction's effect will be determined by its specific nature and location. For example, a utility easement prohibiting any construction within the restriction's limits may be easily worked around if the restriction runs along a minor property line. However, a similar restriction running through the center of the property may virtually split the site in two and seriously hinder cost-effective site development.

Legal and physical restrictions that limit the site's development potential should be assigned priorities and separated into those conditions that can be worked around and those that cannot. The cost of such adjustments must then be added to the cost of the site.

Environmental Impact

Regardless of whether an environmental impact report (EIR) is required, the degree to which the new facility affects the existing community and landscape needs to be addressed. Both the building itself and its related structures and noisy activities (for example, roads, pathways, sewage disposal, and traffic) should be considered. If the facility is to be considered a beneficial element by the community, its appearance also should be of concern to the planning team. (See chapter 8, "Design Concepts.")

Neighborhood organizations in opposition to a development project can add considerable delays and expense to the regulatory review process. Such delays can even require a project to be abandoned. When possible, neighborhood groups should be approached as allies, not adversaries.

Waste disposal is of special concern for imaging projects. The manner in which film-processing chemicals, radioactive substances, and medical supplies are disposed of must conform to current codes and regulations. Frequently, local requirements are more restrictive than federal standards.

Another condition that may have a significant impact on both the environment and site development is the previous use or uses of a land parcel. For example, a property used previously as a gas station may require significant investigation and monitoring to determine whether gasoline has contaminated the soil and groundwater. Additional remedial work may be in order to reverse the situation. In many cases, an environmental survey is required by lending institutions as a condition of financing.

One effective method of site selection is to develop a comparative site selection matrix. (See figure 9-1.) The matrix should list three or four of the preferred sites being examined. Each of the above selection criteria should be listed and ranked in terms of its relative importance in the final selection process. Then, each site will be ranked for each of the weighted criteria. A final score will incorporate not only the strengths of each site, but also the importance of each strength relative to the entire selection process.

Site Analysis

Site analysis is a two-part process that begins as part of site selection. First, a brief site analysis is performed early on to provide data necessary for site selection. Later, after a preferred site is selected, a more thorough site analysis—a site evaluation—is conducted as an instrumental first step in the design process.

Figure 9-1. Site Selection Matrix

Selection Criteria	Importance	Site 1	Site 2	Site 3	Comments
1. Proximity to patients and referring providers					
2. Major road access					
3. Accessibility to public transportation					
4. Direct access					
5. Size and usable area					
6. Configuration and orientation					
7. Zoning restrictions					
8. Legal and physical restrictions					
9. Environmental impact					
Total points					

Site analysis helps identify opportunities and constraints that will affect facility design and placement. It also gives credence to the project schedule and budget by uncovering to the degree possible any site-specific factors that could delay the construction schedule or budget.[7]

Site analysis involves verifying the ability to balance the building program with the site. The building program consists of:[8]

- *The building footprint,* including total gross area, number of floors, and building configuration. (This may assume a variety of forms.)
- *Parking requirements,* including the number of parking spaces required per unit of occupancy, the total number of parking spaces required, average amount of area allotted per parking space (usually 325 to 400 NSF, including circulation, for surface parking and 300 to 375 NSF, including circulation, for parking garages).
- *Circulation and open space requirements,* including pedestrian and vehicular circulation, space required for accessibility, and common open space. Circulation and open space requirements may account for 35 to 60 percent of the total site area on suburban sites, considerably less in urban areas. This is determined by the governing zoning ordinance.

  Sites used for imaging facilities should be able to accommodate a mobile imaging technology dock, which may be used initially or in the future for new procedures that can be accommodated in temporary or mobile structures. If a technology dock is to be used, adequate circulation space for installation, removal, and access to the dock and the associated mobile units must be provided.
- *Special constraints and requirements,* such as utility easements, rights-of-way, floodplains, and ecological preserves.

As mentioned previously, the second part of the process of site analysis is site evaluation. A site evaluation summary (figure 9-2) lists many factors that should be considered. Site evaluation includes:[9]

- *Physical factors,* such as climate, topography, geotechnical characteristics, utilities and services, and site character
- *Cultural factors,* such as site history, surrounding land uses, and economic value
- *Regulatory factors,* such as zoning; planning and site plan reviews; and building, life safety regulations, and other construction codes

Figure 9-2. Site Evaluation Summary

Physical Factors

Climate

A. Prevailing winds
   1. Direction
   2. Maximum, minimum, and average velocities

B. Solar orientation
   1. Sun angles
   2. Days of sunlight
   3. Shading for adjacent structures

C. Temperature
   1. Ranges of variation
   2. Maximums and minimums

D. Humidity
   1. Ranges of variation
   2. Maximums and minimums

E. Precipitations
   1. Peak period totals
   2. Annual and seasonal totals

Topography

A. Site survey maps
   1. Legal property description including limits of property, easements, rights of way, and north indication

B. Topographic maps and aerial photos
   1. Contours and spot elevations
   2. Slopes: percentage, aspect, orientation
   3. Escarpments
   4. Erosion channels
   5. Extent, location, and general configuration of rocks, ledges, outcrops, ridges, drainage lines, and other unique features
   6. Visual characteristics
   7. Potential problem areas during construction: situation, erosion, etc.

C. Analysis of physical features
   1. Major loci and vantage points and their relationships within, into, and out from the site

D. Existing access and circulation
   1. Vehicular
   2. Pedestrian

E. Vegetation

F. Existing water bodies
   1. Location, size, depth, direction of flow
   2. Water quality: clean, polluted, anaerobic conditions, etc.
   3. Use seasonal, year-round
   4. Wetlands: ecological features

G. Drainage canals, rivers, streams, marshes, lakes, ponds, etc.
   1. Natural and built
   2. Alignments and gradients
   3. Pattern and direction

H. Existing waterway easements
   1. Surface
   2. Subsurface

I. Surface drainage
   1. Patterns on and off site (location of streams and marshes)
   2. Proximity of floodplains
      a. Maximum flood levels
      b. Frequently flooded areas
   3. Local watershed areas, amount of runoff collected, and location of outfalls
   4. Swampy and concave areas of land without positive drainage and other obstacles that may interrupt or obstruct natural surface drainage
   5. Potential areas for impoundments

J. Unique site features

Figure 9-2. (Continued)

Geotechnical/Soils

A. Basic surface soil type: sand, clay, silt, rock, shale, gravel, loam, limestone, etc.

B. Rock and soil type, character/formation and origin
   1. Geologic formation process and parent material
   2. Inclination

C. Depth to bedrock
   1. Bedrock classification

Utilities

A. Potable water

B. Electricity

C. Gas

D. Phone

E. Sanitary sewer service

F. Storm drainage (surface, subsurface)

G. Fire protection

General Services

A. Fire and police protection

B. Trash/refuse removal services

Cultural Factors

Site History

A. Former site uses
   1. Hazardous dumping
   2. Landfill
   3. Archaeological grounds

B. History of existing structures
   1. Historic worth
   2. Affiliations
   3. Outline
   4. Location
   5. Floor elevations
   6. Type
   7. Condition
   8. Use or service

Land Use, Ownership, and Control

A. Present zoning of site and adjacent property

B. Adjacent (surrounding) land uses
   1. Present
   2. Projected
   3. Probable impacts on the development of this site

C. Type of land ownership

D. Function and pattern of land uses: public domain, farm type, grazing, urbanized
   1. Present
   2. Former

E. Location, type, and size of pertinent community services
   1. Churches
   2. Shopping centers
   3. Parks
   4. Municipal services
   5. Recreational facilities
   6. Banks
   7. Food services
   8. Health services

(Continued on next page)

Figure 9-2. (Continued)

Economic Value

A. Political jurisdictions and land costs

B. Accepted ''territories''

C. Future potential

D. Size of surrounding lots and approximate price ranges

Regulatory Factors

Zoning Codes

A. Permitted uses
   1. By variance
   2. By special use permits
   3. Accessory structures

B. Minimum site area requirements

C. Building height limits

D. Yard (setback) requirements
   1. Front and rear yards
   2. Side yards

E. Lot coverage
   1. Floor area ratios (FAR)
   2. Percentage lot coverage
   3. Open space requirements

F. Off-street parking requirements

G. Sign requirements

Subdivision, Site Plan Review, and Other Local Requirements

A. Lot requirements
   1. Size and configuration

B. Street requirements
   1. Widths
   2. Geometry: grades, curves
   3. Curbs and curb cuts
   4. Road construction standards
   5. Placement of utilities
   6. Dead-end streets
   7. Intersection geometry
   8. Names

C. Drainage requirements
   1. Removal of spring and surface water
   2. Stream courses
   3. Land subject to flooding

D. Parks, open spaces, natural features
   1. Open space requirements
   2. Park and playground requirements
   3. Screening from adjacent uses

Building Codes and Requirements

A. Site-related items
   1. Building separation
   2. Handicap parking and access
   3. Service and emergency vehicle access and parking

B. Building design requirements

Reprinted, with permission, from Zimmerman, F., Terusaki, S., Mingle, E., and Lombardo, J. A. *The Project.* Vol. 2, *The Architect's Handbook of Professional Practice.* Washington, DC: American Institute of Architects, 1987, pp. 4–5.

Often, the maximum height and size of structure(s) permitted on the site are defined in local zoning ordinances. Usually, this is governed by specific limits such as maximum lot coverage, maximum gross floor area, street setbacks, height restrictions, and bulk plane restrictions defined for the particular zone in which the lot is located. The maximum buildable floor area may be defined as a floor-to-area ratio (FAR) that limits the gross floor area as a proportion of the total lot size. Bulk plane restrictions describe an imaginary three-dimensional envelope beyond which building and parking structures may not extend. (See figure 9-3.)

Before design concepts are developed very far, a site survey and a soils report should be obtained. The *site survey* will precisely define the size and configuration of the site. In addition, it will identify special features such as prominent vegetation and components of existing utility systems. The survey also should locate existing building structures. The *soils report* identifies physical geologic characteristics of the soil. Core samples are taken at several locations through various depths. The soils report provides information about the structure-bearing capacity of the land. This information is necessary for the structural engineer to design a proper structural system.

Additional components of the site to be analyzed include:

- *Site utilities:* electric power, water supply, sewage disposal, telecommunications, natural gas, and other systems that lead to and from the building
- *Site circulation:* pathways of patients, visitors, and staff, public transit routes, and emergency and service routes (pedestrian and vehicular) that run through the site
- *Parking:* parking, loading, and waiting zones for each of the types of traffic
- *Landscaping:* ground cover, trees, shrubs, gardens, outdoor furniture, and play areas
- *Drainage:* surface and subsurface drainage systems for rainwater and floodwater

References

1. Rostenberg, B. *Design Planning for Freestanding Ambulatory Care Facilities.* Chicago: American Hospital Publishing, 1986, pp. 35–40 [out of print].
2. Lifton, J., and Hardy, O. B. *Site Selection for Health Care Facilities.* Chicago: American Hospital Publishing, 1982 [out of print].
3. Lifton and Hardy, p. 15.
4. Lifton and Hardy, p. 18.
5. Lifton and Hardy, p. 14.
6. Lifton and Hardy, p. 18.
7. Zimmerman, F., Terusaki, S., Mingle, E., and Lombardo, J. A. *The Project.* Vol. 2, *The Architect's Handbook of Professional Practice.* Washington, DC: American Institute of Architects, 1987, pp. 1–14.
8. Zimmerman and others, pp. 1–3.
9. Zimmerman and others, pp. 3–8.

Figure 9-3. Bulk Plane Limits and Other Zoning Restrictions

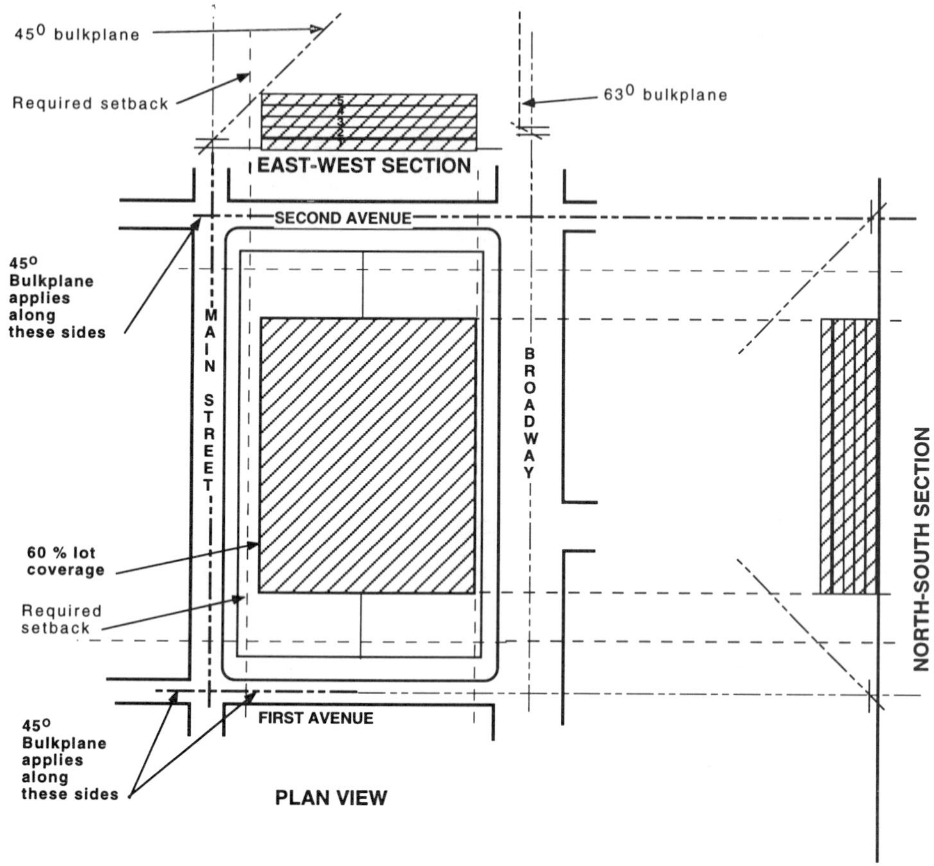

The massing shown above represents 5 levels and approximately 447,000 BGSF (assuming 5 floors, each 13.5 ft. high.)
Note: parking levels would actually have a lower floor-to-floor height.

1. GENERAL ZONING REQUIREMENTS

Three factors determine the maximum allowable building envelope:

1. Maximum Allowable Lot Coverage
2. Maximum Allowable Gross Floor Area
3. Bulkplane Restrictions (see diagram)

In H-2 zones, the bulk limits are restricted by a 45° angle where the site is adjacent to residential lots not owned by the Hospital, and less restrictive at other sides of the site.

Site Data

Approximate Lot Size:	149,000 SF
Existing Zoning:	R1, R3
Assumed New Zoning:	H-2 Hospital District Or possible application for H-1-A with some restrictions
Maximum Lot Coverage: (includes parking structures)	89,400 SF (60% of lot area)
Maximum Gross Floor Area: (excludes parking)	447,000 SF (3 times the lot size. May be further reduced by bulkplane limits).
Parking Requirements:	1 space per 300 BGSF of building (assume 350 SF per parking space).
Floor-to-floor Height Assumptions:	13.5 feet for Ambulatory Care Building 10.0 feet for parking structure

2. PARKING REQUIREMENTS BASED ON BUILDING SIZE

BLDG SIZE	REQ'D. # OF PKG. SPACES	REQ'D. PKG. FLOOR AREA	TOTAL FLOOR AREA REQUIRED
100,000	334	116,900	216,900
125,000	417	145,950	270,950
150,000	500	175,000	325,000
175,000	584	204,400	379,400
200,000	667	233,450	433,450

3. PROGRAM REQUIREMENTS

200,000 BGSF is desired for the Ambulatory Care Building.
NOTE: A 200,000 BGSF building would probably yield approximately 150,000 NFS of usable space.

4. CONCLUSIONS:

A building of 200,000 BGSF and its required parking will fit within the H-2 Zone bulk and lot coverage restrictions of the site. If parking and the Ambulatory Care Building are combined as one structure, the building could be as low as 5 levels. However, it would be more desirable to separate the two structures, which can also be done within the bulk plane and lot coverage restrictions.

Courtesy of Stone Marraccini Patterson, San Francisco. Used with permission.

Chapter 10

Work Flow and Circulation

Work patterns and the highly repetitive movement of staff between different activity areas is a major driver of department layout. Internal traffic patterns to consider include those of:

- Patients
- Technologists
- Radiologists
- Film librarians
- Radiologic nurses
- Other support staff

In addition, the flow of films, images, information, and supplies will influence traffic patterns between the imaging department/facility and related departments and facilities.

This chapter identifies the work flow and circulation principles that influence facility design and layout. Work flow *constants* are described to illustrate the primary functional needs of imaging facilities. Work flow *variables* illustrate the numerous variations to work flow that must be accommodated through flexible design. Finally, transport and communications systems are discussed to demonstrate how imaging services can be linked to other health care service areas.

Work Flow and Circulation Principles

For purposes of both efficiency and convenience, circulation routes should be short and direct. Patient and staff traffic should be separated from one another, to the extent practical. Inpatients and outpatients also should be separated, but not to the extent that procedure rooms cannot be used by either group when necessary.

> The primary planning should be based on patient traffic, which includes accessibility, promptness of attention, comfort, convenience, privacy, thoroughness of examination or treatment, and courteous assistance to the exit. The objective is to provide the patient with a prompt and accurate examination or treatment in pleasant circumstances. . . .
>
> The secondary planning is based on film [or image] flow. The efficiency and speed with which the films are processed is reflected in the promptness with which reports are delivered to the staff members and in the dispatch with which patients are handled. [Note: Planning based on film or "image" flow is changing significantly as filmless imaging redefines much of radiology work flow.]

> The tertiary planning is based on [technologist] traffic to allow a minimum of personnel to expedite the examinations and treatments with maximal efficiency and minimal fatigue.
>
> The quartan planning is based on achieving the most effective traffic pattern for the radiologist and professional staff, that they may interview, examine, and treat patients quickly and thoroughly.[1]

An efficient layout provides clear circulation paths for patients, staff, equipment, and supplies. Therefore, most commonly used and high-volume procedure rooms, such as chest, mammography, and general radiography rooms, are best located close to the waiting area and department entrance. (See figure 10-1.) This reduces the distance that most patients need to travel and limits the amount of traffic entering the more complex procedures areas.

It may be desirable to segregate rooms for special groups such as women's services (for example, mammography, ultrasound, or bone densitometry) into separate activity clusters to provide additional privacy and a special identity. Similarly, in practices where pediatric patients are seen frequently, a separate children's waiting alcove, removed from heavy traffic areas, is helpful. Patient examination and dressing areas should be screened from the view of waiting patients.

Some imaging modalities have unique traffic requirements. For instance, circulation near a magnetic resonance imaging (MRI) exam room may be restricted by the forces emitted from the magnet, particularly if it is not magnetically shielded. (However, recent developments in actively shielded MRI systems have simplified design for MRI rooms to some extent.) Also, the gamma cameras used in nuclear medicine should be kept some distance from MRI systems because the cameras are very sensitive to magnetic fields. For the same reason, they should not be located close to power transformers.

As another example, nuclear medicine patients often leave the department after being administered a low-level radioactive dose and return a short time later for their examination. Therefore, nuclear medicine functions should be organized so that dose administration rooms are easily accessed from the waiting area and are near the dose preparation room. In addition, nuclear medicine procedure rooms and uptake rooms should be isolated from isotope injection, hot lab, and isotope waste holding areas to prevent low-level radiation in these areas from disturbing procedure results. Similarly, the hot lab and isotope waste areas should be located together. Often, nuclear medicine functions are organized as a distinct department, separate from other medical imaging services. Traffic patterns can be mapped on preliminary plan drawings to identify potential areas of congestion or conflict. (See figure 10-2.)

Figure 10-1. Conceptual Department Layout Based on Work Flow and Circulation

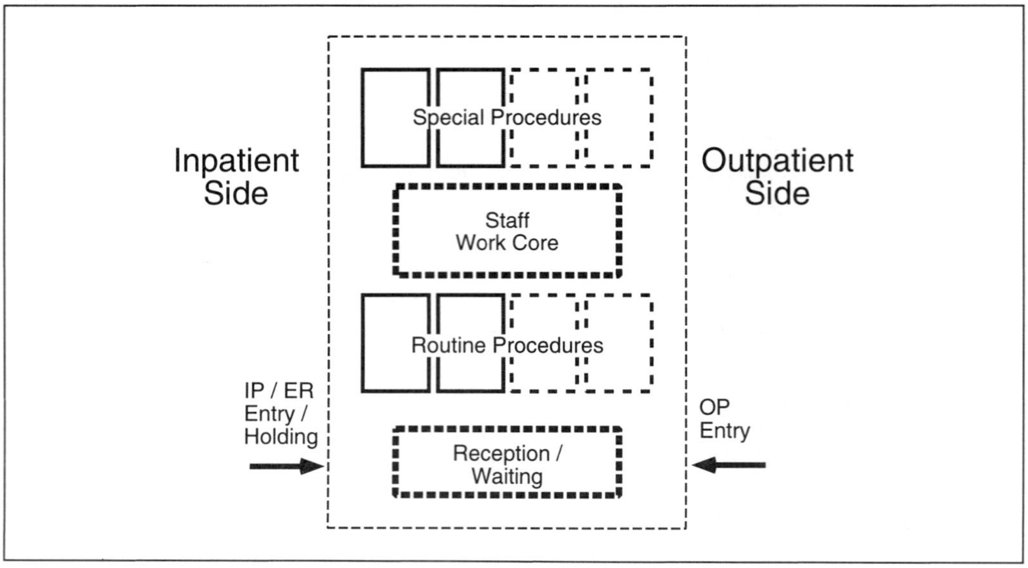

Figure 10-2. Traffic and Circulation within the Imaging Facility

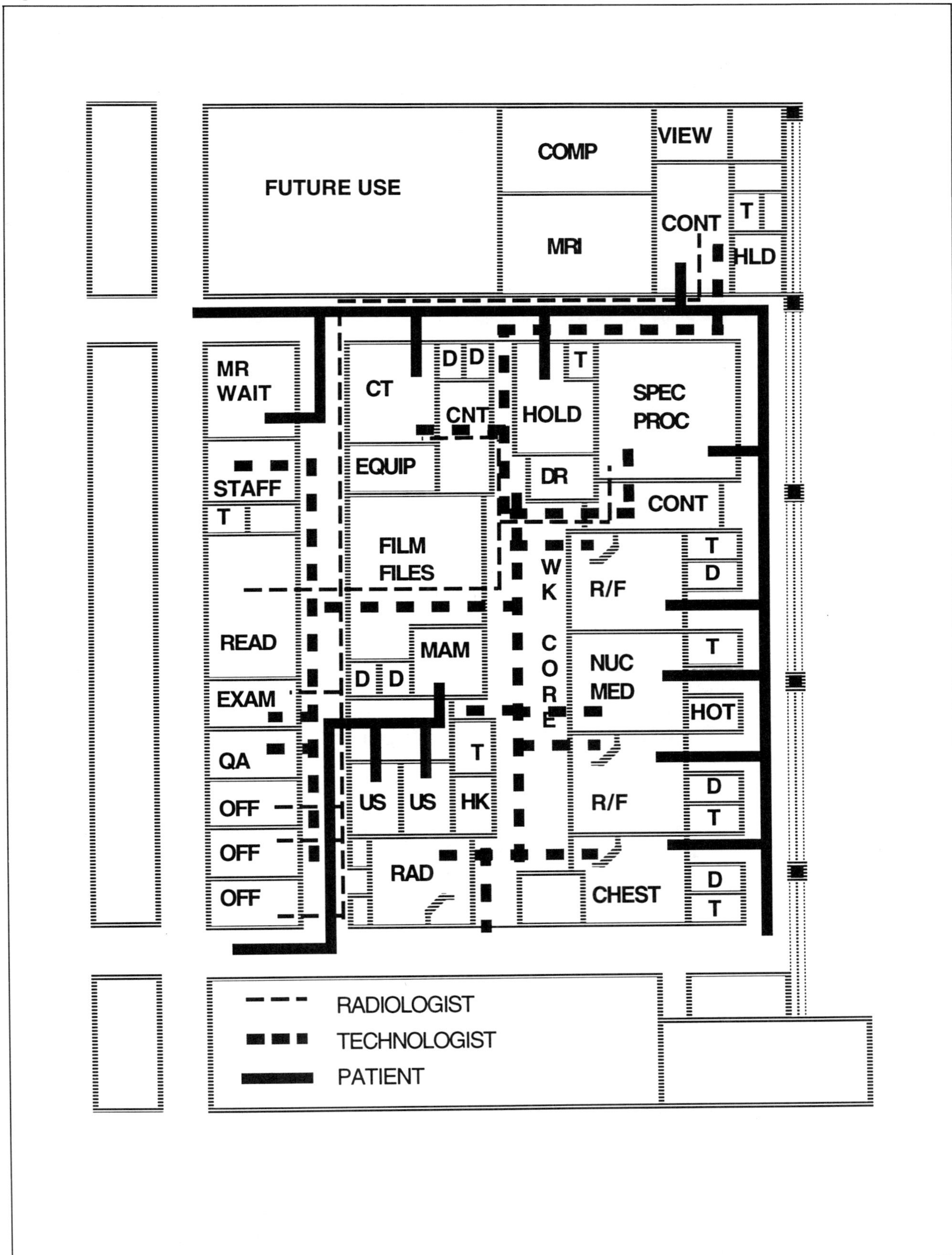

One planning concept known as functional zoning (described in chapter 11, "Department Location and Configuration") suggests a staff control corridor running parallel to a patient corridor. This arrangement enables separation of staff and patient traffic, provides the staff with direct access to the image-handling zone, and allows the technologist to greet the next patient in the exam corridor once the previous exam is completed. As filmless imaging becomes more fully integrated into medical practices, the distance between decentralized image-handling zones can be greater, but the relationship—and thus the circulation—between staff and patients will remain strong.

In many practices, a radiologic technologist may have most of the patient contact. This will depend, in part, on the degree of invasiveness of imaging procedures. Typically, for basic imaging procedures, the technologist greets patients at the reception area, escorts them to the procedure room, positions them on the table, proceeds with the examination, assesses image quality, and either takes additional images or directs the patient back to the dressing or waiting area. Because the technologist frequently passes back and forth between the procedure room and the image-processing and quality assurance viewing areas, these distances should be kept to a minimum. However, the transition to digital imaging is changing the relevance of this proximity relationship.

In some facilities, dedicated processing equipment is located within heavily used procedure rooms or even docked to the imaging unit, to minimize the technologist's travel time. In other cases, the optimal layout incorporates a series of procedure rooms encircling a *work core* that includes image processing, sorting, quality control, and cleanup, with direct access to image storage and file areas and radiologists' offices. This *core layout* implies that each procedure room has two doors—one for patient access and egress to and from the main corridor and one for staff circulation to and from the staff work core. (See the section entitled Plan Typologies in chapter 11, "Department Location and Configuration.") Where film processing that requires a darkroom is still used, lighttight, through-the-wall cassette passboxes can be installed between the darkroom and the procedure rooms or other work areas to further reduce travel time. In addition:

> The traffic patterns produced by technologists and radiologists are of primary importance. Both must be minimized to obtain maximum efficiency. [Some] radiological technologists spend most of their time in the examining room, but also must have ready access to the patient preparation area, the radiographic supply storeroom, the darkroom, and the professional staff. . . .
>
> [Some] radiologists spend most of their clinical time in the examining room, the reading room, or the consultation area. Often the reading room and consultation area are combined. Office space must be provided for the radiologist. If the radiologist's activities are strictly clinical, an office should be located within the radiology area so that technologists and other physicians have easy access to it. On the other hand, if the radiologist is involved in teaching and research, then the office should be located in another part of the hospital so that the radiologist will be free of interruptions when not on clinical assignment.[2]

In 1977, B. G. Brogden, M.D., of the University of New Mexico School of Medicine, summarized the importance of radiology planning that is sensitive to the various traffic patterns inherent to medical imaging. His description remains relevant today:

> . . . there is an inseparable interdependence between the basic external configuration of the department and the final layout, that is, the assignment, design and juxtapositions of confined space to the various operational and support activities of the department.
>
> Within configurational limitations, the layout should be based, insofar as possible, on the anticipated traffic patterns within the department, of which five are the most important:
>
> *The patient traffic pattern* should allow for central reception and control, convenient outpatient waiting or monitored inpatient holding areas, and easy dispersal to on-deck waiting or dressing areas (for outpatients) and examining rooms.

Rooms for rapid, routine examinations (chest, abdomen, extremities and skull) should be nearest the entry port to reduce this maximal patient flow. Examination rooms for more time-consuming procedures (G.I. examinations, ultrasonography, CT scanning, . . . and urography) can be somewhat removed. Rooms for long-duration examination (angiography, neuroradiology, . . .) should be most distant from the patient entry point since this traffic, as a function of the time–distance relationship, will be minimal.

A separate access to the department for emergency suite patients is highly desirable. These patients can then be [brought] into, and out of, the department without seriously imposing upon any other traffic patterns. When facilities for fluoroscopy, CT scanning and film processing can be placed in immediate proximity to the emergency radiographic examination room or rooms, this sub-unit will make an ideal "mini-department" for after hours radiologic services.

Radiology personnel traffic (radiologists and technologists especially) should be isolated from other patterns within the department. [Facility layout] should reflect the internal operational network of activity, emphasizing rapid response, short time and distance requirements and convenience. This pattern should encompass all equipment control and film processing areas and, preferably, should parallel—or be internally concentric to—the patient flow pattern.

Non-radiologic physician traffic should be restricted to specified areas—the film check-out counter, the staff viewing area, the consultation area or reading room and the conference room—and need not utilize the central entry port.

Film traffic must go from the exposure rooms to dispersed processing facilities to central sorting and make up. Processed, made-up examinations, in folders, should then be limited to the file room, the reading room, the staff viewing room or the conference room. [Note: Electronic image management and communications systems will significantly change many of these functional relationships.]

Administrative traffic can be entirely separated from other patterns and relatively far-removed from the central entry point of the department.

All traffic patterns must be isolated from one another, insofar as possible. Intersections and common pathways should be kept at a minimum.[3]

Work Flow Variables

The work flow of a basic imaging examination is subject to many variations. However, almost all imaging procedures involve the following steps in one form or another:

1. The need or indication for the examination is determined.
2. An appointment is scheduled unless the clinical problem is of an emergency nature.
3. The patient's prior records are prepared or retrieved.
4. The patient is received in department (or equipment and staff are transported to patient).
5. The examination is conducted.
6. The image(s) is processed and reviewed for quality and completeness.
7. The patient is either sent home, sent to the inpatient nursing unit or another department, or detained to wait for further instructions.
8. The image(s) is interpreted; diagnosis is made and findings are reported.
9. Results are transmitted and reported to referring physician; the patient record is held, filed, and/or distributed.
10. Follow-up imaging evaluation or treatment is scheduled as necessary.

Although these 10 steps may appear to be a simple linear succession of events, many complex subsets of activities are involved in each step. For some activities, patients are intimately involved; for other activities, patient involvement is limited or nonexistent. Some procedures require detailed interaction among patient, radiologist, radiologic nurses, and support personnel, whereas other procedures may be performed entirely by the technologist. The work flow activity matrix in figure 10-3 illustrates the relationships of space and personnel to each of the basic steps that are part of medical imaging work flow.

Regardless of how each step is carried out, the basic activity can be referred to as a *constant,* whereas the various means by which it is carried out can be referred to as *variables.*[4] Each activity will vary according to the operational philosophy of the institution, the type of institution (teaching hospital, community hospital, freestanding imaging center, health maintenance organization, physician's office, and so on), the type of examination and equipment involved (routine versus special procedure), and the type of patient (emergency, acutely ill, stable, inpatient, or outpatient). Another important variable in facility design is physical organization, such as centralized versus decentralized image processing. For each constant, hundreds of variables may exist, all of which have architectural implications. For example, in the case of an emergency department (ED) patient who must be transported to the main imaging department for examination, it would be desirable to have the two departments located near each other and connected by a circulation route that is short and direct. The appendix at the end of this chapter illustrates some of these variables and their architectural implications.

Corridors and Exitways

Corridors designed for movement or circulation seem to have a way of becoming a home for equipment and supplies whose assigned storage space is either inadequate or poorly located. Sometimes corridors become temporary holding areas for patients prior to, and after, imaging procedures. Such inappropriate use of corridors is both unsafe and contrary to aesthetic goals. Additionally, life safety codes have strict requirements limiting the use of exitways for equipment holding or storage. Thus, ample equipment storage must be provided to prevent instruments from ending up along corridors and in unassigned alcoves. Ideally, supply storage rooms should be located near all patient and staff areas.

Although hospital corridors generally are required to be at least 8 feet wide, the required width of corridors in outpatient imaging facilities is not so clearly spelled out and may vary by jurisdiction. Life safety codes usually require that exit corridors in a medical office suite or clinic be at least 44 inches wide. However, this width is too narrow for maneuvering patients and equipment within an outpatient imaging facility. In outpatient imaging facilities, dedicated staff passageways with *no* patient or equipment traffic should be at least 4 feet wide (although 5 feet is preferable). Outpatient corridors with ambulatory patient traffic but no gurney traffic should be at least 5 feet wide (6 feet is preferable), and outpatient corridors with some equipment or stretcher traffic should be 8 feet wide, although a width of 6 feet may be acceptable in some jurisdictions.

The installation and replacement of large pieces of equipment may influence corridor width and door sizes. In many cases, removable access panels or door panels are installed to adjust for installation of large equipment components.

Some jurisdictions have special occupancy classifications for outpatient facilities, depending on the type of procedure performed and the degree to which the patient may become temporarily "nonambulatory." Each classification has special exiting requirements, including minimum corridor widths. In addition, licensing agencies often have their own requirements. Although these requirements may not appear in the building codes, they must be adhered to if the facility is either to be licensed or certified or to receive certain levels of reimbursement.

Additionally, the facility should be provided with a back door or service door, especially if deliveries are scheduled during patient treatment hours. A back door also allows staff to come and go without passing through the waiting area and provides a direct route if emergency transport of medically unstable patients becomes necessary.

Both the size of the facility and its occupancy classification will determine the minimum number of required exits. Exiting requirements often are subject to interpretation by various regulatory agencies.

Figure 10-3. Work Flow Activity Matrix

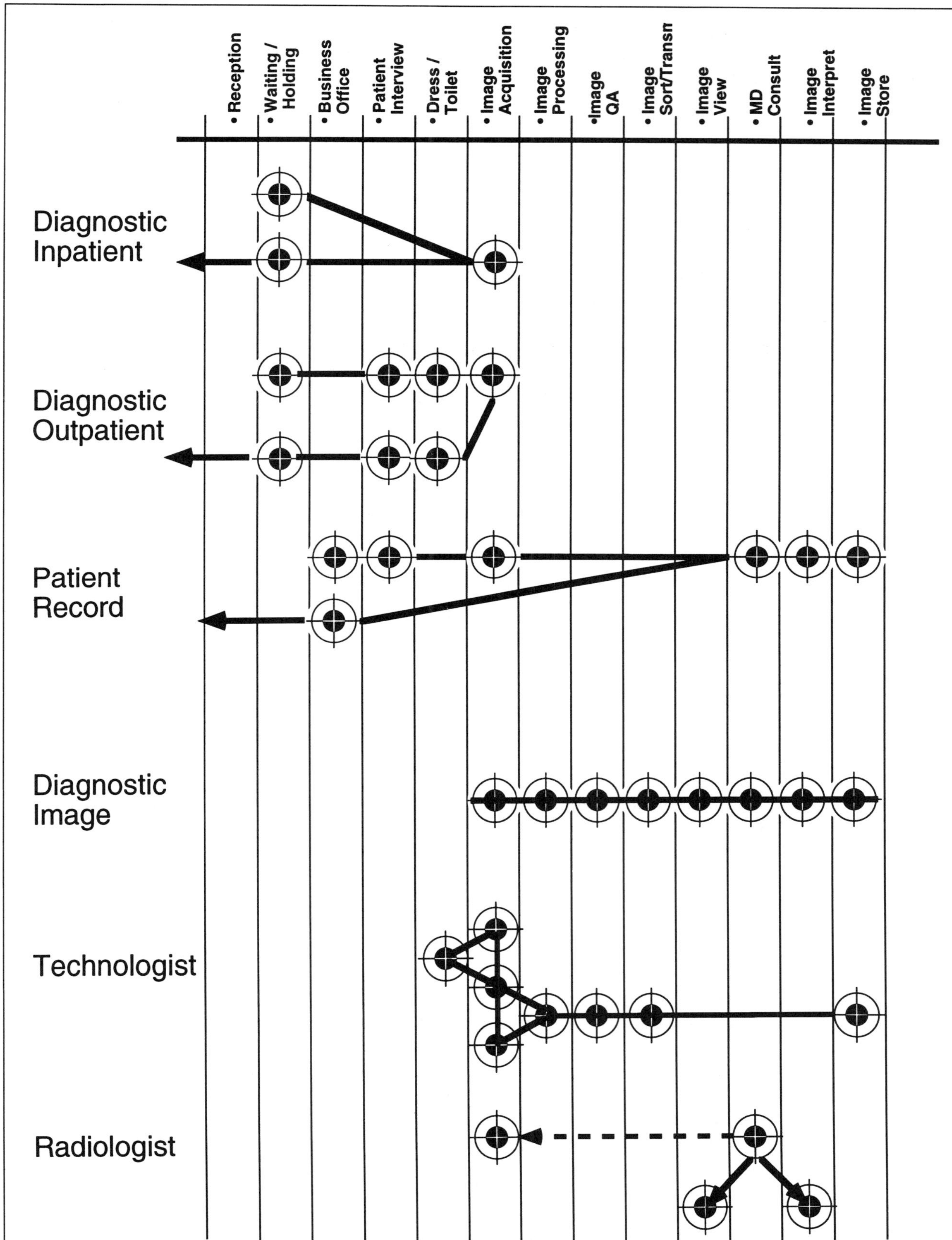

Adapted from S. C. Bushong. *Radiologic Science for Technologists: Physics, Biology, and Protection.* 5th ed. St. Louis: Mosby-Year Book, 1993.

Transport and Information Systems

Imaging services interact with numerous other components of the hospital and health care network. (See chapter 11, "Department Location and Configuration.") Systems that help link the various activity centers include material management systems and information, communication, and conveying systems.

Material Management Systems

The delivery, disposal, and reuse of supplies and equipment for imaging services will be part of a larger system of material management, if the imaging service is hospital based. If the facility is freestanding or independent, the material management service may be less complex. In either case, the flow of material and the space required for its storage, staging, and holding must be considered.

A number of supply systems may be employed: exchange carts, topping-up carts, just-in-time delivery, or any combination of these. Each system has its own space, scheduling, staffing, and cost implications. (It is beyond the scope of this book to discuss them in detail.) To select the appropriate supply systems and to understand their associated space requirements, it is important to identify the material needs of the imaging services provided.

Linens, reusable supplies, and disposable items will all be used. Generally, a linen cart is preferred over fixed shelving for holding clean linens. The cart should be located in a clean supply room or at its point of use, rather than in a space where circulation is heavy. Soiled linens must be stored in a separate area, preferably near a service corridor and away from the main entrance. Typically, ultrasound and interventional procedures are heavy users of linen.

Clean reusable and disposable supplies are typically stored on movable carts, which can be located in a central clean supply room, at their point of use, or within a series of decentralized storage areas. Secured holding areas for biohazardous waste and contaminated linens should be provided, ideally near a service corridor away from unauthorized traffic. Some special procedures will require packaged sterile instruments similar to those used in the surgical suite. Initial cleaning of these instruments may be performed in cleanup rooms in the imaging department, whereas terminal sterilization will likely take place in a central sterile department. The initial cleaning area should be located convenient to the special procedures rooms.

Bulk film and chemicals should be stored in separate lockable rooms with special ventilation and temperature control. Film storage also must incorporate radiation protection to prevent unexposed film from fogging, due to gradual exposure to even small amounts of ambient radiation present in the immediate environment. Bulk film and chemical storage should be located along the perimeter of the department, preferably near a service corridor for easy access. Smaller amounts of film may be stored in a darkroom, if necessary.

Nuclear medicine services have special material-handling requirements due to the use of radioactive substances inherent to that imaging modality. Typically, a hot lab will be used for the receipt, preparation, and storage of radioactive substances. A cold lab, which is usually adjacent to, or part of, the hot lab, is where these materials are later processed and prepared prior to administration to the patient. In addition, a locked isotope waste room, adjacent to the hot lab, is where radioactive waste and linens are held until they decay to a safe level, after which they can then be safely transported and removed.

The area set aside for nuclear medicine should be configured in such a way that the hot lab, cold lab, and isotope waste room are located together and separated from nuclear medicine scanning rooms and public areas. In addition, special ventilation, exhaust, and gas-scavenging systems should be used in rooms where gases such as radioactive xenon are used. Nonabsorbent, easily cleanable surfaces should be specified for corridors and procedure rooms throughout the nuclear medicine area.

Information, Communication, and Conveying Systems

Interdepartmental and intradepartmental transport of films, reports, supplies, and information may be accomplished through a number of specific systems. (Image management and communication systems [IMACSs], picture archiving and communication systems [PACSs], teleradiology, telemedicine, radiology information systems [RISs], and hospital information systems [HISs] are described in chapter 7, "Image Management and Film Processing.") Most advanced systems rely on transmission of images and data via fiber-optic cable, coaxial cable, satellite, and telephone networks to one degree or another. However, some also use wireless cellular fax and telephone technology. Imaging facilities that do not envision immediate use of advanced information technology should, at a minimum, plan for future incorporation of these electronic data communication systems, even if they are to be slowly incorporated into daily routines. Planning should include location and selection of network components as well as identification of space requirements for data storage units, communication closets, and workstations. It is likely that for some interim period, both electronic and manual communication systems will be used, and therefore space requirements during this interim period will be greater than for either system alone.

A number of communication subsystems need to be considered. These include:

- Film transport and tracking systems
- Picture archiving and image management and communication systems
- Film digitization systems
- Telephone and intercom systems
- Paging systems
- Digital dictation systems
- Pneumatic tube systems (PTSs)
- Room "in-use" scheduling and tracking systems
- Scheduling and patient-tracking systems
- Accounting and inventory control systems
- Code blue and nurse call systems
- Facsimile systems for receiving and transmitting exam reports
- Interactive teleconferencing systems to accommodate remote observation of imaging procedures and remote interpretation and/or consultation regarding medical images

Regardless of how many information and communication systems are incorporated into facility design, there will still be a need for both staff and patients to physically travel to and from imaging areas. Therefore, these areas should be located near stairwells and elevators. Where possible, staff, service, and public elevators should be separated and the staff, service, and public components of the department should be located accordingly. (Physical relationships between imaging services and other health care services are discussed in chapter 11, "Department Location and Configuration.")

References

1. Blumenkranz, J. *Planning Guide for Radiologic Installations—Fascicle 4a: Basic Concepts: Layout Considerations—Planning X-ray Facilities.* Chicago: American College of Radiology, 1977, p. 13.
2. Bushong, S. C. *Radiologic Science for Technologists: Physics, Biology, and Protection.* 5th ed. St. Louis: Mosby-Year Book, 1993, pp. 621–23.
3. Brogdon, B. G. *Planning Guide for Radiologic Installations—Fascicle 4a: Basic Concepts: Layout Considerations—Diagnostic Departmental Planning: Location, Configuration and Layout for Diagnostic Radiology.* Chicago: American College of Radiology, 1977, pp. 32–45.
4. Lindheim, R. *Uncoupling the Radiology System.* Chicago: Hospital Research and Educational Trust, 1971, p. 57 [out of print].

Appendix. Work Flow Constants and Variables

1. Constant: The Need or Indication for the Exam Is Determined.

Variables

- Emergency patient is rushed to the emergency department (ED). If the ED has radiographic capabilities, an imaging staff is either based there or will be called in. If comprehensive radiographic capabilities do not exist in the ED, or if more sophisticated imaging capabilities are needed, the ED staff will have the patient transported to the main imaging department. Scheduled imaging patients may be delayed because of the emergency patient. Based on the results of plain radiographs, computed tomography (CT), ultrasound, and so on, the patient may be returned to the ED or brought to other locations such as the operating room (OR), the ICU, or the medical nursing unit.
- An inpatient is identified as needing an imaging examination. The referring physician requests the next available examination time slot.
- An outpatient is identified as needing an imaging examination. An outpatient clerk or manager schedules an appointment when it is convenient for the patient and imaging department.

Architectural Implications

Adjacency between emergency and radiology departments is desirable; the circulation route should avoid busy public areas such as lobbies and waiting areas. To some degree, the importance of this adjacency depends on the extent of radiographic capabilities in the ED. Radiology staffing also will be affected by the extent of radiographic capabilities in the ED. It should be assumed that most seriously ill emergency patients will require CT or other special exams (even MRI), which might necessitate transporting patients to the radiology department or a special imaging unit.

2. Constant: An Appointment Is Scheduled.

Variables

- Appointments are scheduled manually.
- Appointments are scheduled via automated scheduling system.
- Some appointments are accepted on a drop-in basis.
- Billing and payment methods may be determined during appointment scheduling.
- Patient is given preparation instructions.

Architectural Implications

If a large percentage of appointments are unscheduled (for example, a drop-in or emergency basis), room utilization may be inefficient. This should be considered when calculating the number of procedure rooms, waiting areas, and dressing booths to be provided and determining overall space requirements.

3. Constant: The Patient's Record Is Prepared.

Variables

- This is the patient's first imaging exam; his or her record needs to be assembled, if possible. Faxing the patient's most recent clinical examination and the indications of old imaging examinations may be adequate.

- The patient has been seen before but for a different medical problem. The old record is retrieved and held until the exam.
- The patient has been seen before for the same medical problem. The old record is retrieved and held until the exam. Just prior to the exam, previous images are displayed for comparison with the new image. The old record may be either in an active file or stored in a remotely located archive file.
- If an automated hospital information system (HIS) or radiology information system (RIS) is in place, record preparation is highly facilitated, because the pertinent information is readily located and continually updated. If not, the information needed by the radiologist will be documented manually.

Architectural Implications

Space should be provided for record assembly. Where hard copies of films and written information are handled, storage space for this information and some type of conveying system (carts, hand delivery, pneumatic tube, and so on) are needed. Where electronic information systems are used, computer workstations are needed. (See the section entitled General Considerations for Computer Workstation Environments in chapter 13, "Room Design.") Digital information can be transmitted electronically at determinable rates (instantaneous and slower). In some instances, hard copy can be transmitted electronically via fax or teleradiology devices.

4. Constant: The Patient Is Received in the Department

Variables

- An acutely ill patient is brought from the ED to the radiology department; his or her family members arrive later in the ED. The patient is accompanied by the medical team and is brought directly into the procedure room once it is available and has been prepared.
- An inpatient, already dressed in a hospital gown and accompanied by his or her medical chart, is transported from the nursing unit and kept in the inpatient holding area prior to the procedure. He or she may require monitoring, oxygen, and supervision prior to and during the exam. The transporting supervisory team may transfer its monitoring responsibilities to the radiology monitoring team, which includes radiologic nurses.
- An outpatient accompanied by family and/or friends arrives in a registration and waiting area. Registration and waiting areas may be either within the radiology department or combined with other outpatient functions. Additionally, outpatient waiting may be separate from, or combined with, inpatient waiting (separation is desirable). Individual waiting areas may be designated for special populations such as women's health or pediatrics.
- Copayment may be required when the patient arrives. In that case, the billing representative may be needed to determine the amount of copayment required.
- A patient requires preexam preparation. With a nuclear medicine exam, for example, the patient receives a low-level radioactive dose and returns either minutes or hours later for the exam.
- A patient gowns and either remains in a subwaiting area or goes directly to a procedure room. His or her valuables and street clothes are stored in a locker area or remain in a locked dressing room.
- Educational information may be provided while the patient is waiting. Television and video may be used to facilitate patient education.

Architectural Implications

Waiting areas should be provided for inpatients, outpatients, and friends and family members. At least one area should be designated where patients, and those accompanying them, can ask questions confidentially. Consideration also should be given to providing an "education alcove" near the waiting area. Additionally, secure places should be made available to store patients' valuables and, in the event that cash payment is required upon arrival, to temporarily store money that has been collected. For MRI exams, metal objects, magnetic data storage media, and other similar items need to be separated from the patient and the staff and temporarily stored away from the procedure room. Dressing areas should be located so that gowned patients can move discretely to and from the examination room.

5. Constant: The Exam Is Conducted.

Variables

- Exams may be simple and brief or complex and lengthy. A patient may require considerable assistance to be properly positioned for an exam. In some cases, young children might be accompanied by a family member as long as his or her presence does not pose a safety hazard. For example, during an MRI exam, a friend or family member may wait in the MRI procedures room reading or comforting the patient.
- Patients may undergo one exam or a series of exams. In the event of a series, some exams may need to take place before others. For example, if the patient has had a barium enema and is then referred for an intravenous pyelogram or a gallbladder examination, the exam may not be possible because residual barium is likely to obscure the region of interest. Thus, the next examinations may be delayed for days because of this error in sequencing. (Source: G. S. Lodwick, and E. Kovisto, Radiology space requirements in the computer age. In: M. Kormano and F. E. Stieve, editors. *Planning of Radiological Departments.* Stuttgart, Germany: Georg Thieme Publishers, 1974, p. 112.)
- An exam may cause considerable or no discomfort to the patient.
- An exam may involve considerable or no risk to the patient.
- A patient may become nauseated, vomit, or develop a skin rash or anaphylactic shock in response to the required radiologic medication. (Immediate medical treatment must be available.)
- Some imaging procedures, such as a barium enema or an abdominal ultrasound, require that a bathroom be directly and immediately accessible from the procedure room.
- A patient may require monitoring, life support, and medical supervision. In the case of MRI exams, only ancillary equipment made of special materials may be brought into the procedure room.
- Exams may be conducted by either one technologist, one radiologist, one nurse, or a team of health care professionals.
- An exam may need to be repeated if the acquired image quality is not acceptable.
- An exam may involve a conventional film-screen (roentgenographic) or phosphor plate (digital) acquisition of images.
- Some procedure rooms may accommodate various imaging procedures; others may be equipped only for specific procedures (for example, a dedicated chest room).
- Some exams may yield single images that are "fixed in time"; others may yield a series of images that represent a continuum of "real time." Some images represent a two-dimensional view; others are manipulated to form three-dimensional models.
- Facility layout may provide imaging control areas within the procedure room or may separate the two.
- Facility organization may include one large, centralized imaging department or may provide multiple satellite imaging areas located near inpatient care areas.
- Inpatient and outpatient exam areas may be combined or separate.
- Some modalities may be provided via mobile trailers. These may be permanently located at one campus or may be shared and travel among numerous institutions.

Architectural Implications

Special facility requirements for different imaging modalities are discussed in chapter 13, "Room Design."

6. Constant: The Image(s) Is Processed and Reviewed for Quality.

Variables

- Image processing may occur in one central area, multiple decentralized areas, or some combination of the two.
- Some imaging equipment may have dedicated and automated film processing that is directly attached. Networking of laser cameras is popular.
- Some methods of image processing require a lighttight darkroom; others can take place in daylight.
- Some methods of image acquisition and processing utilize photostimulable phosphor plates in lieu of film. (See chapter 7, "Image Management and Film Processing.")
- For some imaging techniques, image acquisition and image processing are simultaneous (or within a fraction of a second).
- Some facility layouts and some imaging techniques require the technologist to leave the exam room in order to transport films to processing areas; some do not.
- Some imaging techniques, such as MRI, CT, and digital subtraction angiography (DSA), involve complex manipulation of the image as part of image processing.

Architectural Implications

Special facility requirements for different image processing are discussed in chapter 13, "Room Design."

7. Constant: The Patient Is Sent Elsewhere.

Variables

- A patient is held for further observation. Usually, this occurs somewhere other than in the imaging department, for example, in the nursing unit or the ED.
- A patient is rushed to surgery.
- A patient is returned to the ED.
- A patient is returned to the nursing unit.
- A patient returns home.
- Payment at cashier/billing office may be due prior to departure, or the patient or his or her insurance carrier or health plan may be billed later.
- A follow-up appointment may be scheduled prior to departure.

Architectural Implications

A direct path of travel should be provided between the radiology department and the emergency, surgery, and nursing units. If possible, the route of travel should avoid busy public areas. Inpatient, outpatient, and emergency traffic should be separated, where practical. Family waiting areas should be located so that they can be supervised but screened from patient areas.

8. Constant: The Image(s) Is Interpreted and a Diagnosis Made.

Variables

- Some diagnoses will appear obvious; others will require collaboration and consultation among various specialists to develop.

- Most imaging diagnoses will be defined in terms of anatomical topography and will denote likely, if not specific, pathological entities. Nuclear medicine studies usually will present information in terms of metabolic activity. Similarly, some diagnoses will relate to what has already happened to the patient; in some cases, future risk can be of greater importance therapeutically.
- If teleradiology, teleconferencing, or other means of automated information management and communication are in place, image interpretation and diagnosis can occur rapidly and simultaneously from remote locations.

Architectural Implications

Image-reading areas and instruments (film illuminators, alternators, computer workstations, and so on) should be provided within radiologists' offices and/or in reading rooms, based on the particular requirements of the institution. Film illuminators also are needed in most procedure rooms. In addition, group viewing areas should be provided for radiology staff and physicians from outside the department. If teleradiology, teleconferencing, or other means of electronic image management and communications systems are in place or are anticipated, special cables and transmitting devices may be required. In general, special indirect variable lighting is needed for viewing images, either electronic or on film. (See the section entitled General Considerations for Image-Reading/Viewing Rooms in chapter 13, "Room Design.")

9. Constant: Results Are Transmitted, Reported, and Stored.

Variables

- The reporting, transmission, and distribution of information may be automated, manual, or some combination of the two.
- Digital image viewing stations located in the ICU, the operating room(s), or the ED will allow rapid transmission of images when time is of the essence.
- Hospital information systems (HISs) may be integrated with, or separate from, comprehensive radiology information systems (RISs). Multimedia diagnostic workstations are in use and are being refined to simplify access to data on other systems.
- Information may be stored as hard copy (film); on magnetic disks, optical disks (within electronic jukeboxes), or magnetic tapes; or as a combination of archival media.

Architectural Implications

Physical requirements for image transmission, distribution, and storage will vary greatly depending on the medium. Manual and electronic image management are discussed in chapter 7, "Image Management and Film Processing."

10. Constant: Follow-up Imaging Consultation or Treatment Is Scheduled.

Variables

- An infinite number of variables exist.

Chapter 11

Department Location and Configuration

The numerous activities surrounding an imaging examination intertwine to form a complex, almost-choreographed sequence of events. For hospital-based imaging services, department location and configuration must be coordinated with the hospitalwide flow of patients, staff, supplies, and material. At the same time, however, because the movement of people, information, and equipment involves peaks and lulls in workload, a variety of patient types, and a range of procedures, the imaging department must be adaptable and capable of change. For freestanding imaging facilities, issues of location will differ from those for hospital-based departments, although issues of configuration and layout may be similar.

This chapter considers criteria for the location and configuration of imaging departments and facilities relative to both interdepartmental traffic and intradepartmental work flow. It also discusses special considerations for freestanding imaging facilities. Additionally, the chapter illustrates various layout typologies.

Department Location and Access

Frequently, imaging departments are located on the lower floors of hospitals, often without access to natural daylight. The weight of imaging equipment and film files, the need for radiation protection, and desired adjacencies to other departments frequently located on the lower levels (such as the emergency department) are some of the reasons typically cited for a basement location.

Departments located below grade can be difficult to expand unless excess unfinished space or "soft" space also is provided, or unless major expansion (in which expansion of the imaging department is one component) is planned. Additionally, many basements contain industrial functions, such as material management and central processing, which are incompatible with patient activities. It is desirable to have those spaces remote from patient traffic routes.

Usually, a grade-level location is preferred for imaging services if it provides the proper functional adjacencies and accommodates future expansion. The ability to expand the department or to allow for future conversion of areas within the department should be a primary consideration in determining location and configuration. Another advantage to a grade-level location is access to natural daylight. Natural daylight can be helpful in brightening and softening the image of interior spaces, particularly in facilities planned with perimeter patient corridors. A perimeter corridor also allows light into the department and provides a direction for future expansion. (See figures 11-1 and 11-2.)

Where the imaging department should be located within the hospital depends on two important factors: (1) who will be using the department's services and (2) what the facility's overall organizational philosophy is with regard to the provision of imaging services.

Figure 11-1. Perimeter Patient Corridor

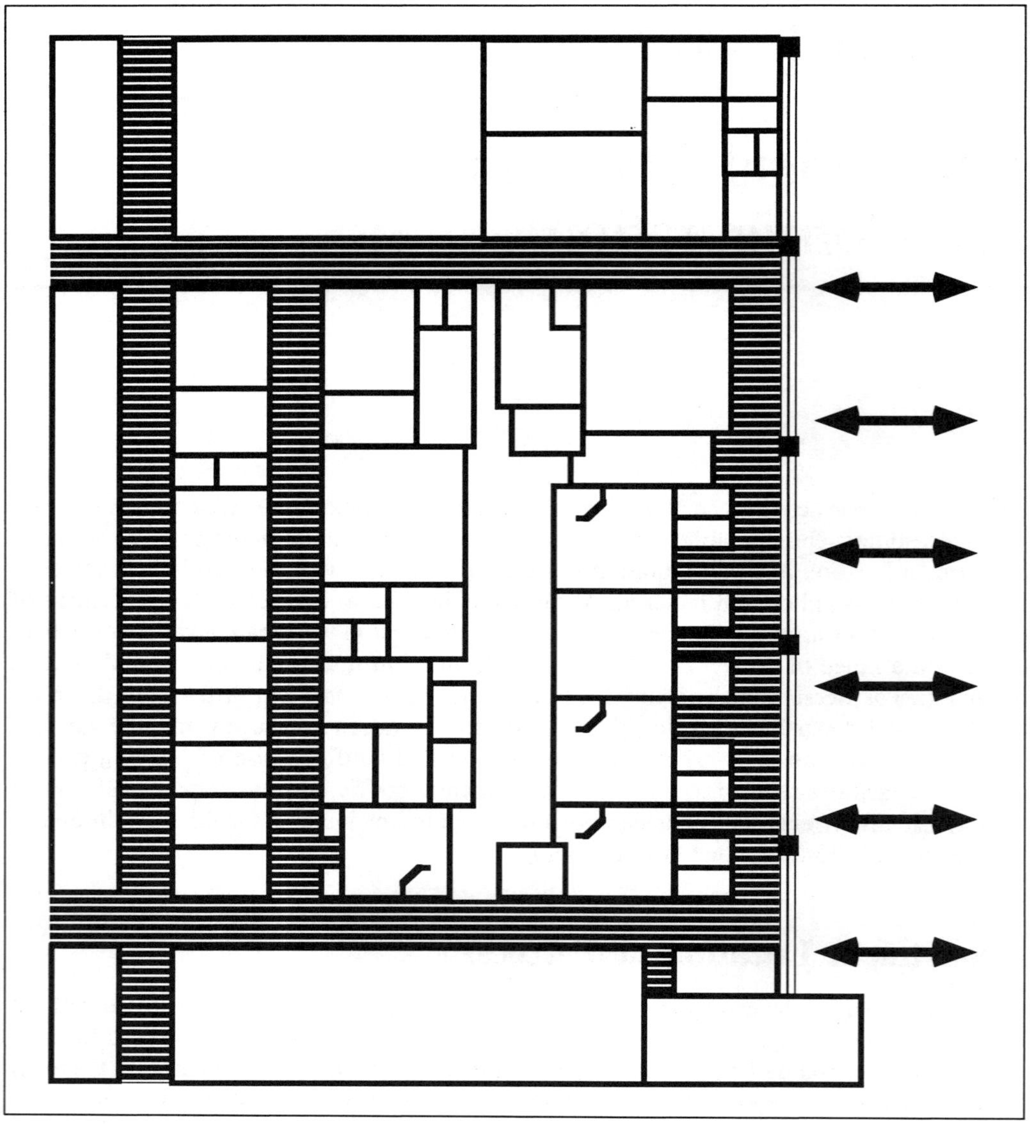

Courtesy of Stone Marraccini Patterson, San Francisco. Used with permission.

Users of Imaging Services

Imaging services often comprise at least three components: basic imaging, special imaging, and nuclear medicine (although nuclear medicine sometimes is physically separate from the other forms of imaging). *Basic imaging* includes routine procedures (for example, basic radiography and fluoroscopy) that are of short duration and in frequent demand. *Special imaging* includes procedures (for example, magnetic resonance imaging [MRI], computed tomography [CT], and interventional imaging) that are of longer duration and often require specialized equipment. *Nuclear medicine* is a unique form of imaging that measures radiation emitted from an internal source of radioactivity. Specialized forms of nuclear medicine include single-photon emission computed tomography (SPECT) and positron emission tomography (PET). Sometimes all three components are organized to form a central imaging department; sometimes basic imaging is decentralized whereas special imaging and nuclear medicine are centralized; and sometimes nuclear medicine is organized as a department separate from the other forms of medical imaging. Additionally, in some cases, special zones within the department are dedicated to certain patient groups—for example, a women's screening area

Figure 11-2. Example of Perimeter Patient Corridor

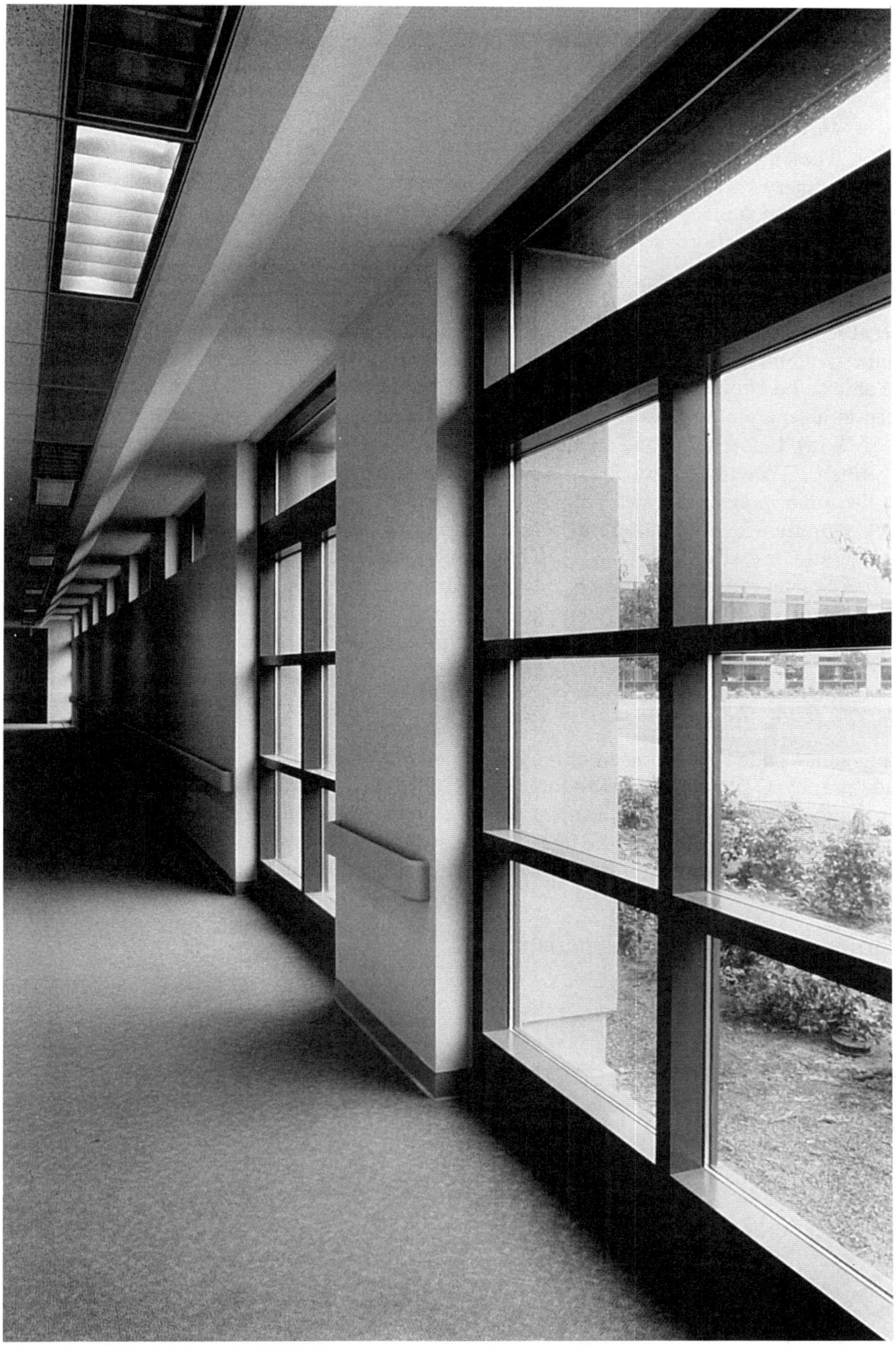

Courtesy of Stone Marraccini Patterson, San Francisco. Used with permission.

with ultrasound, mammography, and bone densitometry. (The types of imaging are described in chapter 6, "Imaging Modalities.")

Certain adjacency requirements are critical for a centralized imaging department. (See figures 11-3 and 11-4.) These include:

- Outpatient registration and clinic areas
- The emergency department (ED)
- Surgery
- Nursing units

Access from Outpatient Areas

Because more imaging functions are performed on an outpatient basis, ambulatory patients make up an increasing majority of imaging procedures. Thus, the imaging department should be able to be conveniently accessed by ambulatory patients, regardless of whether they are seen in a separate outpatient facility. In many cases, outpatients will be required to have a chest X ray, blood work, and an electrocardiogram (EKG) prior to other forms of outpatient treatment. Therefore, basic X-ray services, as part of either an outpatient imaging facility or the main imaging department, should be near each of these functions, which often are located in the vicinity of an outpatient entrance or main hospital entrance. Imaging services also should be easily accessible to specialty clinics, such as orthopedic clinics (which frequently utilize general radiography, MRI, and CT), obstetric/gynecological clinics (which use ultrasound), and oncology clinics (which use many imaging modalities such as MRI, CT, radiography, fluoroscopy, mammography, ultrasound, and nuclear medicine).

Access from the ED

Emergency patients often need immediate access to many imaging services, especially basic radiography, CT, and MRI. Most large EDs (20,000 or more annual visits) have some imaging capabilities within the department. However, even when imaging capabilities are provided in the ED, close proximity to the imaging department is desirable to facilitate additional staff and patient traffic and to improve access to specialty imaging services that are integral to

Figure 11-3. Interdepartmental Functional Relationships

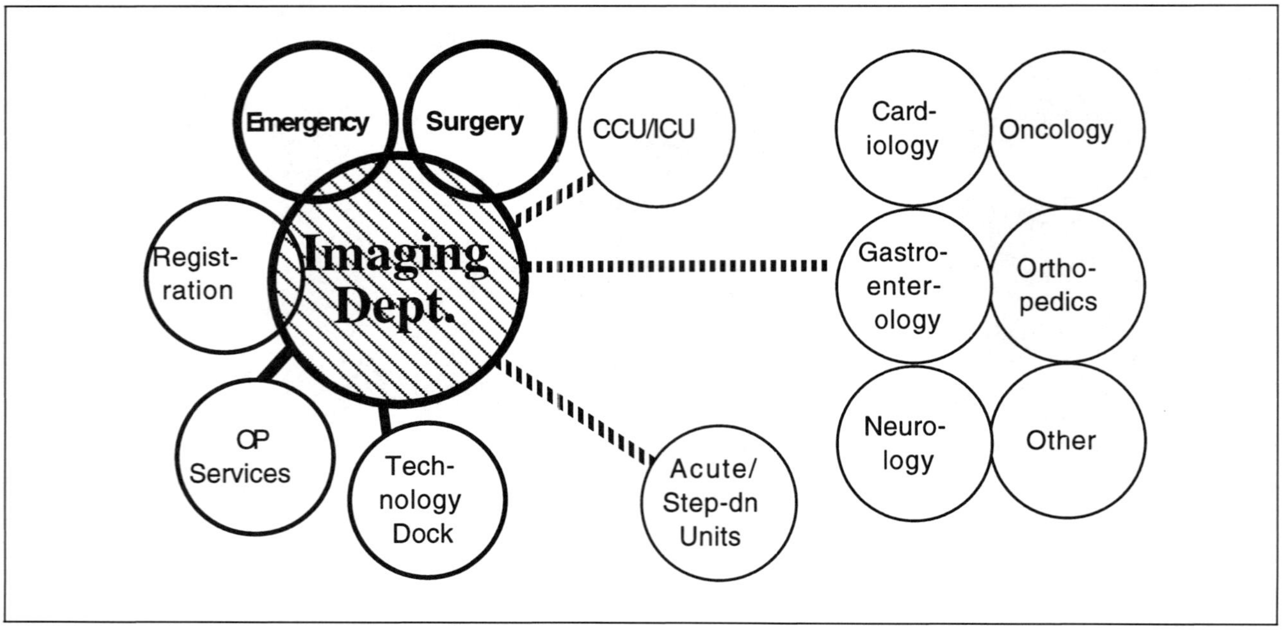

Figure 11-4. Intradepartmental Functional Relationships

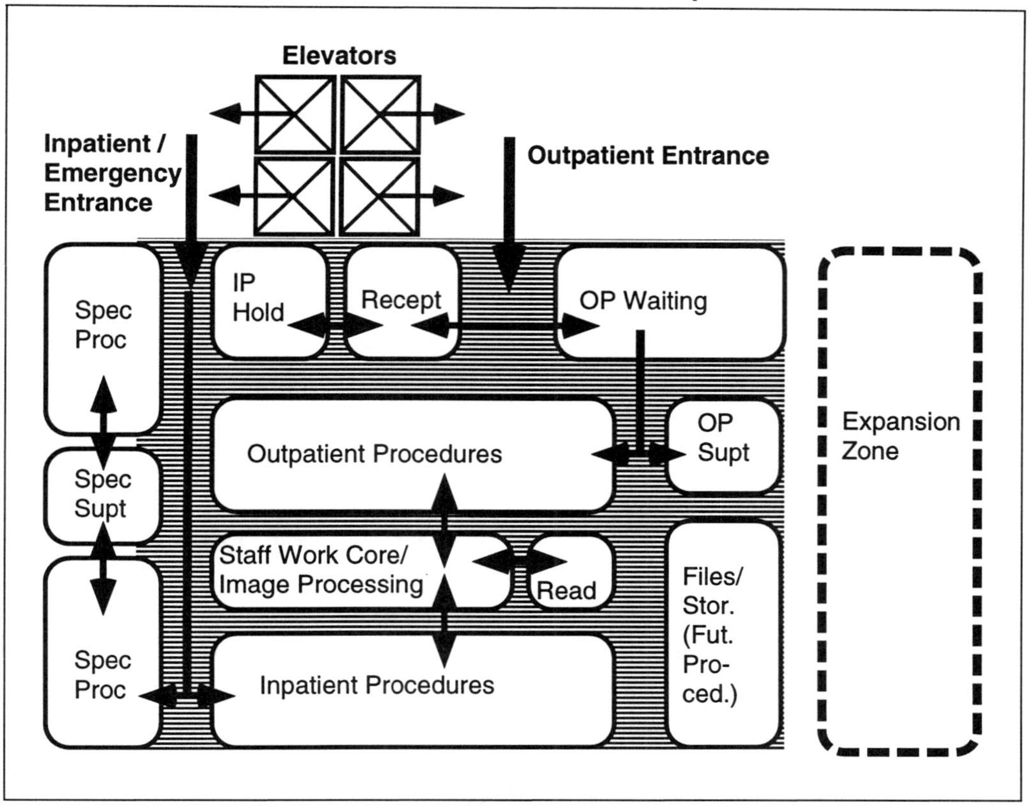

ED care. Additionally, if some imaging services are not staffed at night, the ED may be the only area that is fully staffed. Thus, if the ED is located at grade level, ideally, imaging services also should be located there. (See the section entitled Imaging and Emergency Medicine in chapter 14, "Imaging outside the Radiology Department.")

Access from Surgery

Imaging is becoming an increasingly important component of surgery, and surgical procedures are becoming an increasingly larger component of imaging. Presurgical planning, which utilizes three-dimensional CT and MRI, is useful in the preparation for complex surgical procedures. Various forms of imaging such as ultrasound, fluoroscopy, and even CT also are significant tools used within the operating suite to track surgical progress and location. Imaging itself is becoming more interventional. Surgical procedures such as stereotactic neurosurgery or biopsies may be performed within CT or even MRI suites.

Many imaging procedures now involve invasive treatment, and thus some imaging procedure rooms may require a high level of sterility and additional support spaces for additional personnel and patient observation and holding. Imaging's integral role in surgery suggests that (1) radiologists and technologists need access to surgical suites and (2) surgeons will be performing more procedures in conjunction with radiologic personnel. Therefore, both proximity and advanced communication systems between the two departments are desirable.

Imaging's interventional nature suggests that some patients may need surgical backup in the event of a medical emergency. In addition, observation of imaging patients prior to and after their procedures can sometimes be efficiently combined with the end-stage observation of surgical outpatients. (See the section entitled Imaging and Surgery in chapter 14, "Imaging outside the Radiology Department.")

Access from Nursing Units

As inpatient census declines and much of the emphasis of health care shifts to outpatient diagnosis and treatment, the patient population in the hospital generally is more critically ill than it was in the past. Thus, imaging plays a pivotal role in the management of inpatients.

In the intensive care unit (ICU), in particular, rapid turnaround of images and image interpretation is essential to the effective care of patients because their medical condition is likely to change quickly. In addition, it is important to minimize the transport of these patients. One approach is to process, interpret, and hold ICU patients' images within the ICU for the duration of the patients' stay in the unit. Another alternative to help accomplish these goals would be a partial picture archiving and communication system (PACS) connecting the ICU to a centralized imaging department. (See the section entitled Imaging in the Intensive Care Unit in chapter 14, "Imaging outside the Radiology Department.")

The imaging department should have direct access to and from elevators used for inpatient transport. (See the section entitled Transport and Information Systems in chapter 10, "Work Flow and Circulation.") In some hospitals, basic imaging services are decentralized and located near either critical care or acute care inpatient units. Generally, a cluster of approximately 100 beds is required to justify decentralized imaging in the nursing unit. If basic imaging is decentralized, specialized imaging functions are likely to remain centralized. Some of the advantages and disadvantages of decentralized imaging are discussed in the following subsection.

Centralized versus Decentralized Imaging Services

An institution's decision to centralize or decentralize imaging services within the hospital is related to that organization's overall philosophy of providing medical care. As mentioned previously, for centralized departments where both basic and specialized imaging services are located within one zone, vertical and horizontal connections to the various users of imaging services will be necessary.

In contrast, sometimes hospital imaging functions are decentralized and organized around specialty programs. Decentralized imaging usually results in a duplication of routine imaging equipment, which is located close to inpatients, in addition to a centralized imaging department where specialized imaging procedures are performed. (See figures 11-5 and 11-6.) For example, nursing units and diagnostic and treatment functions may be organized by individual

Figure 11-5. Centralized Imaging Services

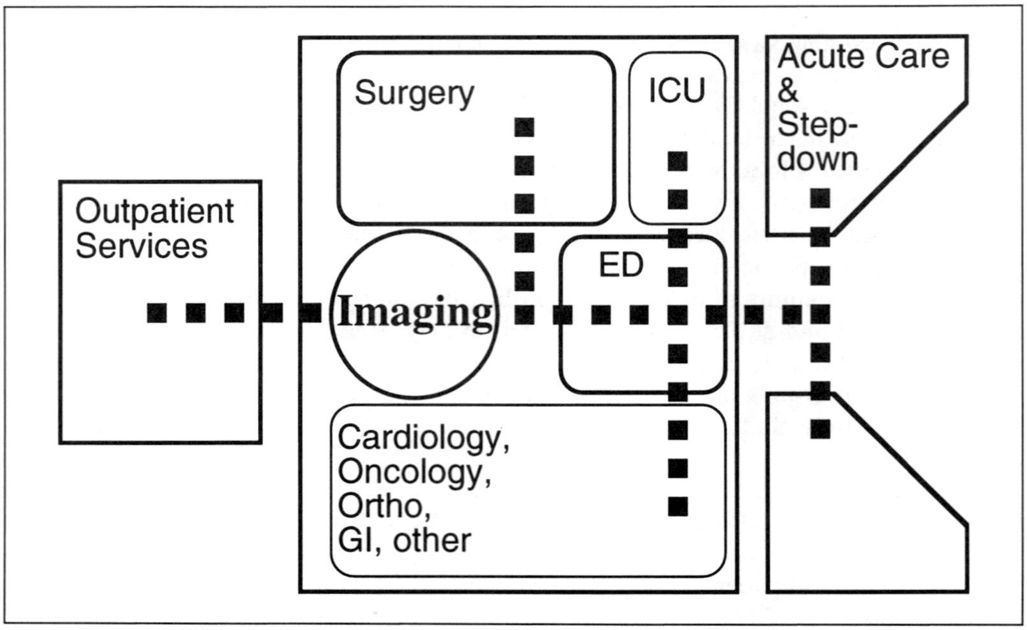

Figure 11-6. Decentralized Imaging Services

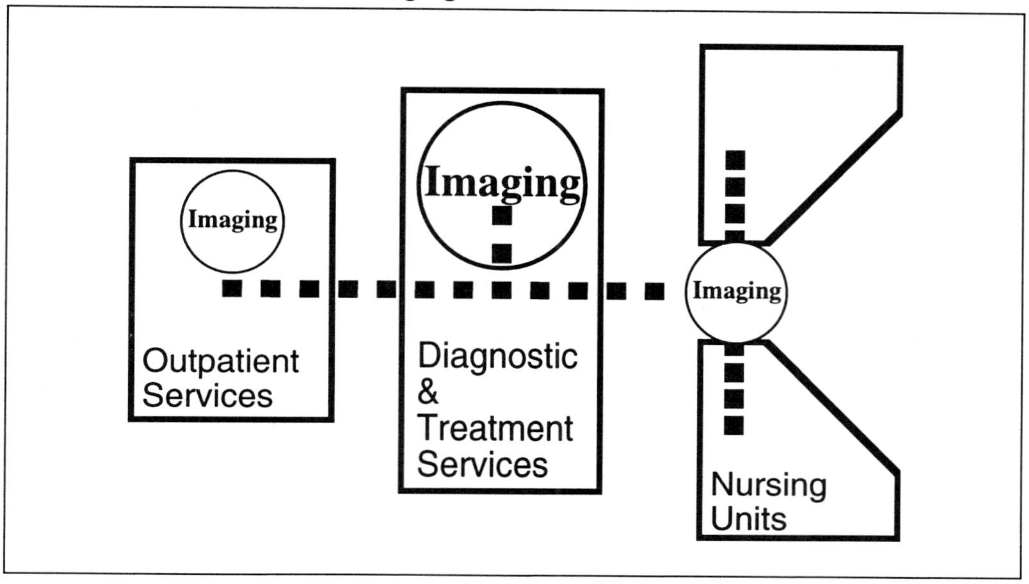

organ-specific or medical subspecialty program floors, such as musculoskeletal programs (providing orthopedic, rehabilitation, and radiology services), neurosensory programs (providing neurology, neurosurgery, and neuroradiology services), and cardiopulmonary programs (providing cardiac and thoracic surgery, cardiology, pulmonary, and radiology services). Organization based on decentralized programs often is found in large teaching hospitals where patients, staff, residents, interns, and medical students would otherwise have to frequently travel long distances between related areas.[1]

Decentralized imaging also is part of the patient-focused health care delivery strategy (discussed in chapter 2, "The Forces of Change in Imaging Facility Design") to reduce the amount of inpatient transport, to simplify the radiography work flow process, and to reduce overall labor costs. (See also the section entitled Work Flow and Circulation Principles in chapter 10, "Work Flow and Circulation.") Another form of decentralized imaging services occurs when outpatient imaging is separated from inpatient imaging. Outpatient services may be provided within a separate zone of the imaging department, a separate outpatient imaging department within the hospital campus, or a physically separate outpatient facility.

Proponents of centralized imaging claim that in a centralized department, quality control is monitored better, radiology personnel are utilized more efficiently, and equipment is not duplicated unnecessarily. On the other hand, advocates of decentralized imaging cite reduced patient transport, decreased waiting time, reduced overall labor costs, a streamlined imaging work flow process, and flexibility as beneficial outcomes of decentralizing these functions.

Decentralized imaging suggests a decentralized system of filing and scheduling that makes patient data accessible wherever they are needed. Decentralized active film can further complicate what traditionally has been one of the most problematic areas of imaging departments—keeping track of patient records and diagnostic images. Decentralized scheduling also can complicate the orderly and efficient utilization of procedure rooms. However, both these processes are areas where electronic PACSs and image management and communication systems (IMACSs) can be real assets once they become more cost-effective.

Department Configuration: The Functional Zone Concept

Numerous systems based on repetitive planning modules have been used to develop the layout of imaging departments. One notable example is a detailed system of modular radiology planning described in 1972 by Dr. Thure Holm of the University Hospital in Lund, Sweden, at the International Symposium on Planning of Radiological Departments in Finland.[2] This concept, sometimes referred to as the *functional (or concentric) zone concept,* was further described in 1982 by Dr. Harry Fischer of Strong Memorial Hospital–University of Rochester (New York) School of Medicine and Dentistry.[3] (See figure 11-7.) It comprises the following activity zones:[4]

- *Patient zone,* where waiting and patient preparation occur
- *Examination zone,* where the primary activity of imaging examination occurs
- *Central image-processing zone,* where the three functions of image handling occur
- *Personnel zone,* where staff offices and support spaces are located
- *Long-term file zone,* where inactive files are stored

Although details of Holm's and Fischer's descriptions of modular planning are somewhat dated (for example, room sizes will not necessarily apply to today's equipment and electronic image management was not considered because it was not yet available), the philosophy behind the concept is worthy of review. Their identification of separate functional zones led to a clear planning logic that has since been incorporated into many contemporary design solutions.

Patient Zone

The patient zone includes space for patients prior to and after their imaging procedure(s). Patients have their first contact with the imaging department and staff in this area. First impressions should be positive ones.

If both inpatients and outpatients are seen in the department, the patient zone can be separated into two distinct areas, each adjacent to the examination zone. Functions found in the patient zone include:

- Patient and visitor waiting areas
- Dressing rooms
- Toilet rooms
- Lockers

Figure 11-7. Functional Zone Concept

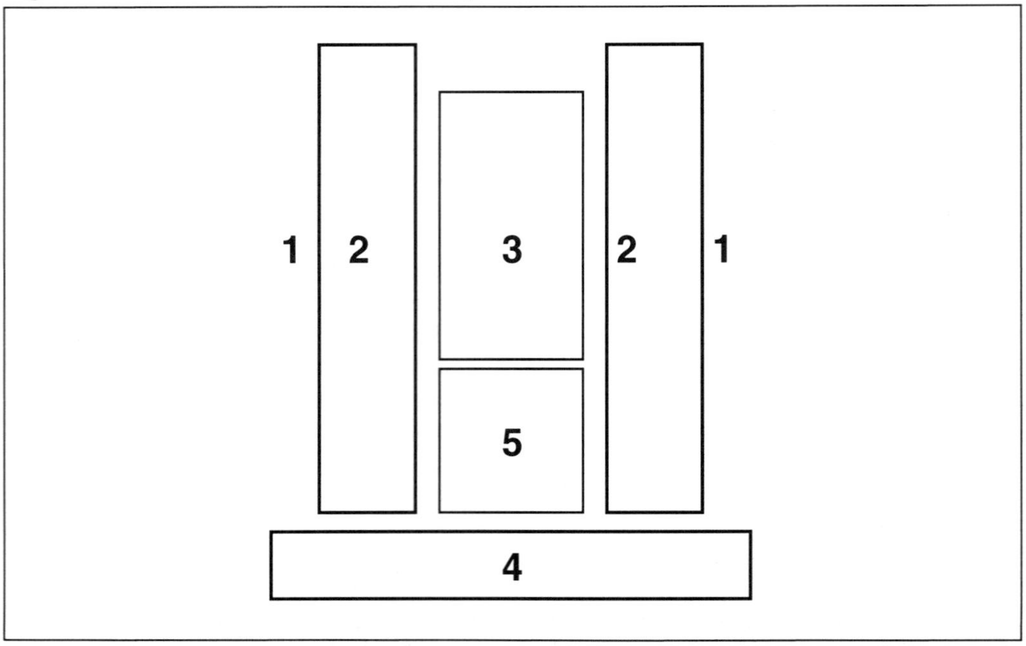

Note: (1) patient zone, (2) examination zone, (3) central image handling zone, (4) personnel zone, (5) image storage zone.

- Education space
- Reception and registration areas
- Patient corridors
- Patient preparation and holding areas

Reception and registration areas should be located in such a way that clerical staff can easily supervise waiting areas and have easy access to patient records and administration areas. A room or alcove screened from the waiting area should be provided for confidential medical or financial conversations and/or as an education space.

Sometimes, dressing areas are clustered together, with each cluster serving a series of procedure rooms, rather than locating a dressing room near each procedure room. A clustered arrangement tends to accommodate variations in work flow and thus more effectively maintain a high volume of patient examinations. Clustered dressing rooms also may accommodate the accessibility requirements of the Americans with Disabilities Act (ADA) more efficiently than do segregated dressing rooms. Additionally, patients and visitors in the waiting area should not be able to see into examination or dressing areas. If clustered dressing rooms are used, the design should preclude patients from having to travel far through public corridors to and from procedure rooms.

Examination Zone

The examination zone consists of two primary elements: examination or procedure rooms and control areas. Both patients and staff enter the examination zone. (See figure 11-8.) Patients are limited to the procedure room and the patient side of the registration area; they are not permitted in the control area.

The control area is where technologists' consoles and other equipment used to "control" the imaging procedure are located. In the functional zone concept, all control functions were removed from the procedure room and placed in a control corridor, running parallel to a series of procedure rooms.

In many facilities, however, the preferred location for control alcoves is within the procedure room. This occurs more often in basic procedure rooms than it does in special procedure rooms. Special procedure rooms often have a large control room directly adjacent to the procedure room, rather than within a control corridor. (Advantages and disadvantages of control corridors, control alcoves, and control rooms are discussed in the section entitled General Considerations for Control Corridors, Control Alcoves, and Control Rooms in chapter 13, "Room Design.")

As mentioned earlier, the imaging department should be arranged so that those procedures that are of short duration and high frequency are located near the waiting area and the department entrance. This configuration will thus reduce the amount of traffic congestion in the patient corridor.

Image-Processing Zone

Imaging departments that have been planned using the functional zone concept often have a staff work core in the center. If the control corridor approach is used, the work core abuts the control corridor. If the control corridor approach is not used, the work core abuts procedure rooms that have internal control alcoves and control rooms adjacent to the procedure rooms.

The image-processing zone provides space for three functions:

1. *Image processing, quality control, and preliminary viewing,* where the image is processed and reviewed for quality prior to being sent to the radiologist
2. *Reporting and consulting,* where the radiologist reviews and interprets the image for diagnosis and/or consults with referring physicians or others
3. *Film sorting and short-term film storage,* where active images are sorted and stored for archiving (active status may last for months or even years)[5]

Figure 11-8. Examination Zone

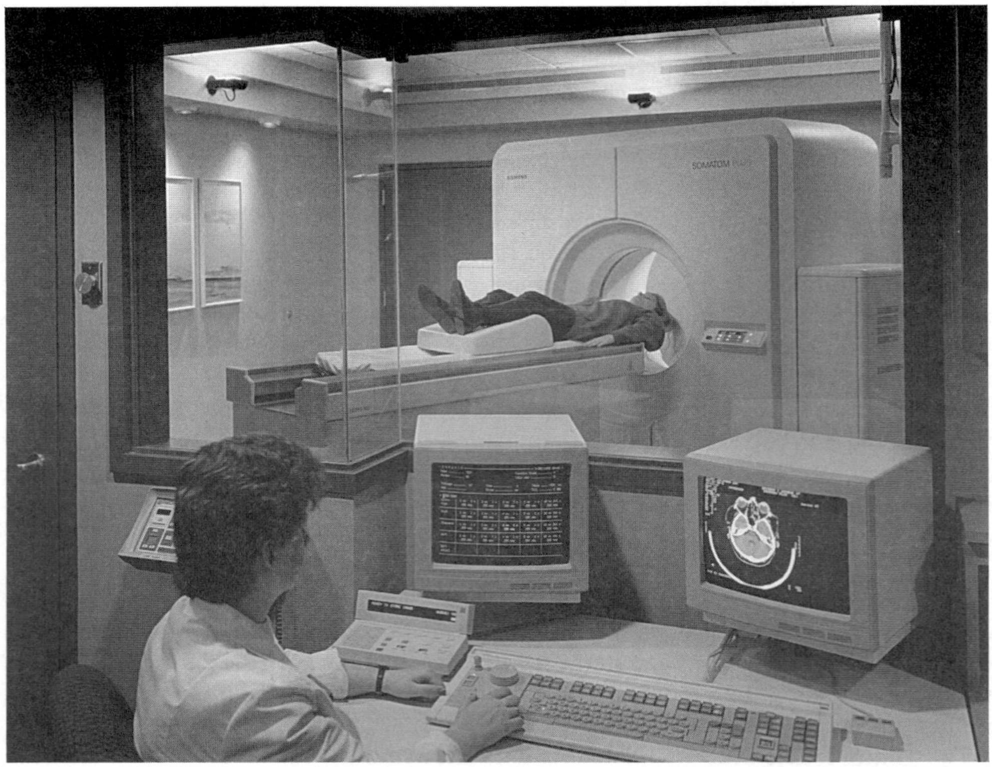

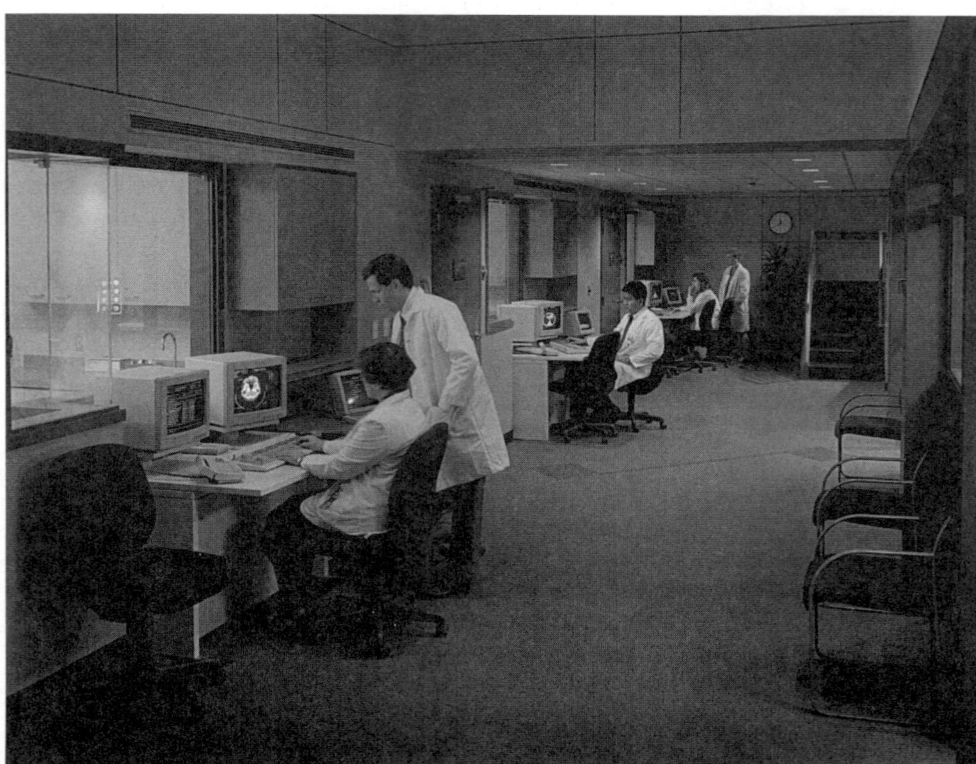

Computed tomography scan suite, Brigham and Women's Hospital, Boston. ©Steve Rosenthal, 1990. Architecture and interior design by Tsoi/Kobus & Associates. Used with permission.

In some practices, reporting and consulting are performed in the personnel zone instead of the image-processing zone.

Image processing may be film based or may utilize photo-stimulable phosphor plates. Film processing may require a darkroom, utilize daylight processing, or both. Image management may employ digital image acquisition, transmission, and archiving systems. Each approach has different facility requirements. (See the section entitled General Considerations for Image-Processing Areas in chapter 13, "Room Design.")

Personnel Zone

The personnel zone includes office space and staff support areas such as lockers, toilet rooms, lounges, and conference space. Beds and showers also may be desired. If staff lounge and conference areas are to be shared by other departments, these spaces should be located along the perimeter of the department to keep nondepartmental traffic away from busy work areas. Some department managers prefer to locate the lounge near the work area for the convenience of the technologists.

Many radiologists review and interpret images in their offices; others review and interpret them in multiviewing rooms complete with film alternators, film illuminators, and multimedia computer workstations that integrate PACS, IMACS, RIS (radiology information system), and HIS (hospital information system) capabilities. (See the section entitled General Considerations for Image-Reading/Viewing Rooms in chapter 13, "Room Design.") Adequate space and equipment must be provided for image review and interpretation to take place effectively. Often, a referring physician reading room is desired to help keep films reviewed by referring physicians in the department. If such a space is provided, it is best located adjacent to the active film filing area, but physically separate to restrict referring physicians from entering the filing area. A passbox or sliding window between the two areas allows films to be sent to the reading room, thus restricting the flow of people into the filing area. Another approach to reducing the number of misplaced films utilizes computer-transmitted images, both digitally acquired and scanned, that can be printed with a laser printer, thus mitigating the problem of lost originals.

Long-Term File Zone

State, federal, and local laws, as well as licensing regulations and individual practice philosophies, all have an impact on the length of time that inactive films must be retained. It is not uncommon for films to be archived for seven years or longer. Inactive film storage often can be located in an area remote from the main department, provided that some means of retrieving old films is practical.

To date, most states require hard-copy storage of archival films. Therefore, a considerable amount of space is still required for film files. However, if archival films are stored in a remote location and the imaging department uses an electronic image management system, archived film images can be digitized and transmitted to the department when needed, thus eliminating some of the need for extensive hard-copy storage within the department.

On the other hand, the eventual widespread use of PACSs and IMACs leads some planners to believe that storage requirements for film files will be drastically reduced—and perhaps eventually will disappear. However, this has not yet been demonstrated. Even if the amount of space required for film files decreases in the future, image-archiving space requirements will first increase, because hybrid systems composed of both film-based and filmless images will be needed during the potentially long transition period during which electronic image management systems become more popular.

Dense racks of film files will generate very high floor loads. Movable shelving units, which utilize space more efficiently than fixed shelving, generate even heavier loads. It is not uncommon for film files to require a greater structural capacity than imaging equipment. (See the section entitled General Considerations for Image and Report Storage in chapter 13, "Room

Design.") Film files that are stacked high are difficult to access and do not meet handicap accessibility requirements. Some facilities file film on only two levels.

Plan Typologies

Over the years, the size and configuration of imaging facilities has evolved in parallel with the evolution of health care facilities and imaging equipment. This section discusses a variety of common plan typologies. Many corridor-based typologies, which lack flexibility, reflect the configuration of early hospitals with long single- and double-loaded corridors. Core and cluster plans improve on their more linear predecessors and reflect an approach to planning that is appropriate for both contemporary hospital-based departments and freestanding imaging facilities. In addition:

> There are . . . [various] . . . basic layouts for diagnostic radiology departments, most related to the basic configuration of the department, each having advantages and disadvantages, all greatly influencing operational management within the department, and all inherently determining the all-important traffic patterns within the department. In large departments, combinations of basic layout schemes can serve to optimize defined segments of the total service.[6]

Many single-corridor imaging department layouts developed as a result of long, narrow hospital wings, which were common in the first three quarters of the 20th century. (See figure 11-9.) Although these layouts may be usable for small departments with small workloads, the single-corridor plan has many limitations.

First, inpatient, outpatient, staff, and service traffic are combined. In addition, there often is little separation between departmental traffic and through traffic.[7] Expansion is inconvenient and usually limited to one end, and travel routes are long, by definition. Many old single-corridor departments needing renovation are better off if they are relocated, especially if they were initially designed with short structural bays (and therefore numerous structural columns), inadequate infrastructure, and floor-to-floor heights that are incompatible with current imaging facility requirements.

The traditional double-loaded corridor plan is a slight improvement over the single-corridor arrangement. (See figure 11-10.) Although there is potential for some traffic segregation, travel distances are still long. Communication among staff and the mixing of different types of traffic remain a problem.[8] In addition, space utilization tends to be inefficient because the increased amount of corridor space is disproportionate to the limited functional advantages it provides.

The core plan solves some of the inefficiencies found in the single- and double-corridor layouts. (See figure 11-11, p. 201.) Based on a concentric arrangement of activity zones, the core plan separates staff and patient areas and allows for the separation of inpatient and outpatient traffic.

As described in the functional zone concept, the core layout allows a discrete division between patient, examination, image-processing, and personnel zones. However, central film filing can be remote. A core arrangement, circumscribed by a patient corridor, can take advantage of natural daylight if it is located along a building's perimeter. At least one edge of the department should remain unobstructed for future expansion. The core plan usually is ideal for small- and medium-sized departments (fewer than 12 procedure rooms).

The cluster plan is a modified form of the core arrangement. (See figures 11-12, p. 202, and 11-13, p. 203.) Cluster plans allow for separation of activity clusters within the examination zone. For example, basic radiography, special radiography, mammography, and ultrasound activity clusters can all be made accessible in a cluster arrangement. This is beneficial when separate zones for special patient groups are desired. In addition, a cluster arrangement usually can accommodate a physical link between the imaging department and a separate imaging dock or relocatable imaging unit.

Figure 11-9. Single-Corridor Layout

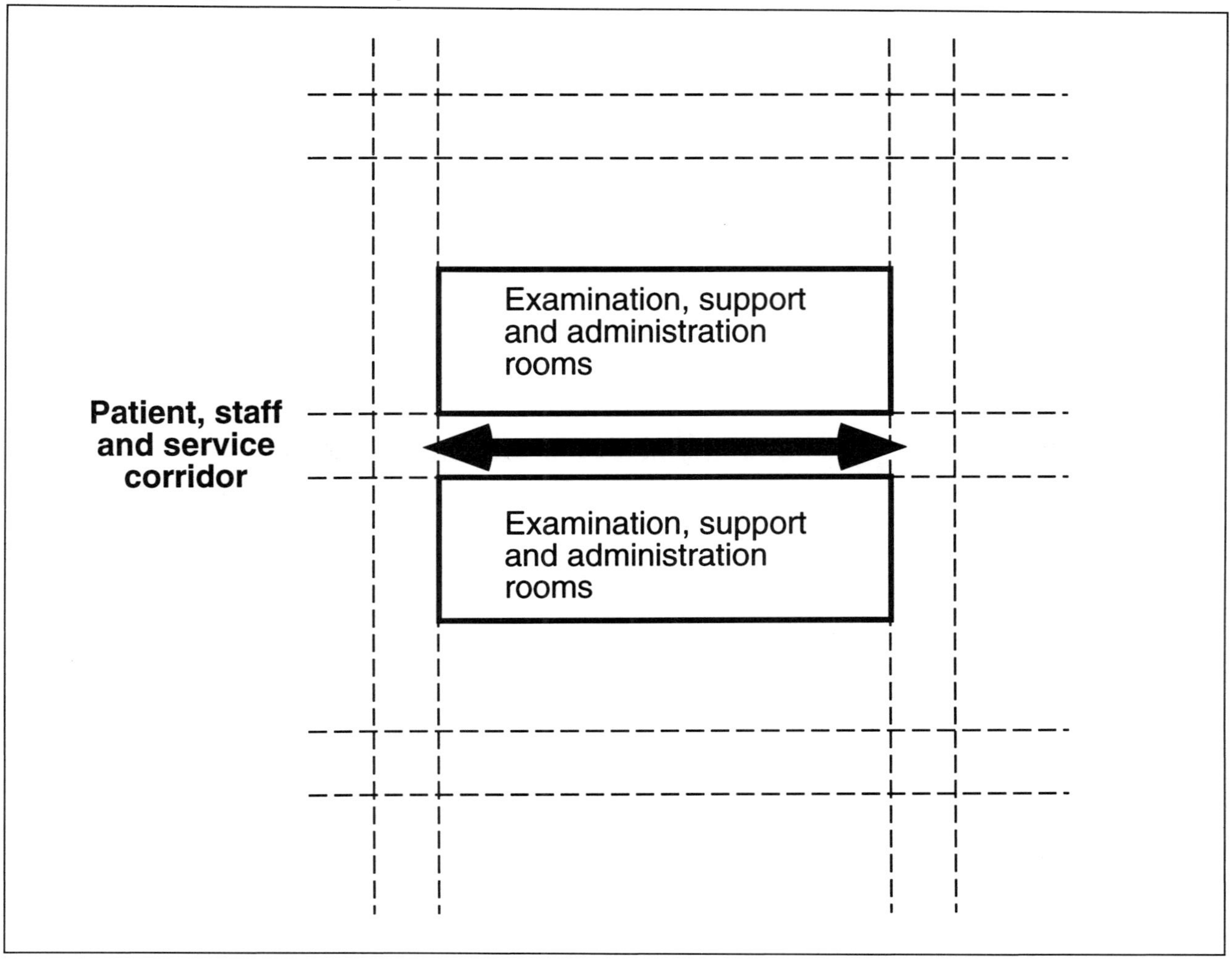

Cluster plans are ideal for most medium- and large-size facilities. They usually accommodate multiple image-processing and viewing areas without creating long travel distances for patients or staff.

Considerations for Freestanding Imaging Facilities

Criteria for the location of, and access to, freestanding imaging facilities will differ from those previously discussed in this chapter because freestanding imaging facilities, by definition, are not physically attached to hospital departments. Location criteria for freestanding centers relate more closely to health care referral patterns, community and regional demographic statistics, and the distribution of services by health plans and managed care networks. (Site location criteria are discussed in chapter 9, "Site Design.")

Imaging services in freestanding centers may be either the sole occupant of a facility or one of many outpatient-oriented tenants of a building or group of buildings. For instance, a medical office complex is likely to have imaging, laboratory, pharmacy, and other medical support services located convenient to medical offices and clinics. However, an outpatient orthopedic, cardiology, or oncology center might have specialized imaging services to support only its needs. Multiple-use facilities also may include both non–health care and health care services.

Figure 11-10. Double-Corridor Layout

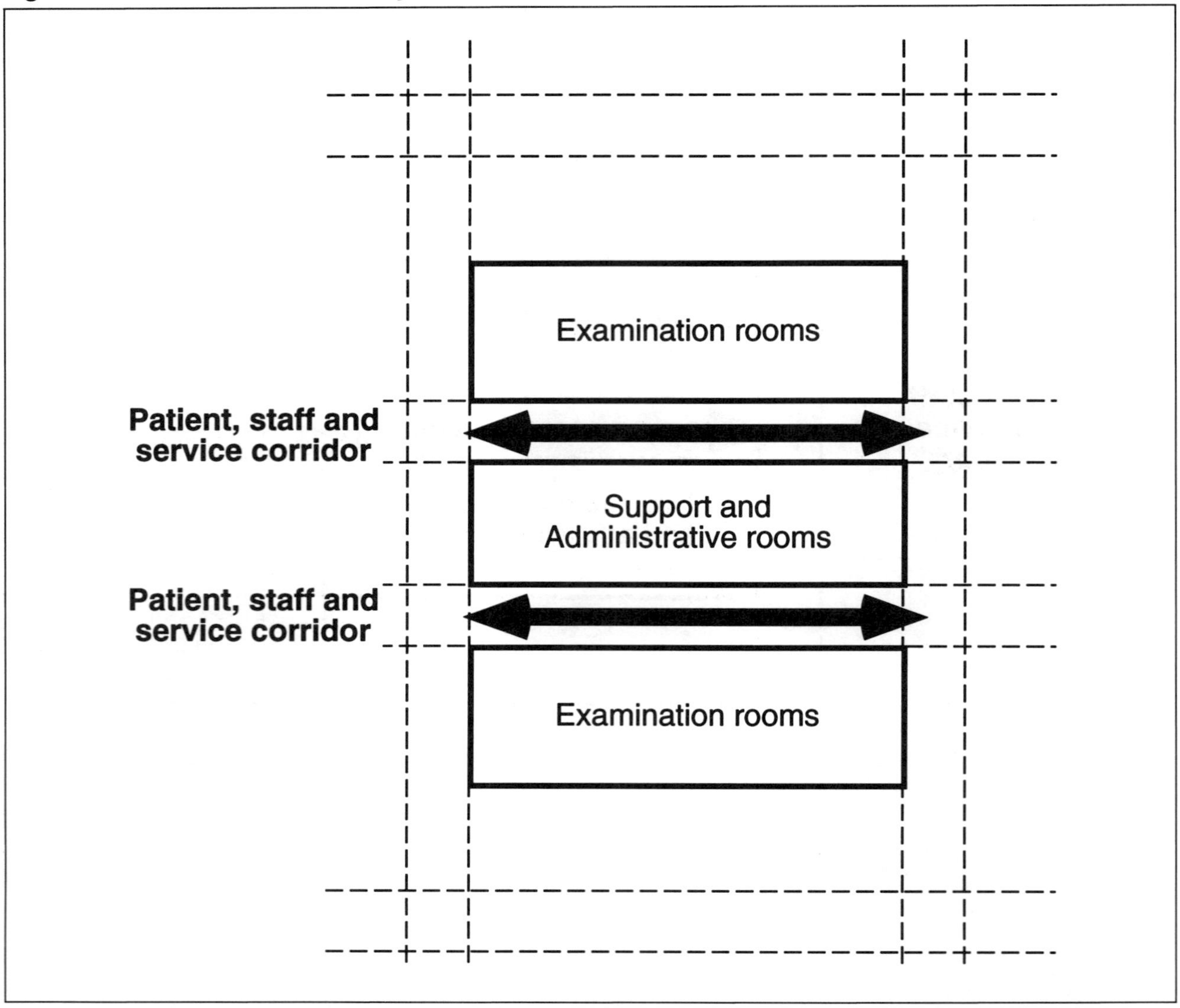

For facilities that house only imaging services, there will be fewer types of traffic and circulation. Thus, flow patterns will likely be simpler. In comparison, for centers with multiple functions, it may be more necessary to separate staff work flow from patient traffic and to segregate users of imaging services from other areas. The degree to which separate traffic routes are needed depends on the size of the facility and the extent to which the various functions within the facility are compatible. However, in any freestanding facility it is a good idea to:

- Allow staff to arrive and leave without having to pass through patient areas.
- Separate service vehicular traffic from patient traffic.
- Provide emergency access and egress routes for patients who may become unstable before, during, or after a procedure. Although freestanding facilities usually provide services to outpatients, some states allow nonambulatory patients to be examined and treated in nonhospital settings. In addition, some ambulatory patients become temporarily nonambulatory during certain procedures because some procedures are more invasive than others. Finally, not all ambulatory patients are in good health. As many aspects of health care continue to move outside the hospital, many patients who are treated in nonhospital settings will require some form of supervision or visual observation.

Figure 11-11. Core Layout

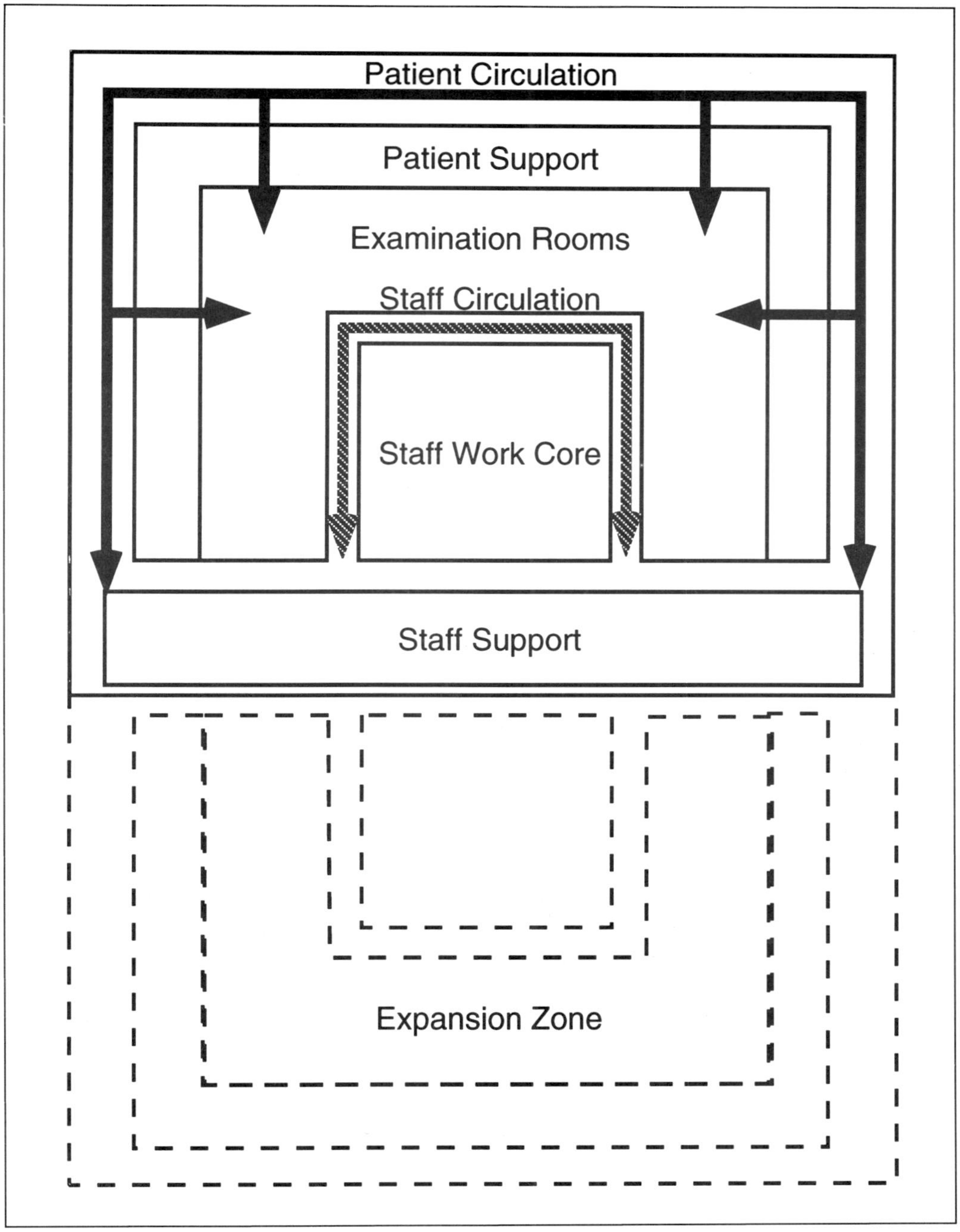

Many of the operational disadvantages of being remote from related services located in the hospital or other freestanding facilities can be mitigated through the use of electronic linkages with other facilities. For example, scheduling and billing services can be remote. Electronic PACS, IMACS, and teleradiology systems allow images and other data to be transmitted to and from remote sites. (See chapter 7, "Image Management and Film Processing.") Thus, radiologists can review images acquired in other locations, and referring physicians can review images and reports sent to their homes and offices. Additionally, remotely located archive images can be digitized and sent on an as-needed basis. Finally, special teleconferencing and interactive communication capabilities can allow real-time consultations to take place and procedures to be observed from remote facilities.

Figure 11-12. Cluster Layout

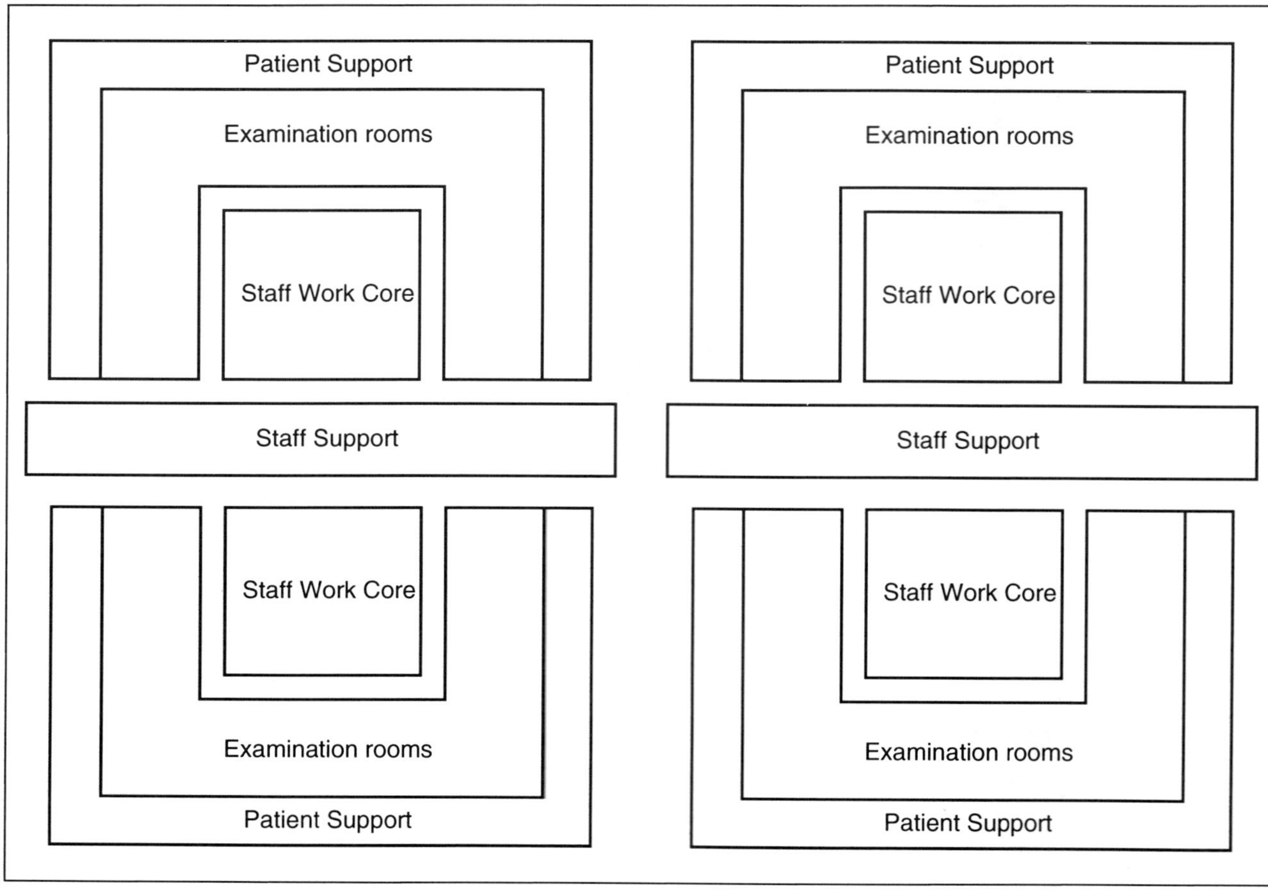

Some people contend that issues of image and appearance are more critical for freestanding ambulatory centers than they are for hospitals. Although ambiance and physical perceptions are essential design considerations for freestanding centers, this logic erroneously suggests that they are less relevant for hospital-based imaging services.

In summary, many design and planning issues are unique to freestanding facilities. Most of them have more to do with the special requirements of freestanding centers in general than with the specific nature of freestanding imaging centers. For more information on design and planning considerations for freestanding health care facilities, readers are referred to *Design Planning for Freestanding Ambulatory Care Facilities: A Primer for Health Care Providers and Architects.*[9]

References

1. Lapayowker, M. S., Kundel, H. L, and Shea, F. J. Planning of a vertically oriented radiology department in a program-floor hospital. In: M. Kormano and F. E. Stieve, editor(s). *Planning of Radiology Departments.* Stuttgart, Germany: Georg Thiem Publishers, 1974, p. 97.
2. Kormano, M., and Stieve, F. E. Planning of radiological departments—international symposium. Dipoli, Otaniemi, Finland, 1974, pp. 126–32.
3. Fischer, H. W. *Radiology Departments: Planning, Operation, and Management.* Ann Arbor, MI: Edwards Brothers, 1982.
4. Fischer.
5. Fischer, p. 6.

6. Brogdon, B. G. *Planning Guide for Radiologic Installations, Fascicle 4a: Basic Concepts: Layout Considerations—Diagnostic Departmental Planning: Location, Configuration and Layout for Diagnostic Radiology.* Chicago: American College of Radiology, 1977, pp. 32–45.
7. Brogdon.
8. Brogdon.
9. Rostenberg, B. *Design Planning for Freestanding Ambulatory Care Facilities: A Primer for Health Care Providers and Architects.* Chicago: American Hospital Publishing, 1986 [out of print].

Figure 11-13. Floor Plan Showing Cluster Layout

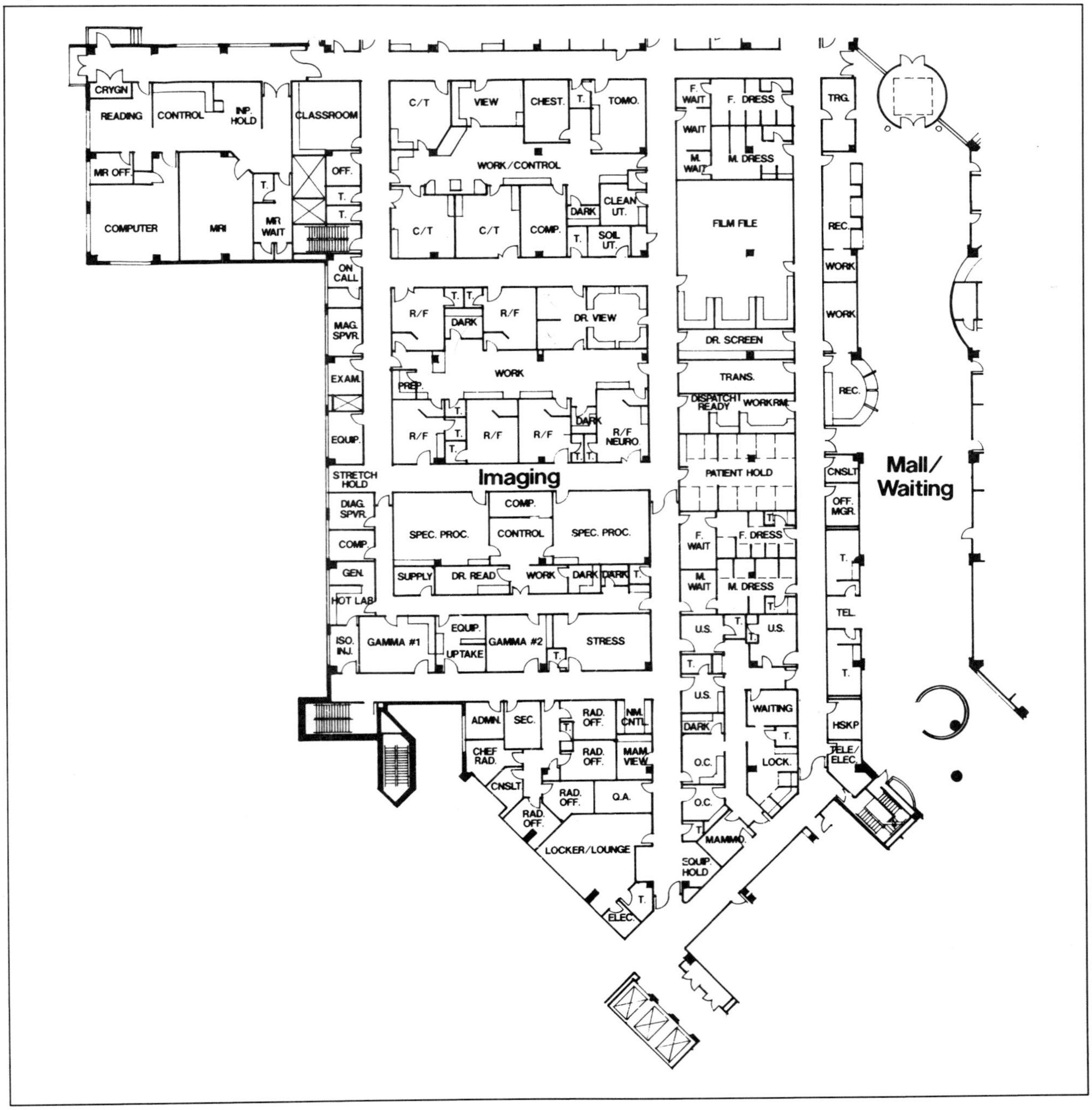

Courtesy of HKS Architects, Dallas, Texas. Used with permission.

Chapter 12

Space Requirements

Planning for too much space costs a lot of money; planning for too little costs even more! With all the complexity and continually changing variables associated with medical imaging, how is it possible to determine the size of an imaging facility, to determine the number and size of procedure rooms needed and their optimum configuration? Because all facilities are unique, there is no single answer to a question such as "How big is a radiology department?" any more than there is an answer to "How big is a house?"

Determining space requirements is a rigorous and complex process that depends on the outcome of other related studies, such as strategic analysis and functional programming. However, some individuals tend to look for quick solutions. Although a broadbrush approach might be acceptable at a project's inception when no more than order-of-magnitude information is needed to see whether it is financially viable, to continue detailed planning without verifying preliminary guesstimates is inappropriate. The penalty paid for bypassing detailed functional and space programming is the creation of a facility that either cannot operate efficiently or will soon require costly renovation.

This chapter describes a general methodology for determining space requirements for any imaging facility and identifies the variables that influence the size of a specific institution. Discussion includes how to project the type, number, and size of procedure rooms required, as well as the amount and size of support space required. Space requirements for any particular imaging facility can be most accurately determined only after conducting a careful analysis of the facility's needs.

Space Determinant Methodology for the Imaging Facility

Planning for the space requirements for an imaging facility requires interaction among facility planners and facility users. Two processes—functional programming and space programming—must precede the design and planning stages. *Functional programming* evaluates historic and present workload data in order to calculate future projections. Thus, functional programming is the first step in the umbrella process of programming. Its end product describes anticipated workloads (quantity, duration, and mix of procedures) in terms of staffing, equipment, and work flow. *Space programming* translates the functional program into area requirements. It includes a list describing the size, number, and spatial characteristics of every room and department in the facility.[1]

Space programming begins with a series of interviews among planners and the administrative and medical users of the facility during which the planning team collects and reviews data, projects anticipated workloads, and calculates requirements. Following are the key components involved in those activities:

- Data collection (provided by facility users)
  - –Existing workload in terms of procedure mix and quantity
  - –Existing staffing requirements
  - –Existing equipment requirements
  - –Historic workload data to determine past trends (where applicable)
  - –Degree of satisfaction with existing space, equipment, and facility
- Workload projections (determined by functional programming team in conjunction with facility users)
  - –Assumptions regarding future trends, based on operational goals, market changes, and changes in technology
  - –Future workload in terms of procedure mix and quantity
  - –Staffing projections to accommodate future workload
  - –Equipment projections to accommodate future workload
- Space and functional requirements (determined by programming and planning team in conjunction with facility users)
  - –Area requirements to accommodate future workload (number and size of rooms to accommodate anticipated patient examinations, consultations, treatment, and so on)
  - –Area requirements to accommodate future staffing
  - –Area requirements to accommodate future equipment
  - –Estimated area requirements to accommodate future expansion
  - –Functional adjacencies
  - –Work flow and traffic patterns

The user group interviews will disclose varying opinions from different individuals within the organization (administrators, radiologists, technologists, nurses, physicists, engineers, housekeeping personnel, clerical staff, patient advocates, and so on). Because the most vocal individuals may not necessarily be those with the most authority, recording individual requests without obtaining some degree of consensus from the group can prove misleading. Thus, the planning team will benefit from having one key individual from each user group first take responsibility for reviewing and verifying the collected data and then become part of the review process all the way through the contract document and construction phases of service.

Key Space Generators

For each type of room or area there usually is a primary driver, or *key space generator,*[2] that best determines its number, size, and shape. Key space generators include units of work (for example, admissions per year), number of staff, and size of equipment.

However, some types of rooms are affected by more than one key space generator. For example, the optimal number of radiographic rooms is determined primarily by the anticipated number of annual exams, whereas each room's size and shape are influenced by the array of equipment and how it will be used. An additional key space generator for a radiographic room in a teaching hospital having the same equipment as its community hospital counterpart might be the need to provide additional space for observers of, or participants in, a procedure.

In contrast to radiographic rooms, which are sized according to workload and equipment requirements, offices are sized according to the number of occupants and their importance within the organization, the number of people involved in consultations, how the office is used, and, therefore, the size and arrangement of furniture. Workload (the number of consultations) has little influence on office size. The number of offices required is based on staffing, which is indirectly a result of both workload and number of procedure rooms. In teaching facilities, the number of offices may be higher than in nonteaching facilities.

Types of Space

Most imaging facilities are composed of three types of space: activity, support, and administration. (See the section entitled Economy in chapter 8, "Design Concepts.") *Activity space* reflects the primary activity of the facility and is the key determinant of department area. The required number of activity spaces (for example, procedure rooms) is determined by the department's anticipated workload.

The size and configuration of imaging rooms often are determined by clearances required for the specific imaging equipment selected. Room dimensions are further influenced by patient flow, staff flow, and ancillary equipment that will be used within the room. It is good practice to size rooms larger than the manufacturer's minimum dimensions. (See table 12-1.)

Support space and *administration space* directly assist the function of activity spaces, whose characteristics determine their number and size. (See table 12-2 for guidelines to be used in determining estimates for support space size.) For example, control rooms assist the

Table 12-1. Procedure Room Size Guidelines

Procedure Room	Minimum Dimensions: Length × Width (ft)	Suggested Dimensions: Length × Width (ft)	Suggested Ceiling Height	Remarks
Chest room without film processor	11 × 10	12 × 11	9′6″	Includes control. (See figure 12-7.)
Chest room with film processor	14 × 12	16 × 14	9′6″	Includes control. (See figure 12-9.)
General radiography	16 × 12	17 × 15 to 20 × 16	9′6″	Includes control. (See figure 12-10; also see Universal Room Design in chapter 13, "Room Design.")
Routine fluoroscopy	16.5 × 12	20 × 16	9′6″	Includes control. (See Universal Room Design in chapter 13, "Room Design.") Remote control also common.
Universal R/F	N/A	20 × 16	9′6″	Includes control. (See Universal Room Design in chapter 13, "Room Design.")
Special procedures/ angiography	26 × 18	28 × 22; varies	10′0″	Excludes control room and equipment room. (See figures 12-11 and 12-12.)
CT	Varies	28 × 19; varies	Varies	Includes operator's console and computer equipment. (See figure 12-13.)
Nuclear medicine with one full-body scanning camera	Varies	18 × 16; Varies	9′0″	See figure 12-14.
Nuclear medicine with two scanning cameras	Varies	35 × 17	9′0″	See figure 12-15.
MRI	Varies	Varies	Varies	See figures 12-16 and 12-17.
Mammography (upright unit)	8.5 × 10	10 × 12	8′0″	See figure 12-18.
Mammography (prone unit)	12 × 12	18 × 12	8′0″	See figure 12-18.
Ultrasound	10 × 12	11 × 14 or 12 × 12.5; varies	8′0″	See figure 12-20.

Note: Minimum dimensions should be avoided. Suggested dimensions vary with specific equipment.

Table 12-2. Support Space Size Guidelines

Area	Space Guidelines	Remarks
Waiting, public	15–17 NSF per seat; allow 20 NSF per seat for areas with fewer than 10 seats	Assume 3–4 seats per routine procedure room.
Waiting, gowned	15 NSF per seat	Assume 1–2 seats per routine procedure room when dressing areas are not adjacent to the procedure room.
Reception	50–65 NSF per position	
Dressing areas	35 NSF for wheelchair accessible; 16 NSF for standard	Assume 1–1.5 dressing cubicles per procedure room for most scheduled routine procedures. Assume 5–6 dressing cubicles per dedicated chest room. Assume 1–2 dressing cubicles per routine fluoroscopy room. Consider clustering dressing cubicles together.
Control alcove	25–35 NSF (usually included as part of procedure room area)	See General Considerations for Control Corridors, Control Alcoves, and Control Rooms in chapter 13, "Room Design."
Control room, special R/F procedures	120–200 NSF, depending on equipment and personal needs	See above.
Control room, CT	Varies	See above.
Control room, MRI	Varies	See above.
Toilet room	50 NSF for wheelchair-accessible, single-accommodation toilet room; 65 NSF if there are two doors into the toilet room.	Assume 1 per R/F or fluoroscopy room; also at least 1 for ultrasound, CT, and MRI.
Darkroom	50–120 NSF; varies with equipment	See General Considerations for Image-Processing Areas in chapter 13, "Room Design."
Light room/image quality assurance	40–60 NSF	Locate near darkroom; also see above.
Image-reading alcove—film illuminators, standing	20–25 NSF/ workstation	See General Considerations for Image-Reading/Viewing Rooms in chapter 13, "Room Design."
Image-reading alcove—film illuminators, seated	30–45 NSF/ workstation	See above.
Image-reading alcove—alternator and film illuminators	70–80 NSF/ workstation	See above.
Image-reading alcove—alternator, film illuminators, and computer workstation	90–140 NSF/ workstation	See above.

Table 12-2. (Continued)

Area	Space Guidelines	Remarks
Image-reading room/private consultation office—film illuminators and computer workstation	80–120 NSF	See above.
Image-reading room/private consultation office—alternator and film illuminators	160–200 NSF	See above.
Group reading room with computer workstations	40–65 NSF per person	See above.
Film files	Approx. 15–20 lineal inches of file per NSF of floor space for static open shelving, 6 rows high; approx. 40–45 lineal inches of file per NSF of floor space for compact mobile shelving, 6 rows high	See General Considerations for Image and Report Storage in chapter 13, "Room Design." Space guidelines will vary by manufacturer and type of filing system.
Housekeeping closet	40 NSF	
Clean supply room	50–100 NSF	Size depends, in part, on how clean linen is supplied and stored.
Soiled utility room	50–100 NSF	Size depends, in part, on how soiled linen is held and removed.
Patient holding/ recovery	80–100 NSF per position; 1–2 positions per invasive procedure, CT, or MRI room	Provide gases and suction, nurse call, and intercom. Consider grouping holding areas together for efficient observation of patients. A nurse's station with medication storage is needed near holding and recovery areas.
Conference room	20 NSF per person	
Staff lounge	10–12 NSF per person	Provide staff toilet room adjacent.
Crash cart alcove	10–20 NSF	
Storage, radioactive decay	40–60 NSF	Varies; radiation protection to be determined by certified health physicist.
Storage alcove, portable X-ray equipment	25–35 NSF/portable X-ray unit; 45–55 NSF/portable C-arm	Assume 1 portable unit or C-arm per 4–6 operating rooms without fixed X-ray equipment.[a] Assume 1 portable unit or C-arm per 6–10 ICU beds.

[a]Laufman, H., editor. *Hospital Special Care Facilities: Planning for User Needs.* New York City: Academic Press, 1981, p. 218.

function of computed tomography (CT) scanning rooms. The number and size of control rooms and computer rooms are determined by the type and quantity of CT equipment, the anticipated CT workload, and the number of staff and equipment in the control room. Similarly, administration space (office and clerical area) requirements are determined by the number and type of staff needed to support and operate the imaging equipment and to assist imaging patients.

Activity Clusters

In most instances, certain types of spaces are grouped together in what can be called an *activity cluster.* The individual spaces in the activity cluster work together to support various functions. In the case of film processing, a darkroom (or daylight processing area), an image quality viewing area, and a film-sorting area form an activity cluster. (See figure 12-1.) Separate tasks are performed within each space, and yet if one of the spaces is not provided, the entire film-processing activity cannot be accomplished. Thus, a film-processing room usually is supported by a viewing area to verify image quality before the patient dresses again. A film-processing activity cluster can be centralized (supporting many procedure rooms), decentralized (supporting a select group of rooms with imaging equipment that can all share the same type of processor), or dedicated (located within the procedure room and attached to an individual piece of imaging equipment. When film processing occurs in the procedure room, image quality can be checked without a separate viewing area. With some image acquisition techniques such as MRI and CT, image quality is reviewed on computer monitors.

Figure 12-1. Activity Cluster: Film Processing

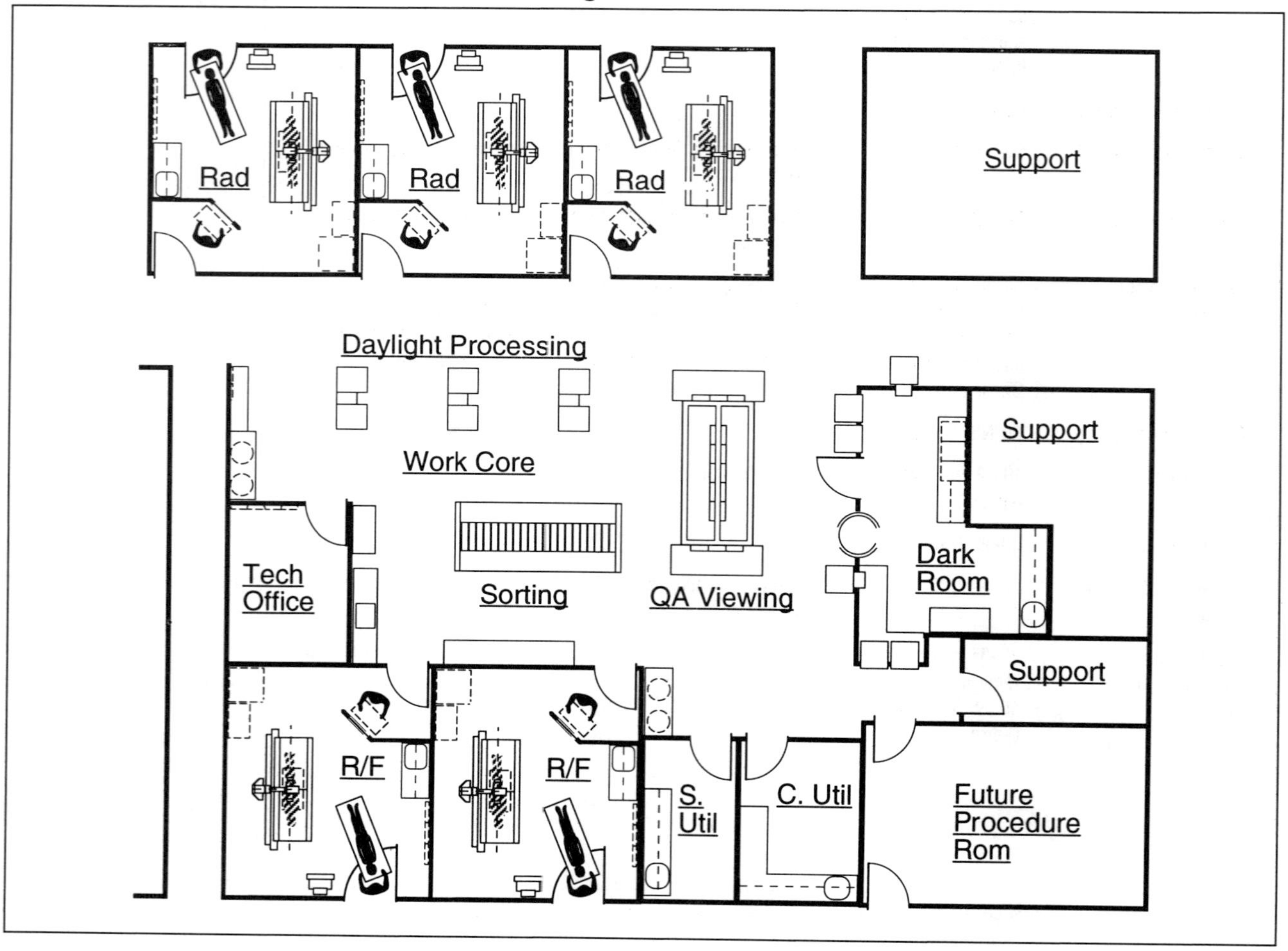

Other examples of activity clusters include:

- Fluoroscopy room/toilet room (so that patients can eliminate immediately following the exam in the event barium enemas are used)
- Ultrasound room/toilet room (so that patients undergoing abdominal ultrasound can eliminate large quantities of water consumed prior to the exam)
- Radiography room/control area/dressing area (see figures 12-2 to 12-5, pp. 211–14)
- CT scanning room/patient prep and holding area/control
- Nuclear medicine scanning room/toilet/dressing/holding/dose room (figure 12-6, p. 215)
- Positron emission tomography (PET) scanning room/cyclotron/dose room

Sometimes one support room within an activity cluster can support multiple activity rooms. For instance, two multicubicle dressing areas (one for men and one for women) can support a group of procedure rooms, rather than one or two dressing cubicles being assigned to each room.

Magic Numbers: Quick Formulas for Determining Facility Size

Over the years, numerous formulas or quick rules of thumb have been developed for calculating the optimal size of imaging facilities. Sometimes they are referred to as magic numbers.[3] Unfortunately, many of these do not take into account the numerous variables involved in developing space requirements. Additionally, many of these formulas were developed years ago and do not reflect recent developments in medical imaging. For example, many older

Figure 12-2. Activity Cluster: Radiography Exam

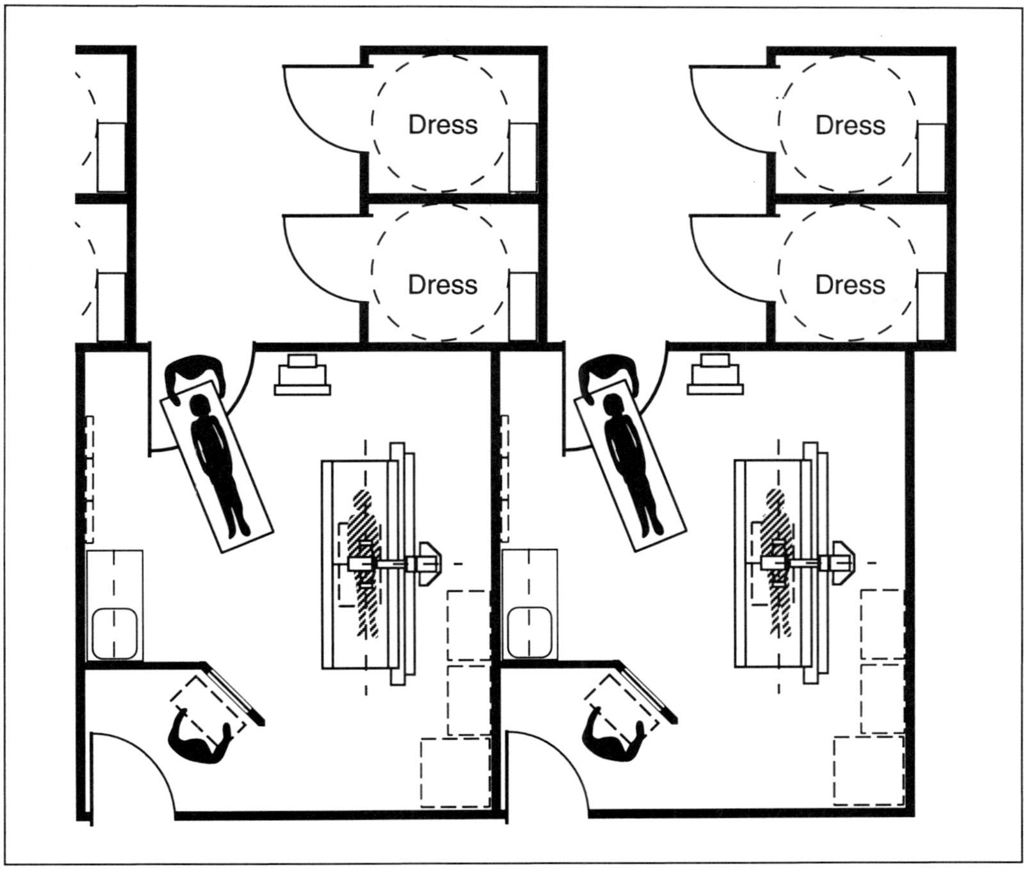

Figure 12-3. Activity Cluster: Radiography or Radiography/Fluoroscopy Exam

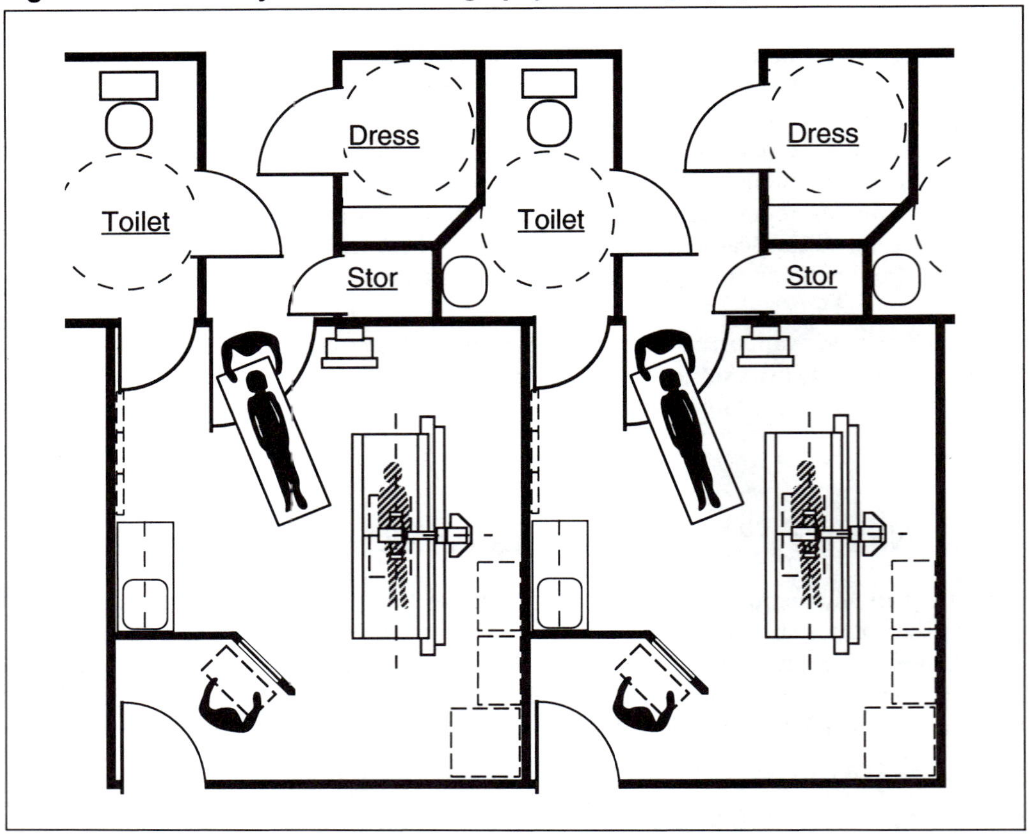

formulas calculate the size of an imaging department by suggesting a certain number of square feet (SF) per hospital bed. Square-feet-per-bed formulas are very misleading because the diagnostic and treatment space needed relative to the number of inpatient beds has changed dramatically over the past 10 years. Other formulas may be useful for undertaking feasibility studies and deriving very broadbrush estimates. (See chapter 3, "Organization of an Imaging Project.") However, they should not be used for facility planning unless their accuracy has been verified by preparing a detailed functional and space program. The following quick formulas (many of which are out-of-date) should be used only to derive the most preliminary order-of-magnitude estimates of space, if they are used at all:

1. Assume 3.4 to 4.5 annual procedures per departmental gross square foot (DGSF), or the projected number of annual procedures ÷ 3.4 to 4.5 = DGSF. For example, 50,000 annual procedures ÷ 3.4 to 4.5 requires a department of approximately 11,111 to 14,705 DGSF.[4]
2. Assume 40 DGSF per hospital bed.[5]
3. Assume 1.3 to 1.5 procedures per hospital bed occupancy day, or 0.18 to 0.20 procedures per bed occupancy day + one procedure for every 5 to 6 outpatient visits + one procedure for every 2.5 to 3.0 emergency patients, and assume each procedures room can handle between 5,000 and 7,000 procedures per year. For example, a hospital performing 50,000 annual procedures would require 50,000 ÷ 5,000 to 7,000 = 7 to 10 rooms.

Using the average 6,000 per year figure, a hospital performing 50,000 procedures would require approximately eight rooms.

(50,000 ÷ 6,000 = 8±).

For non-teaching hospitals, one diagnostic room for each 20 daily procedures [was considered] an accepted guideline. Using a 250 work-day year, a hospital performing 50,000 annual procedures would be doing 200 procedures a day

(50,000 ÷ 250 = 200)

and would require 10 diagnostic rooms (200 ÷ 20 = 10).[6]

4. Assume 4.1 to 4.6 annual procedures per departmental gross square foot (DGSF), or projected number of annual procedures ÷ 4.1 to 4.6 = DGSF. For example, 50,000 annual procedures ÷ 4.1 to 4.6 requires a department of approximately 10,870 to 12,195 DGSF.[7] (Note: Compare these numbers to those in example 1.)
5. Assume that the DGSF for radiology departments in nonteaching hospitals is 4.5 to 5 times the total net square footage (NSF) of all the X-ray procedure rooms and that the DGSF for teaching hospitals is 6 to 7 times the NSF of all the X-ray procedure rooms. For example, if 8 X-ray rooms at 350 NSF are programmed, the size of the department for a nonteaching hospital would be approximately 12,600 DGSF = ([350 × 8] × 4.5) to 14,000 DGSF = ([350 × 8] × 5). For a teaching hospital, the size of the department would be approximately 16,800 DGSF = ([350 × 8] × 6) to 19,600 DGSF = ([350 × 8] × 7).[8]
6. Assume that the DGSF is equal to 1,100 to 1,300 DGSF times the number of procedure rooms in the department.
7. Assume that the approximate number of procedure rooms needed = the projected annual procedures ÷ 6,000 to 8,000 annual procedures per room.

Figure 12-4. Activity Cluster: Radiography Exam

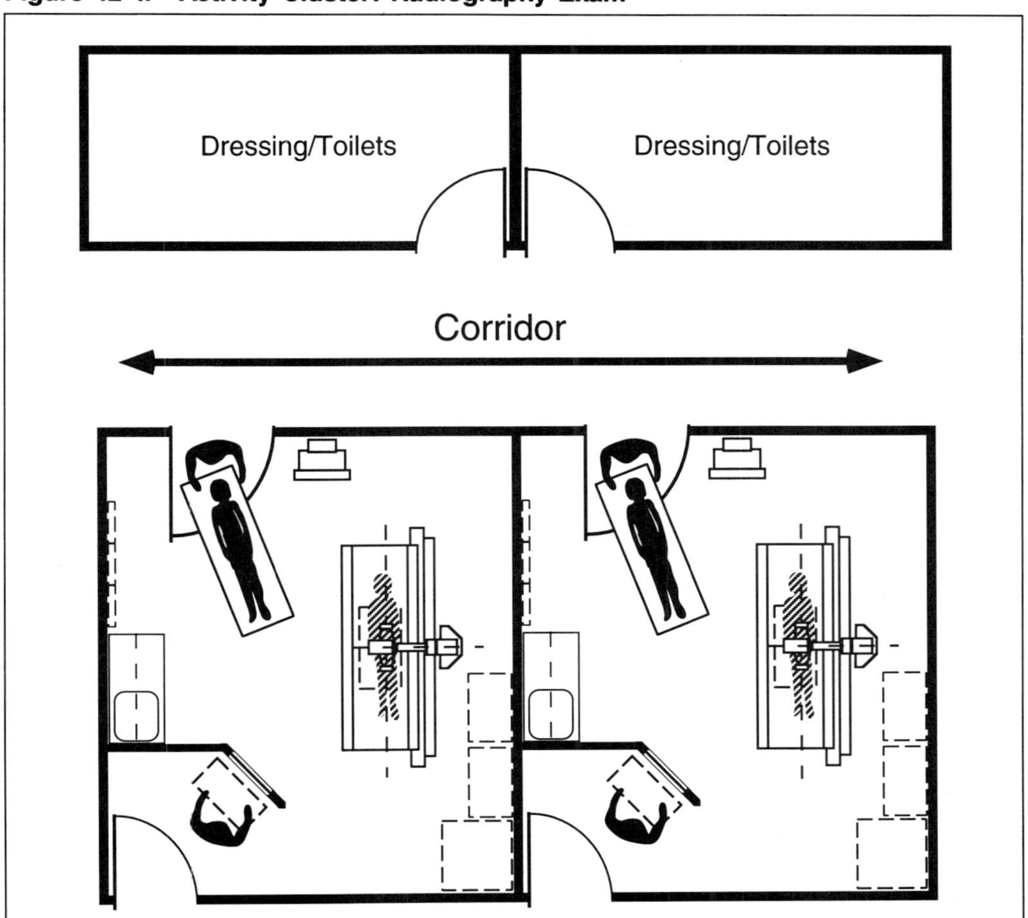

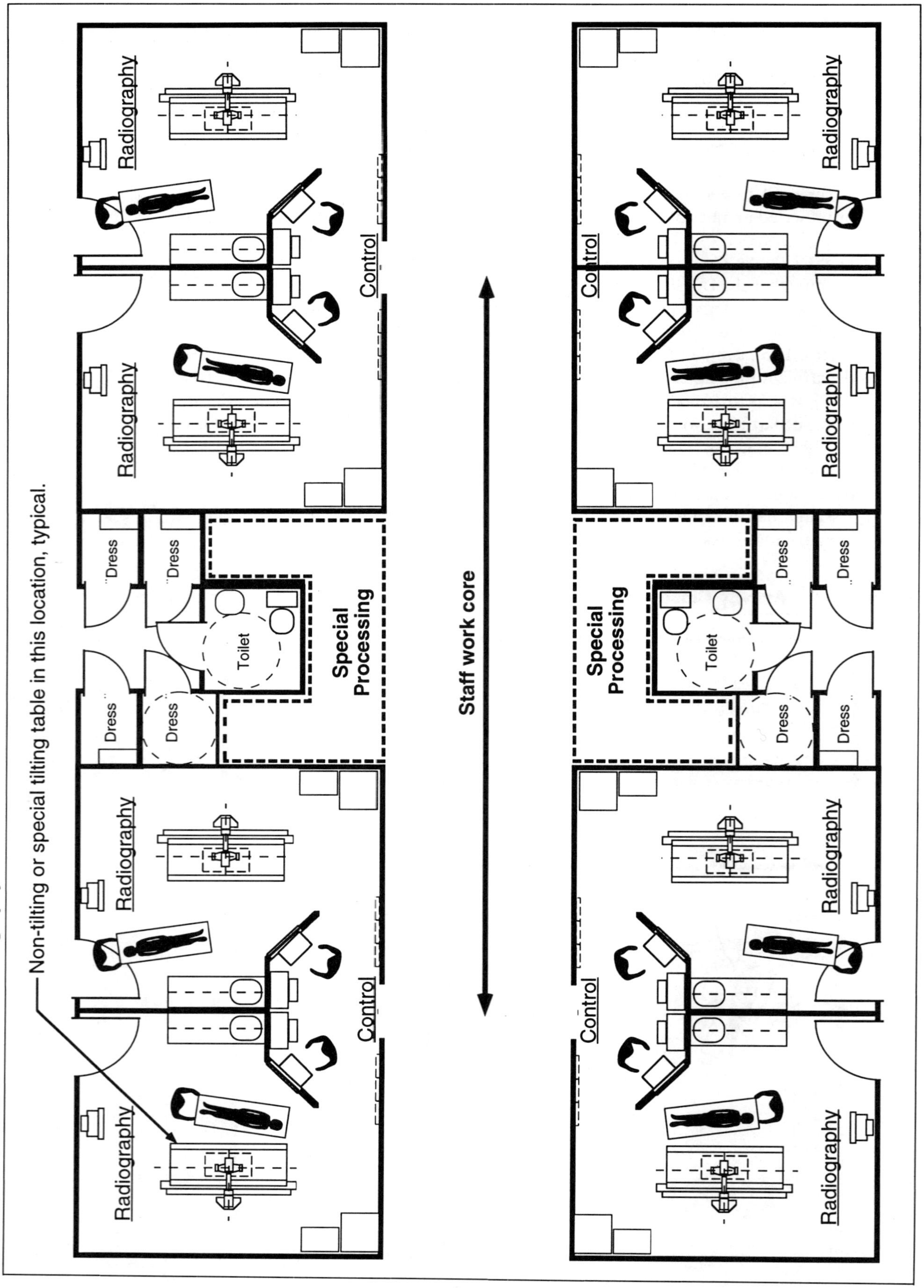

Figure 12-5. Activity Cluster: Radiography Exam

Figure 12-6. Activity Cluster: Nuclear Medicine Exam

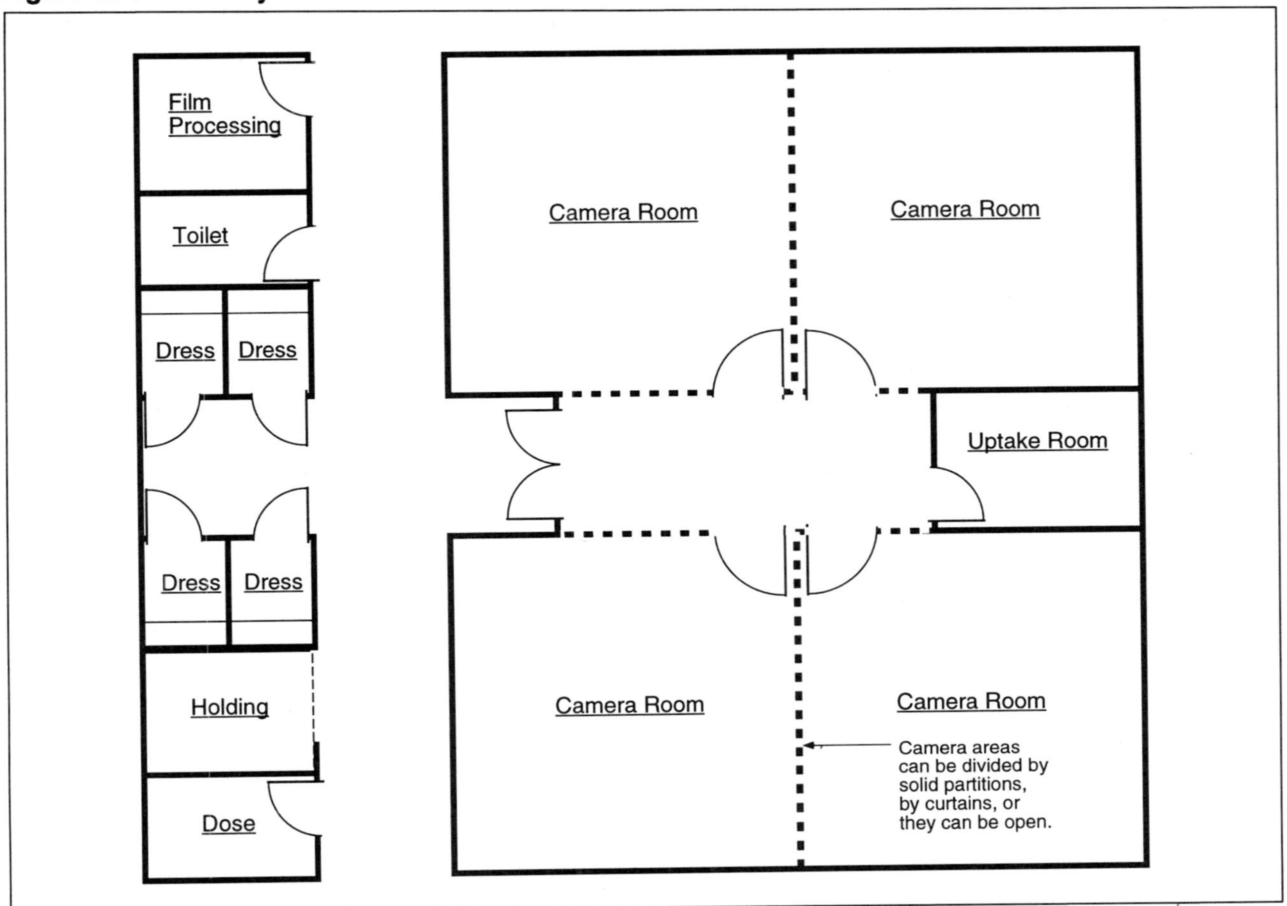

8. Assume that each room can accommodate the following range of annual procedures:

Room Type	*Approximate Annual Procedures*
Routine radiography	10,000–12,000
Routine fluoroscopy	4,500–5,500
General R/F	5,000–7,500
Angiography	800–900
CT	3,000–4,000
Nuclear medicine	2,000–2,500
Ultrasound	3,000–3,500
MRI	2,500–3,500
Mammography	6,500–8,000
Dedicated chest room	25,000–30,000

Variables Affecting Facility Size

It is easy to see that the preceding formulas do not take into account the numerous variables that affect the space requirements of any facility. Although some of the formulas include variables for both teaching and nonteaching hospitals, many other variables are not included. The following also should be considered:

- The number of annual operating hours differs among institutions. Workload projections must be based on stated assumptions regarding operating hours per day and operating days per year. Additionally, at most hospitals the imaging workload varies dramatically from one shift to another. The night shift has peaks and lulls, depending on the workload of emergency cases. In contrast, the day shift may be heavily scheduled and will be subject to staff efficiency and the frequency of emergency cases disrupting the schedule.

- Renovation projects are likely to require more space than a newly constructed facility with the same workload capacity, because planning may not be able to be as efficient as with new construction.
- If radiographic capabilities exist in the emergency department, they should not be counted as part of the primary radiology workload. However, radiology staffing may be inefficient if the same personnel are used to staff the two departments.
- Although some imaging equipment is getting smaller, many imaging procedures are becoming more complex and more people and ancillary equipment are involved; thus, some room sizes are getting bigger and additional patient holding areas are required. Equipment throughput capabilities are increasing; thus, in some instances, the number of annual procedures per examination room is getting larger. Automated image processing and image management and communications systems can reduce average procedure durations, thus also increasing the number of annual procedures per examination room.
- Imaging workload is determined by the *type* of patients in an institution and not just the *number* of patients. For example, a hospital with a large obstetric program is likely to perform more abdominal ultrasound examinations than one without a significant number of such patients. Similarly, a major heart center is likely to perform more cardiac imaging than a hospital that does not focus on cardiology. Magic numbers that simply convert patient beds to procedures per year do not reflect the fact that all patient beds are not equal.
- Outpatient imaging centers, as compared to hospital imaging departments, are likely to perform more routine procedures of short duration. Thus, an outpatient facility is likely to accommodate more procedures per room per hour than a hospital. However, the outpatient facility may not be open as many days per week or as many hours per day as a hospital department. Thus, each room might accommodate relatively fewer procedures per year as compared to hospital procedure rooms.
- Some institutions include nuclear medicine as part of radiology, others do not. Some even include radiation therapy as part of the radiology department. Some institutions have MRI within the imaging department; some have MRI in a separate facility or modular enclosure. A clear description of what is to be included in the department is necessary before determining department size.
- Some institutions have one central imaging department; others decentralize routine imaging rooms and locate them near the various inpatient nursing units. Special procedure rooms usually are placed within one central location. Some institutions combine inpatient and outpatient imaging; others have two (or more) separate facilities. Each of these variables will influence the amount and type of space required.
- Archival film files frequently are stored in a location that is remote from the main imaging department or even off-site. Department area calculations will be affected by whether remote file storage is included or excluded from the total area calculation.
- Filmless imaging departments eventually may require less space for film files than film-based imaging departments. However, to date, most states require hard-copy storage of images (for legal reasons). Filmless imaging departments eventually may require less space than film-based departments for image reading and interpretation workstations, although, initially, more space probably will be required because both film-based and filmless workstations will coexist until the latter become fully integrated into daily routines. Therefore, the degree to which a department utilizes filmless imaging technology will influence space requirements.

Intelligent Numbers: Workload Analysis for Determining Facility Size

Because of the many variables that influence space requirements, a detailed analysis of workload and staffing is needed before design and planning begins. This analysis, which relies on "intelligent" rather than "magic" numbers, should include workload projections for each type of procedure presently performed, as well as the anticipated future workload. Future workload projections might increase because of the development of more rapid technology than that which presently exists; conversely, they are more likely to decrease because imaging referrals will be more closely controlled under managed care as compared to past practices. Other factors that will influence future workload include additional changes in reimbursement and new alternatives to imaging.

The analysis also should consider whether some rooms should be dedicated to only one type of examination or used for a variety of procedures. As an example, chest examinations usually make up a large percentage of the department's total workload. If the number of chest exams is high enough to keep one or more rooms busy all the time, a dedicated room probably will be warranted. A dedicated chest room may be able to be smaller than a general radiography room (which can be used for chest X rays as well as other procedures) although the dedicated chest room may not be as flexible as the general radiography room.

As mentioned earlier, the purpose of the detailed workload analysis is to identify the facility's key space generators. The next steps include determining the types and number of procedure rooms required, as well as the amount and size of support and administration space required, and the proper size of each procedure room.

Determining the Types and Number of Procedure Rooms Required

After deciding what types of procedure rooms should be provided, the optimal number of rooms can be projected. The number of required rooms for each type of procedure (for example, basic radiography, angiography, ultrasound, CT, and so on) is derived from the following basic formula:

Projected annual procedures ÷ projected annual procedures per room
= number of procedure rooms needed

It is assumed that the number of projected annual procedures per room is a function of the average procedure duration, including setup time and the number of hours per day for which the room is used.

For example, assuming that the average duration of a basic X-ray exam is 15 minutes, or 0.25 hours (including setup and cleanup), and that 70 percent of basic X-ray exams are performed Monday through Friday (250 days a year) during the daytime 8-hour shift, even though the facility is open 24 hours a day, 360 days a year, utilization projections should be based on the period of high demand. Thus, on the basis of these figures, the average number of potential procedures per prime shift per basic radiography room is calculated as follows:

8 hours/day ÷ 0.25 hours/procedure = 32 procedures/prime 8-hour shift

Even allowing for downtime, setup, and cleanup, scheduling will not be 100 percent efficient. An 85 percent efficiency factor can be used to account for time in which the room is available but not used. Therefore, the projected number of prime-time annual procedures that the room is capable of is as follows:

32 procedures/shift × 0.85 efficiency factor × 250 days/year
= 6,800 procedures

Because these calculations were based on 70 percent of the basic X-ray procedures anticipated, the total number of annual procedures that one room can accommodate is as follows:

6,800 ÷ 0.70 = 9,714 procedures

Referring back to the original formula, assume that 20,000 basic annual procedures are projected:

$$20{,}000 \text{ annual procedures} \div 9{,}714 \text{ procedures/room} = 2.05 \text{ procedure rooms}$$

Therefore, two basic radiography rooms should be programmed. If the actual workload exceeds the estimate, variations in staffing or hours of operation can accommodate much of the difference.

Similar calculations should be performed for each type of procedure room. The calculations should be adjusted based on the degree to which rooms are to be used for multiple types of procedures. The variables in the formulas should be adjusted because the duration of each type of procedure will vary; some complex procedures may last several hours. Some special studies, such as those requiring that the patient not eat prior to the procedure, might always be performed in the morning. The rooms used for these special studies might be available for basic examinations in the afternoon.

Table 12-3 shows hypothetical average procedure durations that might be used as starting points for the duration variable in the above formula. However, it should be noted that each average can represent a wide range of actual durations. Because the technology and complexity of procedures change rapidly, these figures may not be current or appropriate for some applications. Current data should be examined before factoring this information into space-programming formulas.

Determining the Proper Size of Procedure Rooms

The proper size of an imaging procedure room is determined by understanding the function of the procedure, patient flow, staff flow, and equipment needs. Usually, the most important key space generator is the imaging equipment. The space required for other fixed equipment, movable ancillary equipment, the patient, and staff also must be taken into account. Additionally, consideration must be given to the area required for movement or extension of equipment, including clearances needed when the units are swiveled, tilted, or rotated.[9]

When determining the proper size of each procedure room, three trends must be kept in mind. First, some types of imaging equipment are getting smaller. In some instances, the associated electrical and data components (transformers, generators, computer processors, and so on) also are getting smaller. Second, and in contrast to the shrinking size of equipment, is the tendency for imaging procedures to become more complex. This means that more people and ancillary equipment may be required in the procedure room and that additional patient support spaces may be necessary. Third, sometimes imaging equipment is upgradable by purchasing new software and hardware packages. This means that today's equipment may be capable of more complex examinations in the future. This supports the second comment

Table 12-3. Hypothetical Average Procedure Durations

Room Type	Duration Including Setup and Cleanup
Routine radiography	0.25 hours
Routine fluoroscopy	0.75 hours
Angiography	2.00 hours
CT scan	0.50 hours
Nuclear medicine	1.00 hours (does not include time between administration of dose and scan)
Ultrasound	0.50 hours
MRI	Varies
Mammography	0.25 hours
Chest exam	0.10 hours

Note: These durations are rough estimates and, therefore, will not apply to all equipment or to all situations. Each should be verified with the most recent data available.

that more people and ancillary equipment may continue to be present in the procedure room. Therefore, although some equipment is getting smaller, there often is a need for additional space and surplus capacity of utility systems.

Most equipment vendors list both recommended and minimum room dimensions for their major imaging equipment. Minimum dimensions should be avoided because they usually refer to the absolute least amount of space in which the equipment will function. Often, significant functional sacrifices will be made if minimum dimensions are used instead of recommended dimensions. Minimum dimensions often take into account only the space required for the major fixed imaging equipment but not the needs of ancillary equipment.

Most equipment will require additional clearances for servicing and access. Usually, these dimensions are provided by the equipment vendor.

The area requirements for accessibility by disabled persons also must be included when determining room size and configuration. These dimensions, including those prescribed in the Americans with Disabilities Act, are often omitted in vendor-supplied data. The fact that many functions in the procedure room may not be able to be performed by individuals with mobility impairments does not eliminate the need to incorporate mandated accessibility standards. Usually, a minimum clearance of 36 inches is required in front of all fixed objects. In addition, maneuvering clearances for wheelchair-bound persons are required.

Vertical clearance also must be considered in procedure rooms. For many modalities, imaging equipment is designed for a finished ceiling height of 9 feet, 6 inches, above the finished floor. A lower ceiling might not accommodate the movement or focal angles of ceiling-mounted equipment; a higher ceiling might require the equipment to be modified for proper installation. Ample space is required above the finished ceiling for primary structural beams, air supply and return ducts, lighting fixtures, fire protection piping, and, in some cases, a "unistrut" structural assembly. (See figures 8-15 [p. 152] and 8-16 [p. 153] in chapter 8, "Design Concepts.") These items should have their own dedicated "horizontal zone" above the ceiling so that they do not run into each other. This requires careful coordination during the design and construction phases of the project. Usually, a clear floor-to-floor height of at least 16 feet is recommended (for buildings without interstitial floors) to provide a finished ceiling height of 9 feet, 6 inches, and to accommodate the various subsystems required above the ceiling with some additional flexibility for future modifications. A building designed with a full interstitial space between floors might require a total vertical height of 19 to 20 feet, including both the functional and interstitial zones.

The space requirements for similar equipment supplied by different manufacturers may vary somewhat. Until equipment selections have been finalized, it is best to plan for equipment that requires the greatest amount of space. (See figures 12-7 through 12-20, pp. 220–31.) However, equipment vendors are the preferred source for this information.

References

1. Rostenberg, B. *Design Planning for Freestanding Ambulatory Care Facilities.* Chicago: American Hospital Publishing, 1986, p. 26 [out of print].
2. Hayward, C., and others. *A Generic Process for Projecting Health Care Space Needs.* Washington, DC: American Institute of Architects, 1985.
3. Hayward and others.
4. Porter, D. R. *Hospital Architecture: Guidelines for Design and Renovation.* Ann Arbor, MI: AUPHA Press, 1982, p. 237.
5. Porter, p. 216.
6. Laufman, H., editor. *Hospital Special Care Facilities: Planning for User Needs.* New York City: Academic Press, 1981, pp. 426–27.
7. Laufman.
8. Laufman, p. 428.
9. Jenkins, S. *Planning Guide for Radiographic Installations—Fascicle 7: Functional Design of a Radiographic Room.* Chicago: American College of Radiology, 1981, p. 2.

Figure 12-7. Chest Room without Film Processor

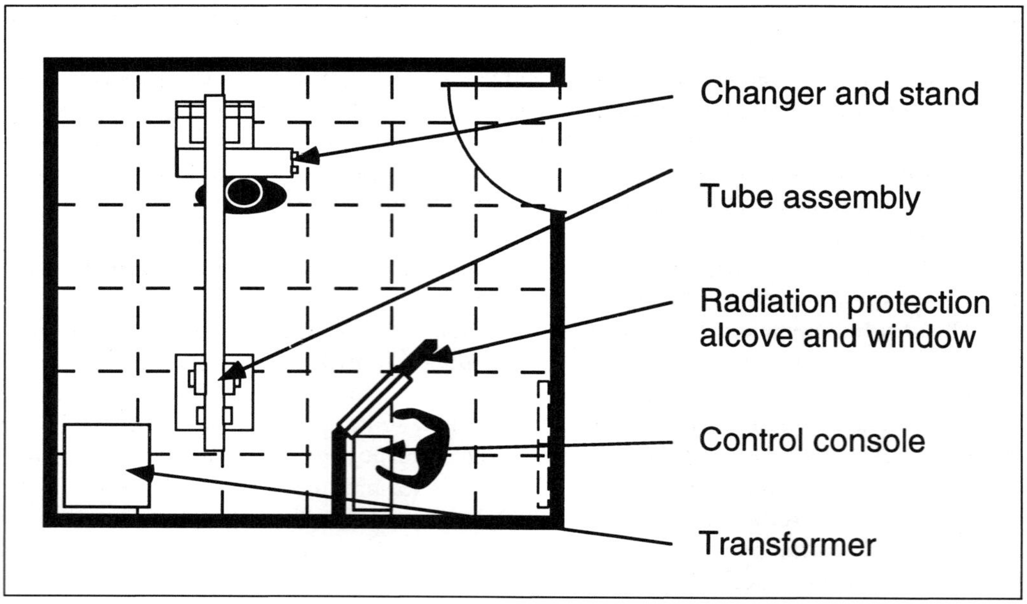

Figure 12-8. Patient Positioning in Chest Room

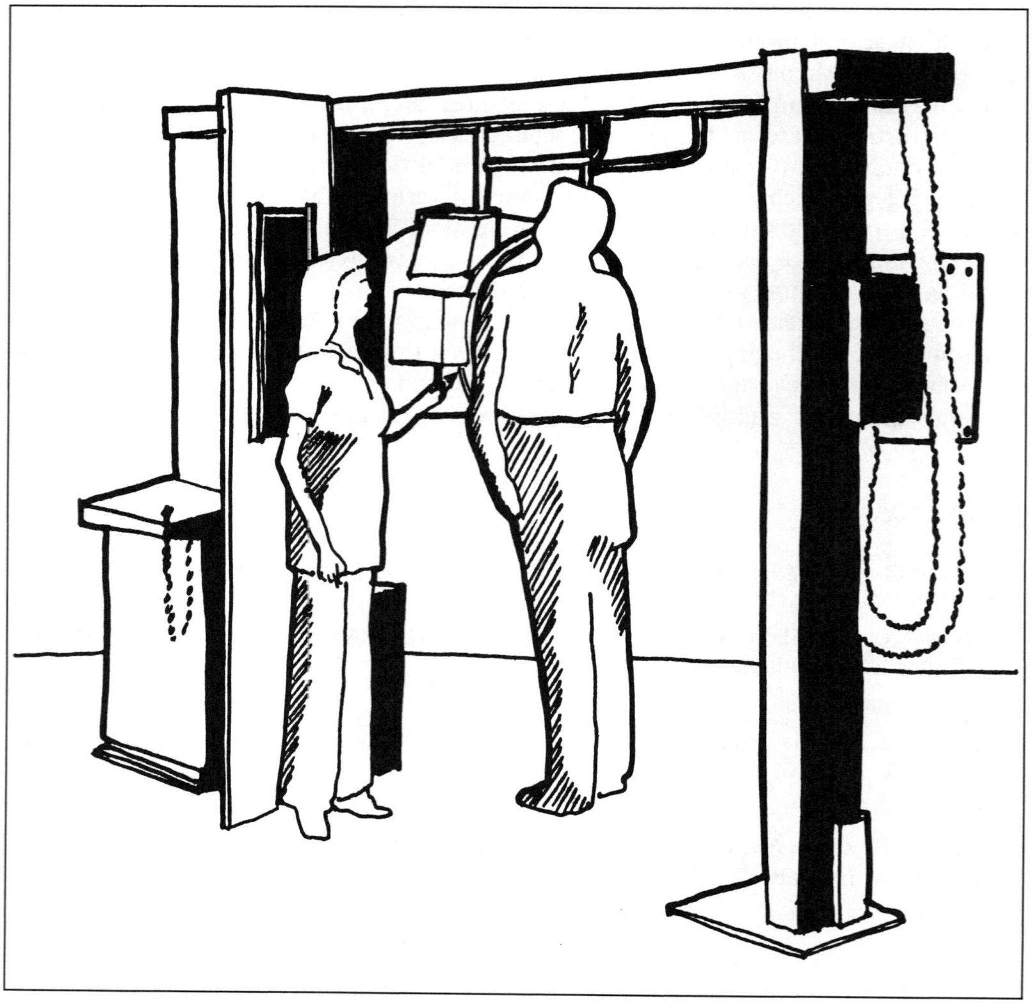

Figure 12-9. Chest Room with Film Processor

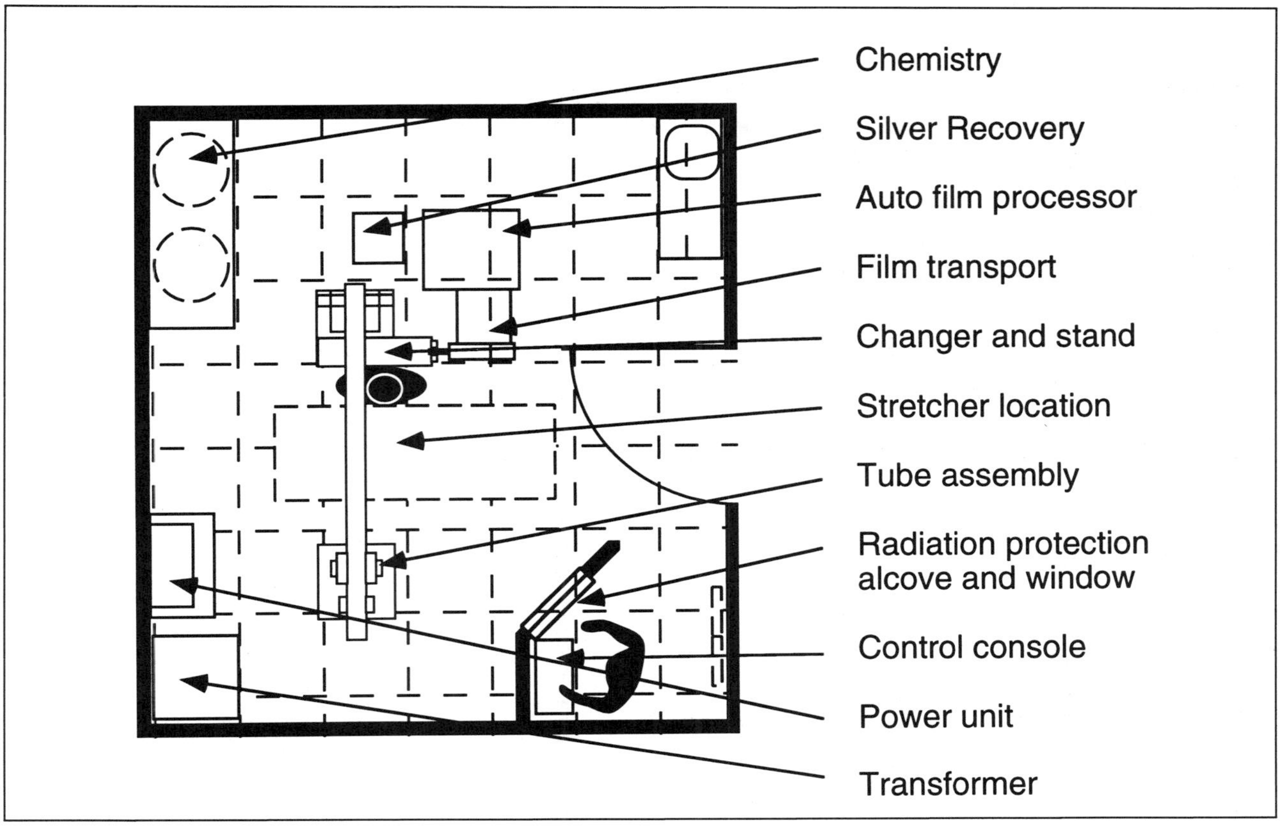

Figure 12-10. General Radiography Room

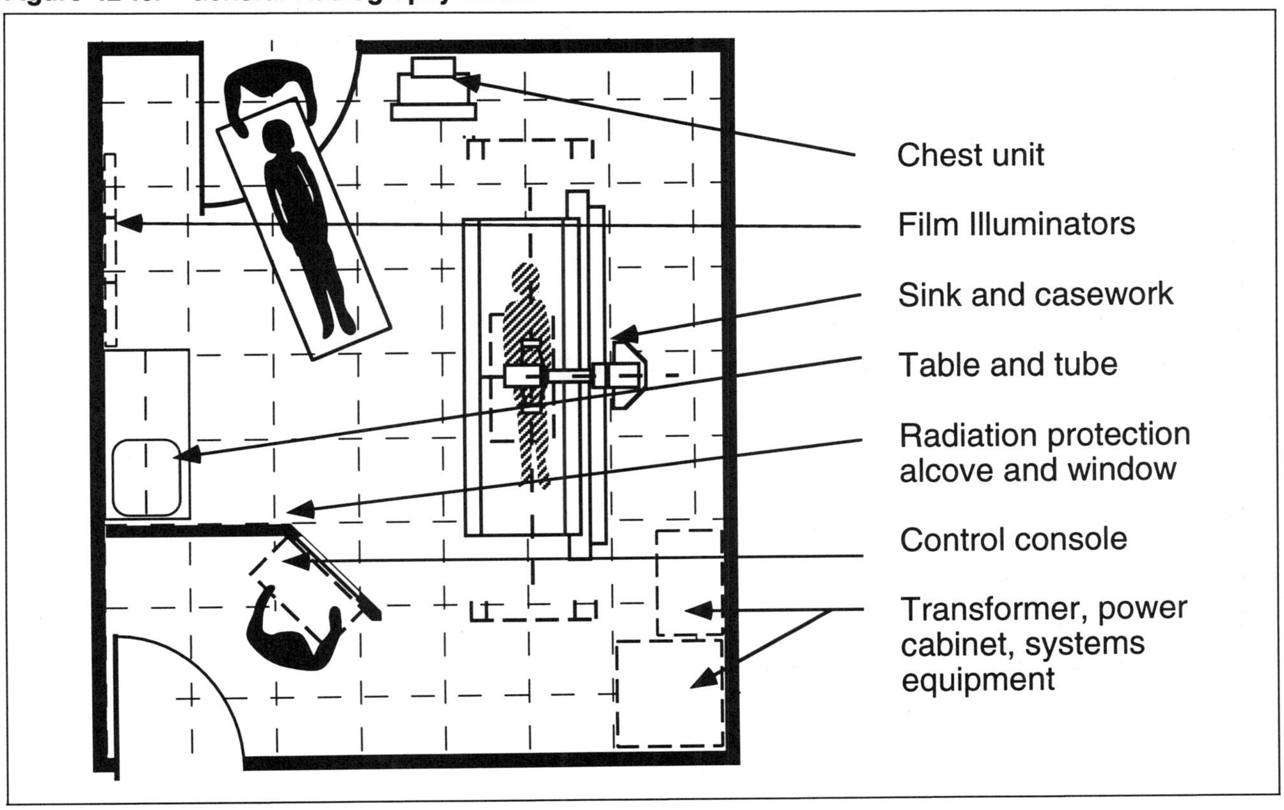

Figure 12-11. Special Procedure/Angiography Room

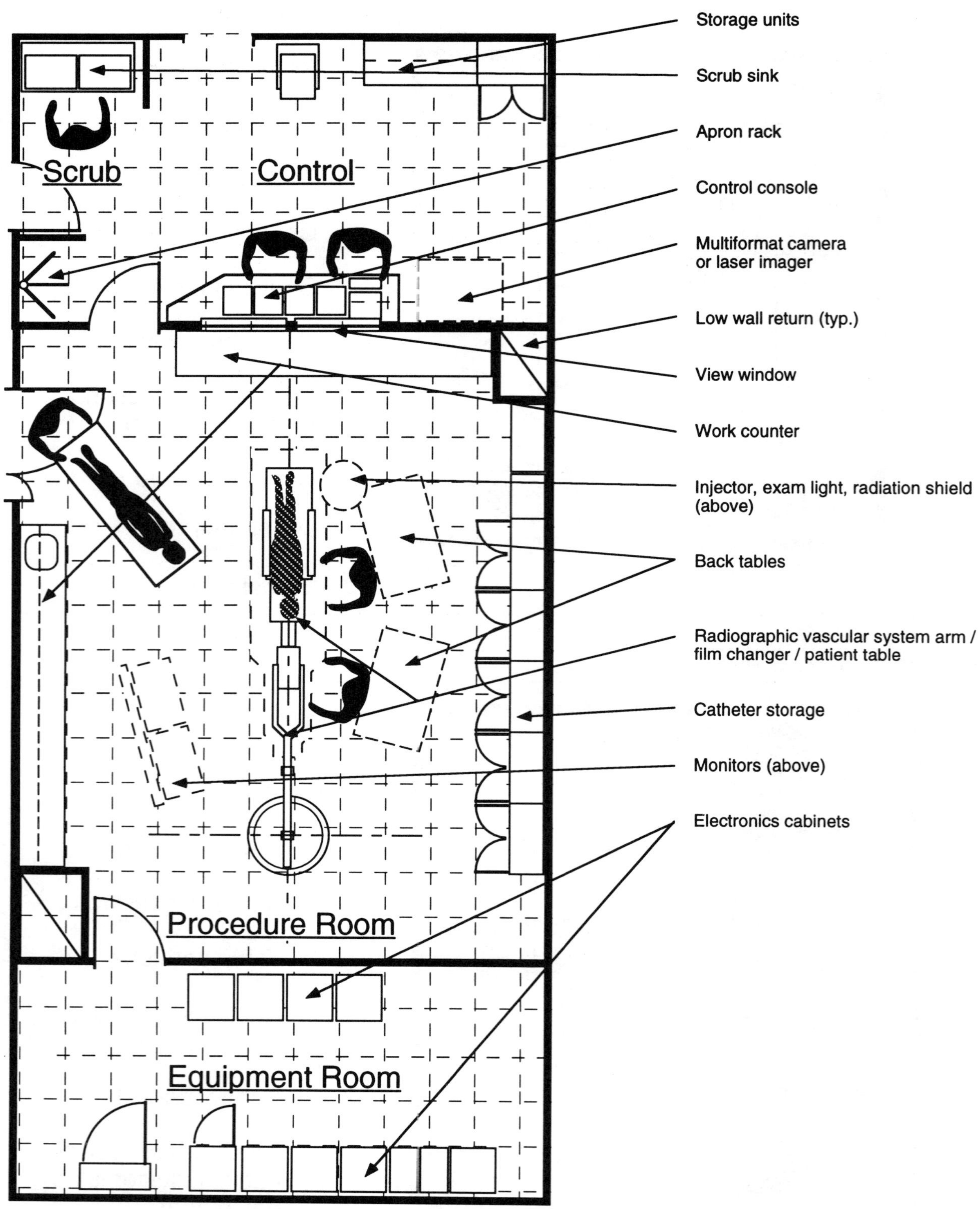

Figure 12-12. Special Procedure/Angiography Room

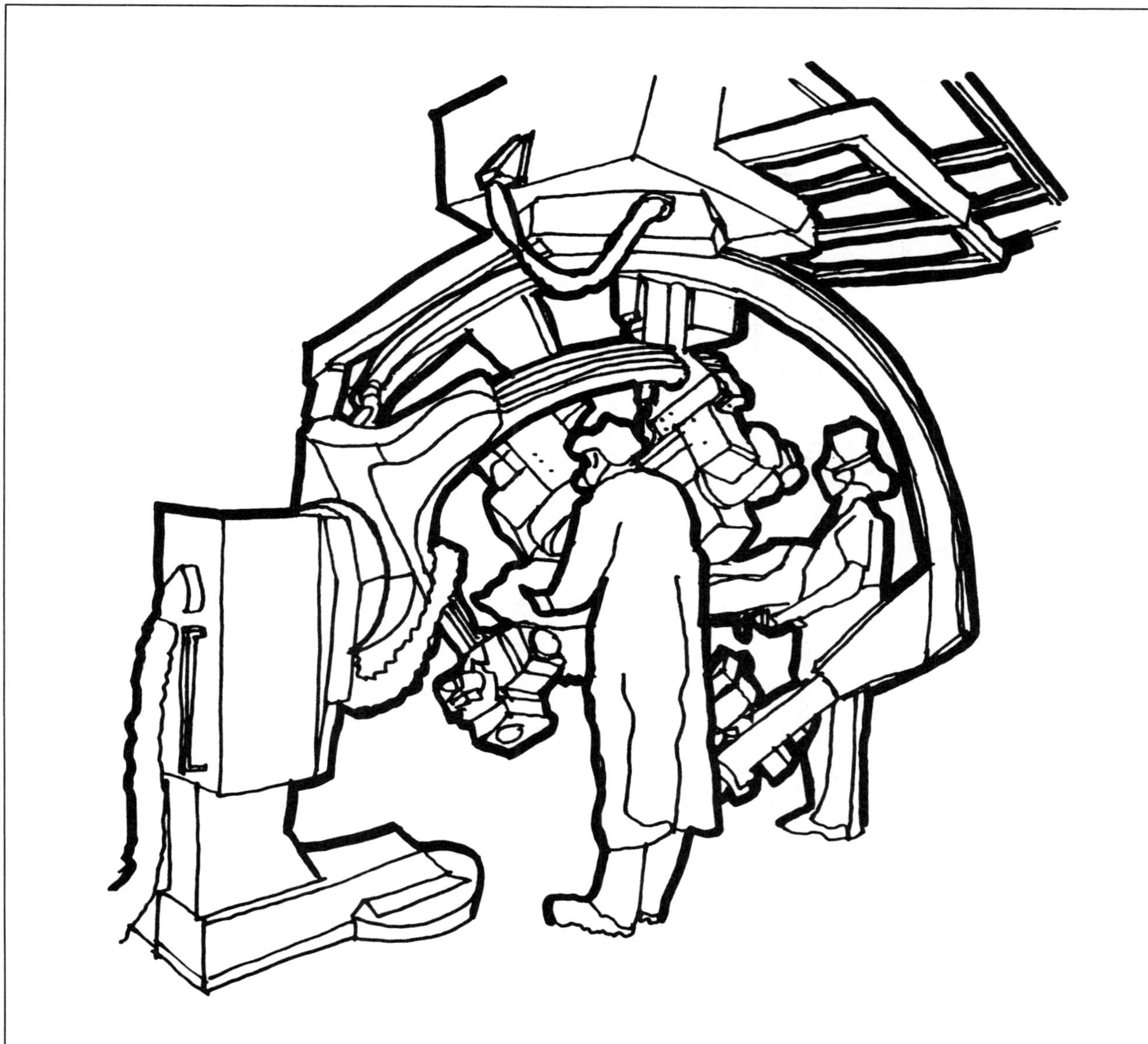

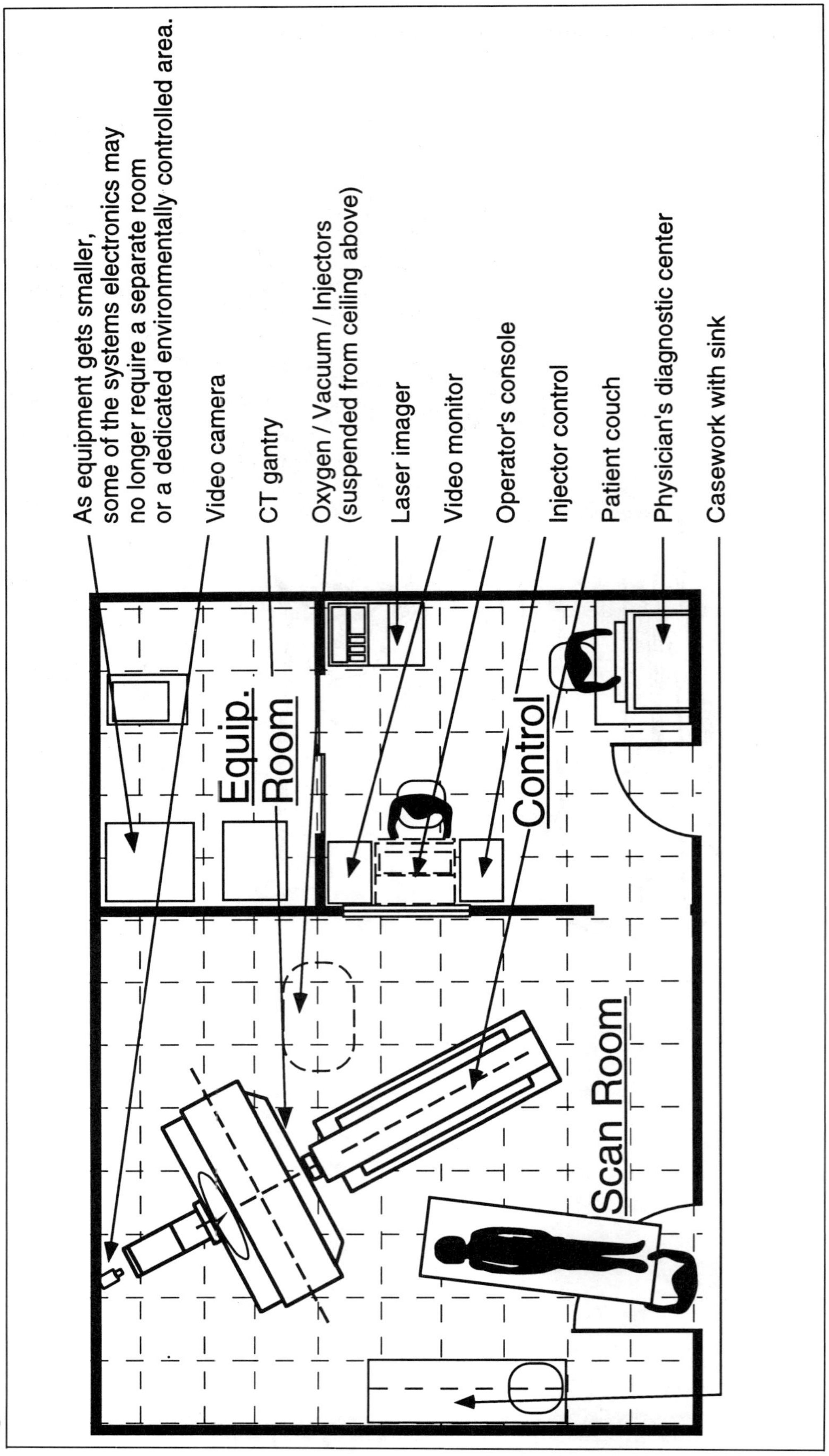

Figure 12-13. CT Room

Figure 12-14. Nuclear Medicine Room with One Full-Body Scanning Camera

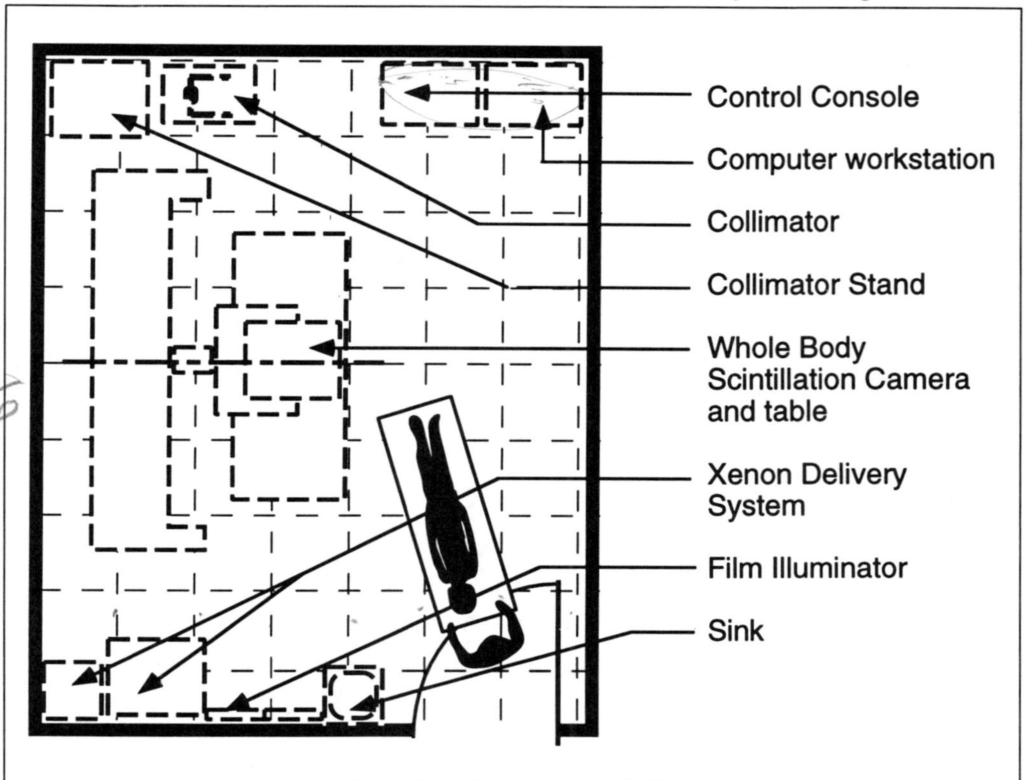

Figure 12-15. Nuclear Medicine Room with Two Scanning Cameras

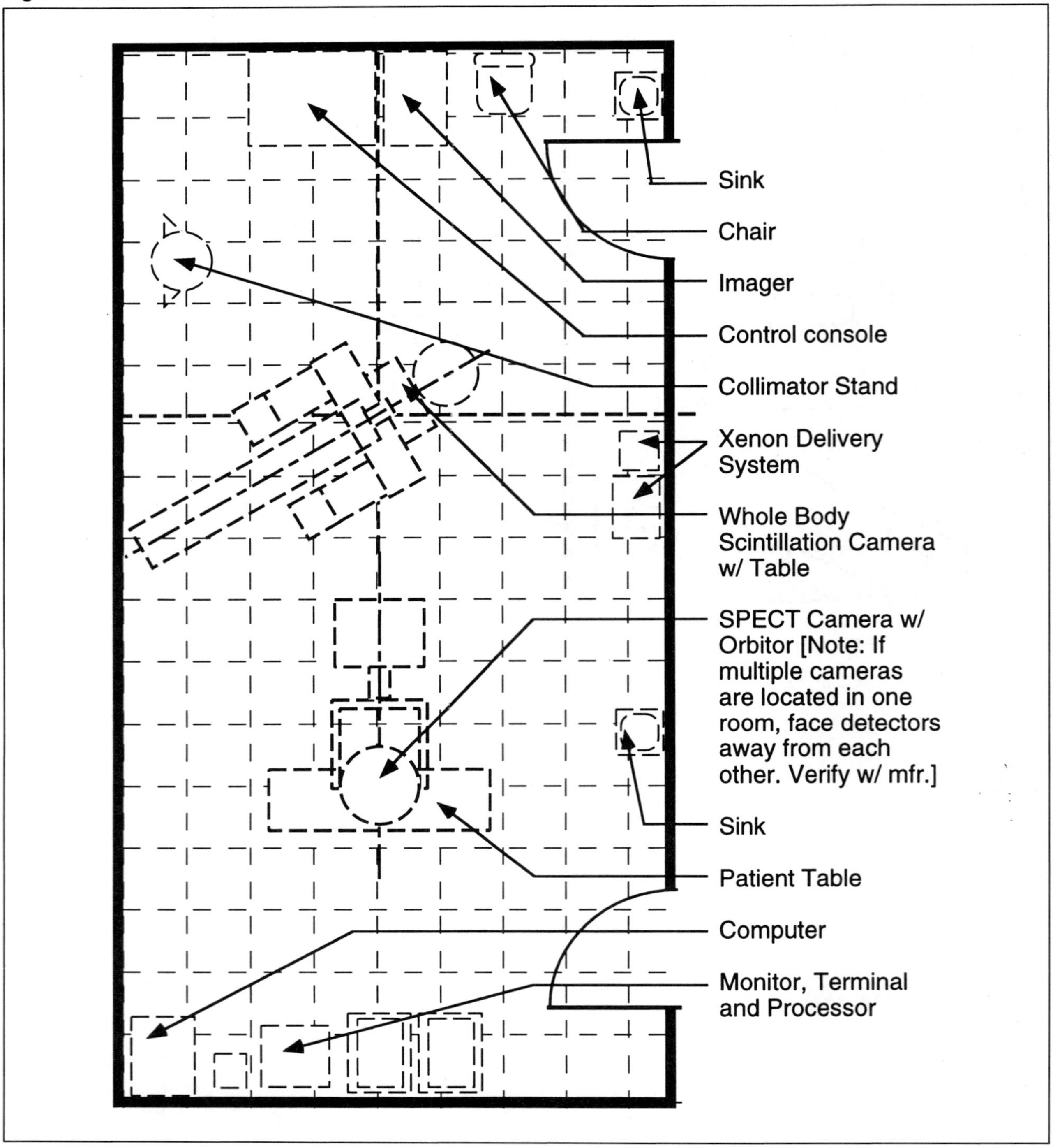

Figure 12-16. MRI Room

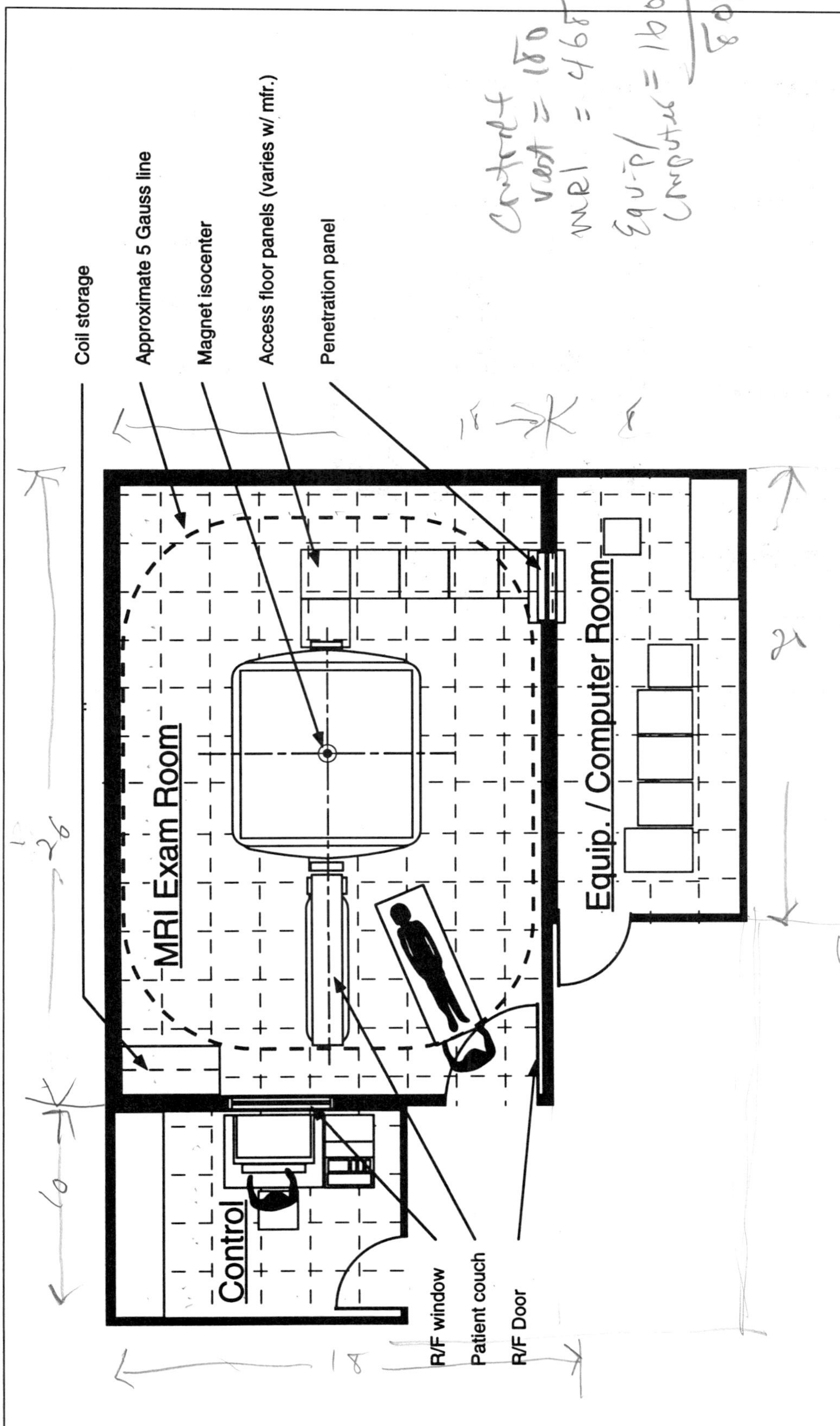

Figure 12-17. MRI Room

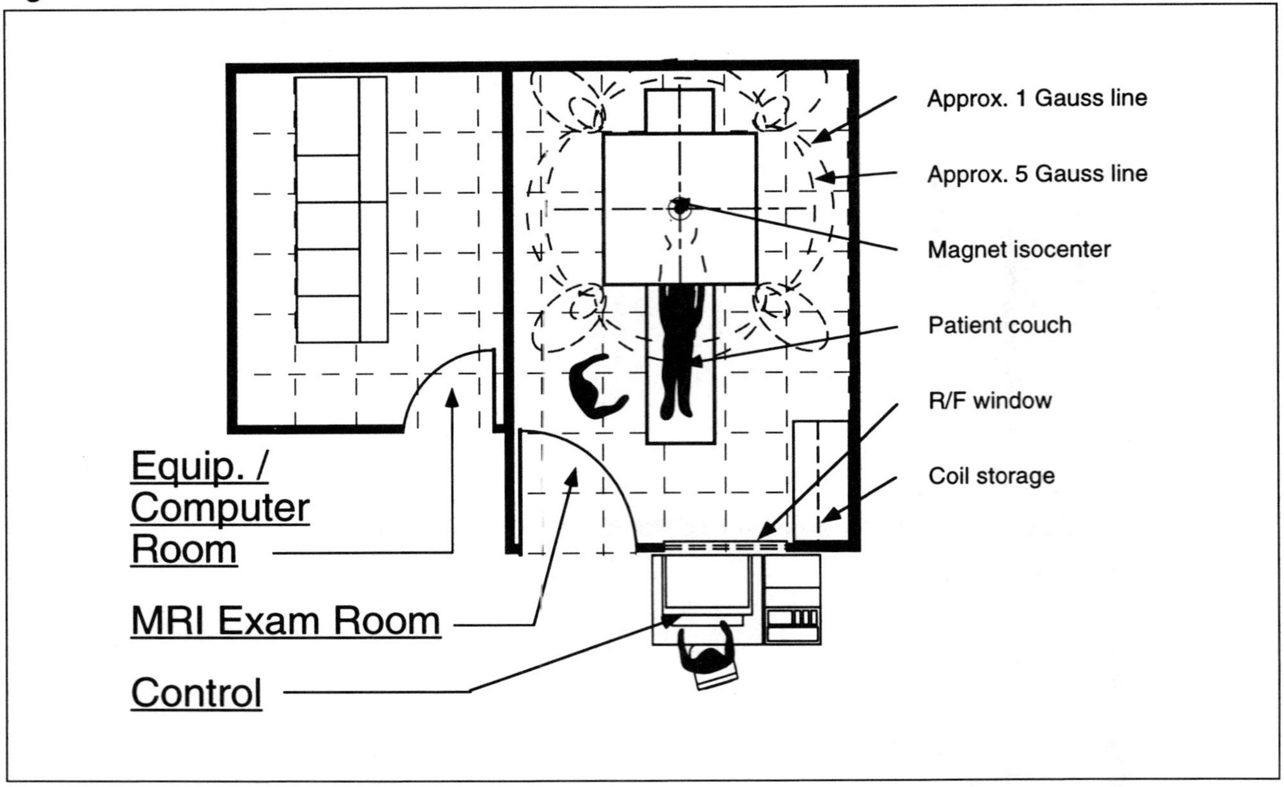

Figure 12-18. Mammography Rooms: Upright Unit (top), Stereotactic Needle-Biopsy Unit (bottom)

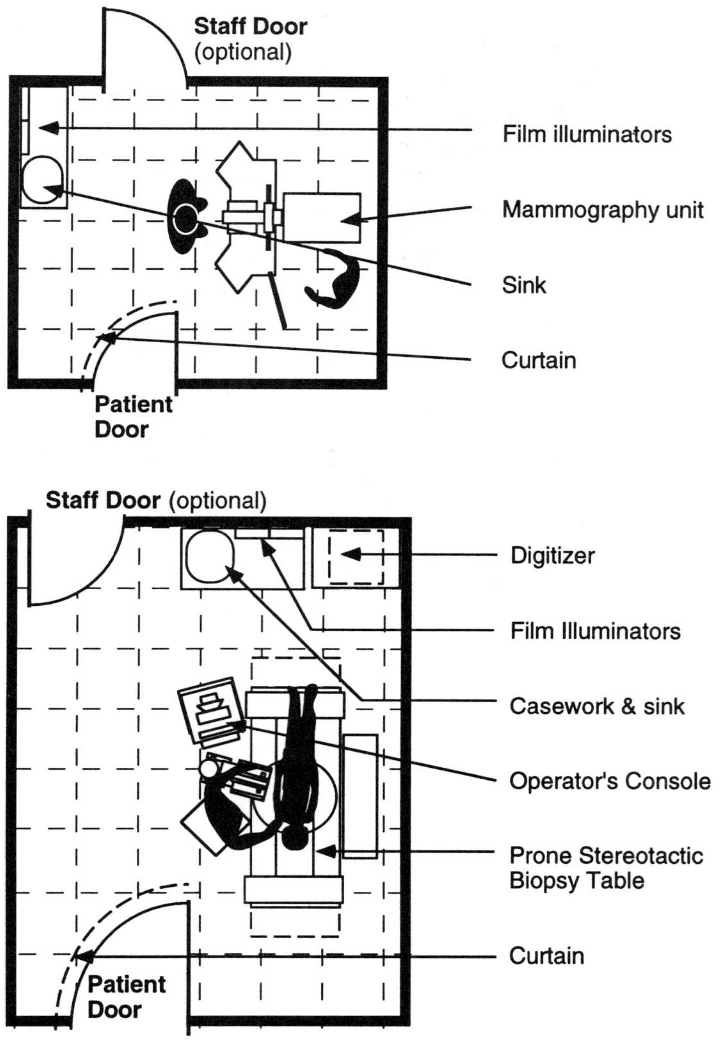

Figure 12-19. Patient Positioning for Mammography Exam

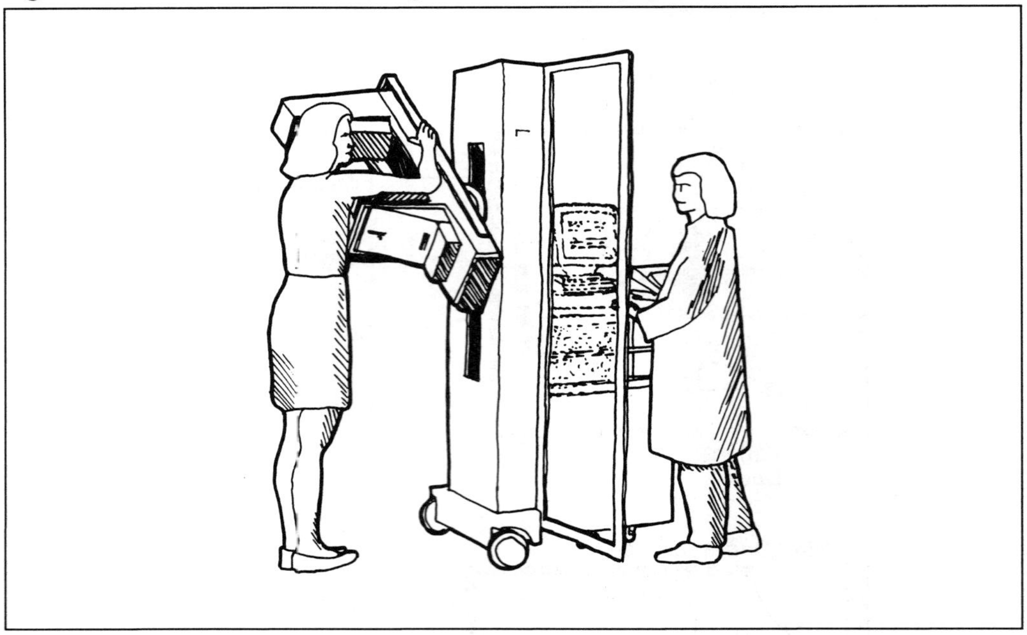

Figure 12-20. Ultrasound Rooms

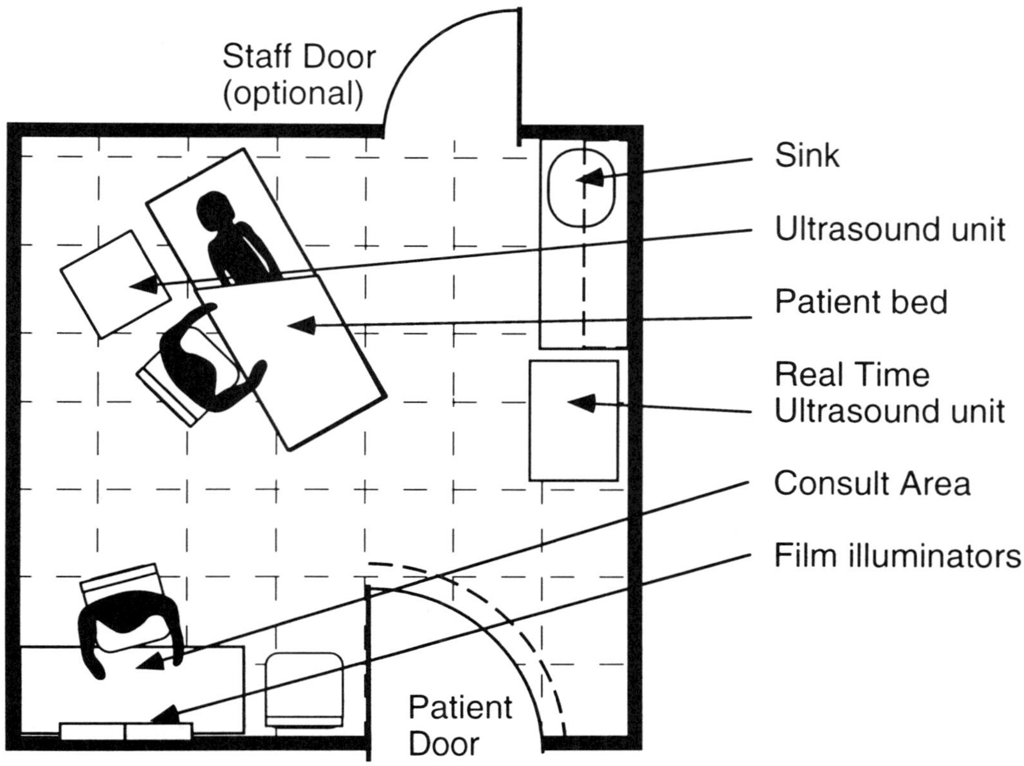

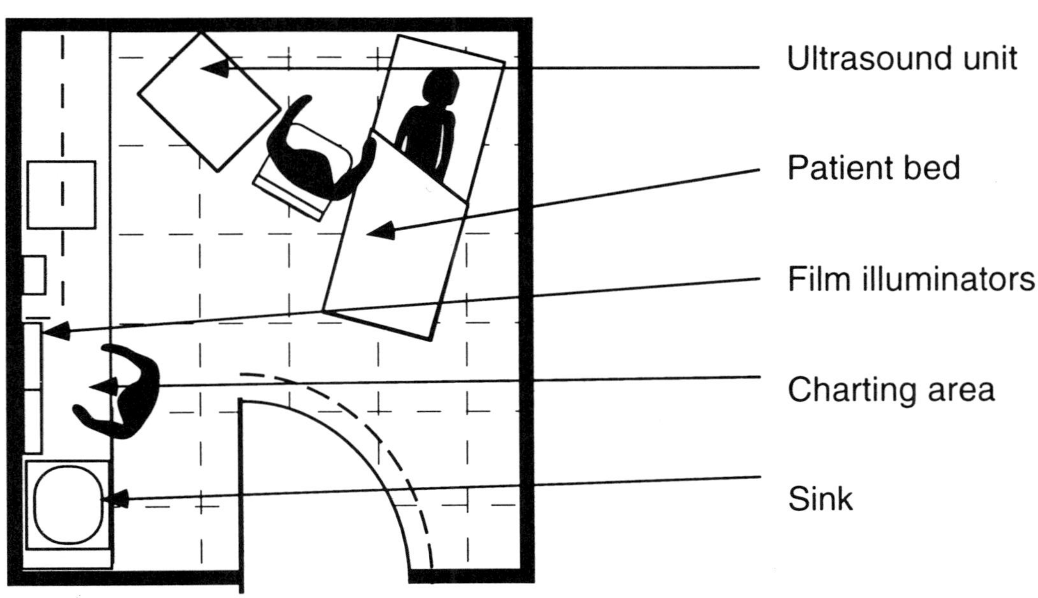

Chapter 13

Room Design

Room design is closely related to both the people who use the room and the equipment that is used in it. There are many possible design approaches. Like the imaging department itself, each room must be designed in concert with work flow; patient, staff, and supply traffic; and the spatial perceptions of the individuals using the rooms. Additionally, primary design drivers, or key space generators for many rooms, are the placement, size, movement, and access requirements of equipment.

This chapter identifies basic criteria to be considered when planning particular types of rooms. The intent is not to describe every room component in detail nor is it to describe any single best design solution for a specific type of room but, rather, to provide general guidelines for the design of procedure rooms, control rooms, image-processing areas, reading rooms, and film file areas. In addition, special sections on universal room design and computer workstation environments supplement the more general text. Finally, the appendix at the end of the chapter outlines specific guidelines for room design based on the unique requirements of individual imaging modalities.

General Considerations for Procedure Rooms

Because the complexity and characteristics of many procedures are evolving rapidly, the number of personnel in the procedure room and the acuity of patients are increasing. And because the size, sophistication, type, and quantity of equipment to be found in many rooms are changing equally rapidly, the dimensions, physical characteristics, and infrastructure requirements of some room types are not necessarily fixed. This applies more to special procedure rooms, such as angiography and catheterization labs, than it does to most basic procedures room, such as general radiography/fluoroscopy (R/F) rooms.

With few exceptions, formulas for complex procedure room design are of limited value. Even those for basic procedure rooms need to be modified for single-corridor, double-corridor, core, or cluster department configurations. (See the section entitled Plan Typologies in chapter 11, "Department Location and Configuration.") This is because single- and double-corridor layouts tend to combine patient and staff traffic (and thus suggest one door into the room), whereas core and cluster plans tend to separate the two types of traffic (and thus suggest two entrances into the procedure room). Therefore, considerable modification is needed to apply a standard room layout to both a control corridor and a control alcove philosophy, as discussed in the next section.

The ability of staff to easily observe patients is another key consideration affecting room design. For example, the technologist should be able to see the patient's face at all times from the control area. If the patient table is accessible from only one side and tilts from horizontal to vertical, this establishes a physical relationship between the placement of the control area and the placement of the patient table within the procedure room. In addition, if the radiologist (or invasive cardiologist) needs access to the patient's right side, an unobstructed view of ceiling-supported monitors, and the assistance of others who can reach catheters and other supplies with minimal movement at the same time that the technologist in the control area needs an unobstructed view of the patient and physician, the equation becomes more complex. Maximum lengths of preassembled equipment cables also influence room design.

Trends

Two trends regarding imaging procedure rooms are worth noting here. The first is that the complexity of outpatient imaging procedures continues to increase. The second is that many procedures, both inpatient and outpatient oriented, are becoming more invasive.

Facility implications of the increasing complexity of outpatient procedures are numerous, especially for facilities other than acute care hospitals. First, floor-to-floor heights in nonhospital buildings are traditionally lower than they are in hospitals. The ability to construct functional and flexible procedure rooms without adequate vertical clearance may be compromised where vertical clearance is inadequate. Similarly, power; heating, ventilation, and air-conditioning (HVAC); plumbing and fire protection systems typically designed for nonhospital buildings may be inadequate for complex procedure rooms and their equipment. Separate, redundant systems may be required just for the imaging component of some outpatient facilities. Structural systems in nonhospital facilities must be able to support the load created by imaging equipment. Additional structural reinforcing may be needed for outpatient renovation projects. Floor-loading capacities that are greater than for other types of nonhospital buildings may be needed for new construction. Finally, much of the construction criteria that apply to complex procedure rooms may be listed in building codes that primarily govern hospital projects, whereas building permits for many outpatient buildings are issued by local agencies that may follow other types of building codes and regulations. Therefore, some local building jurisdictions may be unfamiliar with the construction criteria that are appropriate for procedure rooms and associated building systems.

The implications of increasingly invasive imaging procedures also are numerous. Some procedure rooms require higher levels of infection control, greater emergency and uninterruptable power supply, emergency equipment, medical gas outlets, and more space than was previously required. To accommodate infection control criteria, special wall, floor, and ceiling finishes may need to be specified. Special methods of assembling these materials to limit the growth of organisms and to simplify cleaning procedures also may be necessary. In addition, exhaust, ventilation, and air-filtration specifications may need to be upgraded for these procedure rooms. In some states, special requirements regarding tuberculosis and HVAC systems in imaging procedure rooms have been proposed. (See chapter 16, "Utility Requirements," for specific criteria.)

Details

A broad array of fixtures and accessory equipment is needed in most procedure rooms. Some notable examples follow:

- A hand-washing fixture should be provided in the room.
- Some special procedure rooms need to have scrub sinks located nearby.
- Some rooms, such as cardiac catheterization labs, need an additional sink located nearby for cleaning catheters.
- Many procedures that emit radiation require that patients and personnel wear lead-lined aprons or other forms of protective clothing. Therefore, apron racks are required in or near those rooms. Additionally, radiation protection is integrated into the room construction itself.
- If conventional film processing is used, a lighttight, through-the-wall cassette passbox should be installed, ideally directly between the control portion of the procedure room

and the darkroom. (However, this will become less necessary in the future as the use of darkrooms diminishes.)
- Film illuminators of the proper orientation and configuration should be placed where they are accessible for easy viewing.

Coordination of the numerous accessory items and fixtures required in the procedure room should begin early in the design development phase. If it is not, last-minute decisions regarding seemingly minor items can severely compromise a workable procedure room layout. Wall thickness should be increased where flush-mounted accessories are used and where major conduits pass through wall partitions. Usually, it is advantageous to increase the wall thickness around the entire procedure room.

Finally, various types of special construction are required to accommodate the unique physical properties of many imaging processes. (These specialties—including radiation protection, magnetic shielding, and radio-frequency [RF] shielding—are described in chapter 15, "Physical Properties Influencing Design.")

General Considerations for Control Corridors, Control Alcoves, and Control Rooms

The control area is the space from which the technologist or physician (and sometimes other personnel) monitors and observes the patient while conducting an imaging examination. Many examinations simply involve "making an exposure" or acquiring an image while a relatively healthy patient sits or lies still. However, other procedures are much more complex.

Some procedures involve infants, young children, or elderly patients who cannot hold still without assistance or sedation. For some procedures, radiologists and other medical professionals are in the procedure room attending to the patient. Sometimes the patient's life functions are being supported by respirators, medical gases, and so on; sometimes the patient is injected with contrast material in order to acquire a diagnostic-quality image; and sometimes the patient is undergoing a surgerylike procedure under the guidance of imaging. Procedures such as electrophysiology (EP) studies can last up to six hours, and the nature of the study can subject the patient to potentially life-threatening conditions. In such situations, danger to the patient must be mitigated by close monitoring and immediately accessible life support and stabilization capabilities.

Three types of control areas—control corridors, control alcoves, and control rooms—are described in this section. Although each type requires specific design considerations, the following criteria should be considered when designing any one of the three types:

- Visibility of the patient from the control area
- Ability to communicate with the patient from the control area (often compromised in shared control rooms)
- Ability to communicate with other staff from the control area
- Impact of equipment on the control area location and configuration
- Ability to quickly and efficiently carry out image acquisition and image-processing activities
- Immediate access to the patient from the control area
- Adequate space for (initial and future) personnel and equipment needs
- Adequate space for maneuvering
- Lighting, acoustic, humidity, ventilation, and temperature control appropriate for the activities that will take place and the equipment that will be used in the space (see the section entitled General Considerations for Computer Workstation Environments in this chapter, as well as chapter 16, "Utility Requirements")
- Sound control to avoid disturbing personnel in the control room and the procedure room and to prevent the patient from overhearing confidential conversations

- Protection of medical personnel from physical effects inherent in different imaging modalities, such as radiation protection (see chapter 15, "Physical Properties Influencing Design")
- Proper functioning of special equipment that may be disturbed by, or cause disturbance to, other equipment due to physical effects inherent in different imaging modalities, such as magnetic and RF interference (see chapter 15, "Physical Properties Influencing Design")

Three different approaches to planning control areas were discussed briefly elsewhere. They are:

- A control corridor alongside a series of procedure rooms
- A control alcove within the procedure room (figure 13-1)
- A control room adjacent to a procedure room or between two procedure rooms (figure 13-2)

Control Corridors

The control corridor concept is based on a planning philosophy in which the department is arranged with a series of procedure rooms, each adjacent to a continuous control corridor.

> A feature of [this philosophy] is the control corridor, or technologist's corridor, where all x-ray control [consoles] are located instead of having control [consoles] located in a partitioned area or booth within the x-ray room itself. Radiation protection is simplified by the provision of large glass windows for the technologist and radiologist to see into the x-ray rooms from the control corridor, and the technologist makes the exposure from the control corridor, and the individual room door is closed. Cassette storage and a limited source of supplies are contained in the corridor. This control corridor is mainly for the use of the technologists, and to some extent the radiologist. . . . Patients do not penetrate to the control corridor. The control corridor is the flow path of the technologist to and from the [image-processing area] and other radiographic rooms. . . . Generally, the control corridor is located parallel to the patient zone [waiting, dressing, patient toilet area, etc.] with the x-ray rooms in between, all three areas being of the same length.[1]

Proponents of the control corridor concept[2] claim that this system provides better communication among staff, simplified radiation protection, better separation of patient and staff traffic, and easy supervision of image-processing and procedure areas. In addition, proponents claim that the control corridor concept provides additional flexibility for modifying the facility over time when a modular approach to planning the procedure rooms is used. However, this modular approach requires that all procedure rooms be of approximately equal depth.

Some critics of the control corridor concept question the efficiency and functionality of uniform room depth for all procedures, question its practical (versus theoretical) benefit for flexibility and adaptability, find the control corridor to be noisy, and feel the separation between the procedure room and control corridor hinders communication between patients and staff and compromises the patients' privacy, thus leaving patients feeling isolated. However, all three approaches—control corridors, control alcoves, and control rooms—have been successfully incorporated into imaging facility design.

Control Alcoves

A control alcove located within the procedure room is a popular approach to providing a control area for a simple, basic X-ray procedure room. This approach is ideal when a small and limited amount of control equipment is involved and where the technologist needs to attend to the patient directly and frequently. This often is the case for procedures that are of short duration and high frequency.

Figure 13-1. Control Alcove

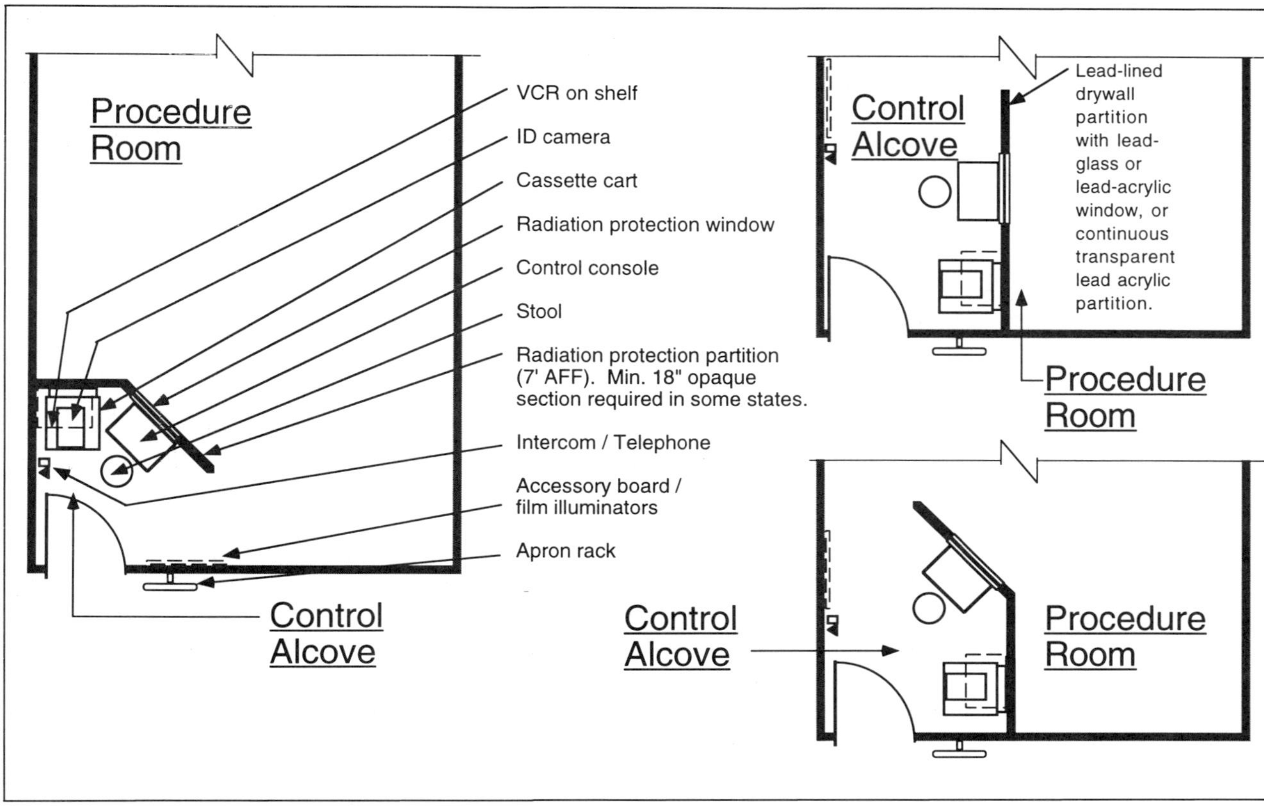

Figure 13-2. Control Room for Angiography

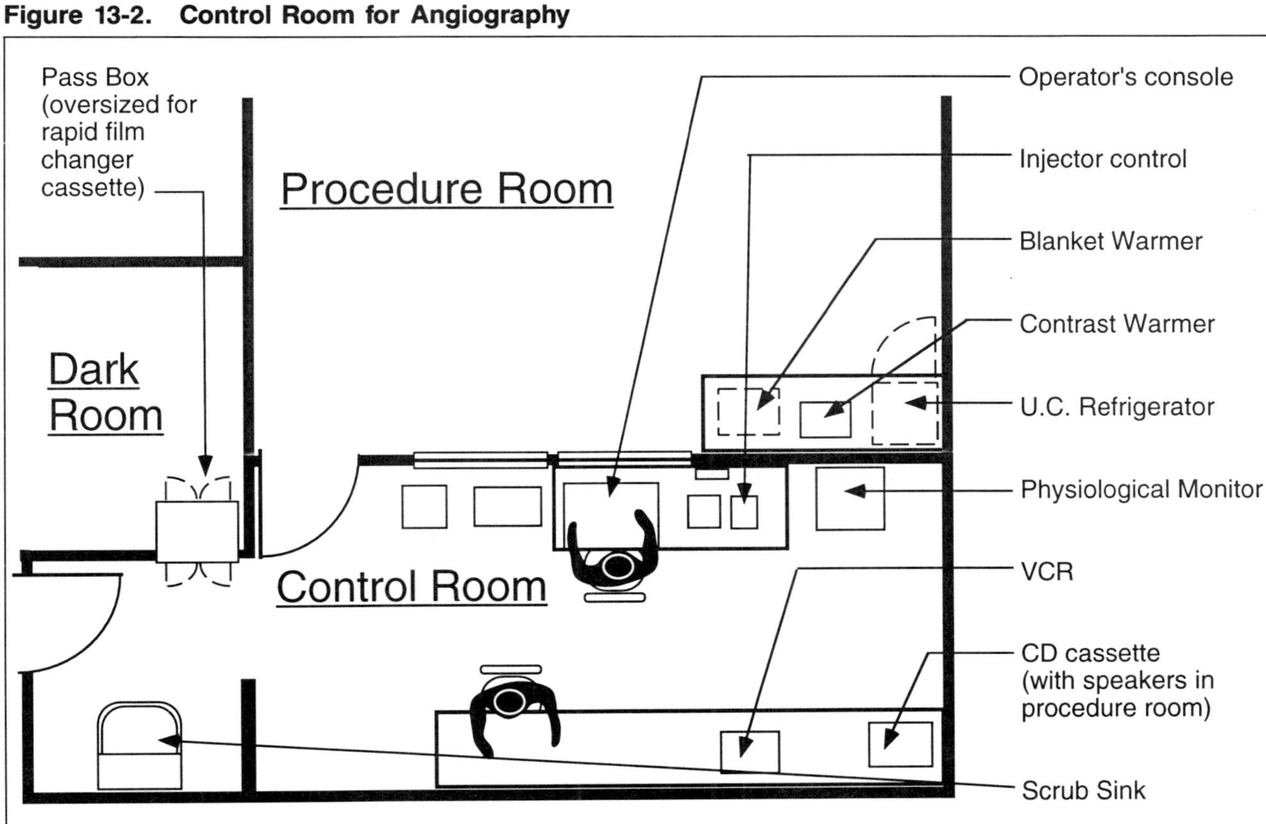

The control alcove is an integral component of universal room design (described later in this chapter). Typically, lead-lined barriers in front of the control alcove extend approximately seven feet above the finished floor surface of the examination room. This allows overhead ceiling-mounted equipment to pass above the control area without unnecessarily restricting its movement. Control consoles are located in the alcove in such a way that the technologist can see the patient through a radiation-shielded but visually transparent window or module.

Some alcoves are constructed with a door separating the alcove from the staff work area; others have a door opening but no door. Some procedure rooms that do not separate patient and staff traffic locate the control alcove at the back of the room, away from the patient/staff door.

The decision as to whether to provide a door (instead of just a doorway) depends on a number of factors. These include:

1. Whether radiation protection is required at the opening (which, in turn, will depend on a number of variables such as the location and movement of radiation-emitting equipment relative to the door opening, whether the control alcove itself shields the door opening, whether there is adequate space for a radiation maze [an arrangement of protective partitions that block scatter radiation], and so on)
2. Whether noise control is determined to be more important than the ease of technologist movement into and out of the procedure room
3. The amount of equipment that will be transported between the staff work area and the procedure room
4. Whether there is adequate space to accommodate both the door swing and staff and equipment movement

(Note: Even though physically disabled individuals may not be able to perform all the tasks required of X-ray technologists, both the procedure room and the control area must meet the requirements of the Americans with Disabilities Act [ADA], which specifies minimal clearance dimensions.)

Sometimes two control alcoves are placed back-to-back to form a double-control alcove that serves two procedure rooms. (See figures 13-3 through 13-5, pp. 239–40.) Advantages of this arrangement are:

- It opens the possibility of sharing one generator. At one time this arrangement meant cost savings, but it is becoming less common because most new imaging systems require their own dedicated generators.
- It easily accommodates an image-processing area that can be accessed directly from both control console areas.
- It provides space for toilet rooms between the two procedure rooms.
- It simplifies staff traffic between the two procedure rooms.

However, double-control alcove configurations often result in one "right-hand room" and one "left-hand room" rather than a consistent standard room arrangement. This is because a patient lying supine on a table is often approached from his or her right side and some tables only tilt in one direction, as shown in figure 13-5. There also may be problems associated with mirror-imaging the placement of X-ray equipment. The right-hand room will have good visibility between the control area and the patient table, but the left-hand room may have compromised visibility because the patient table may block the technologist's view of the patient's head. Thus, when planning a double-control alcove, it is important to verify that the patient table and imaging equipment assembly to be installed will allow adequate view of the patient from the control area. Some imaging equipment does not come in right- and left-hand models. Therefore, when the table tilts, the patient may be visible only if the control alcove is located to the right and at the "foot" side of the table.

Some procedures do not require a separate control area. For example, most mammography units incorporate a radiation-protected control space into the design of the imaging equipment itself. In ultrasound rooms, the control areas may simply consist of a chair located near the equipment console.

Control Rooms

For special procedure rooms such as angiography suites, cardiac catheterization labs, and other rooms used for interventional studies, a separate control room, rather than a control alcove, usually is necessary. The separate room is desired because of:

- The amount of equipment and personnel that need to be in the room.
- The special environmental (cooling, ventilation, electrical power, and so on) requirements of the equipment.
- The need for acoustic control that prevents noise from disturbing the medical team and prevents the patient from overhearing confidential conversations.
- The increasing need for infection control and sterile conditions in the procedure room. A separate control room allows personnel to enter and exit without passing through the procedure room. It also allows for separate ventilation, humidity, and air-filtration conditions within each space. (For further discussion of HVAC systems, see chapter 16, "Utility Requirements.")

Figure 13-3. Double Radiography Control Alcove

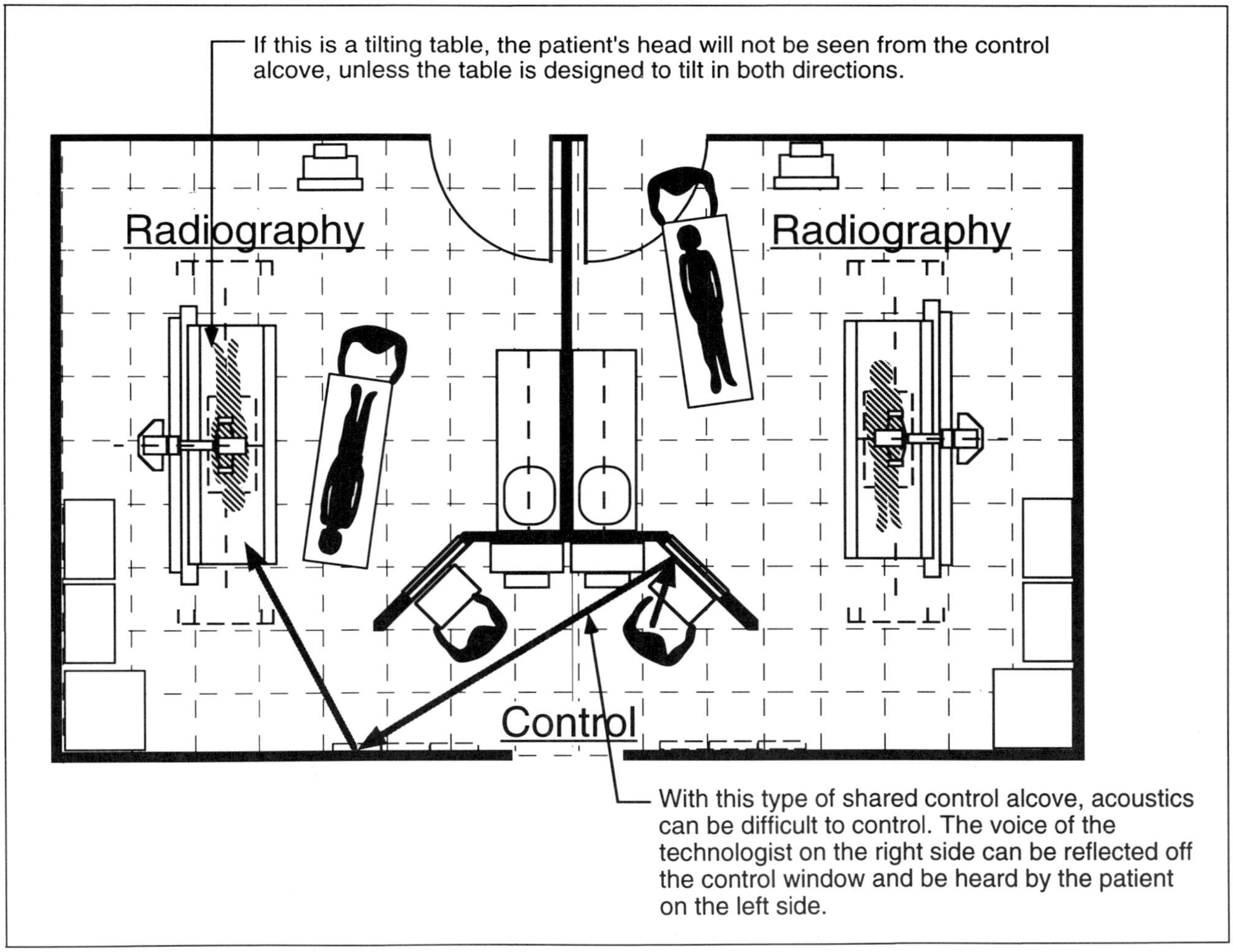

Figure 13-4. Double Radiography or Radiography/Fluoroscopy Control Alcove

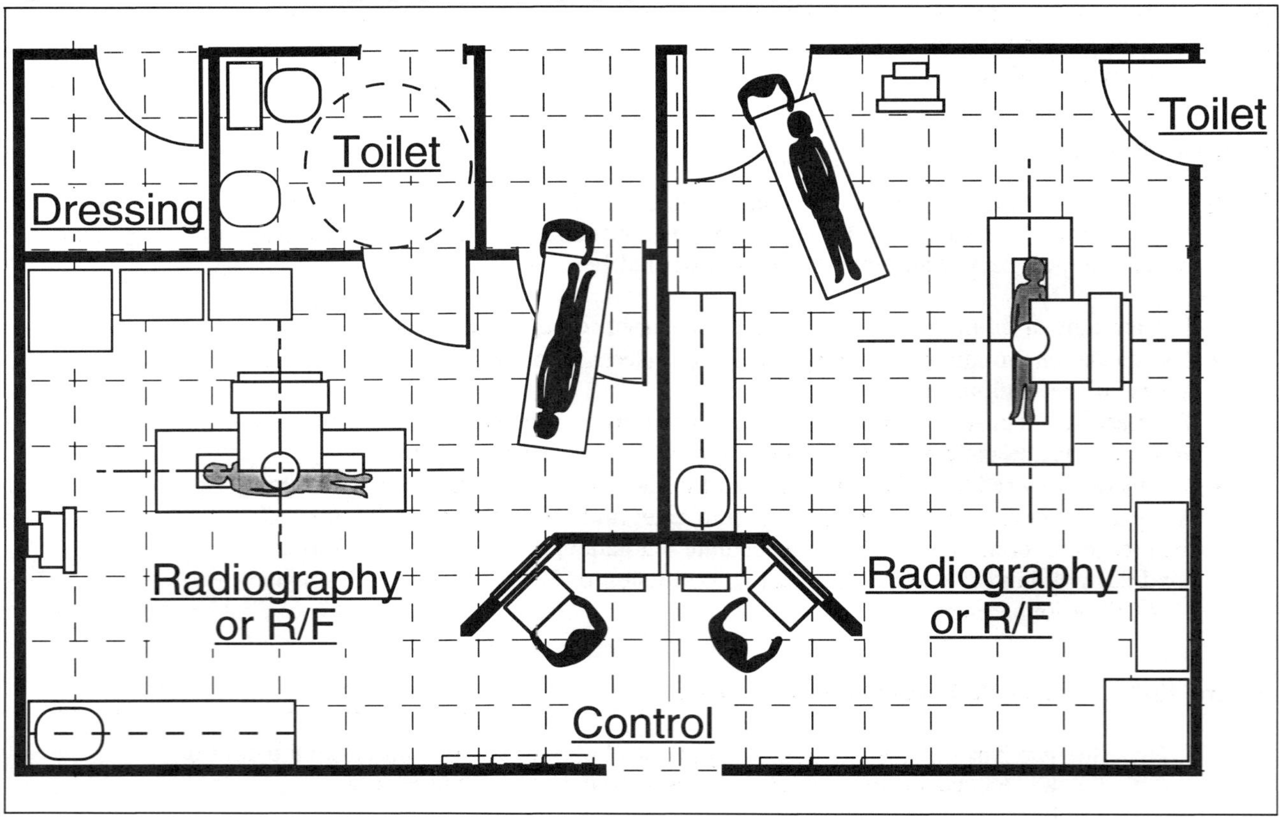

Figure 13-5. Double Radiography or Radiography/Fluoroscopy Control Alcove

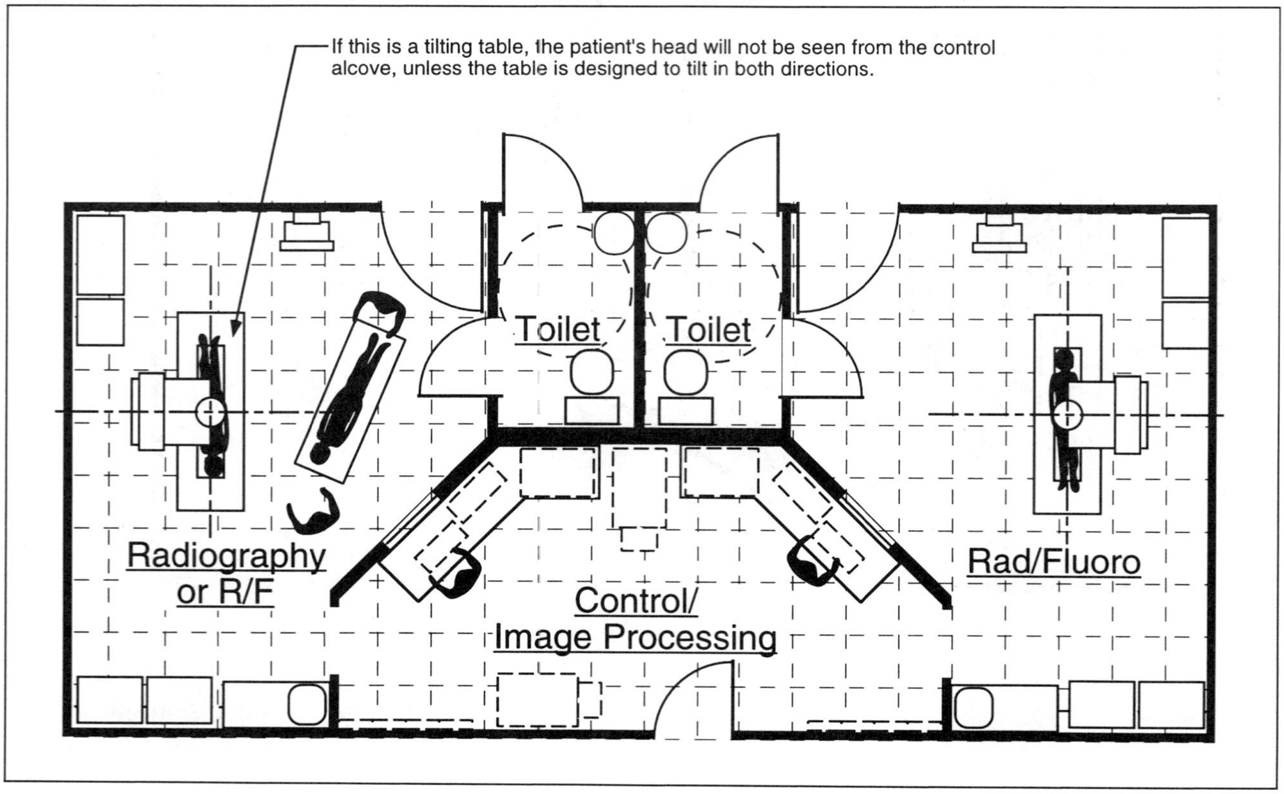

Sometimes one large control room is used for two special procedure rooms. Although in some instances this arrangement can reduce space requirements, it has become less popular for angiography and other interventional suites because of requirements for sterility assurance when two medical teams are present, the need for acoustic control, and the limited opportunities for two procedure rooms to share generators. However, digital printers, scrub sink alcoves, and some ancillary equipment can be shared effectively by two procedure rooms. These can be located just outside the control rooms.

Computed tomography (CT) suites often have a control room and a computer room adjacent to, but separate from, the procedure room. However, some recent CT units do not require the same computer equipment or the same environmental features they did in the past and thus may not require a separate computer room. The control consoles of these units also are becoming simpler than they were in the past; sometimes much of the equipment is incorporated into a simple computer workstation configuration.

Magnetic resonance imaging (MRI) control areas must be physically separated from the procedure room because of magnetic and RF interactions. (See figure 13-6.) In addition, only MRI-compatible equipment can be used within certain distances of the magnet's isocenter. (Planning requirements based on magnetic and RF interactions are discussed in the section entitled Special Considerations for MRI Installations in chapter 15, "Physical Properties Influencing Design.")

Universal Room Design

Frequently, it is desirable to design *universal rooms,* that is, rooms that can accommodate similar equipment from a variety of vendors with few modifications to the space. (See figure 13-7.) There are several reasons for this:

1. Equipment is changing rapidly.
2. Similar equipment from different vendors often requires special infrastructure and design features.
3. Most imaging facilities are expected to outlive the current generation of equipment.
4. It often is difficult and inappropriate for radiologists and administrators to commit to a specific make and model of equipment years before the building is to be occupied.

Figure 13-6. MRI Control Room

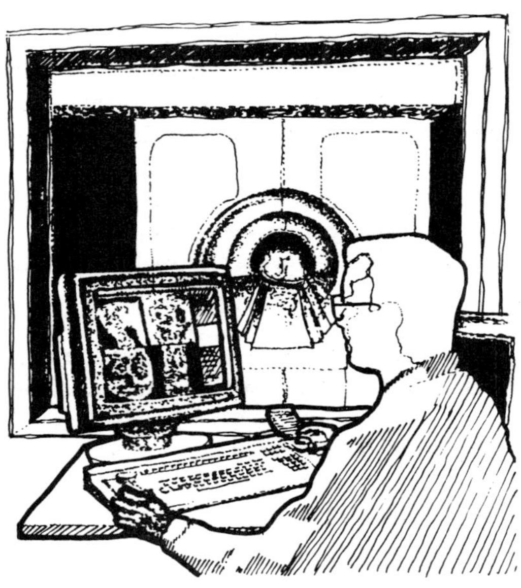

Figure 13-7. Universal Room

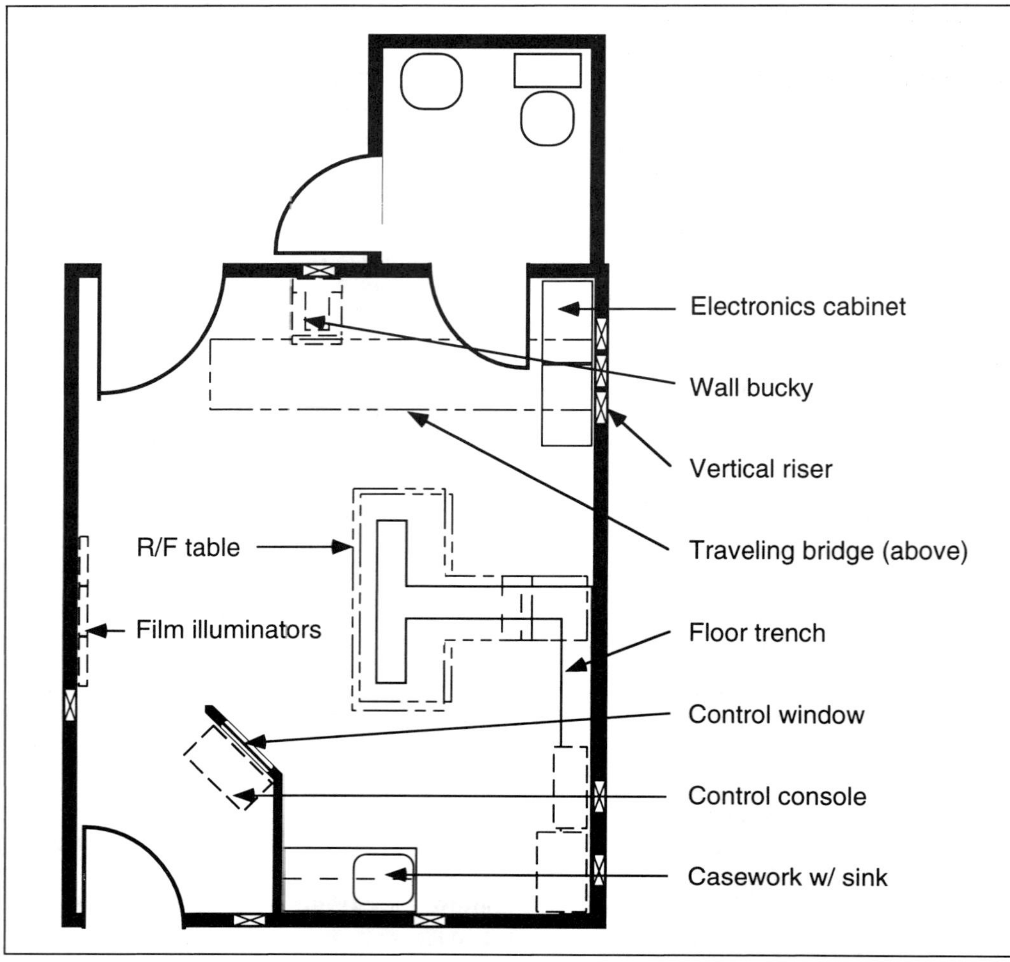

However, even if universal rooms are incorporated into the planning concept, there should be an initial equipment selection to determine baseline electrical loads, heat dissipation, and other criteria.

Generally, universal rooms are appropriate for basic radiographic and fluoroscopic equipment such as that found in general radiography or radiography/fluoroscopy (R/F) procedure rooms. For highly specialized procedures such as angiography and cardiac catheterization, universal room design is less appropriate because variations among the different equipment configurations and their space requirements are greater.

To provide flexibility, control costs related to equipment changes, and minimize the scheduling impact of equipment changes, universal rooms contain special ceiling systems, floor systems, and utility distribution components. In particular, the characteristics of a universal room might include:[3]

- *Slightly more space than equipment-specific rooms:* The additional space accommodates the space requirements of various vendors, and often the room is sized for worst-case conditions.
- *A universal ceiling support system as compared to individual equipment-specific ceiling supports:* Individual manufacturers and individual equipment models require ceiling supports in specific locations. A universal system locates ceiling-mounted supports evenly spaced (usually about ±26 inches on center) along the entire ceiling or a major portion of it. Because the supports are perpendicular to the equipment rails, they can support rails placed in almost any location. (See figures 13-8 and 13-9.)

- *Electrical ducts and troughs provided at various locations in the wall, ceiling, and floor:* Often, vertical riser ducts are located in the walls on all four sides of the room. Typically, they are placed near the control alcove, the power supply, and the likely locations of other fixed equipment, such as generators and transformers. Raceways also are located in the floor connecting the power supply and other equipment to the table and other floor-mounted imaging equipment. For new construction, floor slab thickness should be increased and coordinated with the depth of these flush raceways set into the floor. This may not be practical in renovation projects with suspended floor slabs (that is, for those that are not on grade). In this case, raceways sometimes are

Figure 13-8. Universal Ceiling

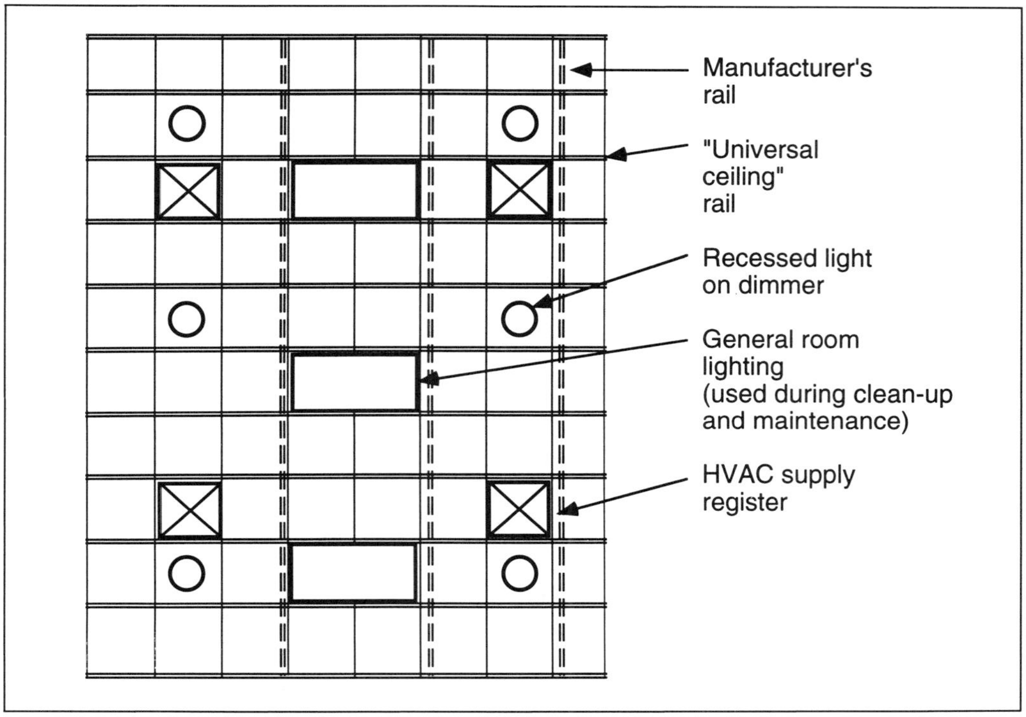

Figure 13-9. Universal Ceiling Support System

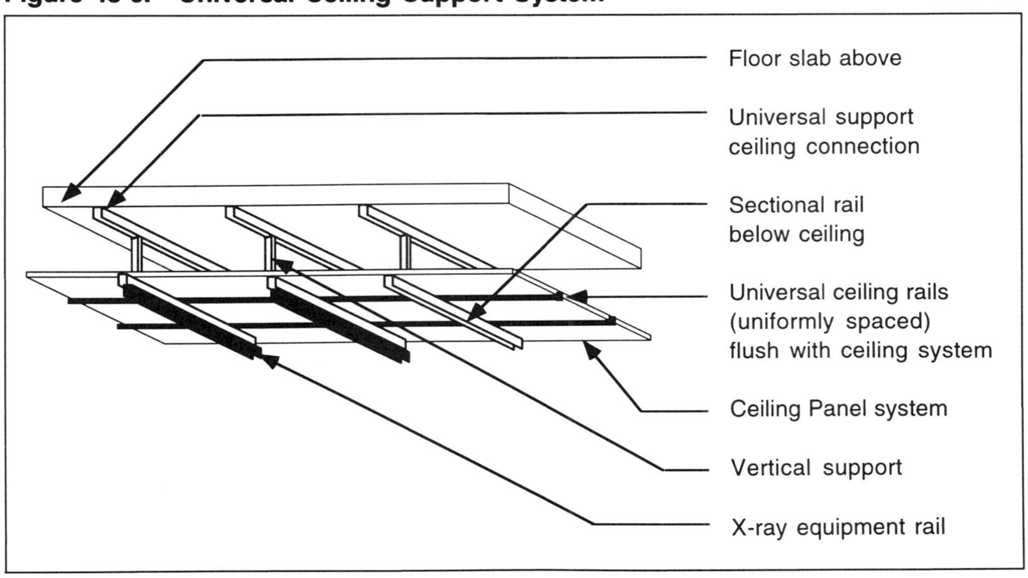

placed beneath the floor slab, if possible. However, running cables through subfloor raceways can be difficult because longer cable runs and numerous bends and turns are required. Finally, a cable tray above the ceiling may be located along the room perimeter. Wires and cable are "pulled" from a power source to the various pieces of equipment. Universal raceways are designed and placed to accommodate wires and cable provided by a variety of manufacturers. In equipment-specific rooms, cables are often run through channel ducts or conduit that is specifically located by the vendor supplying the equipment. (See figure 13-10.)

The universal room approach offers several advantages. They include:

- Ability to accommodate a variety of makes and models of imaging equipment. (Because the universal room is designed for this flexibility, the contract documents [drawings and specifications] can be drafted even if equipment selections change later. However, universal room design does not imply that equipment selections should be deferred. It simply is an attempt to reduce the cost premium that may result if equipment selections change.)

Figure 13-10. Electrical Duct and Trough Layout for Universal Rooms

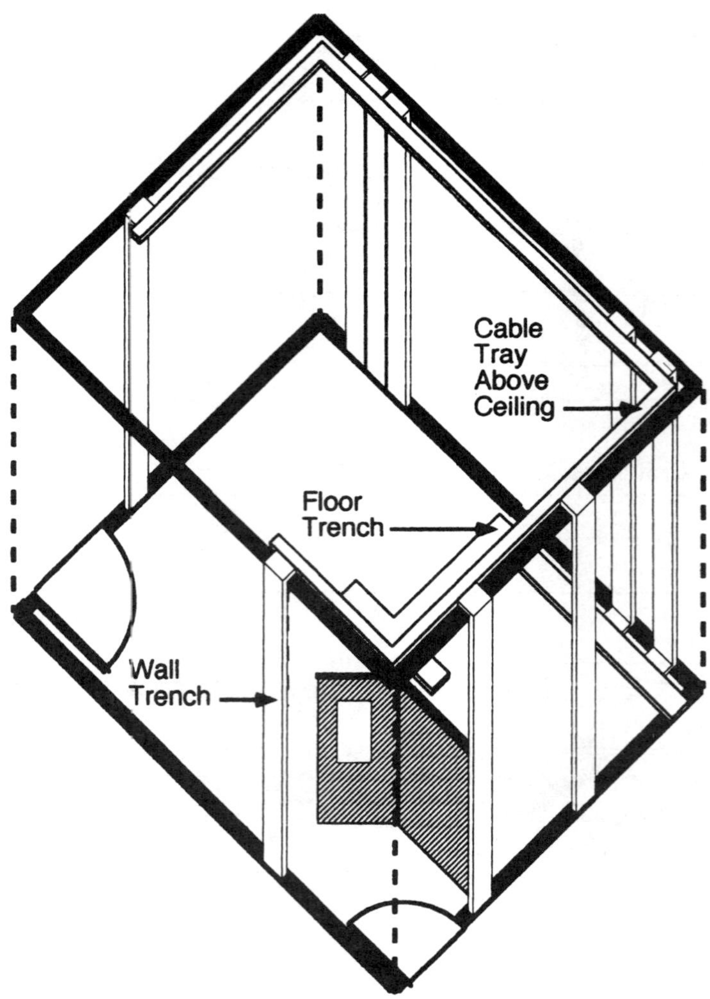

- Ability to modify and/or replace equipment in the future with minimal remodeling or demolition.
- Preservation of the project schedule, which might otherwise be significantly delayed by last-minute equipment changes.
- Preservation of the construction budget due to fewer architectural, electrical, and structural change orders.
- Reduction in additional professional fees that might be warranted by owner-initiated equipment changes.

However, the universal room approach also has a number of disadvantages. They include:

- Cost premiums due to slightly oversized space. (However, this additional space may provide additional operational efficiencies and adequate space for future modifications.)
- Cost premiums for installing universal structural supports. (In addition, as new equipment is selected, additional structural calculations may be necessary, depending on the loading conditions of that equipment. Universal room design implies providing some excess structural capacity. It is likely that not all the excess capacity will be used. However, the alternative of having to increase structural capacity after the room has been built can be prohibitively expensive.)
- Cost premiums for excess electrical, plumbing, and HVAC capacity, as well as placement of additional raceways and ducts.
- Possibility that the flexibility provided by the universal room design will not accommodate all equipment selections and configurations. (This is particularly true as certain imaging technologies go through significant changes within brief periods of time. Therefore, the particular characteristics of universal rooms may need to be evaluated and refined periodically. For this reason, universal room design is most appropriate for basic procedure rooms, where physical needs are relatively constant.)
- Requirement that specific equipment must be identified before the regulatory review process can begin. (This might suggest that the equipment that represents the worst case for structural, HVAC, and electrical conditions should be selected for the purpose of the review process. However, the worst case may be represented in one piece of equipment for some conditions [such as structure] and in another for other conditions [such as HVAC and electrical systems].)

The theory behind universal room design is that of investing a little extra money initially in order to avoid greater costs that would be required by future changes. Because the likelihood of future changes is high, the advantages of universal room design for most basic imaging rooms generally outweigh the disadvantages. There should always be some reserve capacity in the building systems. The difficulty is in defining and justifying the optimal amount.

General Considerations for Image-Processing Areas

Image processing can be centralized, clustered, or dedicated to specific equipment. *Centralized image processing* requires less duplication of processing equipment but may require more staff travel time. Thus, it is most appropriate for small- or medium-size departments, where travel distances are relatively short. *Clustered (or decentralized) processing* is effective for medium- and large-size departments or facilities that have clustered or decentralized imaging services. Clustered processing may require some duplication of processing equipment, but that cost usually can be offset by shorter travel distances for technologists.

Equipment-dedicated processing is appropriate for high-volume imaging modalities, such as chest X rays, general radiography, and fluoroscopy, and sometimes for mammography systems that require films to be processed at special speeds. In equipment-dedicated processing, the processing equipment is attached directly onto the image acquisition unit or at least close by. Equipment-dedicated processing allows the technologist (or other personnel) to process the image without leaving the patient or the procedure area.

There are three types of image-processing areas, some of which may be combined—darkrooms, daylight areas, and digital equipment areas—and each of which has specific design guidelines. (These three image-processing areas correspond to the image-processing techniques discussed in chapter 7, "Image Management and Film Processing.")

Darkrooms

The conventional darkroom traditionally has been the area in which images are processed and, although alternative image-processing methods are evolving rapidly, it is unlikely that the darkroom will soon disappear altogether. Often, a light-sensitive darkroom is desired at least for backup capabilities.

Darkroom size is affected by the number of processors provided and the number of personnel working in the room at one time. Sometimes two film processors are provided in busy darkrooms to increase workload capacity. "The greatest inefficiency occurs when the technicians can unload films faster than an automatic processor can accept them. To remedy this, two processors may be installed instead of one to double the film-feeding rate."[4] The darkroom should be sized for peak workload capacity.

Automatic film processors usually are located just outside the darkroom (although alternative arrangements are possible), with a film feed tray passing through the wall into the darkroom. (See figure 13-11.) The lighted side of the wall where the processor is located is used for quality control review of films as they come out of the processor. The through-the-wall connection must be lighttight. If possible, the lightroom side should be designed so that it can be completely darkened. This will facilitate recovery of films that may become trapped in the processor.

Adequate clearance should be provided next to the processor to allow for maintenance access. Typically, a clearance of 24 inches is recommended on all sides. Silver-recovery instruments should be placed low in the room so that the system will not be forced to pump against the force of gravity. Additionally, a service sink should be located nearby for cleaning the processor's rollers.

Figure 13-11. Darkroom with Automatic Film Processor

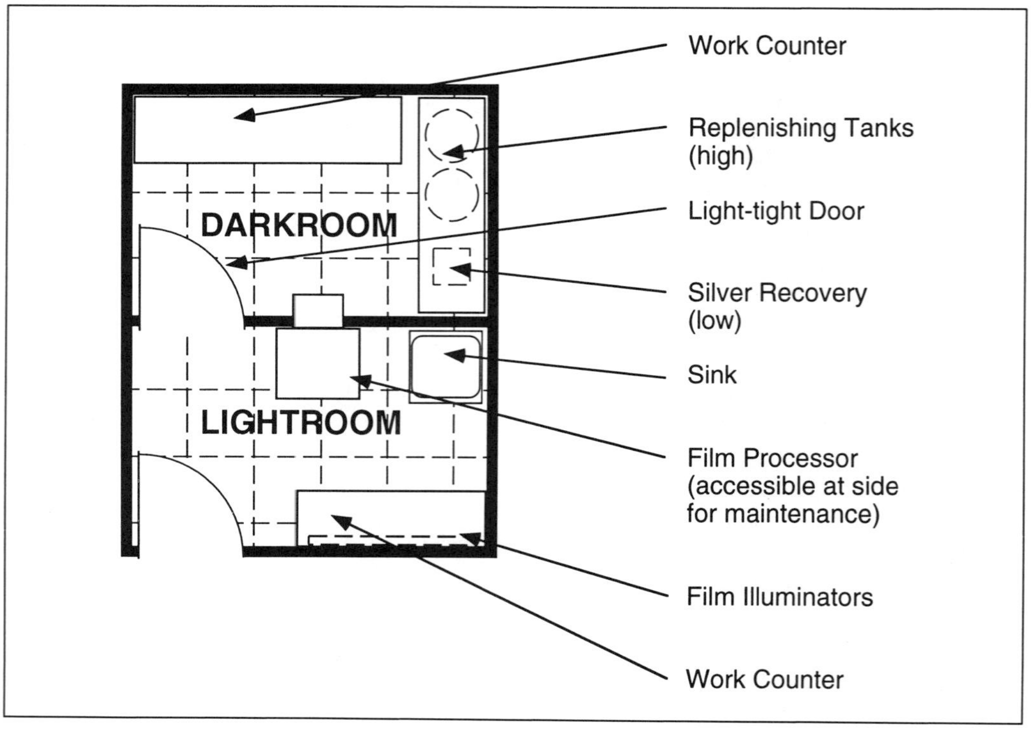

X-ray film is highly sensitive to many physical conditions, including light, radiation, static electrical discharge, and so on. Details and methods employed in darkroom design must reflect the sensitive nature of radiographic film processing:

> Radiographic [X-ray] film can be affected by heat, light, humidity, static electricity, pressure, chemical fumes, and radiation. Since so many things can alter radiographic film, the darkroom must be considered a scientific laboratory.
>
> The most common cause of unsatisfactory radiographs is fog. Fog is noninformational density, or blackness from silver deposits that occur in the wrong place, masking the visibility of detail. . . . Many energy levels cause radiographic film to become exposed and, after processing, to become black. Once radiation exposure has been made, the radiographic film becomes at least twice as sensitive to all energy levels, and thus extreme care is required in working within the darkroom laboratory.[5]

Doors

A variety of lighttight doors is available for darkrooms. Rotary doors may not comply with accessibility requirements unless they are very large. Although lighttight mazes can be used, they require more space than swinging or hinged doors. Lighttight hinged doors with lighttight speak holes are available to aid communication between the darkroom technician and personnel outside the darkroom. Intercom systems also should be considered.

Safety and emergency egress also need to be planned. Alarm systems, smoke alarms, fire extinguishers, and other fire protection systems should be installed:

> Darkrooms pose a particular challenge to designers and contractors, because the people who will use them must work in subdued light or . . . darkness. . . . Sharp corners on workbenches [should be eliminated; wall cabinets typically have open slots and no doors]. Recesses for waste cans, unobstructed safety exits . . . [and] locks that can be defeated from the outside in case of an emergency [should be provided].[6]

Optional interlocks also may be provided to turn room lighting off when a film storage bin is opened.

Lighting

Two types of room lighting should be provided. *Safelighting*—illumination that does not fog or cause other visible changes to light-sensitive material—is used when the darkroom is operational.[7] *Incandescent white lighting* is provided for cleanup and equipment maintenance. Incandescent lighting is preferred over fluorescent lighting because fluorescent lights tend to glow after they are turned off.[8] Switches for each type of lighting should be located away from each other so that the wrong switch is not inadvertently activated. In addition, the white lighting switch should have a lock or cover to prevent accidental activation. Another problem is the following:

> Oftentimes, too many safelights are used or they are too close to the work surface, resulting in exposure to the film. Safelights mounted over a processor feed tray should be connected to the processor so that they turn off when the film is fed into the sensor switch. Some special films, which are generally called new-modality films (for computerized tomography, ultrasound, nuclear medicine, magnetic resonance, and lasers), are based on cine emulsion technology and are sensitive to red light and thus require a dark green filter or no lights at all. The dark green filter is very dark.[9]

A light-colored ceiling surface will maximize the reflectance of overhead safelights, as will walls painted an off-white or cream color. Darkroom walls and ceilings do not need to be painted black.

Gypsum board ceilings are preferred over lay-in ceilings. The latter are not lighttight and seams may need to be masked to prevent light leakage. Additionally, lay-in ceilings can allow dirt and other particles to drop from above.[10]

Finishes and materials that allow static energy charges to build up should be avoided. Static discharge can affect film images. For example:

> Static energy occurs in nonconductive material such as plastic (film base, synthetic-fiber clothing) and build up until it reaches a potential to allow rapid discharge in the form of a spark. Film is made of [a] nonconductive base (a good static producer) and emulsion layers on each side. The emulsion layer contains gelatin that is a semiconductor and a mild static producer. Static generated in the base as the film is banged around inside the cassette can escape only through the gelatin layers, which also contain the recording media (silver halide crystals). Thus the discharge is recorded as a pile of silver in the form of a tree, a crown, or smudge static markings. To prevent the rapid discharge (the spark), it is important to provide as many avenues as possible for the electricity to dissipate (bleed off) gradually. [Film holders, if used] must be grounded, as must the passbox (which cannot be lined with rubber or plastic) and the darkroom work bench. . . . In addition the relative humidity in the darkroom should be 40 to 60% at all times.[11]

HVAC

Air filtration and ventilation systems for darkrooms must prevent excessive amounts of dust from settling, which can affect film image quality. In addition, personnel who work with potentially harmful chemicals must be protected from illness and injury. "A typical darkroom should have a [lighttight] ventilator in the lower portion of the entrance door or in the wall near the floor. At the opposite end of the room, there should be an exhaust fan in the ceiling. Fresh air should flow past the worker, then move on past processing areas to the exhaust. There should not be any pockets of stale air or fumes."[12] (For further discussion of HVAC systems, see chapter 16, "Utility Requirements.")

Temperature and humidity should be kept within ranges recommended by film processor manufacturers. For example, high temperatures can shorten the shelf life of unexposed film and therefore affect image quality. Low humidity may result in film artifact from static electricity discharges.[13]

Daylight Processing Areas

Daylight film processors allow for greater flexibility in the design of the image-processing area because the processing equipment does not require an enclosed lighttight room. In particular, the design of central work cores has been greatly simplified by the advent of daylight systems. Often a series of procedure rooms will be arranged around an open work core with daylight processors, image quality viewing stations, and film-sorting areas. (See figure 13-12.) Sometimes conventional darkrooms also will be located near the work core. Because daylight systems can be placed in open work areas, these processors can be placed close to control areas without the need for lighttight, through-the-wall cassette passboxes.

The overall turnaround time for processing images can be shorter with daylight systems, and access to the equipment usually is easier. Space requirements for some daylight processing areas are less than those for darkrooms, although this is not always the case. Compact daylight systems are available for use as equipment-specific processors or to be shared among multiple-image acquisition devices. Daylight systems can be used for most types of imaging, including radiography, fluoroscopy, ultrasound, mammography, CT, MRI, and nuclear medicine.

Temperature and humidity control are as important for daylight systems as they are for conventional darkroom processing. The discharge of chemicals (for both darkrooms and daylight systems) is highly regulated, and requirements are becoming increasingly strict. A service sink should be located nearby for cleaning processor components.

Figure 13-12. Open Work Core with Daylight Film Processors

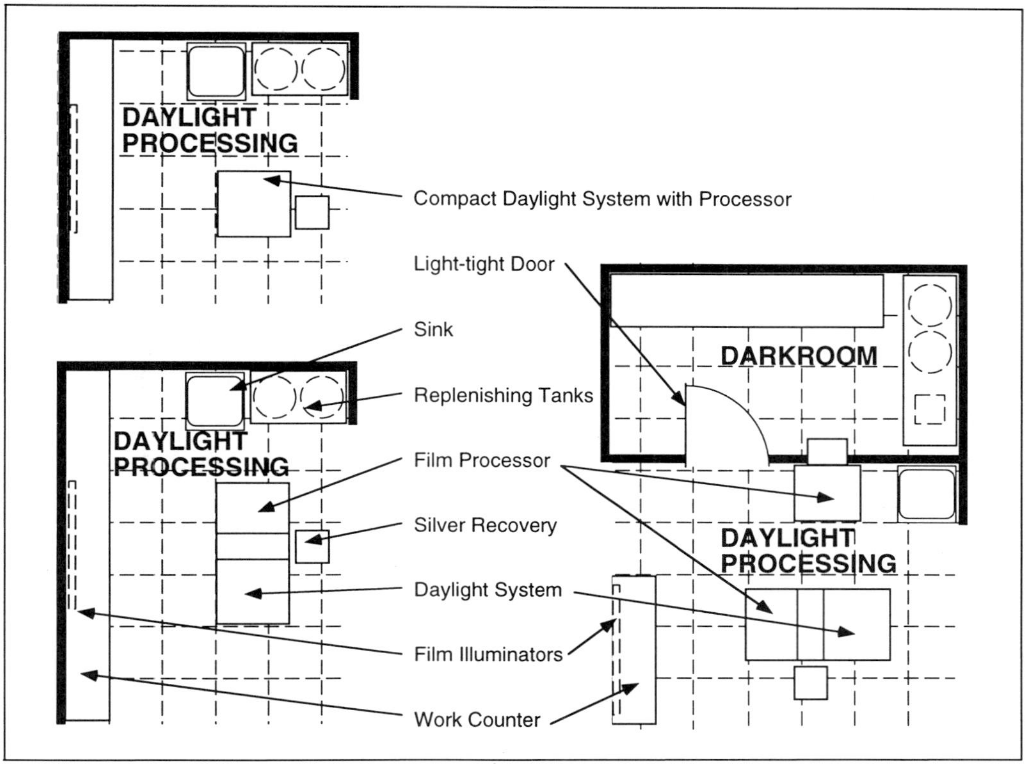

Chemicalless film-processing systems have recently been introduced. With increasingly stringent chemical disposal regulations, it is likely that such systems will have a significant impact on medical image processing in the future.

Digital Image-Processing Areas

Two approaches to digital image management are gaining in popularity. One approach, *film digitization,* converts film images to a digital format by digitizing the hard-copy image. The other method, *digital image acquisition,* acquires the image digitally, either directly or on photo-stimulable phosphor plates instead of film-screen (X-ray-sensitive film sandwiched between X-ray-excitable phosphors) cassettes. (See figure 13-13.)

Film Digitization

Film digitization occurs when light (either focused or laser) is transmitted through the film image and onto a light detector, which usually is a form of video camera or photomultiplier tube. The detector records the image, converts the information from analog to digital format, and transmits the digital data for storage, display, or future retrieval.[14]

In addition to requiring space for film-processing equipment and personnel, this approach requires space for a film digitizer. Additional space should be provided for:

- Computer workstations
- Printers
- Digital image storage devices
- Computer systems equipment
- Various other components of the image management and communication system network

Figure 13-13. Digital Image-Processing Area

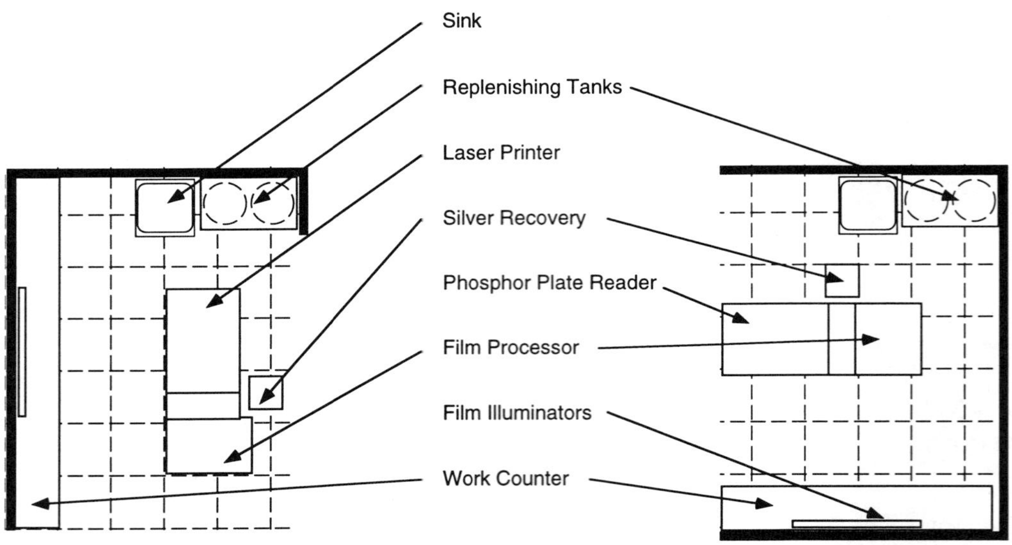

Digital Image Acquisition

Truly filmless image acquisition utilizes a reusable, light-sensitive (or photo-stimulable) phosphor plate (or other type of reusable medium) rather than film to capture the image. The plate can be reused in much the same way that a magnetic disk used with personal computers can be reused after data stored on the disk are erased. (Some imaging equipment, such as CT and MR, has inherent system components that capture the digital image directly without ever converting it to film or phosphor plate.)

The digitally acquired image is then read by a laser scanner, where a direct digital image is obtained. Delivery of the latent image can be automated, or the phosphor plate can be carried to the processor manually in much the same way that it is done with conventional film-screen image processing. Once the digital image is obtained, it can be stored, transmitted, or displayed throughout the digital network. In addition, hard-copy images can be printed on paper or film.[15]

Digital image management systems may involve a number of components, including:

- A computed image acquisition device(s) that includes a direct digitizer or a laser film digitizer (to convert film images to digital format)
- An image-viewing monitor (to verify image quality)
- A data compression unit (to reduce the quantity of storage space required)
- Data storage devices (to provide both intermediate storage and archival storage)
- Image display workstations (to be located in a variety of places such as the imaging department, the intensive care unit, the emergency department, operating rooms, physicians' offices and homes, remote reading areas, and so on)
- A laser film printer (to produce hard-copy images)
- An image transmission network
- A teleradiology unit (to transmit images to remote locations)
- A radiology information system (RIS) and/or hospital information system (HIS) interface (to combine image data with other patient information)
- Multimedia workstations (to allow the user to access PACS, RIS, HIS, and other systems from one location)

Special electrical, ventilation, heat dissipation, acoustic, and space requirements are necessary. However, each is likely to change as the technology develops further.

General Considerations for Image-Reading/Viewing Rooms

Medical images are viewed or read by individuals as well as groups. They serve a number of purposes and are useful tools in:

- Initial diagnosis
- Follow-up review
- Peer discussion and consultation
- Communication of second opinions
- Discussion and consultation with referring physicians
- Consultation and education with patients (usually done by the referring physician rather than the radiologist)
- Student/resident teaching
- Quality control

Images may be read in a number of different areas, including:

- The physician's private office or home
- A referring physician's viewing alcove or room
- The procedure room
- A group reading room
- A large conference room
- An auditorium
- Various remote locations simultaneously

Additionally, images may be viewed using a variety of equipment, including:

- Conventional film illuminators
- Alternators or multiviewers
- Computer workstations
- Video monitors
- Projection screens

In private or group reading rooms or alcoves, medical images are viewed primarily on film illuminators, alternators, and computer workstations, or some combination thereof. (Guidelines for determining space requirements for these areas are listed in table 12-2 [pp. 208–9], chapter 12, "Space Requirements.")

Film illuminators (sometimes referred to as *view boxes* or *light boxes*) provide a translucent surface where film images can be placed temporarily and viewed. (See figure 13-14.) Each film illuminator is slightly larger than, and roughly the same shape as, a film image. Film illuminators are typically arranged in one or two horizontal rows. For example, two rows of four illuminators each are said to be in a four-over-four configuration. A configuration of multiple film illuminators should provide consistent lighting intensity and color throughout the entire configuration. Film illuminators can be flush or surface mounted on walls and can be arranged for use by standing or sitting personnel. Often, a continuous shelf is placed below the illuminators to hold individual films.

Alternators or *multiviewers* allow several films to be viewed simultaneously and allow groups of films to be viewed in rapid sequence. Large numbers of films are placed in transparent panels or belts and held in place within a relatively compact area. Each group of films is quickly placed over a large translucent panel where the assortment of images can be viewed by small groups of personnel.[16] Frequently, a movable, high-intensity "hot" spotlight is provided to illuminate areas of detail.

Computer workstations enable electronic images to be read. These include both images that are captured on computed image acquisition instruments (for example, computed radiography, CT, and MRI) and film images that are later digitized. Computer workstations may have multiple monitors configured similarly to multiple film illuminators. (See the section entitled General Considerations for Computer Workstation Environments later in this chapter.)

Reading rooms should have indirect lighting that is capable of being dimmed. The general level of room illumination should be similar to that of the image-viewing surface, and glare should be limited to the extent possible. Film illuminators, alternators, or computer workstations should not face each other directly because the light emitted from these devices can cause significant glare. The control of glare in offices that have exterior windows or direct lighting can be difficult. (Specific guidelines for lighting are discussed in the section entitled General Considerations for Computer Workstation Environments in this chapter and in chapter 16, "Utility Requirements.")

Acoustic control should be provided in any reading area to help contain conversations within the room and to keep distracting noises outside. Additionally, acoustic control will help keep conversations about viewed images private and confidential. This is particularly important when image display workstations are located within patient care departments, such as intensive care units, where patients and family members might be nearby.

Some computer equipment can generate considerable noise in group reading rooms in which computer workstations are located and used. Thus, it would be preferable to locate the noisy computer equipment in an acoustically isolated room separate from the computer viewing stations.

As mentioned previously, group reading rooms are likely to contain three types of viewing equipment: film illuminators, alternators, and computer workstations. Each type of equipment should be arranged to permit small groups of three to six individuals to view images together. Some stations might be configured to accommodate only one or two individuals. Reading areas should have a calming environment, and secluded sections should be provided

Figure 13-14. Conventional Film Illuminators

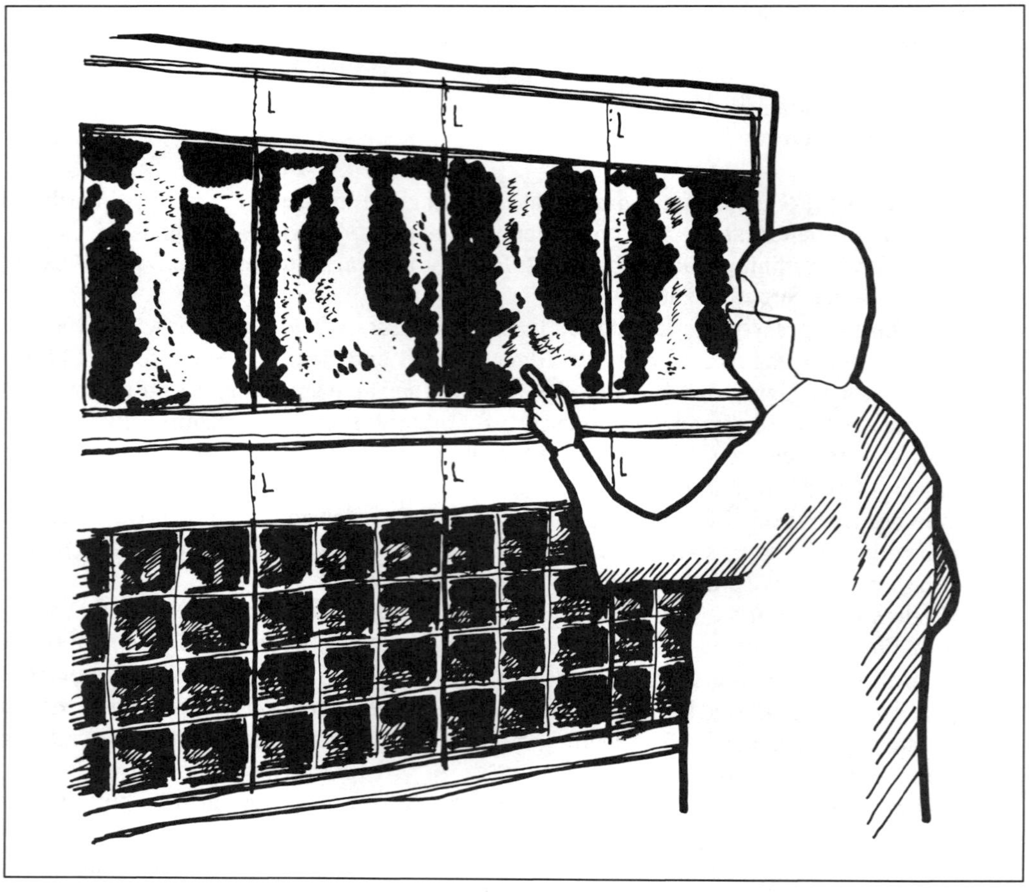

so that staff members can discuss difficult cases in privacy. Reading rooms also will contain computer equipment for other information systems such as HISs and RISs. Along with PACS workstations, HIS and RIS workstations are currently becoming more fully integrated into multimedia consoles.

Images read in radiologists' offices are viewed on either film illuminators and/or computer workstations. Because of their size and service clearance requirements, alternators are less commonly used in private offices. Office furniture should be arranged so as to allow the radiologist to view images from his or her desk and to consult with other physicians.

Because most imaging exams are the result of referrals from other physicians, it often is desirable to provide a special room in which referring physicians can view images. This room is best located next to the active film file room but entered in such a way that referring physicians do not have to pass through the working areas of the imaging department. A pass-through between the viewing area and the film file room allows referring physicians to view films without taking them out of the department. This can help reduce the number of lost or misplaced films. The viewing room also can be connected to selected procedure rooms by closed-circuit television so that referring physicians can observe procedures in progress. In addition, all radiologists' work areas can be connected to a central dictation system, if desired.

General Considerations for Image and Report Storage

Although the comprehensive use of electronic image management systems has the potential to eventually replace hard-copy film and report storage systems, it is unlikely that file rooms will completely disappear, at least not in the near future. In fact, the overall space requirements for image and data storage will first increase as electronic image management systems become more popular. This is because, initially, two types of storage systems will be needed—hard copy (film and paper) and electronic (magnetic or optical media). Because the transition to filmless imaging will be slow for most facilities, a *dual* or *hybrid* system will be in place during this period. It would be prohibitively expensive to convert all previous analog film images to digital media, even though this is technically possible.

For a number of years after filmless imaging becomes widespread, older images on film will still need to be recalled to compare current with previous images. In addition, hard-copy images must be kept as legal records. This is presently required by law in most states.

Two types of files are necessary: active and archive. *Active files* are located in the department or freestanding facility where they can be easily accessed by medical staff. *Archive files* (or inactive files) can be placed in remote locations, and old films and records can be retrieved as needed.

Hard-Copy Storage

Either fixed or movable shelving may be used for film files. In addition, movable and other forms of compact systems that allow a greater quantity of films to be stored in the same amount of space as is required by conventional file systems are available. (Space guidelines for film storage files are indicated in table 12-2 in chapter 12, "Space Requirements.")

Film storage systems can be extremely heavy. Compact systems generate higher, concentrated floor loads than do conventional systems. It is not uncommon for the structural capacities required to support film files to be greater than those for many types of imaging equipment.

Most hard-copy storage systems contain only the original image produced from a patient examination. If that film original is lent out for review, there is no additional backup copy. The frequency with which film originals become lost is quite high and has a significantly detrimental effect on the entire operation of the imaging department or facility. One of many benefits of electronic image and information management systems is the reduction in the number of lost films.

Electronic Storage Systems

A variety of electronic storage media are available. These include magnetic or optical storage devices for temporary, intermediate, and long-term storage of images and patient data.

Temporary storage is the storage of an image on a reusable phosphor plate (typically stored for less than four hours) until the latent image is processed. *Intermediate storage* is similar to a department's local film library, where data from patient examinations are stored for a specified period of time before being transferred to long-term storage. Intermediate storage units hold many gigabytes of data (where one gigabyte can record approximately 1,500 to 2,000 images depending on image file size).[17] *Archival storage* is used for long-term storage. Archival storage systems can hold several terabytes of data (where one terabyte is equal to 1,000 gigabytes). If active files are electronic and remote archive files are stored as hard copy, old images can be digitized and electronically transmitted to the active file as needed. This eliminates the need for manual delivery of old images to the active file system.

Computer storage devices have very specific utility requirements for uninterruptable and "clean" power, as well as temperature and humidity control. Although archival jukeboxes are small relative to their storage capacity, additional ancillary equipment is usually required as part of the long-term storage system. Because computer rooms can be noisy, acoustic damping of the room is recommended to prevent the transmission of noise into adjacent areas. Computer data storage rooms are relatively large; providing 600 to 800 net square feet (NSF) of space is not unrealistic for a totally filmless department in a large teaching hospital. Additional space may be needed for future expansion. However, the amount of data that can be stored in high-density storage devices is rapidly increasing. Therefore, if storage capacity increases more quickly than does the amount of data to be stored, the overall space requirements for archival storage will eventually decrease.

Electronic storage devices that contain medical images usually are linked to electronic data systems such as an HIS or an RIS via an electronic information network. In this way, various types of patient and business data can be combined. The network may be composed of twisted-pair wire, coaxial cable, fiber-optic cable, or some combination thereof. Microwave satellite systems also can be used to transmit information. Following is a comparison of these media:

- *Twisted-pair wire* is less expensive than the other media, but transmission speeds are lower and maximum transmission distances are relatively short.
- *Coaxial cable* is slightly more expensive than twisted-pair wire, but its transmission speed and maximum distance are greater.
- *Fiber-optic cable* is more expensive than both twisted-pair wire and coaxial cable, but its transmission speed is significantly greater. In addition, because it is less susceptible to electronic noise and does not emit energy, it offers a greater degree of data security.[18]
- *Microwave satellite transmission systems* are the most expensive of these four media. Their transmission speeds and distance capacities also are the highest.

General Considerations for Miscellaneous Support Spaces

In addition to procedure rooms and image-processing areas, imaging facilities must provide a variety of support spaces. These include dressing areas, patient toilet rooms, and waiting areas. (Guidelines for designing support spaces are listed in table 12-2 in chapter 12, "Space Requirements.")

Dressing Areas

Imaging facilities must provide cubicles large enough to accommodate patients protected under the Americans with Disabilities Act (ADA). Clustered dressing areas—one for men and one for women—tend to accommodate accessibility requirements more effectively than do separate dressing cubicles.

If dressing cubicles are assigned to, and located adjacent to, specific procedure rooms, at least one cubicle within each area is to be made disability accessible, according to ADA requirements. If dressing cubicles are clustered together, where one cluster for males and one for females serve the entire department or area, 5 percent (but at least one per cluster) are to be made disability accessible. However, if dressing areas are clustered together, each gowned patient may have to travel some distance between the dressing area and the procedure room. In addition:

> For new construction, section 4.1.3(21) of the Federal Register (the Americans with Disabilities Act) requires, Where dressing and fitting rooms are provided for use by the general public, patients, customers or employees, 5 percent, but never less than one, of dressing rooms for each type of use in each cluster of dressing rooms shall be accessible and shall comply with [section] 4.35. Examples of types of dressing rooms are those serving different genders or distinct and different treatment or examination facilities [p. 35616].
>
> Sections 4.35.2 and 4.35.4 of the ADA continue, A clear floor space allowing a person using a wheelchair to make a 180-degree turn shall be provided in every accessible dressing room entered through a swinging or sliding door. No door shall swing into any part of the turning space. Turning space shall not be required in a private dressing room entered through a curtained opening at least 32 in. (815 mm) wide if clear floor space complying with section 4.2 renders the dressing room usable by a person using a wheelchair.
>
> Every accessible dressing room shall have a 24 in. by 48 in. (610 mm by 1220 mm) bench fixed to the wall along the larger dimension. The bench shall be mounted 17 in. to 19 in. (430 to 485 mm) above the finish floor. Clear space shall be provided alongside the bench to allow a person using a wheelchair to make a parallel transfer onto the bench [p. 35664].[19]

Because dressing cubicles are small, it usually is desirable to have the surrounding partitions stop well below the ceiling (but above eye level) and to have door bottoms raised 12 to 18 inches above floor level. This allows for ventilation without providing separate air diffusers in each small cubicle. Curtains, in lieu of doors, are not desirable where the door opening leads directly to a departmental corridor or alcove.

Patient Toilet Rooms

Patient toilet rooms should be provided near certain types of procedure rooms, such as fluoroscopy, intravenous pyelography (IVP), ultrasound, MRI, and CT rooms. It is desirable for patients to enter the toilet room directly from the procedure room and exit to the department corridor without having to pass back through the procedure room. With this arrangement, which may require more space than would a toilet room with only one door, the procedure room is available for the next patient when the previous patient is still in the toilet room. The two doors leading into the toilet room may require special hardware to prevent the previous patient from unintentionally exiting through the procedure room and to prevent the next patient from inadvertently entering the toilet room when it is occupied. Acoustic insulation and even music systems will improve the level of privacy in toilet rooms adjacent to procedure rooms. Emergency nurse call systems also should be provided and are required in many states. Specific guidelines for designing toilet rooms that meet federal requirements for accessibility are described in the ADA.

Patient Waiting Areas

Waiting areas should be located and arranged so that they can be supervised by a receptionist who also can attend to other responsibilities. Additionally, natural daylight should be provided where possible, although the lighting level in the waiting area should not be significantly brighter than it is in other parts of the department. If windows or skylights transmit direct sunlight, additional shading or screening may be necessary.

Seating arrangements that accommodate small groups are the most appropriate. Individual seats are preferred over couches or benches. Seat fabric and coverings should be attractive and yet durable and easy to clean. Many jurisdictions have strict requirements regarding fire and smoke rating of materials.

If the number of seats required is large, it may be desirable to subdivide the waiting area into smaller sections to ensure privacy and to control noise. It also may be desirable to have multiple waiting areas to accommodate certain groups of patients, such as children or infectious patients.

If dressing rooms are not located adjacent to procedure rooms, gowned waiting space should be provided in addition to general waiting. Gowned waiting should be located within the patient zone of the department, either adjacent to the dressing area or near the procedure rooms.

Because imaging procedures often are frightening and difficult for some patients to understand, an education alcove near the waiting area may be beneficial. The education alcove should provide some degree of visual and acoustic privacy, a place to read books or pamphlets, and possibly a place to view instructional videos. A consultation room adjacent to the waiting area provides privacy in which personal medical or financial matters can be discussed.

Recently, concerns regarding ventilation and air-filtration requirements for persons with tuberculosis have received much attention. Some states have proposed special design requirements that apply to waiting areas as well as other locations. (See chapter 16, "Utility Requirements.")

General Considerations for Computer Workstation Environments

Although considerable effort and expense accompany design and planning efforts for most examination and treatment spaces in medical imaging facilities, technologists' and radiologists' workstations seldom enjoy the same level of concern and detail.[20] For example, the configuration, arrangement of equipment, and quality of light found in interventional radiographic rooms usually is the result of a comprehensive analysis of imaging techniques; ergonomics; and the flow of people, supplies, and instruments. In contrast, computer workstations in the same department frequently are placed in whatever space is available, with little consideration given to lighting, comfort, and work habits.

However, compared to examination and treatment rooms, the workstation is occupied for a longer duration, and so its design is just as critical to the successful delivery of high-quality medical care. In addition, properly designed workstations can help reduce the incidence of occupational injury and improve efficiency and work performance.

The Workstation Environment

As electronic image acquisition, storage, transfer, and manipulation are slowly accepted as fundamental components of modern medical imaging services, the computer workstation will replace more traditional equipment, such as film illuminators and alternators, as the tool of choice for viewing and—more important—for manipulating medical images. The workstation differs from film illuminators and alternators in that it is more interactive and represents the point of access between radiologists and an entire automated system of radiographic, medical, and demographic information. To date, most computer workstations also differ from film illuminators in their lower spatial resolution and luminance and, therefore, their less-desirable image quality.[21] To some extent, this deficiency is compensated by the ability to adjust the gray-scale value of the displayed image. This is possible only to a limited extent with film (which requires the use of a hot light).

To compensate for the workstation's lower luminance, ambient lighting must be dimmable to increase contrast and reduce glare. Visual display terminals (VDTs) and data input devices (keyboard, mouse, trackball, and so on) also must be arranged for user comfort and so that users do not need to frequently and repeatedly shift their focus.

Because radiographic image interpretation often involves multiple radiologists reviewing and conferring with each other, the room in which diagnostic workstations are located should be designed for acoustic control. It is just as important to contain conversational sounds within the space to maintain privacy as it is to prevent outside noises from disturbing ongoing work.

Finally, both seating and work surfaces must be designed for comfortable use over a long period. This suggests both adjustability (so that different users can work comfortably) and durability (so that equipment and furnishings will continue to provide adequate support for each user over time).

Workstation Uses and Locations

Radiology workstations have many uses and thus may be found in various configurations and locations. Two different types include diagnostic workstations used for primary or secondary diagnosis based on image interpretation and clinical workstations where diagnostic images are reviewed along with other pertinent nonradiographic medical data.

Image interpretation usually is based on comparison of recent images with previous ones. Therefore, most radiographic workstations will contain multiple monitors. Sometimes, the monitors are arranged in configurations similar to those of film illuminators, such as two over two or four over four. For example, the U.S. Army's medical diagnostic imaging support (MDIS) system includes diagnostic workstations with two to eight monitors and clinical workstations with one to four monitors.[22] (See appendix A for further discussion of the MDIS system.)

Multiple computer workstations may be found in reading rooms within the radiology department. Often the problems associated with glare and noise are compounded in such large installations. Individual workstations may be found in the offices of radiologists and other physicians. Here, the challenge is to design a physical environment that accommodates activities performed at the workstation as well as other activities such as reading, writing, and consultation. The ergonomic, lighting, and acoustic requirements for each activity are different. For example, an office with an exterior window might be ideal for reading but presents problems of glare when using the workstation.

As another example, a partial PACS located in a critical care suite should provide adequate acoustic control to prevent consultation conversations from being overheard by patients or their families. The workstation should be located near the activity core so that users do not need to leave the unit but far enough from patient rooms to provide privacy and prevent disruption of ongoing critical activities.

Other workstation locations might include the emergency, surgery, oncology, orthopedic, urology, and obstetric departments, or other locations where medical providers rely heavily on viewing or manipulating medical images. Management of nonradiologic images, such as endoscopy and pathology images, is growing in popularity and will have additional impact on the use of computerized medical workstations.

Ergonomics

Improper design of workstations or improper use of well-designed workstations can lead to myriad health problems, ranging from occasional headaches to chronic orthopedic and neurological disorders. "Most experts agree that three points of contact are the chief concerns in maintaining a healthful workplace: where your eye meets the monitor screen, where your fingers press against the keyboard, and where your body rests in its chair."[23]

Eye Problems

Many eye problems can be avoided by proper work habits and proper ergonomic design. One study reported in the *New York State Journal of Medicine* suggested that eye irritation of workers using VDTs was due to poor ergonomic conditions, such as improper lighting, glare, work materials poorly arranged on the work surface, and improperly corrected vision.[24]

Hand Problems

The incidence of hand- and wrist-related health problems has escalated since computer workstations have become increasingly common. One such type of malady, repetitive strain injury (RSI), is caused by constant repetition of the same physical motion. Multiple adjustments of seating, work surfaces, keyboards, and monitors can help reduce the likelihood of such injuries. The proper height of these workstation components can further reduce injury.

In 1988, the American National Standards Institute (ANSI) and the Human Factors Society (HFS) published a voluntary national standard (ANSI/HFS Standard 100—1988) with recommended VDT workstation dimensions. (See figure 13-15.) Table 13-1, p. 260, shows some of the ANSI/HFS Standard 100—1988 requirements.[25]

Seating Problems

Proper seating should conform to the ANSI/HFS-required dimensions and ranges of adjustability. The ability of workers to occasionally modify their posture and seating position can reduce the likelihood of workplace-related discomfort. "Except for specially designed ergonomic computer chairs, standard office equipment is typically not designed to adjust to the full range of settings required to accommodate the diversity of human beings."[26]

Function

There are two key differences between the medical image management computer workstations used by radiologists and technologists and the text management computer workstations used by administrative and business staff. First, functions performed on image management workstations usually involve less-direct data entry, especially extended amounts of keyboard entry. Second, image management workstations generally are used in rooms with lower light levels than their clerical counterparts. To accommodate these differences, medical workstations require both a work surface large enough to accommodate special tasks, such as graphic data selection and editing, and a special approach to lighting design.

Lighting

One of the greatest challenges facing designers of radiographic workstation environments is the low luminance of most VDTs. An overlighted environment or one in which the lighting is designed for paperwork instead of computer work creates a lighting imbalance between the monitor and the work surface. Ambient lighting for computer workstations must be provided in such a way that the contrast between the screen and surrounding surfaces is not so great that it causes eyestrain, and yet the room must be dark enough and free of glare for the screen image to be readable.

Room lighting that is three times brighter than the display terminal itself has been suggested for text-entry workstations; for image management workstations, ambient luminance equal to that of the display terminal has been recommended.[27] In addition, separate task lighting is advised for such low-light conditions. However, task lighting must be arranged so that it does not result in additional screen glare (excessive brightness reflected onto the screen).

Screen glare not only hinders image interpretation, but also causes unnecessary eyestrain. The amount of glare on the screen results from the physical properties of both the computer monitor and the surrounding environment. Although antiglare filters, screens, and coatings are available for most monitors, their use implies placing an additional element between the screen image and the viewer, further compromising the image.

A better approach is to design the surrounding environment to minimize incidents of reflected light. Neutral-colored surfaces with low reflectivity will help. "Selecting surface finish materials with low reflecting values for work surfaces, keyboards, armatures, shelves, and the like also cuts down on glare."[28] If an exterior window is present, it should be capable of being completely blocked and should have adjustable shades or louvers. Monitors should be placed away from the window or at an angle that will reduce the amount of light reflected onto them, directly or indirectly, from the window.

However, the single most effective way to control glare is with the proper selection and placement of artificial lighting within the room. Dimmable indirect ambient lighting fixtures should be used in conjunction with carefully placed dimmable narrow-beam task lights. Indirect light sources project light that is bounced off wall or ceiling surfaces to soften its intensity. The actual light source itself should be completely screened from the workstation. Where indirect lighting is not practical, recessed lamps with a narrow beam can be used. Controls should be dimmable to limit the amount of ambient light.

Figure 13-15. Ergonomics: Range of Seat and Keyboard Support Heights

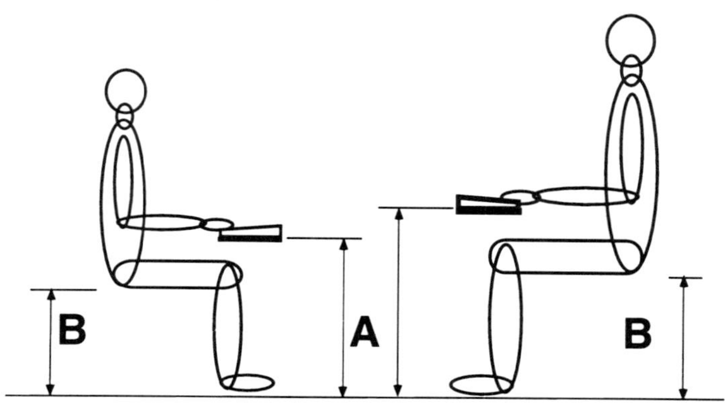

COMPONENT	ANSI/HFS 100–1988 REQUIREMENT
Keyboard Support (see dimension A):	• Keyboard support shall range in height from 23" to 28"
Seat Height (see dimension B):	• Minimum range of adjustment shall be 16" to 20.5"
Seat Depth:	• Seat pan shall provide relief to the back of the knee if seat depth is greater than 16"
Seat Width:	• Seat cushions shall be at least 18.2" wide
Seat Pan Angle:	• Seat pan angle shall allow thighs to be at an angle somewhere between 10° above to 30° below horizontal
Angle Between Seat Back and Seat Pan:	• Fixed back: Angle shall be 90° or more • Adjustable back: Range shall include some part of range 90° to 105°
Backrest:	• A backrest shall be provided • Support in the lumbar region shall be provided
Armrests:	• Inside distance between armrests shall be at least 18.2"

Table 13-1. VDT Workstation Dimensions

Component	ANSI/HFS 100—1988 Requirement
Keyboard support (dimension A in figure 13-15)	Keyboard support shall range in height from 23 to 28 inches.
Seat height (dimension B in figure 13-15)	Minimum range of adjustment shall be 16 to 20.5 inches.
Seat depth	Seat pan shall provide relief to the back of the knee if seat depth is greater than 16 inches.
Seat width	Seat cushions shall be at least 18.2 inches wide.
Seat pan angle	Seat pan angle shall allow thighs to be at an angle somewhere between 10° above to 30° below horizontal.
Angle between seat back and seat pan	Fixed back: Angle shall be 90° or more. Adjustable back: Range shall include some part of range between 90° and 105°.
Backrest	A backrest shall be provided. Support in the lumbar region shall be provided.
Armrests	Inside distance between armrests shall be at least 18.2 inches.

Task lights can be strategically placed to illuminate individual work areas without causing excessive screen glare. Where multiple workstations are provided in one room, low partitions—just slightly higher than the viewer's eye level—on two or three sides of each workstation can help to control both glare and acoustics.

Task lighting fixtures mounted on articulating arms allow the fixtures to be positioned in such a way that ". . . light is projected onto the task from the side instead of from in front of the user. This reduces veiling reflections by bouncing light across a task and not back into the user's eyes."[29] "Veiling glare or veiling reflection results from a source of illumination—such as a light fixture or a window—which is reflected over a glossy surface."[30]

Fixed task lighting can be attached directly to either the wall or a modular workstation. Special lenses are available to minimize glare and reduce fixture brightness. Some fixtures include controls that allow the light intensity to be set at different levels for various activities or for the special lighting needs of different users.

Often, rows of ceiling-mounted light fixtures are integrated into the ceiling system. This is common with lay-in acoustic ceiling systems. Many of these lamps cannot be dimmed. However, if the fixtures have two or more lamps, each fixture can be wired to two switches where each switch controls half the lamps, thus providing variation in the level of illumination.

Where rows of stationary light fixtures are located overhead, computer workstations should be placed perpendicular (rather than parallel) to the rows of lights. In this way, light from the fixtures bounces across the work surface from side to side, rather than from front to back, where it will cause more glare on the screen and in the worker's eyes. (See figure 13-16.)

In reading rooms with both film illuminators and computer workstations, care must be taken to avoid glare from the film illuminators. The two should not be placed directly opposite each other. If such placement is unavoidable, an opaque partition should be placed between the workstation and the illuminator. (For further discussion of lighting issues, see chapter 16, "Utility Requirements.")

Planning for Future Expansion

Increased use of computer workstations suggests the need to plan for future expansion in terms of space and infrastructure requirements. Because computer workstation networks are likely to grow incrementally, it is necessary to identify both initial and future locations for workstations. Typically, a main fiber-optic cable is installed to form a backbone on which to connect various components of an integrated information system. This means that an expansion plan should be established while the first stages of implementation are being designed. Aspects to consider include:

- How many workstations can the network accommodate efficiently? Is it designed for incremental expansion?
- Are initial power, cooling, and ventilation systems adequate to accommodate additional loads?
- Should additional conduit or cable be placed now to limit the need for future renovation?
- Will future communication networks become increasingly portable and capable of wireless connectivity, therefore reducing the need for physical network expansion?
- Will present workstation components be capable of connectivity to other components in the future?
- Will functions located in "soft space" today be able to be relocated so that this space can be used for additional workstations in the future?
- What is the anticipated life of the present network? At what time will it be likely to need replacement?

In addition, a properly designed workstation environment should consider multiple physical aspects. For example, heat generated from computer equipment must be removed for proper functioning of the equipment and for user comfort. Additionally, ventilation systems should not cause a draft over the work area.

Another consideration is the need for clean, uninterrupted power. Electronic circuitry can be easily damaged by slight variations in voltage. Dedicated power circuits and a filtered power supply are recommended. (For a discussion of special power requirements, see chapter 16, "Utility Requirements.")

Figure 13-16. Workstation Location Relative to Overhead Lighting

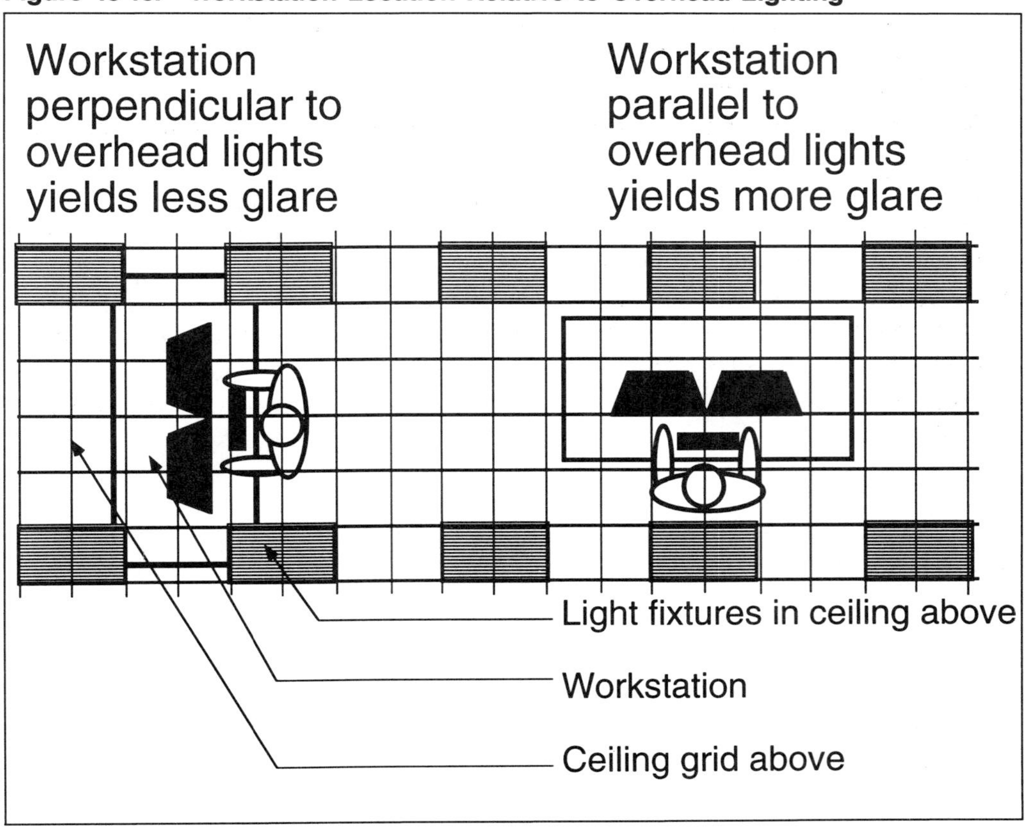

References

1. Fischer, H. W. *Radiology Departments: Planning, Operation, and Management.* Ann Arbor, MI: Edwards Brothers, 1982, pp. 5–6.
2. Fischer, pp. 1–42.
3. Stone Marraccini and Patterson. In-house notes. San Francisco: SMP, 1992.
4. McKinney, W. E. J. *Radiologic Processing and Quality Control—Darkroom/Processing Areas.* Philadelphia: self-published, 1988, p. 2.
5. McKinney, p. 1.
6. Eastman Kodak Company. *Photolab Design for Professionals.* Rochester, NY: Eastman Kodak Company, 1990, p. 30.
7. Eastman Kodak Company, p. 35.
8. Fischer, p. 207.
9. McKinney, p. 5.
10. Eastman Kodak Company, p. 33.
11. McKinney, p. 6.
12. McKinney, p. 3.
13. Fischer, p. 206.
14. Fischer, pp. 299–306.
15. Siemens Medical Systems, Inc. *PACS: Technology in Progress.* Iselin, NJ: Siemens, 1985.
16. Siemens.
17. Siemens.
18. Siemens.
19. *Federal Register,* Architectural and Transportation Barriers Compliance Board, 36 CFR Part 1191, Americans With Disabilities Act (ADA) Accessibility Guidelines for Buildings and Facilities; Final Guidelines, July 26, 1991.
20. Rostenberg, B. Facility design for medical imaging computer workstations. Computer-Assisted Radiology Conference, Berlin, 1993.
21. Horii, S. C. *Electronic Imaging Workstations: Ergonomic Issues and the User Interface—Syllabus: A Special Course in Computers for Clinical Practice and Education in Radiology.* Chicago: Radiological Society of North America, 1992, p. 125.
22. Smith, D. V., Smith, S., Sauls, F., Cawthon, M. A., and Telepak, R. J. *Design Strategy and Implementation of the Medical Diagnostic Image Support System at Two Large Military Medical Centers.* Frederick, MD: U.S. Army Medical Material Agency, 1992.
23. Rosch, W. N. Does your PC—or how you use it—cause health problems? *PC Magazine,* 1991, p. 491.
24. Rosch, p. 492.
25. ANSI/HSF Standard 100—1988.
26. Rosch, p. 494.
27. Horii, p. 131.
28. Herman Miller, Inc. *A Few Simple Facts on the Risky Business of Office Ergonomics.* Zeeland, MI: Herman Miller, 1992, p. 13.
29. Herman Miller.
30. Pile, J. F. *Interior Design.* New York City: Harry N. Abrams, 1988, p. 214.

Appendix. Design Guidelines for Specific Imaging Modalities

The following guidelines identify design considerations for various types of imaging procedure rooms. The room types are presented in the order that each modality is discussed in chapter 6, "Imaging Modalities." Because imaging techniques and equipment change over time, the reader is advised to periodically update these guidelines with current technical information as it becomes available for each modality and room type.

Design and Planning Considerations for Basic Radiography

See figures 12-1 through 12-6 (pp. 210–15).

Functional Requirements

- Convenient direct access from the emergency department (ED) and nursing units (if applicable) would improve patient throughput.
- The control console should be arranged for direct view of the patient's head; if the table tilts, it should not block the technologist's view of the patient.
- Dedicate image processing or computed radiography units should be considered for high-volume procedure rooms such as chest rooms.
- A hand-washing fixture and casework should be provided in the procedure room. (This is required by code in many states.)
- Adequate storage for equipment and supplies in the procedure room and adjacent support areas would help minimize staff travel time and reduce clutter in the procedure room.
- Portable or permanent oxygen and suction services may be needed in the procedure room, depending on the type of patients and procedures intended.
- Contrast agents may need to be available for injection and administration. Crash carts, contrast warmers, articulating exam lights, oxygen, and emergency resuscitation equipment should be provided in areas where contrast agents are used.
- Automated contrast material injectors should be kept near the patient table and installed in such a way that they do not obstruct staff movement.
- Secure holding areas should be provided for biohazardous waste and contaminated linen.
- Space should be provided for hanging multiple radiation protection aprons.
- Space should be provided for film illuminators.
- Wall bucky placement should be convenient for both ambulatory and stretcher patients.
- Two levels of lighting should be provided. Generally, a relatively low light level is adequate for the imaging procedure room and is more comfortable for the patient. A higher light level usually is required for detailed work during biopsy procedures.

Human Factors

- Because direct overhead lighting may cause discomfort to patients facing the ceiling, indirect lighting should be provided.
- Generally, the appearance of the ceiling is important. Patients may spend more time staring at the ceiling than looking at other areas of the room.
- Controlled variable lighting would allow staff to adjust the lighting level and direction to avoid glare and reduce patient discomfort.

Technical Issues

- Radiation protection should be provided as directed by a certified medical or health physicist. State and federal radiation protection requirements often vary. (See the section entitled Radiation Protection in chapter 15, "Physical Properties Influencing Design.")

- Special structural support for floor-, wall-, and ceiling-mounted equipment should be provided per approved structural calculations.
- Adequate access space and structural capacity should be provided for installation and/or replacement of large and heavy equipment.
- If traditional light-sensitive film processing is used, cassette passboxes from the procedure room directly into the darkroom should be considered.
- A variety of methods exist for preventing unauthorized individuals from entering a procedure room during X-ray exposure. These include simply posting notices that warn that X rays are in use and prohibit access of unauthorized personnel (as one extreme) to the use of electronic interlocks that terminate the exposure if the procedure room door is opened (as the other extreme). However, stopping an uncompleted exposure implies that the patient has been irradiated needlessly and that the examination will need to be repeated.

Design and Planning Considerations for Fluoroscopy or Radiography/Fluoroscopy

See figures 6-1 (p. 78) and 12-1 through 12-6. Design and planning considerations for fluoroscopy are the same as for radiography, with the following additions:

Functional Requirements

- A barium preparation or work area should be provided within or near the procedure room. However, as preprepared barium doses become more common, a work area may consist of only a sink and a small counter area. Special barium traps beneath the sink are becoming less common but may be required by code in some jurisdictions.

Human Factors

- An adjacent toilet room with direct connection to the fluoroscopy room should be provided for patients eliminating enemas.
- An enema room should be considered if a large number of cleansing enemas are performed.

Technical Issues

- An air exhaust system and negative air pressure relative to adjoining spaces may be required for the procedure room.
- To reduce the possibility of contamination, clean or dedicated fluoroscopic rooms should be considered for invasive procedures in which barium enemas are used.

Design and Planning Considerations for Mammography

See figures 12-18 and 12-19 (pp. 229–30).

Functional Requirements

- A hand-washing fixture should be provided in the procedure room.
- Adequate storage for equipment and supplies in the procedure room and adjacent support areas would help minimize staff travel time.
- Space and equipment should be provided for quality assurance documentation (patient tracking, equipment monitoring, and so on).
- Two levels of lighting should be provided. Generally, a relatively low light level is adequate for the imaging procedure room and is more comfortable for the patient. A higher light level usually is required for detailed work during biopsy procedures.

Human Factors

- A dedicated dressing area in, or adjacent to, the procedure room should be considered to maximize privacy.
- The exam room should be located so that mammography patient traffic does not need to pass through the entire radiology department.
- The procedure room could be incorporated into a women's health area with a special image (for example, color palette, materials, finishes, furniture, lighting, and so on), if appropriate.

Technical Issues

- Low-dose mammography requires a different film-processing speed than do other radiographic imaging techniques. Sometimes dedicated film processing (often a daylight system) is located in, or immediately adjacent to, the procedure room. Exhaust requirements for the film processor should be verified.
- Due to the low dose of radiation emitted, mammography equipment often does not require external radiation shielding beyond that provided by the equipment itself and the standard materials used in construction of the walls. (The size of the room and the location of the equipment also are factors in determining the need for radiation shielding.) However, some states require that additional radiation protection be installed. A certified medical or health physicist should determine whether additional shielding is needed.

Design and Planning Considerations for Special R/F–Angiography

See figures 12-11 and 12-12 (pp. 222–23). Design and planning considerations for special R/F–angiography are the same as they are for basic R/F, with the following additions. (Note: Additional considerations for cardiac cath labs are listed separately.)

Functional Requirements

- Generally, the procedure room is larger than it is for basic R/F. Room size and configuration will be influenced by types of procedures and equipment selection.
- Often, the control area is larger and contains additional computer equipment. The sharing of one large control area by two procedure rooms has become less popular for angiography because of sterility assurance requirements when both medical teams are present, difficulties in controlling noise during procedures, and the functional limitations of sharing generators.
- Ample space is needed for people and large portable equipment to be brought into and out of the room without disturbing the imaging procedure.
- Consideration should be given to locating a dedicated laser camera or a multiformat camera in the control area.
- The control console should be arranged for direct view of the patient's head. Televised viewing of the patient may also prove more valuable.
- An intercom between the procedure room and the control area should be provided if one is not already provided by the manufacturer. Such systems should allow for good voice modulation to reassure the patient.
- Patient preparation and holding space should be provided, with a nurse's station and lockable medications storage located nearby.
- Clean and soiled work areas should be provided adjacent to the procedure room.
- An area for sterile supplies and storage of large carts and scrubs should be provided.
- Secure holding areas for biohazardous waste and contaminated linen should be provided.
- Contrast agents may need to be available for injection and administration. Crash carts, contrast warmers, articulating exam lights, oxygen, and emergency resuscitation equipment should be provided in areas where contrast agents are used. A floor pedestal

for medical gases and physiological monitoring may work better than wall or ceiling outlets because cables to and from the pedestal are less obtrusive than those connected to the wall or ceiling.

- Angiographic contrast media injectors should be kept near the patient table and installed in such a way that they do not obstruct staff movement.
- Space should be provided for hanging multiple radiation protection aprons.
- Space should be provided for film illuminators in an area where images can be viewed and discussed away from the patient.
- Often, foot-activated lighting controls at the tableside are needed to reduce the light level during fluoroscopy.
- In the past, angiography procedures were recorded almost exclusively on cut film. However, most new installations are being planned or installed with image intensifier-based, film-changerless systems. Close proximity to a laser camera and processor is necessary to facilitate the review of postprocessed images by technologists and radiologists. High-speed digital imaging is an alternative that could eliminate the use of cut film. Multiple film illuminators (six over six or more) should be located just outside the procedure room.
- In addition to the procedure room, at a minimum the following should be provided:
  - Control room
  - Scrub area
  - Imaging electronics equipment room
  - Clean utility room
  - Soiled utility (cleanup) room
  - Technologist work area/office
  - Clean supplies storage area
  - Patient prep and recovery areas
  - Image-processing (darkroom or alternate system), viewing, and storage areas
  - Patient toilet(s) grouped in proximity to prep and recovery areas
  - Staff toilet(s)
  - Staff lockers, staff lounge, patient holding area, and family waiting area (may be shared with other departments)

Technical Issues

- Special environmental conditioning (temperature, humidity, and so on) and electronics rack cabinets may be needed due to additional computer equipment.
- Special air filtration and air pressure relative to adjacent spaces may be required.
- It should be determined whether biplane or single-plane capabilities are desired. Ample space should be provided for future biplane imaging if this option is not selected initially.
- Often, a separate equipment room that allows systems electronics equipment to be stored outside the procedure room is preferred. This allows emitted heat and noise to be isolated and removed. It also preserves the limited wall space in the procedure room to be used for clinical equipment.

Human Factors

- Many procedures are long in duration, and often the patient is awake and acutely aware of his or her surroundings. Therefore, the physical environment should be soothing and sufficiently interesting to take the patient's attention away from the procedure. This is a challenging requirement in a room full of technical equipment. Lighting should be dimmable and indirect, and special audio systems should be available to provide music. However, provisions for the high level of light needed to set up and begin the procedure should also be planned.

Design and Planning Considerations for Cardiac Catheterization Lab

Design and planning considerations for cardiac catherization are the same as they are for special R/F, with the following additions.

Functional Requirements

- Some states classify catheterization labs as one of two types—diagnostic or therapeutic. In some cases, code requirements are different for each type.
- Generally, the procedure room is larger; room size and configuration will be influenced by types of procedures and equipment selection.
- Adequate space should be provided for storage of catheters, guide wires, and so on. A long countertop work surface, sink, and ample wall-mounted cabinets are desirable. Special catheter storage units are available.
- An intercom between the procedure room and control area should be provided if one is not already provided by the manufacturer. Such systems should allow for good voice modulation to reassure the patient.
- Access to surgery, intensive care units, medical imaging, and the ED should be considered.
- Access to operating rooms (ORs), especially a cardiac OR, should be considered.
- In addition to the procedure room, at a minimum the following should be provided:
  —Control room
  —Scrub area
  —Imaging electronics equipment room
  —Clean utility room
  —Soiled utility (cleanup) room
  —Technologist work area/office
  —Clean supplies storage area
  —Patient prep and recovery areas
  —Cine (or digital) image processing, viewing, and storage areas (in addition, two to four film illuminators should be provided for referencing cut films from other procedures)
  —Patient toilet(s)
  —Staff toilet(s)
  —Staff lockers, staff lounge, patient holding area, and family waiting area (may be shared with other departments). (Note that, with the exception of cine processing, this list of rooms is similar to the list described for angiography. In the case of angiography, a darkroom [or alternate type of image-processing area] would be provided instead of cine processing.)
- The radiologist or cardiologist usually will work from the patient's right side. He or she should be able to have direct visual and voice contact with the control room. Both the physician and the technologist at the control console should have a direct line of sight to the patient monitors. Therefore, the control console should be arranged for direct view of the patient's head, when possible. In some installations, this may be difficult to achieve, depending on equipment complexity (for example, biplane versus single-plane capabilities) and physical size.
- The monitors in the cath lab should be located so as to not obstruct the view from the control room.
- If the cardiac catheterization lab also is used for electrophysiological (EP) studies, room utilization may be decreased significantly because of the long duration of many EP procedures.

Human Factors

- Many procedures are long in duration, and often the patient is awake and acutely aware of his or her surroundings. Therefore, the physical environment should be soothing and sufficiently interesting to take the patient's attention away from the procedure. This is a challenging requirement in a room full of technical equipment. Lighting should be dimmable and indirect, and special audio systems should be available to provide music. However, provisions for the high level of light needed to set up and begin the procedure should also be planned.

Technical Issues

- Special environmental conditioning (temperature, humidity, and so on) may be needed due to additional computer equipment.
- Special air filtration and air pressure relative to adjacent spaces may be required.
- It should be determined whether biplane or single-plane capabilities are desired. Ample space should be provided for future biplane imaging if this option is not selected initially.
- Power requirements should be verified with the equipment vendor. In most cases, the cath lab should have its own main feeder line. Additional backup capabilities should be provided. Clean power should be provided to prevent power surges. (See chapter 16, "Utility Requirements.")
- "Light in the catheterization rooms must vary from whole room illumination for general use to [lighting with dimmers] for use during fluoroscopy. Counter lights under cabinets provide limited selective visibility. Fluorescent lighting should be free of interference that can be picked up by [the electrical conducting system of the heart]."[1]
- In cases where the procedure room is used for catheter-dependent EP studies, radiofrequency interference and electrical grounding requirements must be carefully reviewed.

Design and Planning Considerations for Geometric (Linear) Tomography

Design and planning considerations for linear tomography are the same as they are for basic radiography, with the following additions.

Functional Requirements

- Contrast agents may need to be available for injection and administration. Crash carts, contrast warmers, articulating exam lights, oxygen, and emergency resuscitation equipment should be provided in areas where contrast agents are used.
- Adequate storage should be provided.

Human Factors

- A toilet room should be provided nearby or adjacent when the procedure room will be used for intravenous pyelograms (IVPs).

Technical Issues

- Good dimmable lighting should be provided for administering contrast materials.

Design and Planning Considerations for Computed Tomography

See figure 12-13 (p. 224).

Functional Requirements

- A patient dressing and preparation area should be provided in the CT suite.
- The control console should be arranged for direct view of the patient's head. A closed-circuit camera or a mirror may be helpful to allow the technologist to see the patient behind the gantry. Some operators prefer a mirror because it provides a better indication of the patient's color and therefore a truer vision of the patient's medical condition. Others prefer television monitoring to observe the patient and ensure proper

positioning. Some equipment manufacturers may specify the angle of orientation between the table/gantry and the control console.

- An intercom between the procedure room and control area should be provided if one is not already provided by the manufacturer.
- Consideration should be given to locating a dedicated laser camera or multiformat camera in the control area (or nearby for a quieter control area).
- Consideration should be given to locating a dedicated physician viewing console near the control area.
- A hand-washing fixture and casework should be provided in the procedure room.
- Adequate storage for equipment and supplies in the procedure room and adjacent support areas would help minimize staff travel time.
- A ceiling-mounted IV track or a portable IV pole and hangers should be considered.
- Clean and soiled work areas should be provided adjacent to the procedure room.
- Secure holding areas should be provided for biohazardous waste and contaminated linen.
- Contrast agents may need to be available for injection and administration. Crash carts, contrast warmers, articulating exam lights, oxygen, and emergency resuscitation equipment should be provided in areas where contrast agents are used.
- IV contrast storage should be provided.
- Space should be provided for film illuminators to review plain films.
- Storage should be provided for a biopsy setup cart when biopsies are to be performed in the CT room.

Human Factors

- Because direct overhead lighting may cause discomfort to patients facing the ceiling, indirect lighting should be provided.
- Controlled variable lighting would allow staff to adjust the lighting level and direction to avoid glare and reduce patient discomfort.
- Additional high-level lighting may be needed if biopsies are to be performed.
- Large control room windows would improve the technologist's comfort and allow for better observation.

Technical Issues

- Radiation protection should be provided as directed by a certified medical or health physicist.
- Special structural support for floor-, wall-, and ceiling-mounted equipment should be provided per approved structural calculations.
- Adequate access space and structural capacity should be provided for installation, maintenance, and/or replacement of large equipment.
- Special environmental conditioning (temperature, humidity, and so on) may be needed due to additional computer equipment.
- Installation of two dedicated telephone lines should be considered for direct (voice and data) connection to the equipment manufacturer. These lines can be used for remote systems quality assurance monitoring and diagnostics.

Design and Planning Considerations for Electron Beam Tomography

See figures 6-11 and 6-12 (pp. 93–94).

Functional Requirements

- A patient dressing and preparation area should be provided in the suite.
- The control console should be arranged for direct view of the patient's head. Unlike conventional CT, which provides a view of the patient from behind the gantry, the

EBT gantry is closed in the back. Therefore, the only opening for viewing the patient, other than the front of the gantry, is from above. A closed-circuit camera or a mirror may be helpful to allow the technologist to see the patient within the gantry. Often a mirror is preferred because it provides a better indication of the patient's color and therefore a truer vision of the patient's medical condition. The equipment manufacturer may specify the angle of orientation between the table/gantry and the control console.

- An intercom should be provided between the procedure room and the control area if one is not already provided by the manufacturer.
- Consideration should be given to locating a dedicated laser camera or multiformat camera in the control area (or nearby for a quieter control area).
- Consideration should be given to locating a dedicated physician viewing console near the control area.
- A hand-washing fixture and casework should be provided in the procedure room.
- Adequate storage for equipment and supplies in the procedure room and adjacent support areas would help minimize staff travel time.
- Installation of a ceiling-mounted IV track or a portable IV pole and hangers should be considered.
- Clean and soiled work areas should be provided adjacent to the procedure room.
- Secure holding areas should be provided for biohazardous waste and contaminated linen.
- Contrast agents may need to be available for injection and administration. Crash carts, contrast warmers, articulated exam lights, oxygen, and emergency resuscitation equipment should be provided in areas where contrast agents are used.
- A small work area near the scanner should be provided for the equipment manufacturer's field engineer to do paperwork while servicing the unit.

Human Factors

- Because direct overhead lighting may cause discomfort to patients facing the ceiling, indirect lighting should be provided.
- Controlled variable lighting would allow staff to adjust the lighting level and direction to avoid glare and reduce patient discomfort.

Technical Issues

- Radiation protection should be provided as directed by a certified medical or health physicist.
- Special structural support for floor-, wall-, and ceiling-mounted equipment should be provided per approved structural calculations.
- Adequate access space and structural capacity should be provided for installation and/or replacement of large equipment.
- Special environmental conditioning (temperature, humidity, and so on) may be needed due to additional computer equipment.
- Installation of two dedicated telephone lines for direct (voice and data) connection to the equipment manufacturer should be considered. These lines can be used for remote systems quality assurance monitoring and diagnostics.
- Electromagnetic shielding should be provided and/or proper distance from magnetic sources should be maintained. The electron beam may be adversely affected by electromagnetic fields from nearby linear accelerators; MRI units; radio, television, and radar transmitters; or even magnetized equipment such as gurneys.

Design and Planning Considerations for Ultrasound

See figure 12-20 (p. 231).

Functional Requirements

- A hand-washing fixture and casework should be provided in the exam room.
- Adequate storage for equipment and supplies in the exam room and adjacent support areas would help minimize staff travel time.
- A blanket warmer should be provided for patient comfort.
- Ultrasound uses a large volume of linen and/or disposable supplies; thus, adequate supply, storage, and removal systems should be provided.
- A sit-down workstation should be provided for the technologist or physician.
- Good task lighting should be provided for cyst aspiration and other specialized procedures.

Human Factors

- Because direct overhead lighting may cause discomfort to patients facing the ceiling, indirect lighting should be provided.
- Controlled variable lighting would allow staff to adjust the lighting level and direction to avoid glare and reduce patient discomfort.
- For obstetric and gynecological ultrasound examination areas:
  - A dedicated toilet room should be provided adjacent to the exam room because patients will need to empty their bladders after examinations.
  - Consideration should be given to providing a dedicated dressing area to maximize privacy.
  - Consideration should be given to locating the exam room so that patient traffic does not need to pass through the entire radiology department.
  - The exam room could be incorporated into a women's health area with a special image (for example, color palette, materials, finishes, furniture, lighting, and so on), if appropriate.
- Although most patients go home and shower to remove the lubricant that was missed by the technologist, oversized dressing spaces with a hand-washing lavatory should be considered for those patients who cannot go home immediately after the exam.

Design and Planning Considerations for Magnetic Resonance Imaging

See figures 12-16 and 12-17 (pp. 227–28). The following considerations are only general comments; the manufacturer should be consulted for specific requirements. Specific requirements will vary among different magnet types and specific site conditions.

Functional Requirements

- A hand-washing fixture and casework should be provided. However, plumbing lines should be routed and constructed so as not to disrupt the continuous RF shielding. (See the section entitled Special Considerations for MRI Installations in chapter 15, "Physical Properties Influencing Design.")
- A patient dressing, preparation, and toilet area should be provided within the MR suite.
- The control console should be arranged for a direct view of the patient's head.
- An intercom between the procedure room and the control area should be provided if one is not already provided by the manufacturer.
- Adult and pediatric holding areas with medical supervision and lockable medication storage should be provided just outside the procedure room.
- Consideration should be given to locating a dedicated laser camera or multiformat camera in or near the control area.
- Consideration should be given to locating a dedicated physician viewing console near the control area.
- Adequate storage for equipment and supplies in the procedure room and adjacent support areas would help minimize staff travel time.

- Nonferrous oxygen and suction services should be provided in the procedure room. Often, permanent medical gas systems are preferred over portable units because they reduce the risk of having a ferrous metal container carried into the magnet room in response to an emergency. Also, special nonferrous equipment (gurneys and crash carts, for example) must be considered.
- Clean and soiled work areas should be provided adjacent to the procedure room.

Human Factors

- Often, patients placed in the magnet's bore experience fear and claustrophobia. Every effort should be made to alleviate patient stress and anxiety. Sensitive room design, the use of natural lighting, and noise reduction through the use of sound-absorbing materials can contribute to stress reduction. Often, counseling is provided to assist patients in completing an initial exam and returning for follow-up appointments. Some new (low-field) magnets are being designed with an open bore to reduce the incidence of claustrophobia.
- Abrupt loud sounds originating from the gradient coils can be frightening and uncomfortable to both patients and staff. Sound-damping devices can be installed as part of a suspended ceiling or applied directly onto the RF enclosure. Noise cancellation systems programmed to the appropriate frequency have been introduced.
- Audio and video systems should be considered to make the MR environment more pleasant. Various accessories are available to mask noise and combat patient fears generated by claustrophobia. Claustrophobia contributes to patient anxiety that results in a high rate of missed appointments or ineffective exams. Having patients wear prismatic glasses during the procedure and premedication may be helpful.
- Direct overhead lighting (if provided) should only be used for equipment maintenance or room cleanup. It should not be used during the exam because it may cause discomfort to patients facing the ceiling; indirect dimmable lighting should be provided for use during the exam. Controlled variable lighting also would allow staff to adjust the lighting level and direction to avoid glare and reduce patient discomfort. Fluorescent lighting should not be used because it emits RF waves that degrade the MR image. If incandescent lighting is used, special tungsten filaments should be specified; standard ferrous filaments will be destroyed quickly by the magnetic field. Direct-current lighting is recommended by most manufacturers.
- Consideration should be given to providing a room for video patient education prior to the MRI exam.

Technical Issues: General

- Special structural support for floor-, wall-, and ceiling-mounted equipment should be provided per approved structural calculations because some magnets are very heavy.
- Adequate access routes and structural capacity should be provided for installation, maintenance, and/or replacement of large equipment.
- Special environmental conditioning (temperature, humidity, and so on) should be provided to accommodate additional computer equipment.
- Two dedicated telephone lines should be considered for direct (voice and data) connection to the equipment manufacturer. These lines can be used for remote systems inspection and testing.
- Adequate ceiling height should be provided. (See the section entitled Determining the Proper Size of Procedure Rooms in chapter 12, "Space Requirements," and the section entitled Special Considerations for MRI Installations in chapter 15, "Physical Properties Influencing Design.")
- An oxygen-monitoring system should be provided for superconducting magnets.
- Removable access panels should be provided in the ceiling, roof, or walls to enable equipment and magnet gantry installation and replacement.

- A computer equipment room with dedicated air-conditioning should be provided adjacent to the MRI procedure room. Reserve power and air-handling capacity for future expansion and/or equipment upgrades also should be provided.
- Adequate structural support should be provided in the MRI procedure room and along the entire installation route.
- Adequate space must be allocated for dedicated chillers or other types of cooling equipment required by some magnets. These systems are noisy; therefore, acoustic damping should be provided.
- Adequate cryogen venting should be provided for superconducting magnets.
- Wave guides or filters should be installed where the RF enclosure is penetrated. (See the section entitled Special Considerations for MRI Installations in chapter 15, "Physical Properties Influencing Design.")

Technical Issues: Radio-Frequency Interactions

- Radio-frequency shielding should be provided. (See the section entitled Special Considerations for MRI Installations in chapter 15, "Physical Properties Influencing Design.")
- Fluorescent lamps or electronic light dimmers should not be used within the RF enclosure because they generate RF interference.

Technical Issues: Magnetic Interactions

- If the MR unit is not self-shielded, external magnetic shielding may be needed to limit the fringe field. Shimming will compensate, to some degree, for inhomogeneities caused by asymmetrical fixed ferrous objects in the vicinity. However, shimming will not necessarily compensate for moving ferrous objects, such as elevators. (See the section entitled Special Considerations for MRI Installations in chapter 15, "Physical Properties Influencing Design.")
- If possible, the 5-gauss line should be limited to be within the MRI procedure room boundary. This applies to all three dimensions.
- Substantial ferromagnetic objects must be avoided within certain distances of the magnet's isocenter.
- Ferromagnetic structural reinforcement in the floor and ceiling may need to be limited to avoid unshimmable inhomogeneities.
- Consideration should be given to the location of nearby imaging devices (including other magnets and gamma cameras), motors, elevators, electrical transformers, moving steel equipment or vehicles, mechanical equipment rooms, pacemakers, image processors, tape or disk drives, optical drives, credit cards, watches, cameras, and so on. They may affect and/or be affected by the magnet's field.
- Unauthorized traffic within specified distances of the magnet should be restricted by direct supervision and clearly posted warning signs.
- Introduction of metal objects into the procedure room must be restricted. Metal detectors are installed at some sites.
- Incandescent lamps with reinforced tungsten filaments are advised; the reinforced filament mitigates the magnet's effect of shortening the lamp's life span. Direct current is preferred to alternating current.

Design and Planning Considerations for Nuclear Medicine

See figures 12-14 and 12-15 (pp. 225–26).

Functional Requirements

- When locating a nuclear medicine room, it should be remembered that the patient may be administered a radioactive dose either hours or minutes before the exam. He

or she may be asked to remain in the vicinity or return later for a scan that could last from 20 minutes to 3 hours. Ideally, these patients should not be required to traverse the entire radiology department, both for reasons of convenience and because a patient who has been administered a radioactive substance may cause disturbances to certain nearby gamma cameras that are in use.
- Consideration should be given to locating the scanning room near cardio-neuro diagnostics if nuclear stress testing will be performed for cardiac studies. Emergency resuscitation equipment and personnel must be readily available.
- A hand-washing fixture and casework should be provided in the scanning room.
- Adequate storage for equipment and supplies in the scanning room and adjacent support areas would help minimize staff travel time.
- Ample storage space should be provided for multiple collimators, treadmill, EKG, and other ancillary equipment.
- If more than one gamma camera is located in the scanning room, each unit must be spaced a certain distance and angle from the others.
- Gamma cameras should not be placed near MRI rooms or other sources of magnetic interference (such as large motors and major electrical panels) because the cameras are very sensitive.

Human Factors

- Because direct overhead lighting may cause discomfort to patients facing the ceiling, indirect lighting should be provided.
- Controlled variable lighting would allow staff to adjust the lighting level and direction to avoid glare and reduce patient discomfort.
- Patient privacy should be allowed for, especially if more than one gamma camera is located in each scanning room.

Technical Issues: Hot Lab

A radiation-protected hot lab should be provided, including:

- Base cabinets, often with a stainless steel countertop, sink, sliding drawers, and structural reinforcement.
- A lead-lined undercounter refrigerator.
- Lead-lined containers or safe for storing and working with radioactive substances. The work area may include long “extended hands” for holding radioactive vials, radiation shields, and an enclosure of interlocking bricks. The entire work area can sit on the reinforced countertop.
- A 100 percent exhaust radioisotope hood, specially designed for this purpose (optional in some instances).
- An approved system of radioactive waste collection and disposal, including a shielded area for radioactive waste decay.

Technical Issues: Dose Room

A dose room should be considered for the administration of radiopharmaceuticals. This space should include:

- A patient chair
- An exam light
- A hand-washing fixture
- An approved system of radioactive waste collection and disposal
- A small work surface for dose calibration

Technical Issues: General

- Although the floor, walls, and ceilings may not require radiation shielding, radioactivity from the hot lab, radiopharmacy, and even from "hot" patients may disturb sensitive imaging equipment in the immediate vicinity. For this reason, lead-lined partitions are common, especially for separating gamma cameras from incidental radiation coming from the hot lab or dose administration area. Freestanding or mobile radiation shields are useful for shielding the technologist from radiation emitted from the patient. Radiation protection requirements should be provided per the direction of a certified medical or health physicist.
- Special structural support for floor-mounted equipment in the exam room and work spaces in the hot lab may be required.
- Adequate access space and structural capacity should be provided for installation and/or replacement of large equipment.
- An air exhaust system, a gas-scavenging system, and negative air pressure relative to adjoining spaces may be required.
- Special exhaust devices, such as a gas trap or low wall returns, are required when gaseous radiopharmaceuticals (xenon, for example) are used for ventilation scans.
- Easily cleanable, nonporous materials and surfaces that can be readily decontaminated should be used throughout the nuclear medicine suite. Seamless floor covering and work surfaces are preferred.
- Special provisions for receiving, holding, and disposing of radioactive substances must be considered. For example, if radioactive materials are delivered during off-hours, special secure holding containers may be required at the point of delivery. After a certain predetermined time has elapsed, radioactive substances may be disposed of as non-radioactive waste. In all instances, the appropriate regulatory agencies should be contacted to verify current requirements.

Design and Planning Considerations for Positron Emission Tomography Facilities

General Site Planning Considerations

The following describes some room-by-room considerations for PET facilities. These considerations are based on a specific PET center within a large teaching hospital; therefore, readers are advised to review current information on other installations.

- "*Cyclotron Room:* Despite their relatively small size, modern cyclotrons and their associated shielding typically weigh [approximately] 120,000 lbs. For this reason, ground floor installation is [usually] recommended. The concrete slab, upon which the cyclotron rests, is specific to the cyclotron selected. Existing flooring must be completely removed down to the ground. Most manufacturers specify the minimum interior size of the cyclotron room to be 20 ft. × 25 ft. with a 10-ft ceiling. . . . Each cyclotron has specific exhaust, air conditioning, and chilled water requirements. Refer to the manufacturer's site planning guide for these details.

  "It has been found useful to have a cyclotron control console close to the cyclotron. However, because of the noise, magnetic fields, and radiation fields associated with the cyclotron, it is convenient to have the console situated either in a separate room, or within the radiochemistry lab. For ease of troubleshooting, one center has placed a console on a cart which can be rolled into the cyclotron room as needed. [A small sink with hot and cold water for routine target maintenance also is recommended.]
- "*Radiochemistry Lab:* At least 600 sq. ft. of space devoted to clinical radiochemistry is recommended. This is considered a minimum for a diversified, purely clinical program. Significantly more space is required to support research. For greatest efficiency, the radiochemistry lab should be adjacent to the cyclotron room.

- "*Scanner Suite:* The minimum size of the PET imaging room is considered to be 15 ft. × 20 ft. It is preferable, though not required, to locate the imaging area in close proximity to the radiochemistry lab. When this is not practical, a pneumatic tube station (PTS) should be considered for the delivery of unit doses and microbore tubing for delivery of PET gases. [Tubing of some kind may be required for delivery of PET gases, even if the cyclotron and radiochemistry lab are located next to the scanner.]

  "The scanner and computer require rigid environmental control. A monitoring system to alert facilities management personnel to problems in temperature or humidity control is strongly recommended. Several manufacturers recommend the use of a surge protection device for the scanner.

  "The scanner suite should include a . . . control room to accommodate the computer workstation for acquisition and processing. A computer room with raised flooring [used to be required] . . . to house the hardware for the PET computer equipment. [However, most current-generation scanners no longer use computers that must be housed in a separate room with raised flooring.] Space requirements will vary by vendor.
- "*Patient Preparation Room:* One or two prep rooms may be appropriate depending on the anticipated volume of FDG [fluorodeoxyglucose] procedures. This room should be provided with a comfortable stretcher, medical gases and suction. An intercom station and/or nurse call system would also be useful. If the budget allows, it would also be useful to install a remote video camera. [Another alternative would be to provide a semiprivate uptake area with a few comfortable chairs and reading materials. A private exam room could be accessed through a door between it and the uptake area.]
- "*Intercom Stations:* It is extremely useful to install a dedicated intercom system to facilitate communications between key parts of the PET center. Stations [are] useful in the cyclotron room, radiochemistry lab (by the dispensing radiopharmacy hood or PTS), the patient prep rooms, the scanner room and control room, and the reading room. It might also be advisable to install stations in the lab director's and physicist's offices.
- "*Support Space:* Significant economy can be realized if the PET center is physically integrated into an existing nuclear medicine facility. Space for reception and scheduling, patient waiting, rest rooms, staff lounge, storage, reading room, and transcription can all be shared."[2]

Functional Requirements

- "Automated synthesis modules" should be provided in the radiochemistry lab. "Some cyclotron manufacturers provide shielded utility space to accommodate a limited number of synthesis modules. These modules have also been mounted within hot cells; this greatly aids opening and reconfiguring of the unit when another synthesis is required soon after the first since it can be performed without radiation exposure to the chemist. [Hot cells offer flexibility, but require expensive manipulator arms which take up considerable floor space. Shielded synthesis enclosures and hot cells are exhausted similar to fume hoods, due to the potentially dangerous gases produced.]
- "Standard lab furniture is acceptable. Stainless steel bench tops are not necessary but will certainly not be detrimental. It is recommended that utilities on the work counters include vacuum and water (with cup sinks). Two large sinks are also useful. Solvent cabinets for the storage of flammable solvents and acids are necessary unless centralized storage facilities are close by. Generally, possession of more than a few pints of each of several types of solvents mandates an approved [explosion-proof] storage cabinet."[3]
- Bench space should also be provided. "The instrumentation required in the radiochemistry lab will occupy an immense amount of bench space. One active research/clinical center utilizes the following space configuration: [This example comes from a large university research facility. The space requirements for other facilities may vary.]
  - "Cyclotron Room. 8 lineal feet (for target and ion source repair, etc., one radioactive waste storage cave).

– "Cyclotron Control. 12 [lineal] feet (two monitors, printer, logbooks, writing area).
– "Radiochemistry Lab. 55 [lineal] feet plus 20 [lineal] feet of wall space (three HPLCs, GC, dose calibrator, pyrogen testing station, two carrels, two refrigerators, one freezer, two hot cells, two laminar flow hoods, three radiochemical hoods, three sinks, two radioactive waste storage caves).
– "Instrument Lab. 15 [lineal] feet plus 15 [lineal] feet of wall space (TLC plate scanner, electronics shop oscilloscope, multi-channel analyzer, one sink).
– "Clinical Lab. 30 [lineal] feet plus 30 [lineal] feet wall space (two HPLCs, glucose analyzer, blood gas analyzer, two microfuges, one freezer, one refrigerator, one automated gamma well counter, one sink, one incubator, one oven).

"Lab bench utilities should include cup sinks. Standard utilities such as water, air and vacuum should be provided. Generous [distribution of electrical outlets] is necessary since instruments will occupy much of the bench space."[4]

Human Factors

- Because direct overhead lighting may cause discomfort to patients facing the ceiling, indirect lighting should be provided.
- Controlled variable lighting would allow staff to adjust the lighting level and direction to avoid glare and patient discomfort.
- Patient privacy should be allowed for, especially if more than one station is in the patient preparation room.

Technical Issues

- Radiation protection should be provided as directed by a certified medical radiation physicist:

> Dose syringes in pneumatic carriers travel through the pneumatic system at [approximately] 15 ft/sec. At this speed the incidental exposure to personnel is generally considered insignificant: however, it is important to plan for the occurrence of a jammed carrier. A system which has a feedback mechanism to assist in identifying the location of a jam will be very useful. The route of the pneumatic system should be designed to avoid sharp bends in the tubing, as well as areas of potentially prolonged exposure of non-radiation personnel. For example, it would be preferable to route the tube beneath a [corridor] rather than offices or a cafeteria.
>
> Microbore teflon lines . . . , routed through metal conduits, are effective in minimizing personnel exposure during the transit of PET gases. Multiple lines should be initially installed to provide some flexibility for the future and redundancy in the event of problems. Difficulties associated with a line rupture can be minimized if the lines are maintained under a slight negative pressure from the cyclotron room. Ventilation equipment serving the cyclotron room, radiochemistry lab, and scanner room should provide [adequate] fresh air at [the appropriate number of] equivalent air changes per hour. Exhaust from the cyclotron room should be handled through a separate system.
>
> [Specific air exchange and filtration requirements should be identified by a qualified mechanical engineer familiar with PET facilities and applicable codes.]
>
> The manual transport of PET doses can be safely accomplished using a shielding transport cart. This is the same device commonly used to transport therapeutic quantities of radio-iodine. [Another alternative may be to hand-carry the dose for short distances (in a protective nuclear medical dose carrier) to a dose receiving station. Verify applicable code requirements.][5]

- The cyclotron and radiochemistry exhaust stack may require radiation monitoring. The use of charcoal and high-efficiency particulate air (HEPA) filters along with TLD monitors may be another alternative. Verify applicable code requirements.

References for Appendix

1. Laufman, H., editor. *Hospital Special Care Facilities: Planning for User Needs.* New York City: Academic Press, 1981, p. 478.

2. Faulkner, D. B., Kearfott, K. J., and Manning, R. G. Planning a clinical PET center. *Journal of Nuclear Medicine Technology* 19(1):5–19, Mar. 1991.

3. Faulkner and others.

4. Faulkner and others.

5. Faulkner and others.

Chapter 14

Imaging outside the Radiology Department

Continuity of care requires that patients be treated effectively and efficiently within all components of the health care system. Medical imaging is only one segment of a comprehensive medical diagnostic, treatment, education, and preventive care continuum. Thus, imaging systems are not limited to radiology departments. Rather, imaging is an important component of many other departments and services that provide health care, and each of these areas often has unique architectural needs.

This chapter describes the role of medical imaging in three areas outside the radiology department—surgery, emergency medicine, and intensive care—and examines the unique facility requirements that the use of medical imaging generates in each area. In addition, the chapter discusses design considerations for technology docks—docklike structures that allow mobile imaging trailers or modular imaging building components to be "plugged in to" larger facilities.

Imaging and Surgery

The relationship between surgery and radiology can be both cooperative and competitive. As new procedures (made possible by new technology) further dissolve some of the apparent boundaries between the two medical specialties, opportunities for mutual support and understanding are on the rise. As each subspecialty becomes increasingly complex, the need for interdepartmental alliances becomes more necessary.

The imaging procedures associated with surgery can be divided into two categories: (1) those procedures performed on surgical patients presurgically or postsurgically outside the surgical suite and (2) those procedures performed during surgery within the operating environment. An exhaustive list of presurgical or postsurgical procedures is beyond the scope of this book; however, some of the more common modalities are listed in table 14-1.

The focus of this section is on imaging modalities performed within the surgical suite and, in particular, the facility implications of these techniques. It is important to remember that the popularity and efficacy of many imaging techniques used in surgery are in constant flux, in part because of the continuous development of new technologies, and thus the facility requirements for many of these modalities are subject to change.

Although in some cases diagnostic imaging competes with surgery, it also complements it. Various forms of imaging in the operating room (OR)—radiography, fluoroscopy, and ultrasound, with fixed and portable units alike—are integral to many surgical practices and, as the following paragraphs show, help reduce the invasiveness of surgery by providing better visualization and more accurate localization. Furthermore, the coordination of presurgical and postsurgical images with surgical procedures themselves links surgery to other forms of diagnostic imaging that takes place outside the surgical department.

Table 14-1. Selected Imaging Techniques That May Be Associated with the Surgical Patient

Surgical Aspect	Imaging Modality	Remarks
Breast cancer	Screen–film mammography	
	Xerography	
	Ultrasound	Less accurate in distinguishing benign from malignant masses
	Thermography	Less effective in detecting nonpalpable cancers
	Transillumination	Less effective in detecting small nonpalpable cancers
	Magnetic resonance imaging	MR mammography in the early stages of development
Injuries and diseases of the chest and thorax	Chest radiography	Likely to occur in ED or OR
	Computed tomography	
	Bronchoscopy	
Diseases of the lung	Chest radiography	
	CT	
	Bronchography	
	Angiography	
	(Fetal) ultrasound	
Heart disease	Chest radiography	
	Fluoroscopy	
	Echocardiography	
	Radionuclide imaging/ position emission tomography/single-photon emission computed tomography	
	Cardiac catheterization	
	Coronary angiography	
	MRI	
	Magnetic resonance angiography	Not yet clinically competitive with traditional angiography
	Electron beam tomography	Relatively few sites in existence to date
Vascular disease	Echocardiography/ transesophageal echocardiography	
	Radionuclide imaging	
	CT	
	Angiography	
	Interventional angiography	Replacing/competing with certain vascular surgical procedures
	Radiography	
	Fluoroscopy	
	MRI	
	MRA	Not yet clinically competitive with traditional angiography
	Doppler ultrasound	

Table 14-1. (Continued)

Surgical Aspect	Imaging Modality	Remarks
Gastrointestinal disease	R/F	
	Barium enema	
	Endoscopy	
	Radionuclide studies	
	Ultrasound	Used in diagnosis of jaundice
	CT	
Urology	Urography	
	Cystography	
	General radiography	
	Intravenous pyelography (IVP)	
	Ultrasound	
	CT	
	MRA	Relatively new procedure used for kidney studies
	Radionuclide studies	
	Arteriography	
	Lithotripsy	
Obstetrics/gynecology	Ultrasound	Often a procedure of choice due, in part, to absence of emitted radiation
	Genitography	
	Hysterosalpingography	
	Ureterography	
	Urography	
	CT	
	Prenatal ultrasound	Used to detect some malformations in utero
Neurosurgery	CT	Has effectively replaced plain-skull radiography
	MRI	
	Cerebral angiography	
	Digital subtraction angiography (DSA)	
	Myelography	Appears to be on the decline
	Radionuclide brain scan	Almost completely replaced by CT
	Ultrasound	
	PET	
	Arteriography	
Musculoskeletal disorders	CT	
	MRI	
	Myelography	Appears to be on the decline
	Radiography	
	Radionuclide studies	

Source: Eisenberg, R. L. *Diagnostic Imaging in Surgery.* New York City: [publisher unknown], 1987.

The invasiveness of surgeries is not only determined by the direct goal of the procedure (i.e., tumor removal, reconstruction of normal anatomy, etc.), but also by the demand for better visualization, easier access and correct localization.

In order to improve this situation and to reduce the invasiveness of surgery, the use of various imaging modalities (x-ray, fluoroscopy, ultrasound, CT, and recently MRI) has been tested intraoperatively in conjunction with biopsies or surgical procedures. The need for improved visualization calls for special image representation methods such as image reformation or three-dimensional reconstruction. It has been recognized that all the intraoperative imaging techniques, as well as the presentation of preoperatively-obtained images during surgery, rely currently on simple image display methods. However, so far only insignificant amounts of computerized image processing techniques are available to surgeons.

The task of interpretation and integration of multiple image data streams in relationship to surgery (i.e., preoperative and intraoperative imaging information with view of surgical field) is a very demanding mental task for surgeons and would require the support of an imaging specialist. There is an increasing demand for radiologists to participate in the utilization of images beyond diagnosis. The role of radiologists is increasing in preoperative and intraoperative imaging and in developing methods for the planning of surgical procedures. This will result in the redefinition of the role of radiologists in the process of patient care which starts with diagnosis and ends with therapy.

The introduction of advanced imaging and image processing technologies and high speed computing devices in combination with new, minimally invasive therapeutic approaches will eventually change the current role of radiologists. Their work will not be limited to detection and localization but will also include planning and executing various procedures. Eventually there will be a need for an interventional imaging expert who can provide not only a roadmap for the surgeons, but who will participate as an active member of the surgical team in designing, optimizing and controlling protocols.[1]

Ultrasound-Guided Surgery

In recent years, ultrasound guidance has been incorporated into an increasing number of surgical procedures. Miniaturized ultrasound transducers assist and guide the surgeon by visualizing what would otherwise be invisible to even the most highly trained, "unassisted" human eye.

> There is a growing use of high-resolution, real-time ultrasound systems to assist surgeons during operative procedures. This technique has been applied to the neurosurgical localization of brain and spine [tumors, intraventricular evaluation, localization of kidney stones] and surgical procedures involving [the liver] and the pancreas.[2]
>
> Wielding an array of ultrasound techniques, radiologists are plumbing, probing and poking their way into new anatomical territory and directing surgeons about when, where, and on what to operate. Rather than resenting the intrusion, many surgeons request it.
>
> Color Doppler gives surgeons "eyes" to help avoid blood vessels in the laser palliation of patients with unresectable head and neck tumors—a procedure that was previously performed blindly.[3]

Ultrasound was once restricted to neonatal intracranial surgery because the unformed skull of the infant easily accommodates the insertion of an ultrasound probe. However, today, miniature ultrasound probes are being used in conjunction with brain surgery performed on adults. During the operation, ultrasound can help the surgeon to localize intracranial tumors or growths, providing a safe, nonradioactive way to image beneath the surface of the brain. In this way, the characteristics of an intracranial mass can be determined and the trauma associated with the surgery can be minimized.[4] The following paragraphs describe the use of a portable ultrasound unit:

> A portable ultrasound unit is taken into the operating room, and after the skull is opened, the transducer is placed in contact with the brain to locate the tumor . . . some tumors cannot be seen by even the most experienced neurosurgeons. It is imperative that only diseased tissue be removed, otherwise, brain damage could occur. It is equally important that all of the tumor be removed; if not, the tumor could grow back and repeat surgery would be required.[5]
>
> Intraoperative spinal sonography is of value in spinal surgery to resect or biopsy soft tissue masses of the spinal canal or spinal cord. This technique can identify the area of maximum cord enlargement so that a precisely located biopsy can be performed. . . .
>
> Ventricular shunts in hydrocephalic infants are usually positioned in a totally "blind" fashion. Post operatively, a computed tomography (CT) scan is obtained to check the location of the tip of the shunt tube; if the position is incorrect, the infant must be returned to the operating room so that the shunt can be repositioned. Since these infants have open fontanelles, ultrasound can easily be performed during the operative procedure to demonstrate that the tip of the shunt tube is properly positioned. . . .[6]

The use of ultrasound in the OR will continue to grow in the near future. However, the facility requirements associated with intraoperative ultrasound are few in number. Lighting levels in the OR should be designed to facilitate easy reading of ultrasound monitors, without causing glare on the screen and without compromising the light quality required for surgery. Additionally, space should be allocated for storage of portable ultrasound equipment.

Three-Dimensional Image Reconstruction

Specialized ORs, including those used for orthopedic and neurologic procedures, will likely be designed for the use of various forms of image reconstruction to guide and orient the surgeon. The facility requirements associated with imaging will vary according to the type of room and procedure performed. The following paragraphs describe the future applications of three-dimensional image reconstruction in a variety of new surgeries:

> Surgical planning, until now, was used by orthopedic surgeons routinely for prosthesis placement and for reconstructive surgeries. Another example is craniofacial surgery, where usage of 3-D reconstructions for planning has become fairly widespread. In general, we will see an increased availability of computer-generated 3-D reconstructions for the planning of other surgical procedures over the next few years. An important area under development is neurosurgery, where the complexity and the functionality of the anatomy require the use of very careful planning procedures.
>
> Optimally, 3-D reconstructed images should be registered to the patient anatomy, taking motion and deformation due to the motion into account, and provide this integrated display to the surgeon as a manipulatable view. The surgeon should have a stereoscopic display available that is updated while he moves to new vantage points. The position of his instruments will be monitored and updated in the display. He will have the ability to mix the computer-generated renderings with the real-life view. Several computer science groups have been working to introduce the concepts of virtual reality into the medical field.
>
> The first and most crucial requirement is having computer-generated renderings available at an acceptable speed. This means acquiring an update rate of at least several frames per second. In addition, input and output devices must be available. Another essential element of this environment is a computer-controlled mechanical device (i.e., a robotic arm) that can be used to translate actions on the monitor into actions in the real world. Such a device could be utilized to replace the mechanical stereotactic needle positioning device currently used.
>
> Many of the most frequently performed surgical procedures are amenable to the minimally-invasive surgical approach. Cholecystectomies, lumbar disc procedures, treatment of cancer in its early stages and the treatment of metastatic disease are only some

of the most obvious procedures where addition and integration of computer-generated animations will make a significant difference. Most beneficial will be the shortening of procedure times by providing the surgeons with better orientation.[7]

Preoperative CT and MR Images in the OR

Various applications for correlating presurgical and computed tomography (CT) and magnetic resonance (MR) images with the actual surgical procedure are presently in use. As the following paragraphs explain, in some cases neurosurgeons are using this technology in performing brain operations:

> Neurosurgeons at the Cleveland Clinic have begun using a "magic wand" to enhance their craft. Actually the wand is a sonic probe that correlates with magnetic resonance (MR) or computed tomography (CT) images of the brain, enabling the surgeon to point to any spot on a patient's head and immediately identify the location of the probe with respect to anatomic structure.
>
> This revolutionary technology allows surgeons to plan and perform brain operations more precisely and safer than ever before, and it helps prevent surgical errors, which can result in loss of motor or sensory function. Computer guidance also makes it possible for surgeons to remove tumors through a much smaller opening in the skull, which decreases wound complications and speeds recovery time.
>
> With image-guided neurosurgery, the surgeon can target anything in the brain within a millimeter or two. . . . In the brain there are no landmarks. . . . The sonic digitization system provides real-time feedback that is otherwise unattainable. It allows [the surgeons] to remove tumors that are of complex shape and have ill-defined boundaries.[8]

Intraoperative Radiography and Fluoroscopy

Intraoperative radiography/fluoroscopy (R/F) is being used more often in neurologic surgery, where surgeons trying to stop brain hemorrhage can verify their success by performing a contrast study before completing the operation.[9] It also is growing in use in a number of orthopedic procedures. Portable equipment, such as mobile C-arms, are likely to be used in these ORs. (See figure 14-1 for an example.) As an alternative, built-in R/F units may be provided. (See figure 14-2, p. 286.) Built-in imaging equipment was more popular when the image quality of portable equipment was less satisfactory than it is today. However, the image quality of today's portable equipment is noticeably improved, and portable equipment provides greater flexibility than fixed equipment. Where fixed radiographic equipment is provided, it should be installed in such a way that it does not interfere with ceiling-mounted surgical equipment and that enables the imaging tube to be moved away from the center of the room when not in use. Additionally, it must be able to be easily cleaned and serviced.

Regardless of whether imaging equipment is fixed or portable, and even though some portable equipment may emit only low levels of radiation and contain integral radiation protective construction, radiation protection requirements should be determined by a certified medical or health physicist. (See the section entitled Radiation Protection in chapter 15, "Physical Properties Influencing Design.") In some states, lead-lined (or equally protected) wall, floor, and ceiling surfaces and glazing are required by code in ORs that are likely to incorporate radiographic imaging. Radiation protection is especially important when pregnant women occupy adjacent areas.

The surgical staff must be adequately protected from scatter radiation. Often, this is accomplished by wheeled or ceiling-mounted radiation shielding. (See figure 14-3, p. 287.) Both ceiling-mounted shields and those that roll on wheels require space and have the potential to interfere with the movement of other essential equipment.

Although surgical staff often are reluctant to leave the patient's side during surgery, they must be protected from harmful radiation exposure. In some surgical suite configurations, a clean or sterile supply core is directly adjacent to the ORs. Staff sometimes tend to stand in this clean core during X-ray transmission. This is undesirable because any unnecessary traffic into the clean core compromises its degree of cleanliness.

Somewhere near the ORs, space should be provided for storage of portable X-ray equipment, film processing and viewing, and possibly a dedicated X-ray control area. A laser camera or multiformat camera also might be included. In addition, space should be provided for several monitor trolleys and digital image storage devices. Circulation of radiography-related equipment, supplies, and people must be planned in conformance with the special clean and soiled circulation restrictions of the surgical suite. The surgical suite is a good location for considering an electronic link to the imaging department for the purpose of transmitting images electronically between the two areas. (See the section entitled Electronic Image Management in chapter 7, "Image Management and Film Processing.")

Accessories such as overhead monitors, film illuminators, apron racks, and other devices must be incorporated into the OR layout without interfering with the many surgical devices that also are necessary. Often, the specific location of these items is determined by personal preference and is related to the specialized traffic in the OR and the ability to thoroughly clean the surgical suite.

Figure 14-1. Portable Radiographic C-Arm in the OR

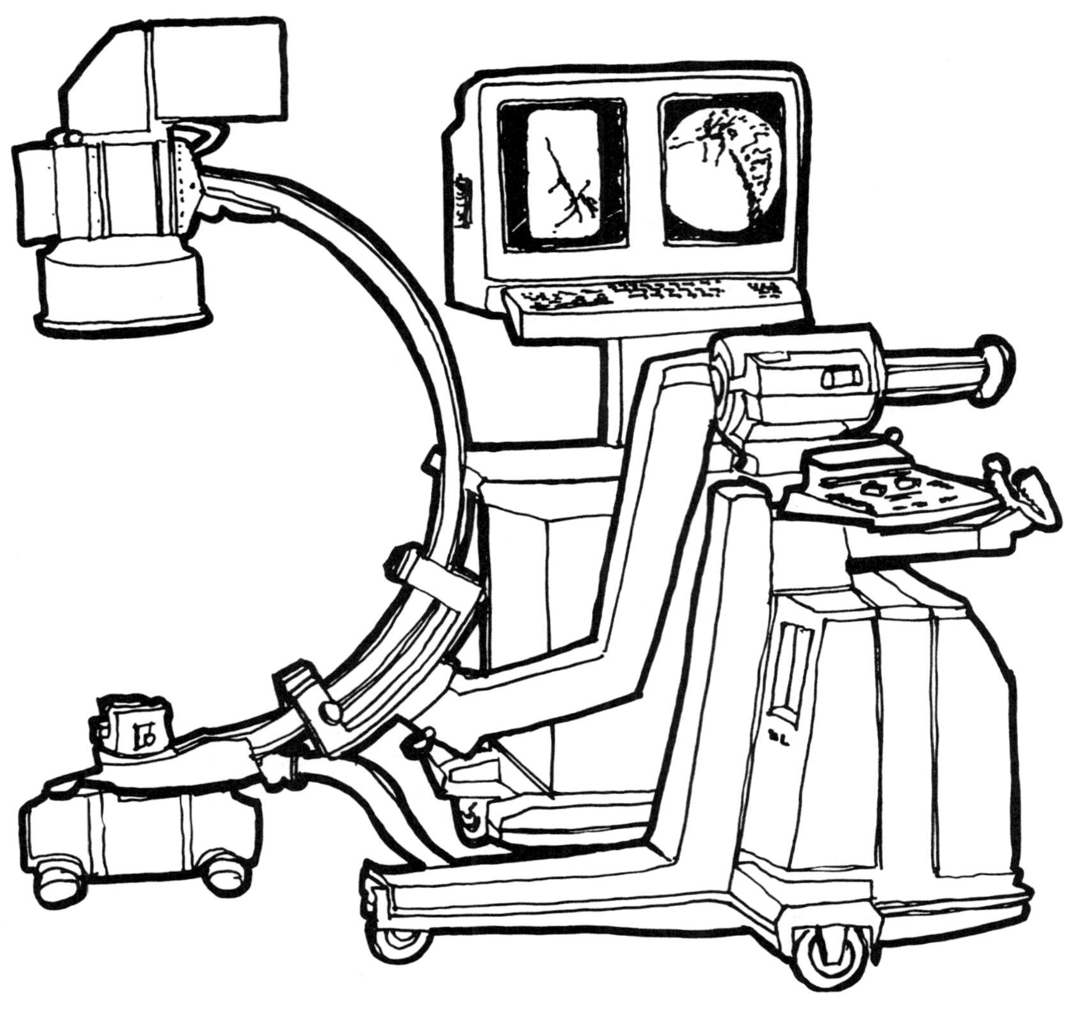

Figure 14-2. Built-in Radiographic Imaging Equipment in the OR

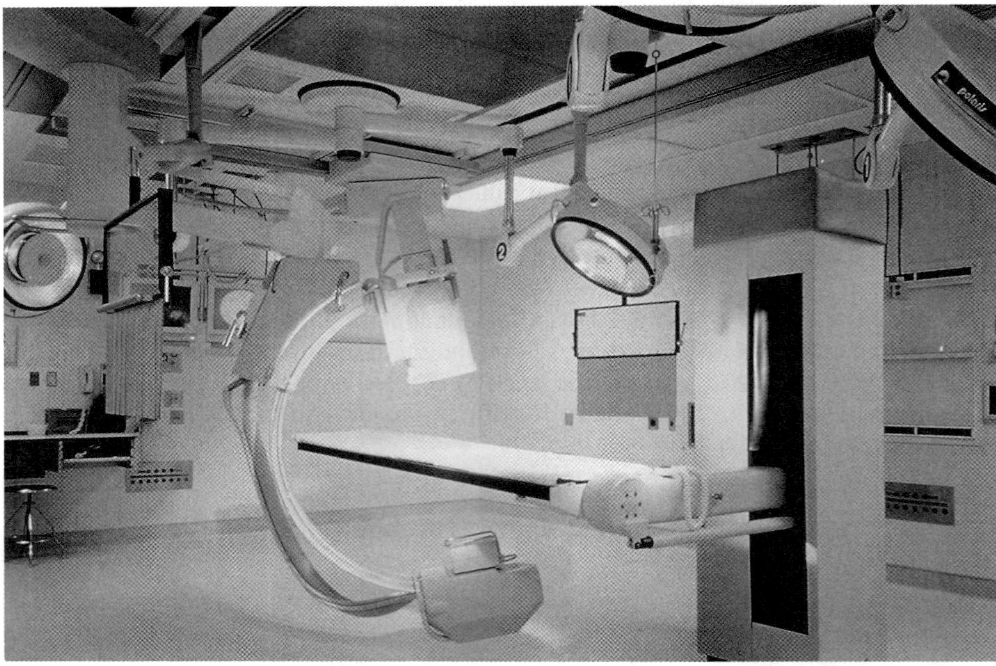

Surgical laser radiography room, Tucson Medical Center, Tucson, Arizona. Photographer: Allen Maertz. Courtesy of Anderson DeBartolo Pan, Tucson, Arizona. Used with permission.

The Cystoscopy OR

Along with surgical treatment, a number of diagnostic procedures may take place in the cystoscopy OR, many of which are performed on an outpatient basis. In addition to the use of cystoscopes (small tubelike optical instruments used to visualize the interior of the bladder), X-ray images also may be obtained. The "cysto room" usually contains special imaging equipment that is constructed as part of the urology table.

One radiographic procedure, "cystography, is a technique in which opaque contrast material is introduced into the urinary bladder through a ureteral catheter. Cystography can demonstrate abnormalities in the shape or position of the bladder and can detect . . . defects within the bladder due to tumors, blood clots and calculi."[10]

A work area—including the X-ray control area, a film-processing area, and a workroom—should be adjacent to, and directly accessible from, the cysto room. The urology table and the cysto room itself require special cleaning capabilities because many procedures involve irrigating the examination site.

MRI-Guided Surgery

Some surgeons and radiologists are focusing attention on the potential for performing surgical procedures within an MRI exam room. The first interventional MR treatment suite in the United States was opened in 1994 at Brigham and Women's Hospital in Boston. (See figure A-1 in appendix A, "Descriptions of Selected Facilities and Departments.") MRI-guided surgery must overcome a number of physical challenges. (Also see the section entitled Special Considerations for MRI Installations in chapter 15, "Physical Properties Influencing Design.") Some of the challenges to overcome include:

- Development of a magnet that provides the surgical team with sufficient access to the patient
- Development of a magnet from which either the patient can be quickly removed or the magnetic field can be quickly terminated if the patient requires emergency stabilization

Figure 14-3. Ceiling-Mounted Radiation Protection in the OR

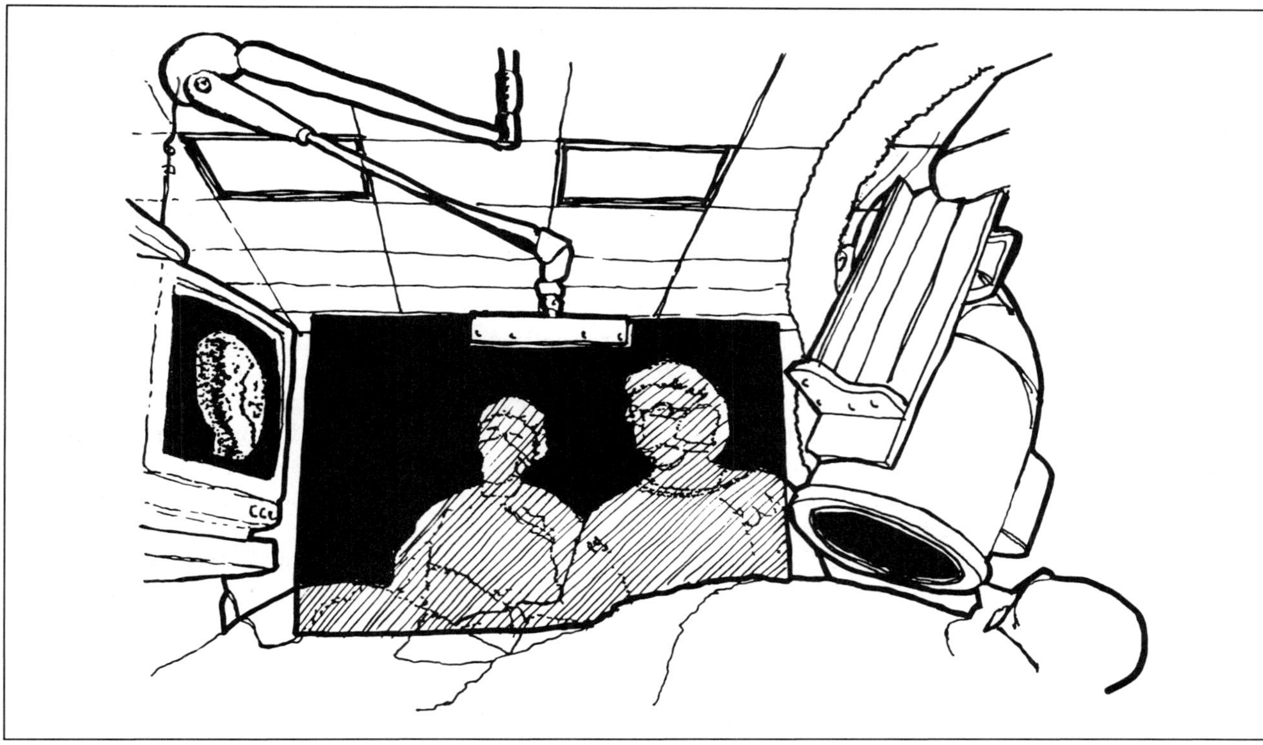

- A magnet that can be kept surgically clean
- Development of nonferrous surgical instruments and life support equipment that can be used in an MRI environment (some of these already exist)
- Surgical lights and other accessories that can be used in an MRI environment
- A radio-frequency shielded enclosure that will enable emergency access to the patient, if necessary
- Development of a quiet magnet or apparatus worn by the surgical team to block noise generated by the gradient coils
- Development of video and cathode-ray tube (CRT) monitors that neither disturb nor are disturbed by the magnetic field

Despite the multiple obstacles, however, there is considerable interest in MRI-assisted surgery. The following paragraphs explain the reasons for that interest:

> MRI may have a unique role in the real-time monitoring of invasive procedures and to control energy disposition or other interventions. Due to the temperature sensitivity of some MR parameters, MR guidance of various thermally-induced therapeutic methods is possible (i.e., hyperthermia, laser surgery, ultrasound heating, radiofrequency heating, cryosurgery). Furthermore, in procedures where the tissue is changing during the intervention (i.e., ethanol injection, embolization, etc.), the excellent tissue characterization of MRI can be utilized for assessing tissue damage.
>
> The introduction of rapid MR imaging techniques and the improvement of spatial resolution makes MR uniquely qualified to be the imaging technique of various high-tech minimally-invasive surgical techniques performed within the environment of the magnet. This imposes some technical difficulties and requires changes of some tools and instruments (MR compatible needles, surgical tools, endoscopes, etc.), but the clear advantages of MRI in localization, target definition and in estimating tissue responses to therapy will justify these changes. The biggest challenge is to design new MRI instruments which provide better access to the patient and can fit into a surgical environment.[11]

Laparoscopy

Numerous surgical procedures are now being performed as minimally invasive surgery (MIS), an approach that is revolutionizing surgery. MIS uses laparoscopic techniques instead of highly invasive incisions.

Although a detailed description of laparoscopic surgical procedures is beyond the scope of this book, a brief explanation of the procedure is worth mentioning here. During laparoscopy, one or two small incisions are made in the abdomen. A laparoscope is inserted through these openings to visualize and manipulate abdominal organs. Some organs, such as the gallbladder, can be removed using laparoscopic procedures. First, the gallbladder is deflated to reduce its size, and then it is removed through the small abdominal opening. Although the laparoscopic procedure often takes longer than conventional surgery, it is considerably less invasive and requires less patient recovery time.

One significant difference between laparoscopy and conventional surgery is that with laparoscopy, the surgeon is viewing anatomy either through the laparoscope or via a monitor rather than directly. Other imaging modalities, such as ultrasound, may be used in conjunction with laparoscopy, further increasing the use of monitors to visualize anatomy. Additionally, the use of intravascular catheters in laparoscopic surgery is enabling surgeons to palpate untouchable organs.[12]

In the future, ORs will rely more heavily on the use of CRTs and other monitors. They also will be more directly linked to picture archiving and communication systems (PACSs), which eventually will be integral to most imaging departments.

Imaging and Emergency Medicine

Most emergency and trauma departments are equipped to perform a variety of emergency examinations. The extent and sophistication of imaging equipment in the emergency department (ED) depends, in part, on both the department's caseload and its proximity to the radiology department and other imaging services.

There are three advantages to providing imaging capabilities within the ED. They are:

1. Emergency patients do not need to be moved away from the department as frequently.
2. Emergency nurses and/or physicians do not need to leave the department to accompany patients.
3. Scheduled nonemergency patients being examined in the radiology department are less likely to be bumped because equipment in the radiology department is not needed as frequently for emergencies.

One disadvantage to providing dedicated imaging equipment in the ED is that additional staff may need to be either stationed there or at least immediately available. This can be inefficient if the demand for emergency imaging is infrequent.

Most basic imaging needs (for urgent care but nontrauma patients) can be accommodated by a single radiography or radiography/fluoroscopy (R/F) room. This space may be used for orthopedic and other patients who can either walk or be wheeled from their exam room into the X-ray room. The imaging area will need its own film-processing and viewing capabilities.

Many EDs with a heavy trauma load use radiographic equipment specially designed for trauma rooms. This equipment can be used in single or multiple trauma bays. For example, a series of trauma bays can be arranged in a row, with a single overhead, ceiling-mounted imaging tube that can be used within each bay. (See figures 14-4 and 14-5, pp. 289–90.) Generally, special radiation protection is required above, below, and at the sides, including the corridor opening. If possible, ob/gyn exam rooms should not be located immediately adjacent to X-ray equipment because of the potentially damaging effect of radiation on the fetus. As mentioned previously, radiation protection requirements should be determined by a certified medical or health physicist.

Figure 14-4. Ceiling-Mounted Imaging Equipment

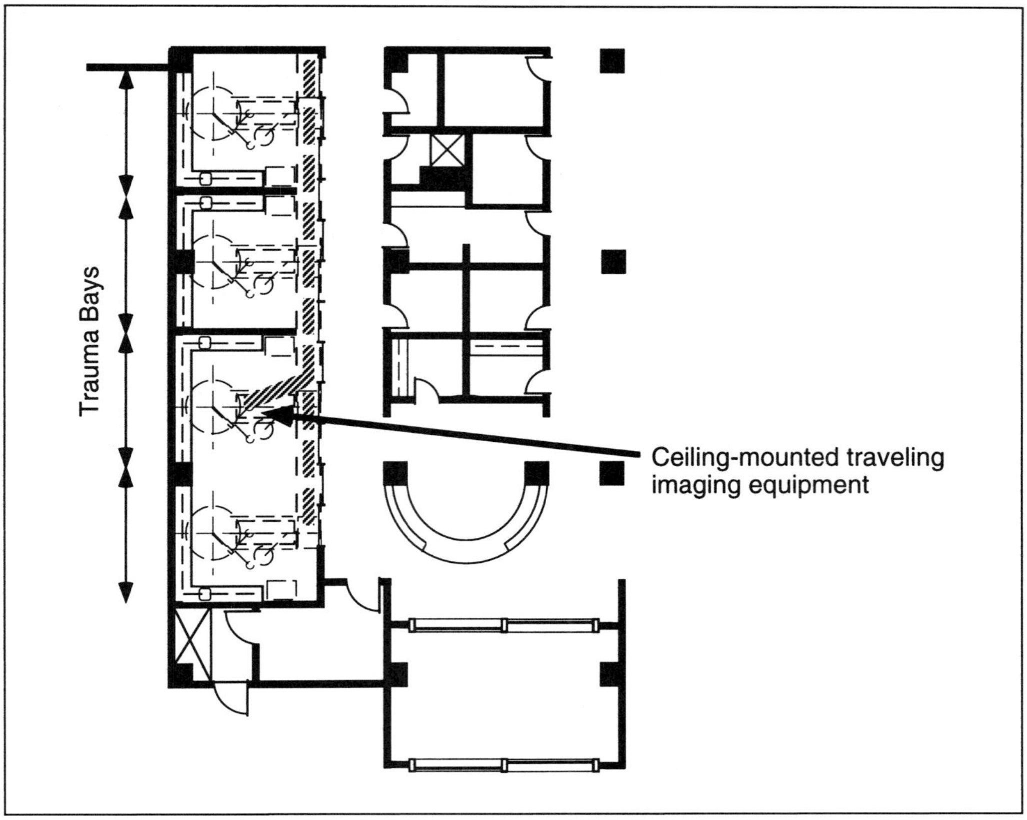

Some busy EDs may include their own CT scanner, although this may seem overambitious. Often, a CT unit in close proximity is adequate. A technology dock (discussed in a later section of this chapter) containing specialized imaging equipment, such as MRI, could be used for some emergency patients if (1) it is located nearby, (2) it is easily accessible, and (3) some provision is made for separating emergency from nonemergency traffic.

Specially designed gurneys or patient beds are desirable in the ED so that patients do not need to be transferred onto the patient table that is part of the imaging equipment. X-ray translucent tables are available, as are special nonferrous tables that can be used for MRI exams. In addition, some equipment designed for trauma use allows the patient table, which usually is designed as part of the equipment, to be removed and replaced by the ED's own gurney. (See figure 14-6, p. 291.)

In addition to (or as an alternative to) special fixed imaging equipment, portable X-ray equipment is useful in the ED. Ample storage space should be provided.

Teleradiology, which transmits medical images to remote sites, can be useful in the ED. It enables one radiologist to interpret diagnostic images for multiple emergency facilities or to interpret films from his or her home or office. (See the section entitled Teleradiology in chapter 7, "Image Management and Film Processing.") Like the intensive care unit (ICU) and the surgery department, the ED is a good location for an electronic link to and from the imaging department.

Imaging in the Intensive Care Unit

Because critically ill patients often require radiographic or fluoroscopic examinations and because these patients should not be moved unnecessarily, some form of imaging capabilities must be integrated into the intensive care unit:

> . . . It is often difficult to obtain an acceptable portable examination not only because the patient is ill and usually encumbered with tubes and other devices but also because respiratory and gross body motion cannot always be controlled. [With traditional] portable x-ray units, kilovoltage and milliamperage are limited, so that exposures are long and image contrast may be excessive. . . . It is difficult to estimate the proper exposure, and an exposure erring by no more than a factor of two causes a noticeable reduction in image quality. Sequential images of the same patient are therefore difficult to interpret because of technical variations (focal film distance, beam alignment and fluctuating exposure factors) and because of the patient's changing volume status and severity of chest disease.[13]

Nonetheless, portable X-ray equipment generally is adequate for most routine needs (especially chest X rays) in the ICU. Ample storage space for the equipment must be provided. "[Another] . . . basic requirement of any radiology system for an intensive care unit is the ability to display the positions of tubes, catheters, and prosthetic valves."[14] Although portable C-arms generally perform adequately for this, a cardiac catheterization lab located in the immediate area can be useful (when available) for inserting and checking the placement of catheters in intensive care patients.

> In the hospitalized population, a significant percentage of [chest] examinations are done at the bedside; in tertiary care hospitals, 30% to 50% of the total chest radiography volume is performed as "portable," with the intensive care unit (ICU) being a common site for these examinations."

Figure 14-5. Imaging in the Trauma Bay of the ED

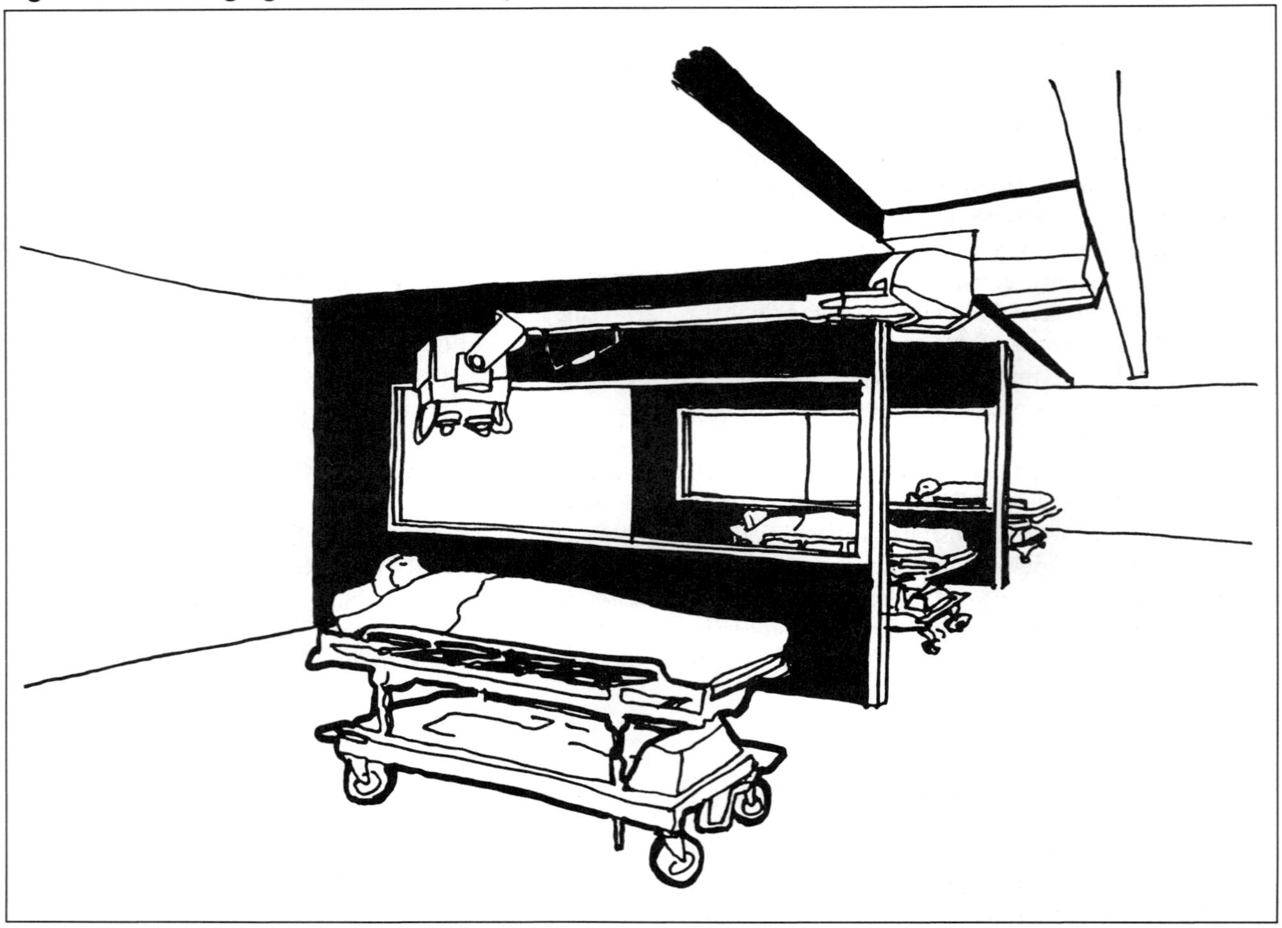

Figure 14-6. Specialized CT Equipment and Patient Gurney for Imaging of Emergency Patients

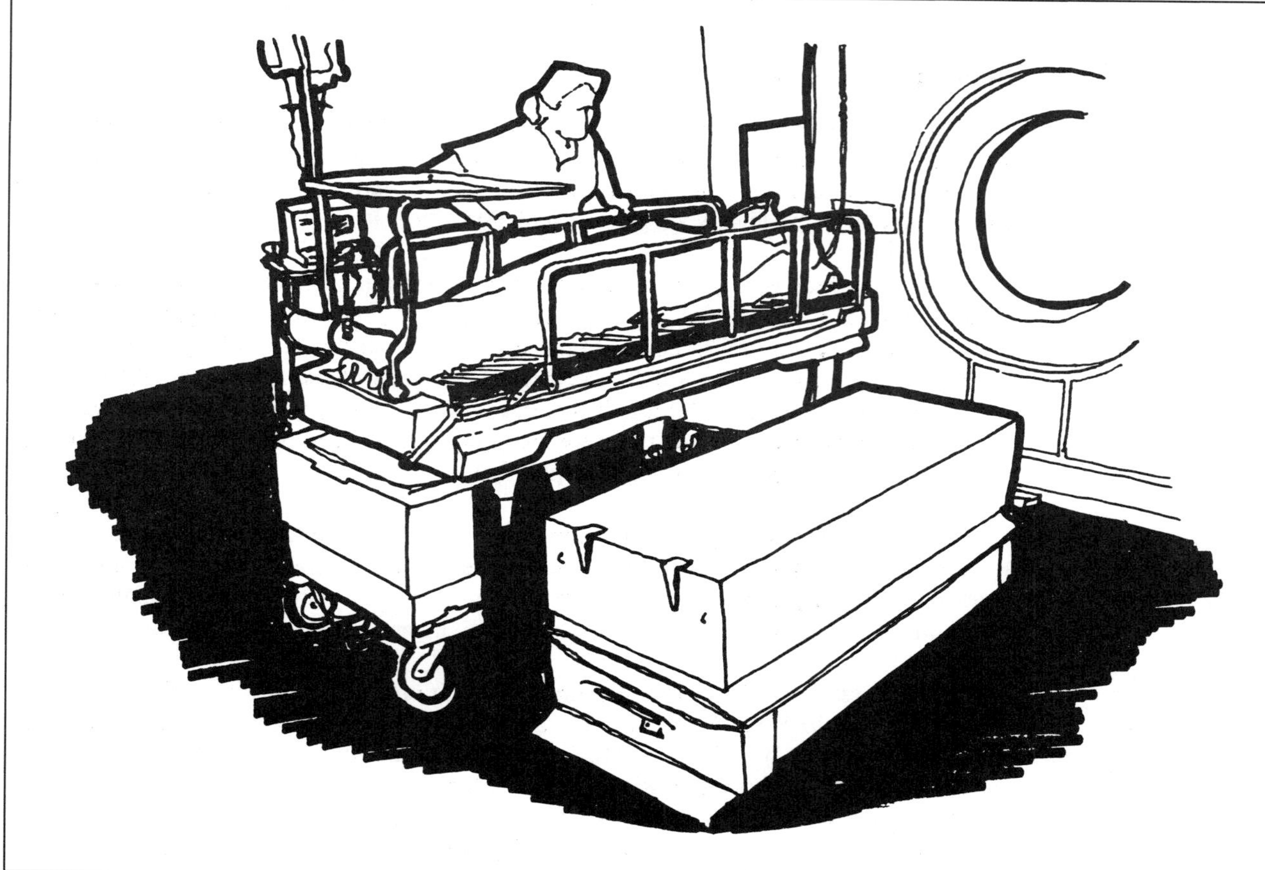

Routine bedside radiographs play an integral role in daily patient management. Prompt radiographs are essential after many invasive procedures. Critical management decisions often are based on image interpretation.

[In several studies[15]] . . . positive radiographic findings including new or worsening cardiopulmonary abnormalities and malposition of support or monitoring devices were present in 45% of all examinations. Routine daily chest radiographs (i.e., those not performed because of an obvious change in medical status or after an intervention) yielded positive findings in 41% of examinations.

[Other studies[16]] . . . found that 39% of routine and 50% of non-routine portable chest radiographs resulted in a change in diagnostic approach or therapy. Excluding catheter and tube adjustments, management efficacy was 24% for routine and 35% for non-routine radiographs. Thus the value of routine bedside chest radiography has been validated in the ICU setting.[17]

Portable X-ray equipment used in the intensive care unit may be similar to the portable equipment used in the surgical suite, except that the imaging tube used in the ICU probably will be smaller. Space should be provided on the unit for portable C-arm storage. In addition, the patient rooms themselves should be configured to easily accommodate a C-arm as well as nonradiologic patient support and monitoring equipment, which also will be in use. If digital imaging equipment is to be used, additional space must be provided for special ancillary equipment. This equipment—and the space required for it—will vary based on the method of acquiring, storing, transmitting, and viewing digital images as described in the following subsection. Image digitizing, processing, storage, and display equipment can be on the unit or in the radiography department depending on the need for rapid image availability, the availability of space on the unit, the budget, the distance between the two areas, and the availability of (manual or electronic) image transmission systems.

Digital Radiography in the ICU

In recent years, digital radiology has been gaining acceptance in intensive care units. Two techniques in particular are applicable for use with intensive care patients. (For a complete discussion of digital image management, see the section entitled Electronic Image Management in chapter 7, "Image Management and Film Processing.")

> Image acquisition in CT, MR ultrasonography, subtraction angiography and nuclear medicine utilizes digital technology. Over the past several years, digital imaging has become a practical clinical tool in conventional radiography, particularly of the chest, as well. In fact, one of the most widely accepted applications of digital radiography has been portable chest imaging. Although there are several different digital radiographic techniques now available, two of these are most applicable to the ICU patient: *film digitization* and *photostimulable* phosphor plates.[18]

Film digitization is the process of converting film images to a digital format by digitizing the hard-copy image. (See the section entitled General Considerations for Image-Processing Areas in chapter 13, "Room Design.") This process requires that space be available on the unit or in the radiology department for a film digitizer, among other equipment.

> Film digitization involves a two-step image acquisition process. First, a conventional radiograph is acquired on film in routine fashion. Second, the image on film is converted to a digital image by a digitizer. Digitizers require transmission of a light source through the film to a light detector (video camera), which records the information in digital format by use of an analog-to-digital converter. Once the digital data for an image exist, the image can be stored, transmitted and displayed on a video screen in the ICU or printed on film. Also, the video display terminal allows the image to be manipulated for desired brightness, contrast and even magnification.[19]

Photo-stimulable phosphor plates are reusable, light-sensitive plates that are used instead of film to capture images. The process is described in the following paragraphs:

> Computed radiography systems utilize photostimulable phosphor plates that allow direct acquisition of a digital image while still using conventional portable X-ray generators. The chest radiograph is acquired in routine fashion at the bedside, except that a reusable photostimulable phosphor plate is substituted for the film-screen cassette. This plate is subsequently delivered to a centrally located processor much as the film-screen cassette would be in a modern radiology department where it is read by a laser scanner, and a direct digital image is obtained. Again images may be stored, transmitted and displayed on video monitors in the ICU or generated on film. This technique has the advantage of eliminating the need for repeat chest radiographs, particularly portable examinations caused by exposure error. The computer will compensate for underexposure or overexposure when the image is displayed. Therefore, underexposure can be routine, reducing the radiation exposure of the patient and nearby personnel. Also, computer algorithms can alter the data to provide, for example, an edge-enhanced image.[20]
>
> To process the latent image, the exposed imaging plate [can be] placed in an automated image reader that opens the cassette, removes the plate, and returns the empty cassette to the operator. . . . [First the data is "pre-read where it is put into digital format, the average exposure level of the plate is determined, and the computer adjusts the sensitivity of its electronics for the actual image reading which follows]. . . . Now in digital format, the data go to yet another component of the image reader, an image processing computer. . . . After the reading is completed, the imaging plate is erased by exposure

to light from a high-intensity sodium discharge lamp. The plate is then sorted and stored for later reuse in the appropriate daylight image plate loader.[21]

Computer Workstations in the ICU

A computer workstation for interpreting images on the ICU should be considered. It should include at least two monitors—one for viewing the most recent image and the other for viewing the image immediately preceding the most recent image. The two images will be compared to each other. The workstation area should be large enough to enable a small group of physicians to discuss the films and should be located away from patient rooms to keep conversations from being overheard. Controlled lighting should be provided to avoid glare on the monitors, and the monitors should be located in such a way that the operator does not need to frequently move his or her head to view the images. Alternatives to a computer workstation for image review include conventional, backlit film alternators and a simple series of film illuminators.[22] These can be used to view laser-generated hard films even from digitally acquired computed radiographic equipment.

Technology Docks

A technology dock is a useful adjunct to most hospital-based or outpatient-oriented imaging facilities. It is simply a structure where mobile trailers or other types of portable imaging enclosures can be incorporated into the facility. The advantages of a technology dock are:

1. It enables the temporary use of imaging equipment during construction or renovation of more permanent facilities. The dock also can be used for temporary placement of expensive equipment that will quickly become outdated, without having to commit to permanent construction to house such equipment.
2. It allows some types of equipment to be accessible at a lower cost because movable equipment can be shared among providers using it at separate locations.
3. It is quick. Compared to a permanent facility, which may take years to design and build, mobile equipment often is more readily available.

If a technology dock is incorporated into the facility plan, special attention should be given to issues of convenience and image. (See chapter 8, "Design Concepts.") For example, is the dock easily accessible? Do users have to walk through the parking lot to reach it? Is it close enough to other imaging procedure areas so that staffing efficiency and patient safety can be maintained? Are patient and staff support spaces provided in the mobile unit of a similar quality to those in other parts of the facility?

The following should be considered when planning a technology dock:

- Site access must allow a large tractor and semitrailer to deliver the mobile unit to the dock. Specific slope and clearance criteria should be available from the manufacturer of the unit.
- The pedestrian connection between the dock and the main facility should be short, level, and protected from adverse weather conditions, if possible.
- The dock's accessibility should be assessed. For example, will it be accessible only from the main facility or will it also have its own entrance? If it has its own entrance, how will this affect patient and staff work flow and circulation? How will having a separate entrance affect patient registration and medical records?
- The degree to which the dock will provide services to inpatients needs to be determined. For example, will the services provided at the dock be needed by inpatients? Will regulatory agencies permit inpatients to be treated in the dock? Will special construction modifications be required for this?
- The regulatory agencies that have jurisdiction over reviewing and approving mobile imaging projects must be verified. In some locations, this is done by the building department;

in others, the department of transportation issues permits. In either case, requirements of the Americans with Disabilities Act (ADA) will apply.

- Some imaging modalities may be adversely affected by excess vibration. Similarly, some MRI units may be affected by large, moving ferrous objects such as trucks, automobiles, and nearby elevators.
- For some MRI units, people will need to be kept out of a 5-gauss exclusion zone that may extend beyond the boundary of the physical enclosure. Required signage should be coordinated with facilitywide signage systems.
- Some imaging modalities will need special service access. For example, superconducting magnets will require storage and access for cryogen replenishment.
- Utility requirements (such as power, water, cooling, sewage, and communication) should be coordinated with the mobile equipment vendor. Clean, uninterrupted power should be made available at the dock. Some units now contain uninterruptable power supply (UPS) systems to ensure uniform power. Required clearances should be verified for adequate airflow. Consideration should be given to providing additional utility hookups and excess capacity that might accommodate additional equipment in the future.
- In cold climates, modifications to the trailer or the trailer site may be necessary to prevent freezing and/or to maintain comfort. Wind breaks may be necessary in windy areas.

References

1. Jolesz, F., and Kinkinis, R. The role of imaging in the operating room of the future. *Administrative Radiology,* Nov. 1992, pp. 43–46.
2. Eisenberg, R. L. *Diagnostic Imaging in Surgery.* New York City: [publisher unknown], 1987.
3. Jones-Bey, H. Ultrasound lights the path for invasive therapies. *Diagnostic Imaging,* June 1992, p. 101.
4. Eisenberg, pp. 814–16.
5. Sochurek, H. *Medicine's New Vision.* Easton, PA: Mack Publishing, 1988, p. 53.
6. Eisenberg, p. 816.
7. Jolesz and Kinkinis.
8. Hunton, N. K. Wandering through the brain: the power of a "magic wand" helps neurosurgeons prepare for complicated procedures. *Computer Graphics World,* Oct. 1992, pp. 71–72.
9. Freiherr, G. *Second Source Imaging,* Jan. 1992, pp. 48–52.
10. Eisenberg, p. 799.
11. Jolesz and Kinkinis.
12. Jones-Bey.
13. Marglin, S. I., Rowberg, A. H., and Godwin, J. D. Preliminary experience with portable imaging for intensive care radiography. *Journal of Thoracic Imaging* 5(1), 1990.
14. Marglin and others.
15. Wiener, M. D., Garay, S. M., Leitman, B. S., Wiener, D. N., and Ravin, C. E. Imaging strategies in pulmonary disease-imaging of the intensive care patient. *Clinics in Chest Medicine* 12(1):169–95, Mar. 1991.
16. Wiener and others.
17. Wiener and others.
18. Wiener and others, p. 172.
19. Wiener and others, p. 172.
20. Wiener and others.
21. Marglin and others.
22. Marglin and others.

Chapter 15

Physical Properties Influencing Design

Physical properties associated with both imaging procedures and imaging equipment must be considered when planning and designing a new facility. Some phenomena, such as the effects of ionizing radiation, are present only after the equipment has been installed and the facility is operational. However, other considerations, such as the size and weight of equipment, come into play during construction as well as after the facility is operational. These physical properties must be taken into account when equipment is being installed and when equipment repair and/or replacement becomes necessary.

Construction specialties, such as radiation barriers, that compensate for unique physical forces protect occupants in adjacent areas from the harmful effects of those forces originating within the procedure room. Other barriers, such as MRI radio-frequency (RF) shielding, prevent external forces from disturbing image acquisition within the procedure room, in addition to preventing those forces that originate in the procedure room from disturbing equipment outside the room.

This chapter examines the key physical properties of imaging procedures and related issues that must be considered when designing an imaging facility. These include the size and weight of the imaging equipment to be used, the type of protection needed from ionizing radiation, and special considerations for magnetic resonance imaging (MRI) installations.

Imaging Equipment Size and Weight

Most imaging equipment is large and heavy. Although it often is delivered in pieces and later assembled in the procedure room, even its smaller components can still be difficult to maneuver. Thus, procedure room design must take into account equipment size and weight. (Guidelines for procedure room size are discussed in chapter 12, "Space Requirements.") Unfortunately, size and weight are not always thoroughly considered when it comes to the route along which equipment is delivered. In some cases, overlooking the delivery route can result in the unplanned partial demolition of a new facility in order to accommodate the installation or replacement of equipment. A series of meetings, first during the early stages of design and then during contract document preparation, involving the architect, the equipment vendor and installation coordinator, and the owner can do much to eliminate unnecessary installation surprises.

Often, special structural systems are required to support assemblies of imaging equipment or ancillary devices such as ceiling-mounted monitors or secondary radiation barriers. Heavy-gauge metal studs are required to support the weight of lead-lined partitions and accessory equipment. Partitions in procedure rooms should be constructed of studs that are thicker than standard studs (typically 6 inches) to accommodate the array of conduit and mounting assemblies that are placed in the wall. Special backing plates often are installed as part of the wall framing and are hidden behind the plasterboard. For ceiling-mounted equipment, secondary structural assemblies often are fastened to the building's structural beams and purlins. Typically, these assemblies are hidden behind a finished ceiling, such as a lay-in ceiling panel system.

Careful coordination is necessary for both wall and ceiling structural supports. In both cases, the support system usually is furnished and installed by the contractor but must meet the precise requirements specified by the equipment manufacturer. All parties must agree on which components are to be part of the contractor-furnished support system for the equipment and which ones are to be provided by the manufacturer as part of the equipment itself. If equipment selections are changed, often the capacity and location of the structural support also must be modified. However, a universal support system will minimize the need for modification for some modalities. (See the section entitled Universal Room Design in chapter 13, "Room Design.")

In addition, most states require a detailed, and often lengthy, review by structural regulatory officials prior to granting a building permit and additional field inspections prior to granting a certificate of occupancy. If equipment is changed after the building permit is granted, the structural review may have to be repeated, causing significant delays. Often, both the structural components and the equipment itself require a long lead time to be manufactured and delivered. Excess capacity designed into the building systems may minimize the potential disruption caused by last-minute equipment changes.

In geographic locations that experience seismic activity, lateral bracing of equipment is required in addition to vertical structural support. Lateral bracing prevents equipment from falling over as a result of vibration or other movement caused by an earthquake. Lateral bracing, when required, usually applies to mechanical ducts, light fixtures, and essential utility lines, in addition to the individual components of imaging equipment and ancillary equipment.

Design of the building's structural system must also minimize excessive vibration, which can be transferred from other components of the building system. Interventional procedures and associated imaging modalities often have more stringent vibration criteria than do other imaging modalities.

Radiation Protection

Patients, staff, and the general public need to be protected wherever ionizing radiation is present. Radiation barriers (such as lead-lined drywall, lead sheets, concrete, lead-lined glass or acrylic, and so on) must be strategically sized and located. Although a basic understanding of the physical principles of ionizing radiation and the specific equipment planned for each room will assist the designer in planning the imaging facility, the exact requirements for radiation protection need to be calculated by a certified medical or health physicist. Often, the physicist is either employed by the owner or contracted as the owner's consultant (rather than as the architect's consultant). The information he or she will need may include:

- The make and model number, intended location, and movement characteristics of each piece of radiation-emitting equipment
- The location of wall-mounted cassette holders and buckys
- The types of procedures to be done in the room
- The average duration of a typical exposure and the room's hours of operation
- The type of occupancy of all adjacent rooms (including those above and below the exam room)
- A floor plan showing equipment, control stations, doors, and room dimensions
- The average number of procedures and exposures each week

Based on this information, the physicist will calculate and prescribe the requirements for radiation shielding. For example, the physicist might prescribe that the north wall requires 2 pounds of lead per square foot, up to a height of 7 feet above floor level, between point A and point B, and 2.5 pounds of lead per square foot between point B and point C as indicated on the floor plans. After construction, a qualified testing agency should test and certify that the room has been built in accordance with the medical health physicist's requirements.

Radiation Protection Regulations

As previously mentioned, radiation protection calculations (based on mathematical formulas that determine the type and amount of protection required) must be made by a certified medical health physicist. *The following is provided for information only and is in no way intended to suggest that anyone other than a certified medical health physicist should perform radiation protection calculations.*

Radiation protection requirements are specified on both the local (state and municipality) and federal levels. Often, local requirements are more stringent than federal requirements, although this varies by location. In 1976, the National Council on Radiation Protection and Measurement (NCRP) published *NCRP Report No. 49—Structural Shielding Design and Evaluation for Medical Use of X-Rays and Gamma Rays of Energies Up to 10 MeV.*[1] Although many new techniques and devices for imaging have been developed since NCRP 49 was first written, the 1976 edition of NCRP 49 still remains the primary regulatory reference for determining radiation protection requirements. Some current aspects of medical imaging, such as computed tomography (CT), are not addressed in NCRP 49. However, various task forces of the American Association of Physicists in Medicine (AAPM) have been working to provide updated information to reflect current practices in diagnostic imaging.

Anyone involved in the design or planning of an imaging facility should become familiar with NCRP 49 and any additional regulations that supersede it. The following paragraph describes the report's intended audience:

> [NCRP 49] . . . includes a discussion of the various factors to be considered in the selection of appropriate shielding materials and the calculation of barrier thickness. It is mainly intended for radiological physicists, radiologists and regulatory personnel who specialize in radiation protection. Sections of the report, [however], should be of interest also to architects, hospital administrators, and others who are concerned with the planning of radiation facilities.[2]

The medical or health physicist's chief charge, as it relates to determining radiation protection barrier requirements, is to protect patients, staff, and public from excessive levels of radiation generated from radiographic equipment. The level of protection for radiation staff is described as a *maximum permissible dose (MPD)* or *maximum permissible dose equivalent.* The MPD is a measure of accumulated radiation exposure and is stated in terms of maximum radiation (or roentgen) equivalent man per week (mrem/wk). Radiology staff (occupational workers) wear personal monitoring devices that keep track of accumulated radiation exposure.

NCRP 49 lists MPDs for patients and the public in a section that refers to noncontrolled areas. Accordingly, they are to be protected not to exceed 10 mrem/wk. Another publication, *NCRP Report No. 91—Recommendations for Occupational Exposure Limitation,*[3] lists new MPDs that will be adopted on a state-by-state basis. These new MPDs are significantly lower than previous listings and are likely to affect architectural protective barrier requirements by requiring a higher level of protection than before.

Modern X-ray equipment generally provides a lower level of radiation than does older equipment. At the same time, however, it is interesting to note that the acceptable level of mrem/wk has been reduced significantly over the years as more knowledge about the biological effects of ionizing radiation has become available. Radiation itself has not changed, but our understanding of it and our philosophy about safety have:

> The concept of Maximum Permissible Dose Equivalent (MPD) as expressed by the NCRP, i.e. the maximum dose equivalent that persons shall be allowed to receive in a stated

> period of time, has been used as the basis for the recommendations in [NCRP 49]. The numerical values of the maximum permissible dose equivalents are such that the probability of adverse biological effects is extremely low and is considered to present an acceptable risk. The MPD values used in [NCRP 49] are those agreed upon by the NCRP at the time of publication of [that] report. They are considered reasonable in light of the scientific knowledge [which was known at that time] concerning the biological effects of ionizing radiation, and constitute acceptable standards for the use of ionizing radiation with safety. They are not limits above which biological damage can be assumed. In addition to specifying values for the Maximum Permissible Dose Equivalent, the NCRP recommendations call for radiation exposure to be kept at a level "as low as practicable" (or at the lowest practicable level).[4]

Radiation protection can be accomplished by a number of methods, each of which provides a means of protecting individuals against excessive radiation exposure. Methods of radiation protection include collimation, filtration, protective apparel, protective barriers, and the selection of appropriate film-screen combinations for imaging. It is the inclusion of protective barriers that the architect will be most closely involved with:

> [NCRP 49] is intended primarily for use in planning and designing new facilities and in remodeling existing facilities. Since corrections or additions after facilities are completed can be expensive, it is important that structural shielding be properly designed and installed in the original construction process. It is also advisable that the planning include consideration of possible future needs for new equipment, higher radiation energies, and increased workloads.
>
> It is recommended that the shielding be designed by a qualified expert [as defined by NCRP] to ensure that the required degree of radiation protection is achieved economically. This objective will be furthered by providing the qualified expert with all pertinent information regarding the proposed radiation equipment and its type of use, type of building construction and occupancy of nearby areas. . . . If possible, the expert should be consulted during the early planning stages; often the shielding requirements affect the choice of location of radiation facilities and type of building construction. It is highly desirable [and often required by law] that final shielding drawings and specifications be reviewed by the qualified expert and by pertinent federal, state or local agencies (if applicable) before construction is begun. While some other aspects of x- and gamma ray facilities, such as interlocks, warning signs and lights, electrical safety and room lighting, are mentioned in [NCRP 49] these aspects are not represented as a complete treatment of these topics.
>
> While specific recommendations are given, alternate methods may prove equally satisfactory in providing radiation protection. The final assessment of the adequacy of the design and construction of structural shielding should be based on the radiation survey of the completed installation. If the radiation survey shows deficiencies, additional shielding or modifications of equipment and procedures are required.[5]

The American Board of Radiology, the American Board of Health Physics, and the American Board of Medical Physics have certification criteria for persons to be considered qualified in radiation protection and in radiation shielding design.

NCRP 49 includes the following appendix titled *Architectural and Equipment Information to Be Supplied to the Qualified Expert for Use in Shielding Design:*

> A. *Architectural*
> 1. Drawings of radiation rooms and adjacent areas; scale preferred ¼ inch = 1 foot, or larger, including position of radiation source, doors and windows.
> 2. Information about occupancy below, above and adjacent to radiation rooms.
> 3. Type of proposed, or existing, construction of floors, ceilings and walls.
> 4. For megavoltage therapy installations, including cobalt, vertical sections and plot plans [note: the use of cobalt therapy is rapidly declining].

B. *Equipment*
  1. Below 150 kV.
    a. Purpose: therapy, radiography, fluoroscopy, special procedures, cystoscopy, etc.
    b. kV and expected weekly workload, if known.
  2. 150 kV and above, including gamma beam apparatus.
    a. kV, or type of gamma source.
    b. mA or R per minute at 1 meter.
    c. Weekly workload, if known, expressed in mA min, or R at 1 meter.
    d. Restrictions in beam orientations without and with beam interceptor, if any.
    e. Use factor for walls and ceiling, if known.
    f. Leakage radiation of source housing with beam "ON."
    g. Attenuation by beam interceptor, if any.
  3. Possible future increases in workload and radiation energy and modification in beam orientation.[6]

In addition to the NCRP requirements, most states—and some local municipalities—have special codes describing radiation protection requirements. These requirements vary considerably from one jurisdiction to another. For example, some states require that protective barriers be installed in the walls of all mammography suites. Others do not require this because of the low level of radiation employed in mammography examinations.

Determination of Radiation Protection Requirements

A number of variables are used to determine requirements for radiation protection that separates a source of radiation from occupants and adjacent spaces. These variables include:[7]

- *Weekly design exposure rate:* Weekly design exposure rate identifies the target level of radiation exposure to which an adjacent occupied area must be reduced. Each adjacent area should be identified as either controlled or noncontrolled. A *controlled area* is limited to radiation staff; a *noncontrolled area* is open to the public.
- *Distance:* Distance identifies how much space (usually expressed in meters) is between the radiation source and the area being protected. The greater the distance, the lower the requirements for radiation protection. Therefore, theoretically, a larger room will require less lead per square foot of wall area. However, the larger room will not necessarily cost less to protect. For one thing, a larger room has more surface area; thus, it may require more (although not necessarily thinner) lead. In addition, the cost of lead is not always proportional to its thickness. Certain thicknesses of lead may cost more because of either their availability or complications in fabricating thin sheets of lead.
- *Workload:* Expressed as milliampere-minutes per week (mAmin/wk[1]), distance denotes the relative activity of the radiation source. Appendix C of NCRP 49 lists typical workloads for various types of procedure rooms.[8] It is difficult to believe that workloads identified in 1976 would be typical for procedure rooms today, especially with new film-screen combinations that require two to four times less radiation than their predecessors. CT is notably absent from appendix C. (If the number of exposures per patient, the number of patients per week, and the average milliamperes per exposure are known, this information should be used instead of NCRP 49, appendix C.)
- *Use factor, or beam direction factor:* Use factor represents the amount of time (expressed as a percent) that the X-ray beam is on, in which the radiation source directly strikes the protective barrier. The use factor for each wall may vary depending on the type of equipment installed and the types of procedures performed.
- *Occupancy factor:* Occupancy factor represents the amount of time (expressed as a percent) in which each adjacent room or space is occupied. This factor suggests that if the occupancy of an adjacent room changes over time, radiation protection requirements also will change. Therefore, if a room's occupancy classification is likely to be upgraded in the future, additional protection might need to be added at that time or a higher-than-actual occupancy factor should be used in the initial calculations.

- *Maximum operating potential of the imaging equipment:* Maximum operating potential signifies the potential power of the equipment. It usually is expressed in terms of kilovolts peak (kVp). The X-ray tube's operating potential determines the intensity of the radiation and its ability to penetrate matter.

Two types of protective barriers—primary and secondary—are considered, based on the characteristics of three types of radiation—primary radiation, scatter radiation, and radiation leakage. A *primary or useful* beam is defined as "radiation which passes through the window, aperture, cone, or other collimating device of the source housing." Of the two types of radiation, primary radiation is more intense. As a result, it usually requires a greater level of protection. *Scatter radiation* is defined as "radiation that, during passage through matter, has been deviated in direction." Scatter radiation is caused by a primary beam reflecting off an object, such as a piece of equipment or the patient. In theory, primary radiation, which usually is collimated or focused, rarely strikes a protective barrier without first passing through the patient and therefore becoming scatter radiation. However, protective barrier design calculations are conservative and often take into consideration the unlikely situation in which the primary beam might be energized without a patient in the room. *Leakage radiation* is defined as "all radiation coming from within the source or tube housing except the useful beam. Leakage radiation includes the portion of the direct radiation not absorbed by the protective source or tube housing as well as the scattered radiation produced within the housing." Scatter radiation and leakage radiation are both considered to be *secondary radiation.*[9]

Protective barriers that are radiated directly by the imaging equipment's primary or useful beam are considered to be *primary barriers.* Barriers that are radiated only by leakage or scatter radiation are considered to be *secondary barriers.* Primary barriers usually require a higher degree of protection than do secondary barriers. This is one reason that a description of the equipment, its movement characteristics, and the frequency of each type of examination should be given to the medical health physicist.

> In a general purpose radiographic/fluoroscopic room, all walls and floors would normally be considered primary barriers. In a dedicated radiographic room, such as one used solely for chest radiography, only one wall would be considered a primary barrier. The control booth barrier is normally considered a secondary barrier, since rarely, if ever is the useful beam directed to that location. Likewise the ceiling is normally considered a secondary barrier.[10]
>
> Lead shielding is not always required for all protective barriers. For example, . . . lead is rarely required for secondary barriers because the computation usually results in less than 0.4 mm Pb. In such cases, conventional gypsum board, glass, or lead acrylic is [often] adequate. Many walls that are secondary barriers can be adequately protected with four thicknesses of ⅝-inch gypsum board. The thinnest available [lead] shielding is 1 lb/ft^2, but because of some difficulties in fabrication, 2 lb/ft^2 sheets are often no more costly.[11]

After the medical health physicist determines the appropriate level of radiation protection required for each barrier, he or she should provide a written report to the owner and the architect. The report should describe the required amount of lead, usually in terms of pounds per square foot. (Tables, found in NCRP 49, listing the equivalent thickness of commercial lead sheets and densities of other commercial building materials as compared to the density of lead are included in appendix B of this book.) For example, approximately 4 inches of concrete provides the same degree of protection as 1/16 inch of lead.[12] However, concrete is typically used for radiation therapy barriers; it is rarely used as a protective barrier in low-energy-level diagnostic imaging facilities. Lead used for radiation barriers in these facilities is most commonly available in the form of sheet lead or lead-lined plasterboard. Where transparency is required, plate glass, lead glass, and leaded acrylic sheets are available. Doors also are available with lead lining.

The recommendations of the medical or health physicist should then be incorporated into the architect's contract documents so that the contractor will be able to include them as part of the facility construction. The physicist's written report should be kept in the architect's file for future reference. If the physicist is acting as the owner's agent, the architect might want to indicate on the contract documents that the criteria for protective barrier design are owner-furnished information. The architect might want to include a clause in the specifications, for example: "The Owner shall engage a qualified radiological physicist certified by the American Board of Radiology or the American Board of Health Physicists to test shielded spaces for conformance with the Contract Documents. In the event that radiation protection fails to meet specification requirements, the Contractor shall remove substandard radiation protection and apply new at no cost to the Contract."

Design and Planning Issues

Radiation protection is just one of many issues that influence design and planning decisions. Such issues affect both the cost and safety of the facility, and often cost and safety are directly interrelated. Increased levels of radiation protection tend to increase construction costs. The goal of both the medical health physicist and the architect is to provide an appropriate level of protection without requiring excessive cost. The architect's ability to understand radiation-related implications of design decisions is key to providing a safe, cost-effective, functional, and aesthetic environment. For example:

> Openings in protective barriers for doors, windows, ventilating ducts, conduits, pipes, etc. may require radiation baffles to ensure that the necessary degree of overall protection is maintained. Whenever possible, the opening should be located in a secondary barrier where the required thickness is less [than that of a primary barrier]. The design of the baffles will depend on a number of factors. These include:
>
> 1. The energy of the radiation.
> 2. The orientation and field size of the useful beam.
> 3. The size and location of the opening in the protective barrier.
> 4. The geometrical relationship between the radiation source and the opening.
> 5. The geometrical relationship between the opening and persons, materials or instruments to be protected.[13]

Because radiation protection is influenced as much by the occupancy of spaces adjacent to the imaging room as it is by the activities within the imaging room, the degree of radiation protection required can be reduced by modifying or controlling the adjacent occupancies. For example, a radiographic room located in the basement will have no occupants below it. Similarly, a radiographic room located on the top floor or at the exterior perimeter of the building also will have limited adjacent occupants.

Sometimes imaging departments are planned solely with the objective of reducing the cost of radiation protection. This is inappropriate. Although lead-lined partitions are somewhat heavier and costlier than standard drywall partitions, the premium paid for this type of construction is minor compared to the cost of other issues, such as adjacencies to interrelated departments, functionally efficient circulation routes, and the optimal size of procedure rooms. As an example, a large office might be located directly adjacent to a procedure room for the purpose of providing a temporary occupancy that could be converted into another radiographic room in the future. In this case, the protective barrier between the two rooms might require more protection than if the room were used for storage. However, the "soft" office space could save considerable expense in the future when it is converted into another procedure room. Radiation protection is one of many important issues that must be considered during design, planning, and construction. It cannot be ignored, but it also cannot be considered in the absence of other crucial issues.

The architect or planner may encounter various conceptually different arrangements for the technologist's control area with respect to the procedure room. One concept locates the control alcove within the room; another locates it in an adjacent but separate control corridor. A third concept provides a separate control room. (See the section entitled General Considerations for Control Corridors, Control Alcoves, and Control Rooms in chapter 13, "Room Design.") The control alcove that is part of the procedure room provides for better personal communication between patient and technologist than the control corridor concept does, but might make it more difficult for the technologist to access the staff work core. It also can provide a reduced level of radiation protection for the technologist, because the barrier between the control area and the radiation source is less obvious than the partition between the procedure room and the control corridor. Even though the control alcove partition usually is a secondary barrier, this is an important consideration because the effects of radiation are cumulative. Some codes require that the solid portion of the partition adjacent to the control alcove viewing window be a minimum of 18 inches wide and 7 feet high.

The planner should be aware of special considerations involved in protecting the developing fetus from ionizing radiation. Whenever possible, ultrasound rooms and other spaces that are likely to be occupied by pregnant women should not be located adjacent to rooms that emit radiation. In the case of radiology staff members who become pregnant, either protective garments can be worn or the staff's daily activities can be temporarily modified without jeopardizing their employment. Because this is such a sensitive issue with respect to health, safety, and equal opportunity employment laws, legal advice on this subject is suggested.

Construction of Radiation Barriers

In addition to lead-lined gypsum board, a number of other materials and products may be used as part of the protective barrier. These include lead glass, acrylic lead glazing, lead-lined viewing windows, lead-lined doors, and so on. Care must be taken when installing the protective barrier over accessories such as wall-mounted cassette holders, through-the-wall cassette passboxes, and even electrical receptacle boxes. Drywall screws set into the lead may require installation of lead disks to maintain a continuous protective barrier; however, some researchers believe that the actual installation of the disks can cause discontinuity of the barrier:

> The shielding of the radiation room shall be so constructed that the protection is not impaired by joints, by openings for ducts, pipes, etc. passing through the barriers, or by conduits, service boxes, etc. embedded in the barriers. Doors (or other means of access to the room) and observation windows also require special consideration to ensure adequate protection without sacrifice of operational efficiency.[14]

Special attention also must be given to wall surfaces that contain multiple sections with different radiation protection requirements because each section may be a different thickness. For example, assuming that one third of a wall's area requires lead-lined plasterboard and the remaining area is adequately protected with standard plasterboard, the difference in thickness of the two materials will be noticeable unless the standard plasterboard is furred out to match the lead-lined material or unless both surfaces are covered with a plasterlike coating to float out the difference.

Although lead usually is placed on the inside surface of room partitions, it also can be placed on the "outboard" side of the wall studs. Sometimes this can simplify installation of room accessories and make future changes easier to achieve, because the radiation protective membrane is less likely to be disturbed when wall-mounted equipment and accessories are removed, replaced, or added.

Special Considerations for MRI Installations

Siting requirements for some MRI units have become simpler in recent years, in part because of the introduction of actively shielded magnets (which can preclude the need for heavy room magnetic shielding in some installations) and lighter magnets. Some 1.0-tesla superconductive magnets now weigh only 7,000 pounds, compared to magnets that weighed more than

20,000 pounds just a few years ago. In addition, the space required for some magnets has been reduced, primarily due to active shield technology and the advent of smaller but more powerful computer systems.

However, siting a magnet is still a complex process. Siting can be further complicated when reconditioned magnets are purchased instead of new units. Due to cost-containment pressures, there is a growing demand for reconditioned MRI equipment. Some of the older MRI units installed in the early 1980s are approaching or have already exceeded their useful lives. Most of the low-field (0.3–1.0-tesla) systems are being abandoned, but many high-field (usually 1.5-tesla) systems are being reconditioned either by the original manufacturers or by third-party suppliers. Reconditioning typically involves replacing the electronics with new computer systems but not necessarily with new magnets.

The main advantage of installing reconditioned high-field systems is their initial purchase price, which can be hundreds of thousands of dollars less than the cost of a new system. The disadvantage is that using older reconditioned systems entails many of the difficult siting concerns that existed in the early 1980s.

Many forces influence the optimal location of MRI units. For instance, the enormous weight of most magnets requires that structural reinforcing be employed not only where the magnet will eventually be positioned but also along the route used to deliver and install it. At the same time, steel beams and other dense ferrous objects distort the *homogeneity* or uniformity of the magnetic field and thus detract from the image quality of the MR system. Finally, the magnetic and radio-frequency (RF) forces emitted from the magnet can disturb, and in turn be disturbed by, other sensitive equipment in the area.

Because MRI does not employ ionizing radiation, X-ray shielding is not necessary. However, RF shielding is required to prevent external radio signals from masking the faint resonating sounds emitted from the patient.[15] If the magnet is not self-shielded and is located near occupied or mechanical space, external magnetic shielding may be necessary to prevent the magnet's force from disturbing, and being disturbed by, objects and signals outside the procedure room. Magnetic and RF shielding enclosures are typically designed and installed by an MRI enclosure manufacturer, not by the architect or contractor.

RF Interactions

Magnetic imaging uses signals of the same frequency as those used for various types of radio and television communications. The MRI unit is a very powerful radio transmitter and is itself a very sensitive radio receiver. To prevent interference from external RF signals, special shielding is required. Radio-frequency shields must completely envelop the imaging volume, which means that the entire area in which the MRI system is installed must be RF shielded. (See figure 15-1.) RF shielding may be prefabricated, modular, or custom applied. It may be a freestanding structure or an integrally shielded room. Freestanding RF structures are common in animal research facilities where appearance is of limited importance. In facilities for patients, however, integral shielding is more common. In either case, the RF shielding must be electrically isolated from all metal structural elements, electrical grounds, and finishes and must maintain its integrity around doors, walls, and mechanical and plumbing penetrations. The RF enclosure is grounded to earth at a single point called a *ground stud.*

Radio-frequency shielding materials need very high conductivity ratings. Although many materials work for this purpose, there are only a few that will provide high conductivity at a reasonable cost.

The most effective and common material is pure copper. Copper is easily shaped and easily soldered to provide good RF seams. It also forms a conductive oxide that protects it from corrosion, thus preserving its RF integrity.

Galvanized steel is also commonly used in the form of thin-gauge sheets. Compared to copper, galvanized steel is inexpensive. However, the zinc surface used in the galvanizing process forms a compound called white rust when it corrodes. This nonconductive rust is the main disadvantage of using steel shielding.

Figure 15-1. RF Shielding

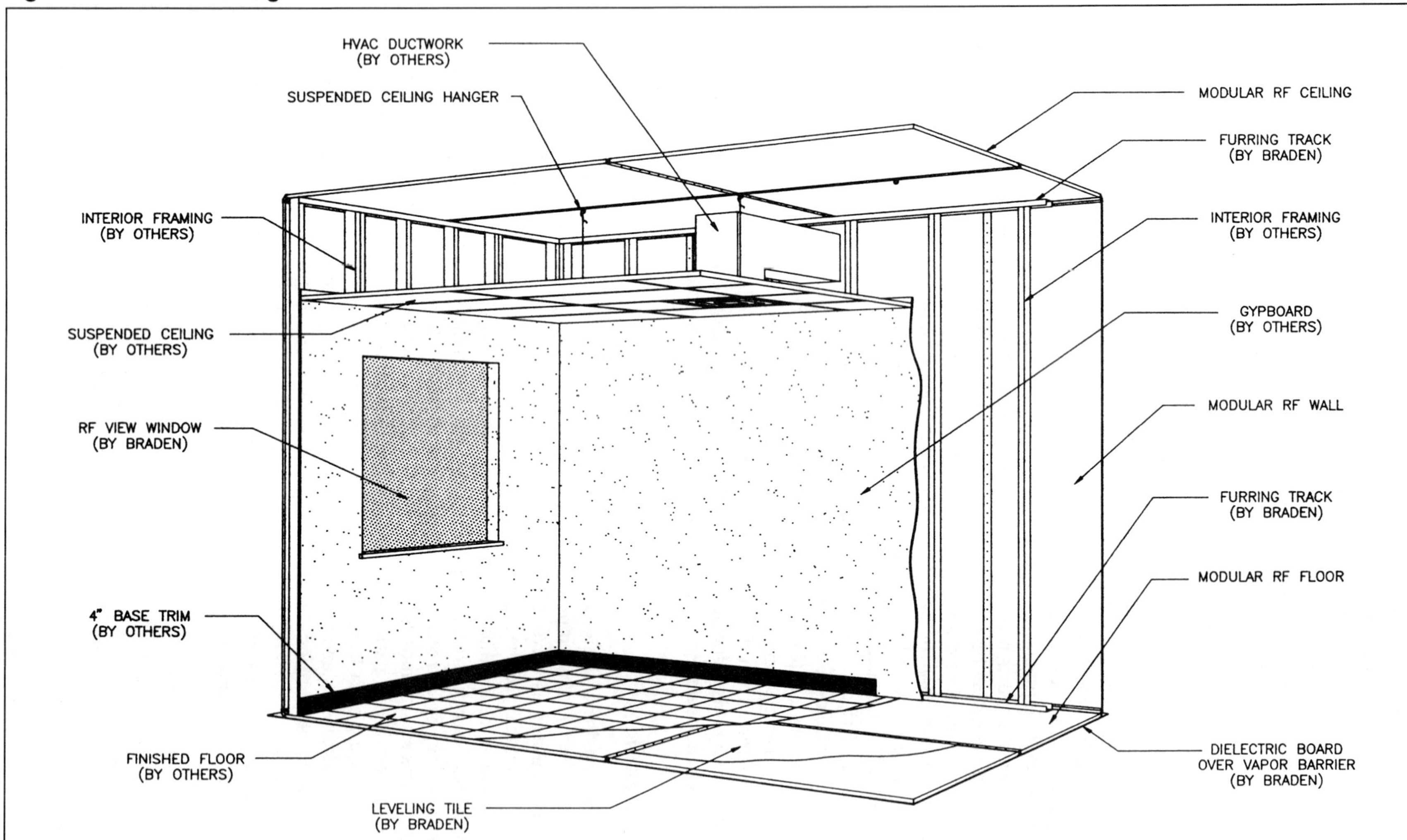

Reprinted, with permission, from Braden Shielding Systems. ©Copyright 1994.

Aluminum is used less frequently for RF shielding. Although aluminum is less expensive than copper, though more expensive than galvanized steel, it corrodes easily and so can become nonconductive.

Another popular way of providing RF shielding is the use of an integrated magnetic- and RF-shielded enclosure. It was found early on that when all the steel plates used to construct a magnetic shield are electrically connected into a monolithic electrical unit, a very effective RF shield results. Electrically connecting an RF flooring system to the magnetic shield creates a complete RF enclosure system. The integrated shield is now used almost exclusively when the site requirements demand some type of full magnetic shield.

In order for the RF shielding to maintain its continuity, special details are required around penetrations in the room enclosure. For example, through-the-wall plumbing lines can degrade the RF enclosure because water running through the pipes may disturb the magnet's RF signal and can cause grounding problems. If a sink is to be installed within the exam room, several precautions need to be taken. A specially tuned, brass-pipe waveguide should be used for each water line as well as the drain line and vent line. For water lines and drain lines, a minimum of 2 lineal feet of PVC pipe should be installed on the exterior end of the waveguide. Local code restrictions and manufacturers' recommendations should be followed.

A large opening in the wall or ceiling will be required for installation and replacement of the magnet. However, once the magnet is installed, this opening will need to be completely sealed with RF shielding. This should be performed by the same company or individual that installs the rest of the RF enclosure to preserve the RF warranty. If the magnet needs to be replaced, the RF shielding surrounding the access opening will need to be removed and replaced in such a way that it continues to provide proper shielding.

Flooring

A number of types of floor construction that provide RF protection are available. Usually, the RF floor assembly is furnished and installed by the RF shielding vendor. However, the finish floor surface may be installed by the contractor.

The RF floor of any enclosure is subject to considerable damage. The magnet's dead load bears directly on it. In addition, it may be damaged by water. (Floors in MRI rooms should be kept dry because water can affect the integrity of the RF enclosure.) Settling of the parent room can also damage the floor. Uneven pavement in the floor can also create problems in RF floor installation.

Two types of RF floor construction are common. They include:

- An epoxy-layered floor that uses an epoxy substrate to both seal the parent floor from moisture and provide dielectric isolation for the enclosure. This type of floor provides a strong surface with high compressive strength.
- A wood core modular system that is constructed of wood panels faced with either galvanized steel or copper. This system, however, is not completely waterproof, and it is difficult to install over an uneven parent floor. It is somewhat easier to install this kind of floor system than it is to install an epoxy-layered floor, and it is slightly less expensive. However, a wood core modular system often requires a greater floor thickness than an epoxy-layered floor. In many cases, the underlying floor surface will need to be depressed in order for the door threshold to meet accessibility requirements.

RF Screens and Glazing at Control Windows

RF-shielded control windows are composed of conductive mesh fabric, usually copper, brass, or treated aluminum. Often, two layers of mesh are provided. Each layer is separated by 1 to 2 inches, and the layers are electrically connected to the primary shield through the window frame assembly. Although glazing is not required for RF shielding purposes, it usually is beneficial to glaze the window opening to provide acoustic, temperature, and ventilation control. Glazing also serves to protect the RF mesh fabric from damage. The optical quality of RF windows from various manufacturers may vary significantly. An RF window that has poor optical quality will have a negative impact on staff. (See figure 15-2.)

The RF screen in the control room window should be blackened. In addition, the two pieces of screen can be rotated slightly to eliminate or minimize the moire pattern that can result from superimposing multiple layers of screen.

RF Doors

"The door is the most critical component of the [RF] shielded enclosure. It is the only component subject to mechanical forces and daily wear and tear."[16] RF doors generally are available in two styles. One has an industrial appearance and is used in research applications where people are not treated. A second architectural style is available for use in areas where human patients are treated. The RF floor leaf has a conductive interior skin, usually made of copper, that provides the RF seal over the door aperture. New "fingerless" RF doors are being developed. This type of door is likely to provide a more durable RF seal than earlier designs. In addition to maintaining a complete RF seal, the architectural-style door must meet the accessibility requirements of the Americans with Disabilities Act and other local requirements. This requires a special handle and a low door threshold. (See figures 15-3 and 15-4, pp. 308–9.)

Waveguides

Although the RF enclosure must maintain its uniformity, certain objects will need to penetrate the procedure room envelope. These include HVAC ducts, electrical cables, and other utility lines. Where ducts penetrate the enclosure, a *waveguide*—a honeycomb cluster of hexagonal tubing that provides maximum open-air space without disrupting RF integrity—is installed by the RF shielding vendor and coordinated with the work of the utility system subcontractors. (See figure 15-5, p. 310.) Usually, the length of a waveguide is four times its diameter.

Utilities that come to the shield in pipes are attached to a pipe penetration waveguide. Power lines are fed into the shielded area via power line filters. A *quench pipe* is a large waveguide connected to the outside in order to provide safe venting of helium gas in the event of a *quench,* a rapid boil-off of liquid helium in which cold helium gas is discharged.

Magnetic Interactions

The magnetic force field has a great deal of influence on facility design because magnetic force can be damaging to both people and objects. The magnetic field extends in three dimensions from the magnet's center. The *fringe field* is the magnetic field extending beyond the magnet. Self-shielding magnets or external *magnetic shielding* of low-carbon steel or iron can be employed to redistribute or reduce the fringe field. The field is measured in *gauss,* an international unit equal to 0.00001 tesla. (Classification of magnets by field strength is discussed in the section entitled Magnetic Resonance Imaging in chapter 6, "Imaging Modalities.")

Because magnetic force can be damaging to people and objects (it can disrupt operation of pacemakers and video monitors, and erase magnetic data from credit cards), gauss lines of an MRI instrument often are plotted on architectural and equipment drawings to locate three-dimensional area boundaries where public traffic should be excluded. A *gauss plot* is available from the equipment manufacturer and should be obtained during the early phases of design. Any area where the magnetic field is greater than 5 gauss is known as the *exclusion zone.* Persons with pacemakers or biostimulator devices must stay out of this area. The 5-gauss line should be contained within the examination room whenever possible. (One exception to this is the use of an unshielded magnet with no external shielding added to the room. Sometimes this is used in research applications to obtain the clearest image possible or when the research program includes chemical shift spectroscopy. An unshielded magnet uses distance instead of magnetic shielding to control the force field. External magnetic shielding, which may degrade the image somewhat, is eliminated and so is the diminished image quality.)

Figure 15-2. RF Shielding—Window Details

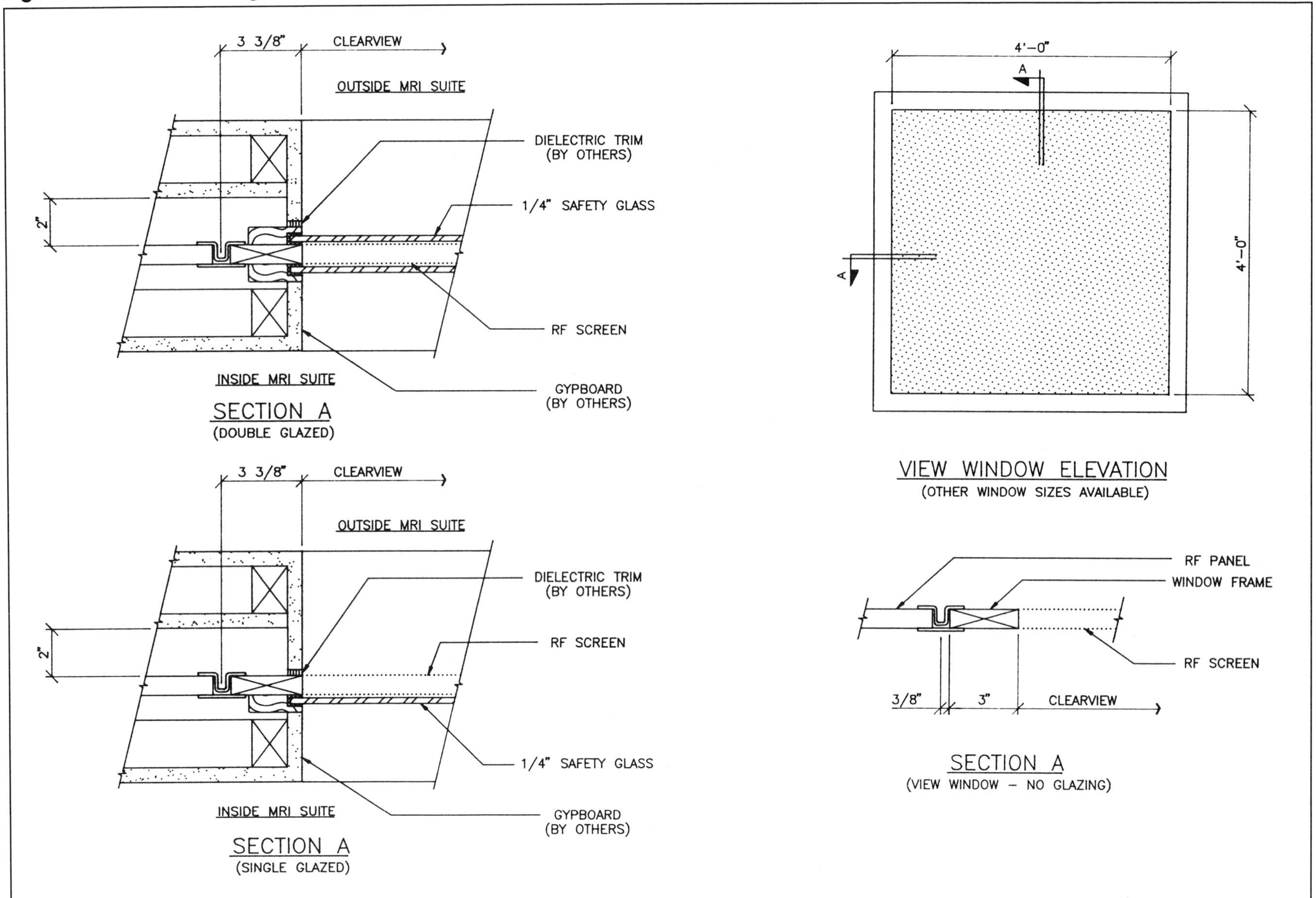

Figure 15-3. RF Shielding—Door Details

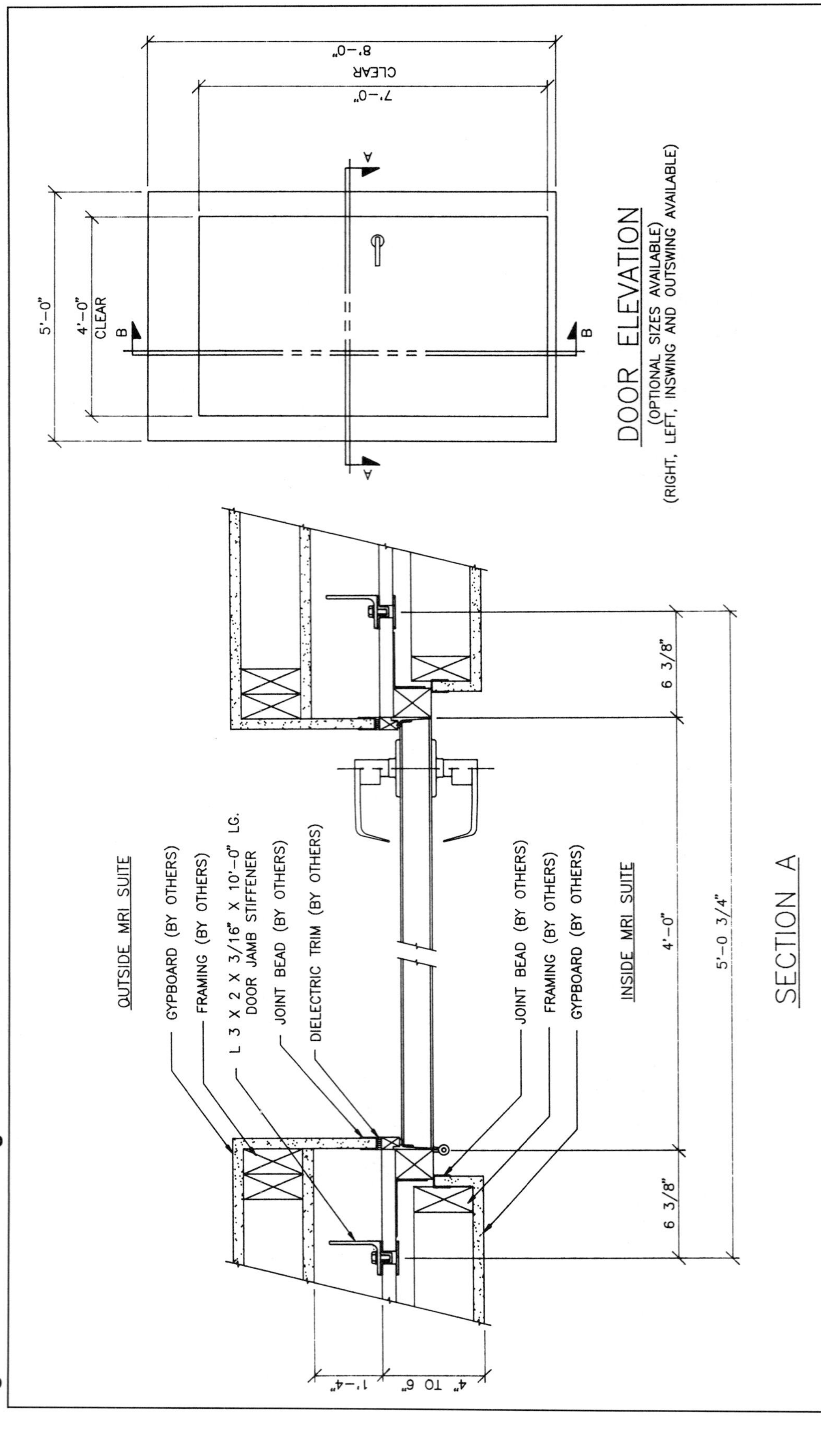

Reprinted, with permission, from Braden Shielding Systems. ©Copyright 1994.

Figure 15-4. RF Shielding—Door Details

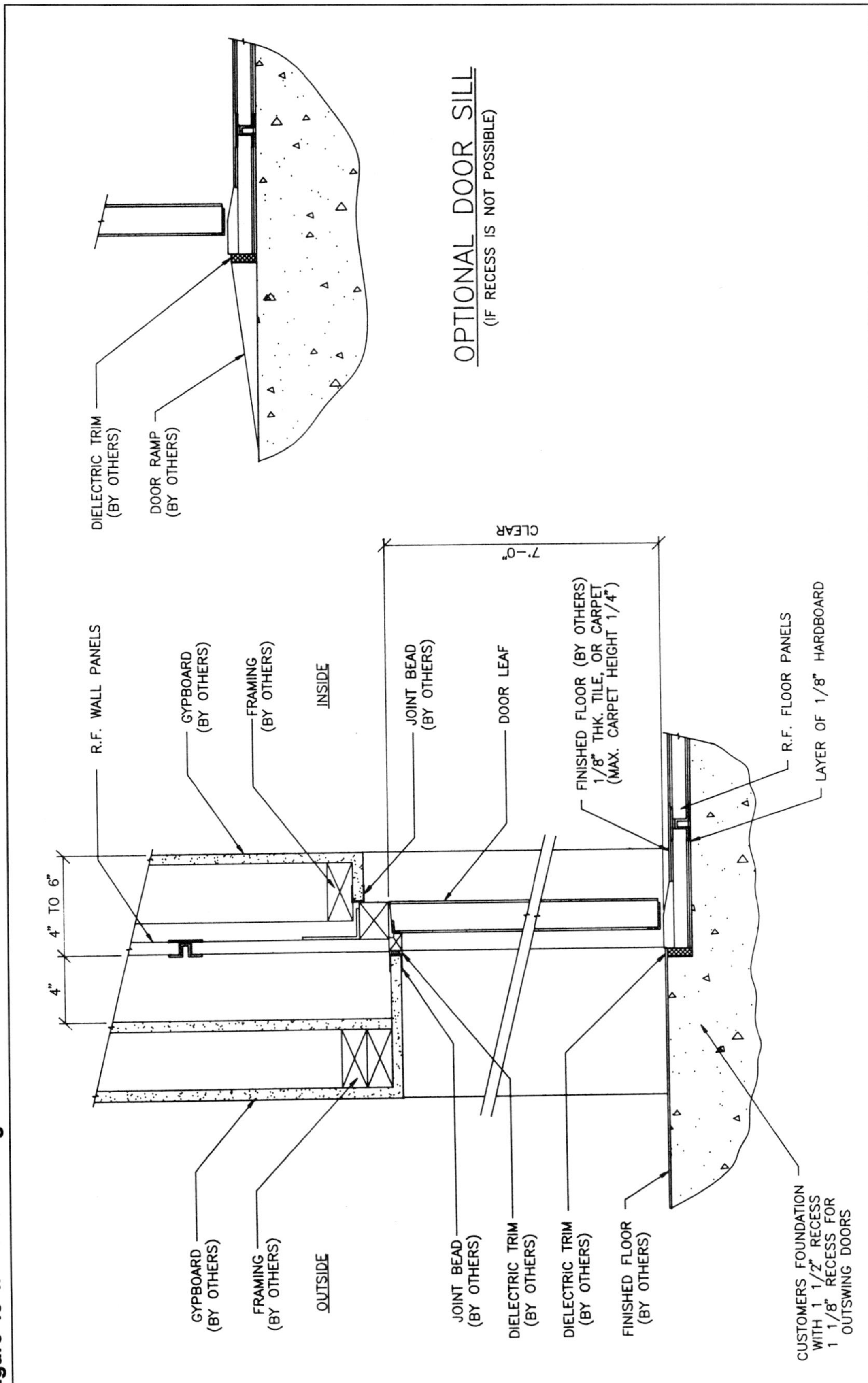

Reprinted, with permission, from Braden Shielding Systems. ©Copyright 1994.

Figure 15-5. RF Shielding—Waveguide Details

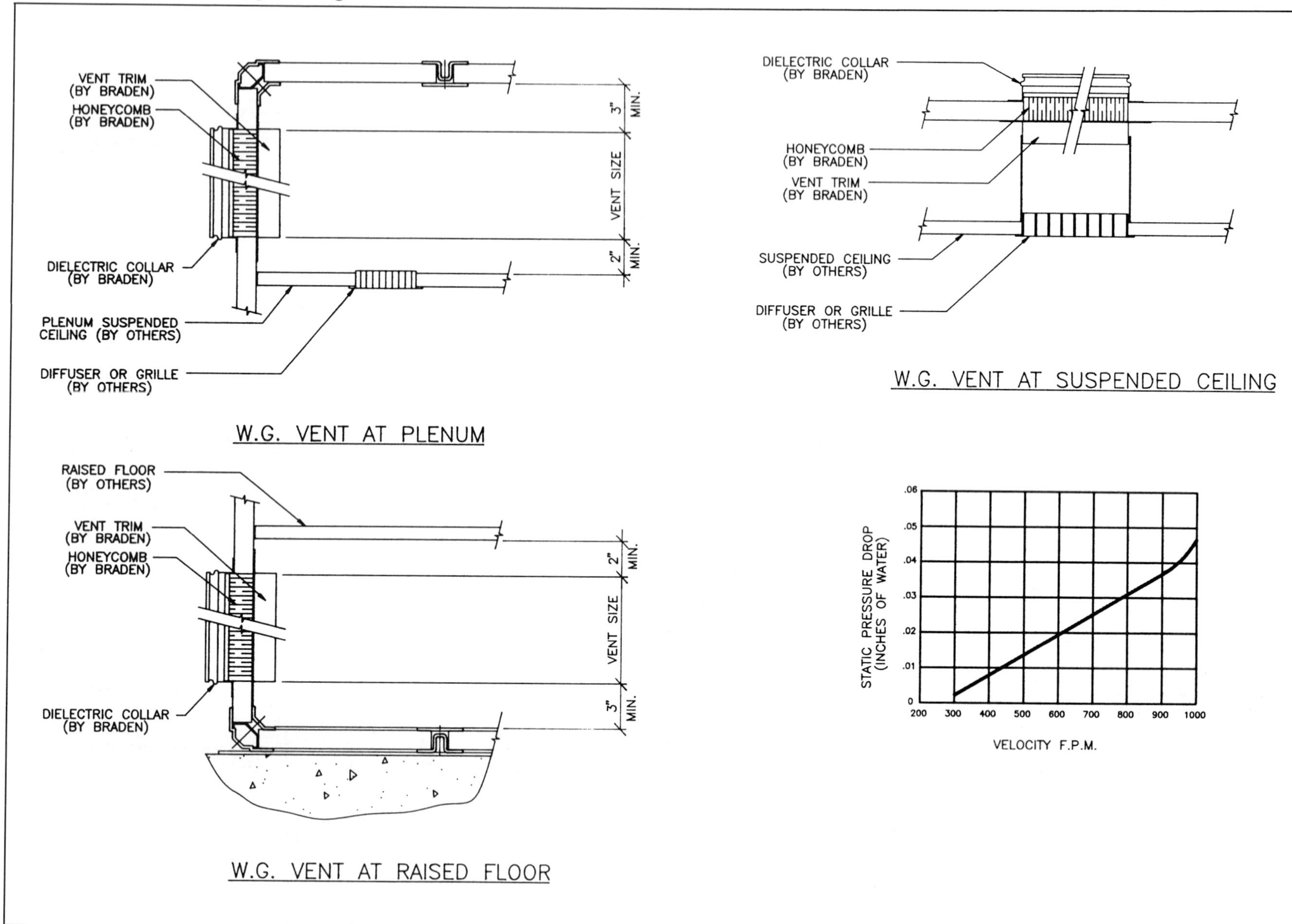

Permanent and resistive magnets tend to be in the ultralow- or low-field-strength group (less than 0.5 tesla) and have tighter, or more compressed, gauss plots than superconductive magnets. In most cases, the force field of permanent and resistive magnets is nearly contained within the confines of the equipment itself. In contrast, the force field of a superconductive magnet that is not actively shielded usually is much larger, often extending beyond the limits of the exam room. Actively shielded superconductive magnets typically contain their 5-gauss field within the exam room. Due to the larger force field, superconductive magnets that are not actively shielded are more challenging to site and require more space than do the other magnet types.

Magnetic shielding, which limits the magnet's fringe field, can either be integrated into the walls of the exam room or be designed as part of the magnet itself. Another alternative is to provide distance between the magnet and other objects in lieu of shielding. A magnet that provides integral magnetic shielding is said to be self-shielded, either actively or passively. In either case, magnetic shielding can cost hundreds of thousands of dollars. A magnet that provides integral shielding adds this cost to the equipment budget; one that is passively shielded adds the cost to the construction budget.

There are four ways that an MR exam room can be magnetically shielded:

1. Passive room shielding made of steel
2. Passive clamp-on ferrous shielding (which is integrated into the magnet's construction)
3. Active electronic magnet shielding
4. Shielding made unnecessary by using distance

Passive room shielding takes on a variety of shapes. When new magnets are shielded, the steel may only need to be installed at the top or along one side of the room. However, older, reconditioned high-field magnets usually need full-room magnetic shielding or a six-sided steel box enclosure. Full-room shields can weigh more than 100 tons. They tend to extend 2 to 4 feet below the finish floor level of the room and up to 12 feet above the floor level. The maximum thickness of the steel box is located normal to the axis of the magnet's bore. From there, it tapers to a thinner construction. When magnetic shielding is placed below the floor level of the exam room, the structural system of the room may need to be modified separately from the rest of the building's structural system.

Passive clamp-on ferrous shielding is made possible by special shielding that is available from the equipment vendor. Unlike the ferrous box integrated into the procedure room walls, clamp-on shielding attaches to the magnet directly. Clamp-on shielding must be precisely constructed so that no electronic shimming problems or gauss distortions are created within the magnetic field. This type of shielding is also heavy, often adding 30 tons to the weight of the magnet. Clamp-on shielding originally was more popular when few alternatives existed. Today, it is used less frequently than either passive room shielding or active shielding.

Active types of shielding available with superconductive magnets incorporate two magnets in one! The imaging magnet is wound around the core in one direction. Then, another magnet is wound around the core in the opposite direction in order to compensate for and cancel out the fringe field of the first. This active shielding can reduce the distance of the 5-gauss line considerably, as compared to a nonshielded magnet. It compresses the magnetic field better than the passive system does, and it does not add as much weight to the installation. Actively shielded magnets were first introduced to the market in the late 1980s and early 1990s. They are available for 0.5-, 1.0-, and 1.5-tesla magnets and are often considered the system of choice when new MRI units are being planned and installed. For some site conditions, an actively shielded magnet and partial passive room shielding might be employed.

As mentioned earlier, an unshielded magnet sometimes is used in research (or clinical) applications where the best possible image is required. Distance is used in place of steel to control the magnetic force field. Special caution (as determined by the magnet vendor) must be used to prevent people and certain objects from entering critical force fields.

In the early days of MRI, distance was thought to be the only way to shield a system. As a result, many of the early units were located in parking lots or remote locations within the facility. This approach led to countless operational inefficiencies and substantial challenges to architectural planners.

Regardless of how the magnet is shielded, both static and moving ferromagnetic objects can influence the homogeneity of the magnetic field. *Shimming,* a process in which the vendor compensates for magnetic inhomogeneity by inserting pieces of iron around the magnet enclosure, can compensate for some imperfections in the magnet and static ferrous objects, such as steel beams. Shimming also can be done electronically, eliminating the need to actually place steel around the magnet. Active shimming does not compensate effectively for moving objects such as elevators, automobiles, and movable medical equipment. These must be kept a distance away unless additional magnetic shielding is installed. Shimming, or for that matter any external magnetic shielding, tends to somewhat compromise the clarity of the MR image.

Certain conditions relating to the facility's construction and its effect on the magnet's performance must be considered. However, as MRI technology improves, siting requirements also change. For each installation, current siting requirements should be verified with manufacturers.

For many magnets no ferrous material can be installed in close proximity to their isocenter, and yet normal construction methods and practices can be followed outside the shielded space. Vendors may specify the maximum amount of iron reinforcement that can be placed in the floor directly beneath or above the MRI unit. Fiberglass structural reinforcement is available as an alternative. If ferrous reinforcement is used in the floor, it should be distributed equally throughout the floor area. Exceeding vendor-specified limits can result in unshimmable conditions.

Often, a detailed analysis identifying the limitations imposed by the magnet's field is performed at the beginning of the design process. This analysis is important for proper magnet placement. It can be performed by either the magnet vendor or a special consultant. However, the service can be expensive. Additionally, the results of the analysis can affect the scope of the equipment purchase. For example, the analysis may result in the desire to compare the cost of an actively shielded magnet with that of a passively shielded installation. If either the magnet or other critical objects in its vicinity are relocated during the design or construction phase, the analysis may need to be repeated.

For systems that require only the installation of an RF shield, the construction of the parent room can be quite simple. However, within the room enclosure some caution should be taken in selecting construction materials. As a general rule, it is best to avoid the use of ferrous materials; however, some items must be made of nonferrous materials. These items include lay-in ceiling grids and hangers, ceiling-mounted lighting fixtures, sprinkler lines and hangers, all cover plates and associated mounting screws, and HVAC ducts and hangers. Aluminum support grids should be used in place of standard metal supports for lay-in ceiling systems. However, items such as steel wall-furring channels and plasterboard screws are generally acceptable. Many ferrous fasteners, which once were eliminated from the MR environment, are now commonly used:

> When MRI was first introduced, it was thought that any ferrous substance would negatively affect image quality. Very expensive construction techniques using nonferrous materials were standard procedure. Wood beams, glued connectors, stainless steel nails, fiberglass, copper and aluminum were considered appropriate construction materials. Now, however, manufacturers generally agree that shimming of the magnet is able to compensate for [many] static ferrous building materials. The use of conventional construction techniques and materials [outside of the shielded room] greatly reduces the expense of constructing an MRI facility.[17]

Electromagnetic fields from power lines, motors, and transformers also can influence magnetic homogeneity. Electromagnetic sources may include nearby medical equipment, including other MR units. Minimum distances must be observed.

Space Required for RF and Magnetic Shielding

When determining space requirements for imaging rooms, area dimensions usually are given in terms of usable net area or the actual space available inside the room excluding wall, floor, and ceiling finishes. For MRI enclosures that require RF and/or magnetic shielding, the exam room is actually a room within a room.

The MR/RF enclosure is constructed within what sometimes is referred to as a *parent room.* The parent room is the space constructed by the general contractor; the enclosure is fabricated (based on the dimensions of the parent room) and installed by the shielding contractor within the parent room. Depending on the type of enclosure used, the inside dimensions of the parent room may be as much as 4 to 10 inches greater in each direction than the inside dimensions of the shielding enclosure. This difference must be accounted for when the space is being planned. If not, the usable area inside the exam room may be smaller than desired. (See figure 15-6.)

Safety

Stories of metal objects transformed into dangerous projectiles probably are more common than the occurrences themselves. Nonetheless, the MRI environment can be a hazardous area when certain safety precautions are ignored or misunderstood. Because magnetic fields are invisible until their effects are made noticeable, these powerful forces of physics often are forgotten.

The minimum distances by which certain objects should be removed from the magnet are available from equipment vendors. However, responsibility for enforcing these requirements is with the owner.

Persons with implants consisting of ferromagnetic material (for example, surgical clips, artificial valves, and some prosthetic devices) should not be allowed near the magnet. Thus, these patients should not be examined by MR. Sometimes, a metal detector is installed near the exclusion zone to prevent unauthorized individuals from entering this area. In most cases, however, proper training, supervision, and signage are just as effective. At a minimum, a clearly visible sign stating "Warning! Strong magnetic field!" should be posted along the 5-gauss line.[18]

Instruments containing ferrous materials (for example, some scissors, gas bottles, housekeeping appliances, and gurneys) also must be kept away from the magnet's field. In addition, magnetic computer disks and credit cards should not enter the magnet's field because information stored on these items can be erased or damaged.

If a patient develops a medical crisis while in the exam room, he or she will need to be stabilized and may need to be removed from the vicinity of the magnetic field. Although many emergency treatment instruments are not permitted in the area, some emergency instruments such as crash carts, pulse oximeters, and vital sign monitors are available in special nonferrous materials for use in the MRI suite. Additionally, aluminum or brass medical gas outlets can be installed to make these gases available in the procedure room. Instruments that are not specially made for this environment should not be allowed near an operational magnet.

In the event that a superconductive magnet must be immediately shut down to allow access to a critical patient, a substantial amount of helium may boil off. As mentioned earlier, this situation is known as a quench. It is a serious problem and may destroy the magnet.

Although helium is nonflammable and nonpoisonous, it is potentially harmful to health because it can dilute the oxygen content of the surrounding air. Ventilation requirements are specified by both the manufacturer and regulatory agencies. Usually, a minimum number of air changes per hour with outside air is specified. In addition, the magnet should be connected to an automatic ventilation system to prevent evaporation of helium into the procedure room. The magnet should never be energized without proper installation of quench venting and exhaust systems.

In many locations, code requires that an oxygen-monitoring system be installed to verify the oxygen content of the air. This is recommended even where it is not required by code.

Figure 15-6. MRI Room within a Room

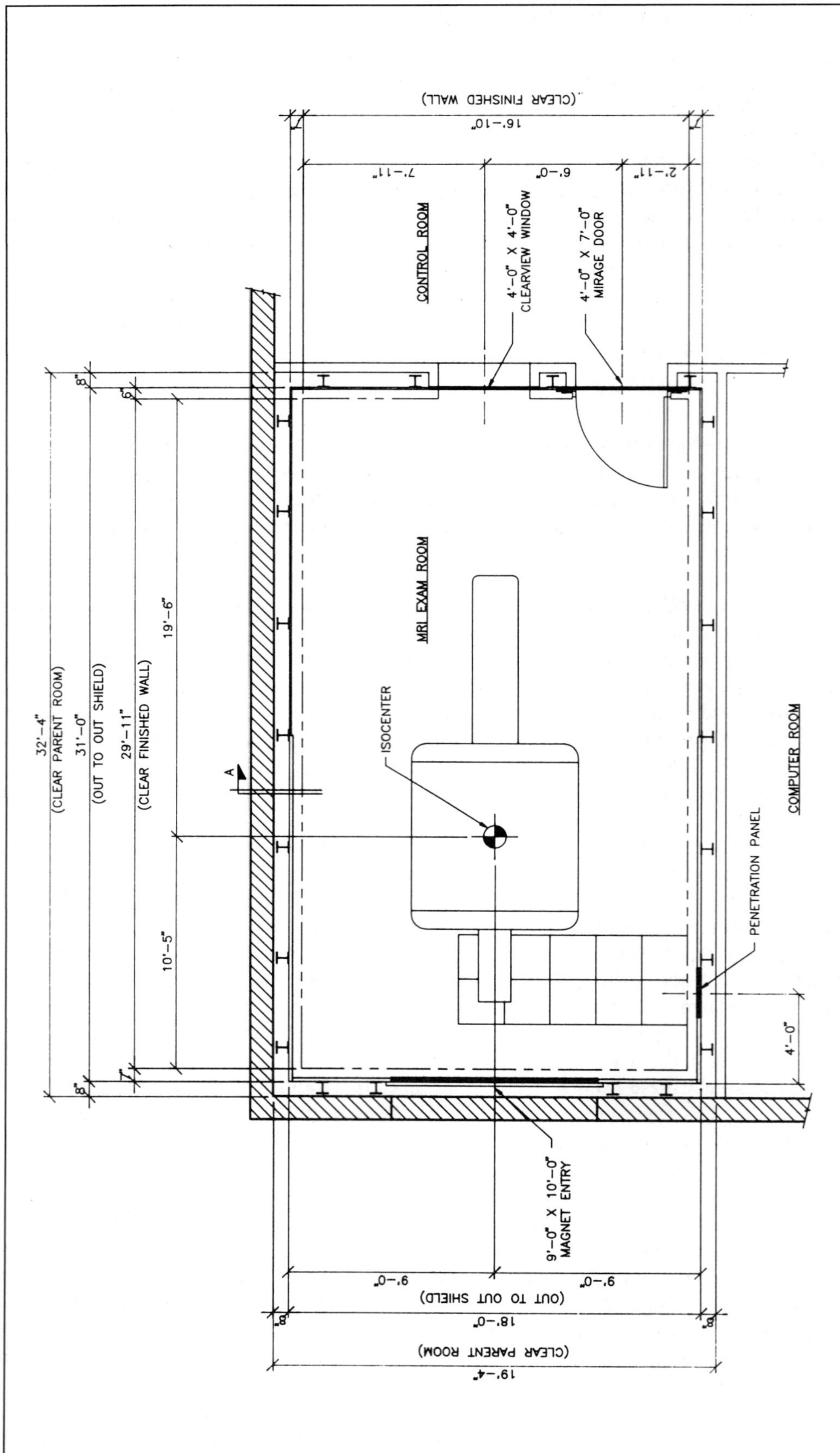

Where possible, the oxygen monitor should be directly connected to the exam room ventilation system in such a way that it automatically turns on the ventilation when the oxygen level becomes questionable.

Prior to bringing a liquid-helium container into the exam room, it should be verified that the container is not made of ferrous material. Special nonferrous containers, which usually are available from suppliers of liquid gas, are labeled as such on the exterior of the container.

Special care must be taken when handling liquid helium and nitrogen. They are extremely cold and can cause severe burns when they come in direct contact with the skin.

Cryogenics

A superconductive magnet consists of an electromagnet with windings composed of a special alloy. The alloy, immersed in liquid helium, is kept cold to eliminate its electrical resistance.[19] Sometimes, liquid nitrogen is used as an intermediate cooling medium to insulate the liquid helium from the surrounding environment. (Using helium alone is the more common practice today.) In other magnets, special shield coolers are used in place of liquid nitrogen. However, shield coolers are very noisy and may elevate patient anxiety levels. Liquid nitrogen is extracted from the atmosphere and generally is less expensive than liquid helium, which is extracted from natural gas deposits. However, liquid helium will maintain a lower temperature than will liquid nitrogen. The magnet must remain at an extremely cold (cryogenic) temperature in order to efficiently produce the high magnetic field required.

The liquid is kept in a vacuum container to isolate it from other parts of the instrument. Once the superconductive magnet is cooled to its cryogenic temperature, it no longer requires an external power supply. Once it is charged, the electric current continues to flow because the magnet's resistance is zero. However, because the ambient temperature surrounding the magnet is some 540°F higher than the liquid helium in the vacuum, the helium evaporates slowly. For this reason, the helium container needs to be replenished occasionally. Older superconductive magnets may need to be filled several times a month; newer instruments may require filling only three or four times a year. This depends on the particular instrument and the type and frequency of its workload.[20]

Although the superconductive alloy coil has no electrical resistance at its operating temperature of below −452°F, a very slight temperature increase above this mark creates electrical resistance, which in turn produces a considerable amount of heat. Increased temperature does not in itself damage the magnet's coils, but because liquid helium boils at −452°F, any increase in temperature will trigger the rapid boiling of the cryogenic helium. In rare circumstances, an excessive amount of cryogen may be caused to boil off, resulting in a quench.[21]

Special venting in the form of a quench pipe must be installed per the manufacturer's specifications to keep helium from discharging into the procedure room. If a quench occurred, it would place very high stress on the ventilation system. Cryogenic vents should have the least number of bends or turns possible. Bends and turns may create back pressure within the ventilation system. In addition, the vent should be supported structurally to withstand increased gas pressure and velocity during a quench. The vent pipe must extend to the building's exterior, and its discharge point should be away from areas accessible to people. In addition, a warning sign should be posted near the point of discharge cautioning people such as maintenance workers not to approach. The warning should be posted at the edge of nearby accessible roofs if the discharge point is below and hidden from view.

Room configuration and ceiling height should provide for easy cryogen replenishment. Often, the exam room has a higher ceiling in the center than along the edges. A place to temporarily store the cryogenic dewar may be appropriate for some magnets. Additionally, ample space around the magnet should be provided because the dewar must be placed directly in front of or alongside the instrument during filling and topping off. A typical dewar may be 3 to 4 feet in diameter and weigh up to 1,000 pounds when full. The width and height of the door leading to the exam room also should be sized to allow passage of the dewar.

Some superconductive magnets utilize water-cooled compressors as part of the refrigeration system. Such installations may utilize either a closed-loop or an open-loop cooling system.

For open-loop systems, special water conditioning may be necessary to ensure a proper pH level. For closed-loop systems, demineralized water should not be used.

Acoustics

The MRI examination is an inherently noisy procedure. In particular, sounds originating from the gradient coils, which are activated during imaging, create a loud banging sound. This adds to the fear and anxiety that most patients already have about their encounter with this mysterious machinery. A significant number of MRI patients either fail to show up for their appointments or are unwilling to return for follow-up exams because of their fear of the noise and claustrophobia induced by the equipment.

Equipment manufacturers have not been entirely successful in reducing the noise generated by gradient coils. Architects and interior designers can mitigate the noise impact within the procedure room somewhat, although the greatest acoustic problems occur within the magnet's bore. Acoustic damping of the walls, floor, and ceiling of the procedure room softens the environment and provides an extra measure of comfort. Proper acoustic detailing reduces the transmission of both airborne noises and those traveling through walls and partitions. For example, consideration might be given to placing fabric-wrapped acoustic panels on the walls and acoustic panels with a high noise reduction coefficient (NRC) on the ceiling. Carpeting acts to control noise levels, but some manufacturers discourage the use of carpeting at the patient couch location or in the path along which dewars will be transported because it impedes their movement. The finish surface of the procedure room floor should not be higher than adjacent floor surfaces or create high thresholds in doorways for reasons of disability access and movement of heavy equipment from room to room. In addition, such floor height differences may make it difficult to create an integral RF enclosure.

A variety of audio and video systems are available to mask noise and distract patients from thinking about the machinery or the medical procedure. Some systems include specially designed headphones and goggles that can be used near the magnet. Others consist of special television monitors on which patients can watch local television stations or their favorite videos. Still others include a mirror either in the form of glasses or mounted on a bracket placed near the patient's chest or feet. The patient then looks down the bore of the magnet to see a pleasant view of either a fixed or video image reflected in the mirror:

> Some centers have purchased special mirrored glasses. . . . Patients who wear the glasses do not face the bore of the magnet; instead, their eyes see the area in the back or front. At many facilities, patients can look at mind-soothing murals that have been placed at the end of the scanner. In other centers, the scanner is positioned so patients see the scanning room's door opening.
>
> [The glasses are] a method used to distract the patient and eliminate the closed-in feeling and make them much more relaxed. [They are particularly well suited for spine patients.] The glasses give the patients the option to look out of the magnet; otherwise, they would just be looking inside at the bore.
>
> Many times a family member will stand in the patient's line of vision for added comfort. When the patient is being scanned, therefore, he or she can look back through the glasses and see a loved one.[22]

Most magnet manufacturers are attempting to design less-noisy machinery. However, sometimes artwork, views to the outside, or other visually interesting objects can effectively compensate for the acoustic disturbances inherent to most magnets by transferring the patient's awareness away from the noise. Many magnets (especially those with ultralow or low field strength) are being designed to have an open bore. Such designs reduce the feeling of claustrophobia for many patients.

Lighting

Proper lighting in the MR exam room is important for both functional and aesthetic reasons. Two lighting levels should be provided. A lower level, for patient examination, is necessary in the area around the magnet's bore and the patient couch. Direct lighting should be avoided in these areas to maximize patient comfort. However, fluorescent lamps and certain types of electronic dimmers cannot be used because they create RF disruption and degrade the MR image quality. At the same time, standard incandescent lamps should be avoided because the magnetic field will quickly destroy their filament. Incandescent lamps with a special reinforced tungsten filament usually are recommended. The reinforced filament extends their life considerably. Direct-current lighting will serve better in the MR environment than will alternating current lighting. Most MR manufacturers specify the use of direct-current lighting.

A lighting level higher than that of the patient areas should be provided around the magnet's perimeter. This is necessary for servicing and routine maintenance and is typically provided by fluorescent lamps in nonferrous fixtures. Its controls should be separate from those used during the patient exam.

The control room adjacent to the exam room also should have two lighting levels that are of equal value to the levels in the exam room. Balancing the level of lighting in the two rooms will minimize glare along the control room window. For the same reason, direct daylight or artificial light should be controlled to minimize glare on the operator's console.

The technical equipment room can have a single lighting level. Preferably, its level should be equal to the service light level in the control and exam rooms.

References

1. National Council on Radiation Protection and Measurement. *NCRP Report No. 49: Structural Shielding Design and Evaluation for Medical Use of X-Rays and Gamma Rays of Energies of up to 10 MeV.* Bethesda, MD: NCRP, 1976, pp. 1–3.
2. NCRP.
3. National Council on Radiation Protection and Measurement. *NCRP Report No. 91: Recommendations for Occupational Exposure Limitation.* Bethesda, MD: NCRP [no date available].
4. NCRP 49.
5. NCRP 49.
6. NCRP 49, appendix E.
7. Archer, B. R. Radiation Design Criteria for Diagnostic X-Ray Facilities: Part 1. A paper presented at the Radiological Society of North America, Chicago, 1991, p. 2.
8. NCRP 49, appendix C.
9. NCRP 49, p. 46.
10. Archer.
11. Bushong, S. C. *Radiologic Science for Technologists.* 3rd ed. St. Louis: Mosby-Year Book, 1984, pp. 514–15.
12. Bushong, p. 515.
13. NCRP 49, pp. 14–15.
14. NCRP 49, p. 13.
15. Bushong, p. 406.
16. Lindgren RF Enclosures, Inc. *MRI Shielded Architectural Site Planning Guide.* Glendale Heights, IL: Lindgren RF Enclosures, 1989.
17. Malkin, J. *The Design of Medical and Dental Facilities.* New York City: Van Nostrand Reinhold, 1980, p. 235.

18. Phillips Medical Systems. *Gyroscan T5 Site Planning Guide.* Shelton, CT: Phillips North America, 1989.
19. Phillips Medical Systems.
20. Phillips Medical Systems.
21. Phillips Medical Systems.
22. Hatfield, S. Glasses look good to MRI professionals. *Advance for Radiologic Technologists,* Oct. 8, 1990, p. 26.

Chapter 16

Utility Requirements

Utility systems—electrical, air-conditioning, and plumbing assemblies—allow for the proper functioning of both building components and medical equipment. Close coordination among all design disciplines (architectural and engineering) is necessary for these systems because each is competing for a place in the limited space above the ceiling of procedure rooms. Therefore, a highly organized system that identifies zones for each utility type is recommended.

Because utility systems must be properly sized to meet current as well as future needs, reserve capacity in all systems is also recommended. Furthermore, the architectural and engineering team can no longer effectively size mechanical, electrical, and telecommunications spaces using traditional rules of thumb because the space requirements for these systems are constantly changing. Mechanical rooms, distribution panels and closets, pipes, raceways, and conduit should be carefully thought out and organized systematically to logically accommodate expansion and increased utility capacities, as needed. Systems for future expansion must integrate both the architectural and engineering components of the building. This can be accomplished through the use of raised computer floor systems, universal room design, or even an integrated building systems (IBS) approach, as appropriate. (See the section entitled Universal Room Design in chapter 13, "Room Design," and the section entitled Flexibility in chapter 8, "Design Concepts.")

This chapter identifies some utility requirements that are unique to medical imaging facilities. These descriptions are not intended to be exhaustive, nor are they assumed to apply to every type of imaging procedure. Similarly, references to codes and standards are not assumed to be comprehensive. Thus, the descriptions that follow should be supplemented with specific utility requirements provided by equipment manufacturers and evaluated by engineers specializing in each discipline discussed in this chapter. These disciplines include lighting; power; heating, ventilation, and air-conditioning (HVAC); and plumbing.

Lighting

Lighting designers should be familiar with both the principles of lighting and the additional requirements necessitated by the unique nature of imaging procedures. Considerable literature on lighting design has been published by the American National Standards Institute (ANSI), the Institute of Electrical and Electronic Engineers (IEEE), the Illuminating Engineering Society (IES) of North America, and other sources. In particular, the following documents should be reviewed:

- *IEEE Recommended Practice for Electric Power Systems in Commercial Buildings,* ANSI/IEEE Standard 241—1990, Chapter 10

- *IES Lighting Handbook,* Reference and Application Volumes, 1993
- *IES Lighting for Health Care Facilities,* 1985
- *IEEE Standard 602—1986, Electrical Systems in Health Care Facilities*

Lighting design influences the way people behave emotionally and physically. Inadequate lighting levels impair their ability to maneuver through space and to perform simple tasks, whereas too much light can create a harsh, impersonal environment. Light that is improperly balanced distorts the qualities of reflected light, which is perceived as color. Lighting systems that are not designed in concert with heating, ventilating, and cooling systems or daily patterns of building use will not utilize energy efficiently.

Special Considerations for Imaging Facilities

Two important considerations regarding lighting design in imaging facilities are: (1) that patients may be lying supine and staring at the ceiling more frequently than they are sitting or standing and (2) that many aspects of imaging involve looking at video monitors, cathode-ray tube (CRT) displays, or film illuminators. As a result, direct downlighting may be uncomfortable for patients looking upward, and direct lighting in general may cause disruptive glare for personnel looking at monitors and computer display terminals (CDTs). Illuminance balance also is critical for comfortable viewing of images on film illuminators and computer workstations. Consideration should also be given to balancing the contrast ratio, which is the ratio between the dimmest and the brightest objects in the field of view. A high level of contrast between the monitor image and the surroundings causes eye strain. Therefore, lighting design that would adequately and comfortably illuminate other types of spaces might be inappropriate for imaging facilities.

Ideally, imaging procedure rooms should be provided with four different lighting conditions. These special lighting design requirements are the following:

1. Low-level indirect ambient lighting should be on when the patient enters the room. Fixtures should be located in such a way that they do not shine into a supine patient's eyes. The lighting level should provide a pleasant transition between the brightly illuminated waiting room or corridor that the patient will come from and the darker space that the procedure room will become during the procedure. For this reason, it may be advantageous for adjacent corridors to be less brightly illuminated than other public corridors.
2. The room's ambient lighting will be dimmed further when the imaging examination begins. Task lighting may be needed for procedures such as biopsies and catheterizations that are performed within the examination room. In fluoroscopy rooms, or any room in which a video or CRT monitor is used, the ambient lighting should remain low and free of glare to make the monitors easy to view. (Note: The use of image intensifiers allows fluoroscopy rooms to be more brightly illuminated than in the past.) If a control room is adjacent to the procedure room, the lighting level in the two rooms should be similar so as to reduce glare on either side of the control window.
3. High-level luminance should be provided for cleanup and setup of the room.
4. Emergency lighting is to be provided for safe egress in the event of an emergency. Additionally, emergency lighting will help staff in their efforts to stabilize a patient in the event of an emergency. (Emergency power is discussed in a later section of this chapter.)

Often, variable lighting in the procedure room is achieved by using indirect wall-washing fluorescent lamps when the patient is waiting in the room and a series of dimmable overhead downlights (either incandescent or low-voltage halogen) that can be dimmed during procedures or brightened during cleanup. Separate lighting may be preset for a variety of lighting scenes, depending on the procedure. Often, the radiologist will want to have a foot control switch located near the patient table. Many fluorescent lamp types are difficult to dim without resulting in annoying flickering. However, this problem is becoming less common over a wide dimming range due to recent improvements in lighting design.

The movement of overhead imaging equipment is another consideration for lighting design in the procedure room. Ceiling lights can be staggered to prevent all the fixtures from being blocked at any one time, regardless of where the overhead imaging equipment is positioned.

Wherever groups of film illuminators are used, lighting should be uniform in both color and intensity. Film-viewing areas are typically dark, and therefore special care should be taken to ensure luminance balance within such areas.

Corridors that are illuminated by equally spaced ceiling-mounted fixtures (typically 2 feet × 2 feet, 2 feet × 4 feet, or 1 foot × 4 feet) can cause unpleasant glare and extremes of brightness and darkness for gurney patients transported beneath their staccato placement. Indirect lighting systems should be considered, where practical.

(Specific considerations for lighting in darkrooms are discussed in the section entitled General Considerations for Image-Processing Areas in chapter 13, "Room Design." Considerations for lighting at computer workstations are discussed in a section entitled General Considerations for Computer Workstation Environments, also in chapter 13. Considerations for lighting in MRI suites are discussed in the section entitled Special Considerations for MRI Installations in chapter 15, "Physical Properties Influencing Design.")

General Considerations for Lighting Design

Certain general conditions must be considered as part of the lighting design for an imaging facility. These include illumination and luminance balance, reflection and glare, the introduction of daylight, lighting consistency, and energy efficiency.

Illumination and Luminance Balance

Illumination is the projection, either direct or indirect, of light on a surface or object for the purpose of seeing the surface or object, performing a task, or safely moving through an area. Different types of lighting usually are present in any given space. Following are definitions of three different types of lighting used in most spaces and of the unit of measurement used to determine lighting levels:

> *Task lighting* is the provision of adequate and suitable light for every activity or task that depends on good vision. General or background lighting provides a comfortable level of light for finding one's way around a space, locating objects, and seeing people and objects. This general or background lighting, often called *ambient* light, should be strong enough to avoid excessive brightness contrast between it and task lighting. Special lighting focuses attention on specific objects or areas and generates variety and contrast to make a space lively and interesting, even to add aesthetic impact. This is often called *accent* lighting [pp. 218–19].
>
> Lighting measurements are based on a unit called a candle power, the amount of light given by a standard candle of controlled size and composition. The level of light delivered to a surface one foot away from such a standard candle is designated as one footcandle [pp. 219–21].[1]

A guide to lighting levels for certain areas and activities is provided in table 16-1. However, it does not take into account that many of the reading, writing, and other activities in an imaging facility take place in a slightly darker-than-normal environment in which lighting levels frequently are adjusted in order to view images on film illuminators or computer workstations. In addition, it does not take into consideration that people of different ages and eyesight need different lighting levels to perform similar tasks.

Luminance balance occurs when the lighting level or luminance of the area in which a task is being performed is relatively close to luminance levels found within the peripheral field. *Luminance imbalance* occurs when bright task lighting exists within a dark environment. Extreme

Table 16-1. Suggested Lighting Levels for Selected Activities

Task or Area	Foot-Candle Level
Movie theater (during a movie)	1
Passages and storage areas	5
Stairways	10
Intermittent reading or writing	20
Reading fine type (such as a newspaper)	25
Typing, bookkeeping, switchboard operation	30
Prolonged reading, study, business machine operation, close work	50
Drafting	50–100
Surgery	2,000

Source: Pile, J. F. *Interior Design*. New York City: Harry N. Abrams, 1988, pp. 220–21.

luminance imbalance or "extreme luminance differences between sequentially and frequently fixated areas, or even only occasionally fixated areas may produce noticeable performance decrements and discomfort."[2] Therefore, high-luminance sources in the peripheral field of view should be avoided in dark areas such as reading rooms, control rooms, and even darkened procedure rooms. High-luminance sources include luminaires (light fixtures with lamps), windows, and reflective surfaces that bounce light from its source. Table 16-2 illustrates illuminance selection and lighting design considerations for selected imaging rooms.

Reflection and Glare

The reflectance of room surfaces affects both visual comfort and the efficiency in which light (and thus energy) is utilized. Unfortunately, reflectance can affect visual comfort and efficiency inversely. For example, highly reflective surfaces on walls, floors, and ceilings sometimes are specified as a means of increasing the amount of useful light emitted from each light source. In doing so, however, excessive brightness—or glare—may result, and the amount and intensity of reflections can be uncomfortably increased. Visual comfort will suffer if brightness levels exceed established limits or ratios, particularly in areas where visual tasks are demanding.[3]

Reflection can be extreme in areas with large expanses of glass (such as control rooms) and in areas where VDTs or CRT monitors are used (for example, in procedure rooms, control areas, reading rooms, offices, and almost any area within an imaging facility). In addition to highly reflective room surfaces, reflections can be extended by reflective furniture and even reflective equipment surfaces. Workstations located near windows also are subject to excessive reflection unless adequate sun control is incorporated. Careful placement of light sources is necessary to avoid disruptive reflectance.

Veiling reflection is a specific type of reflection that occurs when light is bounced off a glossy work surface such as a desktop or magazine page and causes reduced contrast between the background and the subject or material being viewed. Usually, veiling glare is the result of improper geometry between the light source location and the viewer and is most extreme when the work surface becomes a "mirror" bouncing light into the viewer's eyes. For this reason, light sources are better located behind and off to the side of the viewer, rather than directly in front. For the same reason, if ceiling-mounted luminaires are installed in rows, workstations should be oriented perpendicular to the rows, rather than parallel, so that light is bounced from side to side of the viewer and not from front to back. (See figure 13-13, p. 250.) Veiling reflections are reduced when the ceiling is lighted more uniformly.[4] Sometimes, the use of special prismatic lenses will help if the geometrical relationship between the light source and the viewer cannot be modified.[5]

Daylight

The introduction of daylight—through windows or skylights—into waiting areas, corridors, work areas, and sometimes even procedure rooms can have a beneficial effect on patients,

Table 16-2. Illuminance Selection and Lighting Design Considerations

Activity	Target Illuminance Range			Design Considerations						
	LOW	MEDIUM	HIGH	Speed/Accuracy	Room Surface Reflectance	Task Background Reflectance	Visual Comfort	Control Dimming/Switching Multiple Levels	High Color Rendering Index	Remarks
Radiology Waiting Area	2	3	5							
Radiographic/Fluoroscopic Room	2	3	5	■		■		■	■	
Film Sorting	100	150	200	■		■	■		■	
Barium Kitchen	50	75	100	■		■	■			
CT Scanning Room	5	7.5	10	■		■	■	■	■	
Equipment Maintenance Room	50	75	100	■		■	■			

Adapted from ANSI/IEEE Standard 602—1986, Chapter 7, Table 15, p. 254.

visitors, and staff. However, daylight can be more difficult to control than artificial light because of its variety and intensity. Glare, reflection, and shadows can disturb the vision needed for demanding tasks if these aspects of daylight are not adequately regulated. Lighting conditions in procedure rooms that require some degree of darkening during the procedure so that monitors can be easily seen (such as fluoroscopy rooms) can be particularly difficult to control if daylight is abundant. Windows also may call for specially designed solutions to radiation protection, depending on the room's location, adjacent occupancies, and the characteristics of radiation emission in the room.

Consistency

The various sequences of work flow that take place within an imaging facility are discussed in chapter 10, "Work Flow and Circulation." Both patients and staff travel through numerous spaces during the course of a single imaging procedure, and yet each room has very specific and different lighting requirements. Despite these differences, a certain degree of lighting consistency is necessary for people who frequently move between various spaces in the facility.

First, the luminance level between adjacent spaces should be similar, if possible. This is one reason that procedure rooms are brighter when the patient enters than they are prior to the procedure, after the brightness has been gradually reduced.

Second, the color rendition of lighting throughout the facility, or at least throughout the patient areas, should be as consistent as possible. Inconsistent lighting should not cause a patient to appear "healthy" in one room and not in another. Likewise, inconsistent lighting should not cause a patient to appear stable in two different rooms when, actually, his or her condition is changing but goes unnoticed because of lighting variations. Different types of lighting fixtures (fluorescent, incandescent, high-intensity discharge, and so on) have different characteristics and lighting qualities, and each can be fitted with a variety of lamps, which in turn have unique color characteristics. The more often different types of fixtures and lamps are used, the more difficult it will be to maintain lighting consistency. Consistency will also simplify the procurement and storage of replacement bulbs and lamps.

Energy Efficiency

Most states and federal agencies have strict requirements regulating the amount of energy that a building can consume. These regulations usually are based on the building's size and occupancy.

Lighting systems are responsible for a significant portion of overall energy consumption and heat gain. Unfortunately, sometimes the requirements of energy efficiency and optimal lighting conditions oppose each other. Therefore, the approach to lighting design must be comprehensive and consider both individual room requirements and facilitywide issues.

Power

Special considerations must be taken into account when designing the systems that will supply electrical power to the imaging facility. These include the quality of the power supply, the provision of emergency power, the provision of uninterruptible power supplies, and the special requirements of X-ray installations.

Power Quality

Like water quality, power quality varies significantly from location to location. Similarly, power is "cleaner" in some facilities than in others. Common causes of poor power quality include inadequate grounding, disturbances from other equipment, inadequate system capacity, and harmonics. In addition, impurities in power supply sometimes are a result of the power generation process. Clean, uninterrupted power is more critical today than it was in the past because most modern electronic equipment is more susceptible to power line fluctuations than its predecessors were. Serious damage to electronic instruments and medical equipment can result from power line disturbances.

Two main factors are responsible for today's increased need for improved power quality and better electrical grounding of medical electronics systems. First, the increased use of sophisticated electronic systems in almost every aspect of medicine—and particularly medical imaging—has caused these issues to permeate all types of medical facilities. Second, the increased complexity and sensitivity of modern electronics have magnified the impact of previously innocuous power line disturbances.

For example, the average number of transistors packed into each microchip processor grew from only a few in 1971 to more than 1,200 in 1989.[6] Unfortunately, increasingly dense digital circuitry and advanced microprocessors mean that the space separating each transistor is very small—less than one-millionth of an inch. This decreased width, along with other characteristics of contemporary semiconductor technology, makes semiconductors highly susceptible to "electrical noise."[7]

> The horror stories and propaganda to illustrate the detrimental effects of "bad power" on medical equipment are legendary—everything from losing patient data on a telemetry system to power surges causing imaging devices to deliver excess radiation to the patient.
>
> We can't blame the utility company for power disturbances; electrical disturbances have always been a byproduct of the way power is generated and distributed. And even though electrical disturbances generated within the hospital probably create more medical system problems than externally generated disturbances, we can't blame facility management for poor power. The problem is due to *modern electronics*—breakthroughs in technology have increased the susceptibility of electronic equipment to disturbances that have always been a part of the electrical environment.
>
> By correcting improper or inadequate wiring, and developing (or purchasing) a proper power interface between the utility power and sensitive electronic system, several benefits result, including better system reliability, improved uptime and improved throughput. Other advantages include better repeatability of tests, as well as economically measured benefits such as reduced time and costs for servicing equipment.[8]

Power protection solutions should meet four basic requirements. These are:[9]

1. To reduce electrical noise levels to published standards
2. To provide a clean, single-point ground
3. To provide a low-impedance source of power
4. To meet low-leakage current specifications to maximize patient safety (*Leakage current* includes any current that may be conveyed to a patient via exposed metal components of the equipment or the surrounding environment.)

Based on the above requirements, a number of power protection alternatives may be considered. These include:[10]

- Dedicated power lines
- Surge suppressors
- Isolation transformers
- Ferroresonant transformers
- Low-impedance power conditioners
- Uninterruptible power supplies
- Input and output filters

However, it should be noted that each of these alternatives has different cost implications as well as different degrees of effectiveness. The appropriateness of any of these approaches to specific situations should be discussed with a qualified electrical engineer.

Emergency Power

Emergency power should be provided for the purposes of emergency lighting and to keep critical equipment operational in the event that normal power becomes temporarily unavailable. Components of emergency power systems include generator sets, automatic transfer switches, engine generator controls, engine cranking batteries, and battery chargers.[11] Fuel storage for emergency generators should contain enough fuel for at least 24 hours of continuous operation.

Many documents are available that refer to the design of essential electrical systems in hospitals and other health care facilities. These include:[12]

- ANSI/ASME A17.1, *Standard for the Installation of Elevators, Escalators and Moving Walks*
- ANSI/NFPA 20, *Standard for the Installation of Centrifugal Fire Pumps*
- ANSI/NFPA 70, *Standard for the Installation of National Electric Code*
- ANSI/NFPA 71, *Standard for the Installation, Maintenance and Use of Central Station Signaling Stations*
- ANSI/NFPA 72A, *Standard for the Installation, Maintenance and Use of Local Protective Signaling Systems*
- ANSI/NFPA 72B, *Standard for the Installation, Maintenance and Use of Auxiliary Protective Signaling Systems*
- ANSI/NFPA 72C, *Standard for the Installation, Maintenance and Use of Remote Protective Signaling Systems*
- ANSI/NFPA 72D, *Standard for the Installation, Maintenance and Use of Proprietary Protective Signaling Systems*
- ANSI/NFPA 72E, *Standard on Automatic Fire Detectors*
- ANSI/NFPA 75, *Standard on the Protection of Electronic Computer/Data Processing Equipment*
- ANSI/NFPA 99, *Standard for Health Care Facilities*
- ANSI/NFPA 101, *Code for Safety to Life from Fire in Buildings and Structures*
- ANSI/NFPA 110, *Standard on Emergency Power and Standby Systems*

In particular, NFPA 70 and NFPA 99 describe essential electrical systems for health care facilities. Article 517, Part K, and article 660 of the *National Electric Code* (NFPA 70) describe requirements for X-ray installations. Special requirements for portable, mobile, and transportable X-ray equipment also are discussed. Emergency power requirements are also listed in chapter 7.23 of *Guidelines for Construction and Equipment of Hospital and Medical Facilities, 1992–1993 Edition.*[13]

Chapter 8 of NFPA 99 discusses essential electrical systems for health care facilities. Following is a description of those systems:

> Essential Electrical Systems for hospitals are comprised of two separate systems capable of supplying a limited amount of lighting and power service which is considered essential for life safety and effective hospital operation during the time the normal electrical service is interrupted for any reason. These two systems are the Emergency System and the Equipment System.
>
> The Emergency System shall be limited to circuits essential to life safety and critical patient care. These are designated the Life Safety Branch and the Critical Branch.
>
> The Equipment System shall supply major electrical equipment necessary for patient care and basic hospital operation.
>
> Both systems shall be arranged for connection, within [specified] time limits . . . to an alternate source of power following a loss of the normal source.[14]

As NFPA 99 mentions, the life safety branch of the emergency system covers electrical circuits considered essential to overall hospital safety. These include:[15]

- Illumination of exitways
- Exit signs and directional signs
- Fire alarm systems
- Alarms connected to medical gas systems
- Hospital communications systems
- Task illumination and selected receptacles located at the generator set
- Elevator cab lighting, control, and signal systems

The critical branch of the emergency system covers those circuits considered essential to critical patient care. These include:[16]

- Task illumination, all receptacles, and fixed equipment in anesthetizing locations
- Isolated power systems in special environments
- Task illumination and selected receptacles in certain patient care areas
- Additional specialized patient care task illumination and receptacles, where needed
- Telephone equipment rooms and closets
- Task illumination, receptacles, and special power circuits for the following (and other) areas:
  - Angiography labs
  - Cardiac catheterization labs
  - Human physiology labs
  - Selected emergency treatment areas

In addition, hospital authorities may consider "providing and properly maintaining automatic battery-powered lighting systems to provide minimal task illumination in operating rooms, delivery rooms, and certain special procedure radiology rooms where the loss of lighting due to failure of the Essential Electrical System might cause severe or immediate danger to a patient undergoing surgery or an invasive radiographic procedure."[17]

The second of the essential electrical systems for health care facilities is the equipment system. The equipment system includes (but is not limited to):[18]

- Central suction systems serving medical and surgical functions
- Sump pumps and other equipment required to operate for the safety of major apparatus, including associated control systems and alarms
- Compressed air systems serving medical and surgical functions
- Other selected equipment shall be permitted to be served by the equipment system (for example, selected equipment in radiology or other imaging rooms)

Uninterruptible Power Supplies

As the name indicates, an uninterruptible power supply (UPS) is a continuous source of electrical power. The following paragraphs explain how UPSs operate and that they are increasingly being incorporated into electrical system design to provide backup power in vital areas of the imaging facility:

> Uninterruptible power supplies (UPS's) are highly efficient power converting devices that provide a regulated ac voltage at their output terminals regardless of the quality of the source at the input terminals.
>
> In the event of a total power loss at the UPS input, output power is generally provided by means of a bank of batteries. An inherent, additional benefit of the UPS is its [frequent] ability to filter spikes and power aberrations from the ac source between the input and output terminals. These power problems could result from natural causes, buffer line disturbances on the utility power, or they could be caused by disturbances, such as load switching, within the facility itself.

Uninterruptible power is generally not specified by code requirements for hospitals or health care facilities. However, UPS systems are increasingly being incorporated into such electrical designs. Typical applications include backup support for sensitive laboratory and diagnostic equipment, life-support equipment in intensive care units, data processing systems, and for illumination in life-support areas.[19]

Heating, Ventilation, and Air-Conditioning

Guidelines and requirements for heating, ventilation, and air-conditioning (HVAC) system design are specified in both national and local mechanical codes, as well as in life safety codes and voluntary standards. Compliance with these may be required for Joint Commission on Accreditation of Healthcare Organizations (JCAHO) certification and certain levels of reimbursement. In addition, a growing epidemic of multiple-drug-resistant tuberculosis has led to added concern and reevaluation of previous air filtration and ventilation standards. As a result, many revised requirements have been proposed by regulatory agencies governing the design and construction of HVAC systems in health care and other types of facilities.

In addition, air distribution systems must be designed to restrict the flow of smoke in the event of fire. The location of smoke dampers, exhaust fans, and smoke partitions must be coordinated with the facilitywide designation of smoke compartments for both functional and economic reasons. Finally, ample chilled water must be available for the cooling systems in various kinds of complex medical equipment. Cardiac catheterization labs and CT and MRI equipment in particular require significant cooling capacity.

Many HVAC system requirements are specified in the following:

- *The American Society of Heating, Refrigerating and Air-Conditioning Engineers (ASHRAE) Handbook,* 1992
- Model mechanical codes (which vary according to location in the country)
- *Guidelines for Construction and Equipment of Hospital and Medical Facilities, 1992–1993 Edition*

Airborne Infection Control

In many jurisdictions, select imaging procedure rooms are required or at least asked to have air-pressure levels that are negative relative to adjoining spaces for the purpose of limiting the spread of odors and airborne pathogens. Those spaces that are negatively pressurized should be exhausted directly to the outdoors. Recently, many codes have been modified to strengthen requirements that protect against the spread of airborne pathogens that have resulted from the increased incidence of multiple-drug-resistant tuberculosis. For rooms in which invasive or semiinvasive procedures are performed, it generally is desirable for relative air pressure to flow from "clean" to "less-clean" spaces. However, this contradicts the previous suggestion of negative pressurization because it assumes that the procedure room is positive relative to adjacent spaces. Where such codes appear to be in conflict, each situation should be reviewed individually.

High-efficiency particulate air (HEPA) filters also may be required in some rooms with patients who are either contagious or highly susceptible to airborne infection. Ultraviolet lamps located within HVAC system ducts also may be employed in some situations.

As an alternative, waiting areas may be allowed to have special filtration or exhaust systems. For example, some jurisdictions suggest that new or remodeled waiting rooms that are likely to serve tuberculosis patients meet the following requirements:

(a) Negative air balance (air pressure) relative to adjacent areas.
(b) Minimum of 10 air changes per hour if HVAC system is 100% outside air.

(c) Minimum of 2 air changes per hour of outside air and a minimum of 10 total air changes per hour if HVAC system is not 100% outside air.
(d) All air exhausted directly to outdoors.

For existing or new waiting rooms which have recirculating air, if item (d) is not feasible, staff shall recommend that HEPA filter(s) be located within the return duct(s), in an accessible location, and as near to the intake(s) as possible.[20]

It should be noted that waiting rooms are not listed in table 2, Ventilation Requirements for Areas Affecting Patient Care in Hospitals and Outpatient Facilities, in *Guidelines for Construction and Equipment of Hospital and Medical Facilities.*

Procedure Rooms

For purposes of heating, ventilating, and air-conditioning, X-ray procedure rooms may be classified as either surgical/critical care and catheterization rooms or diagnostic and treatment rooms.[21] Based on these classifications, the guidelines described in table 16-3 (which lists basic ventilation requirements for selected rooms in imaging facilities) may apply. (Note: Additional notes are provided in *Guidelines for Construction and Equipment of Hospital and Medical Facilities, 1992–1993 Edition.* Readers are encouraged to review the guidelines directly.)

Darkroom Ventilation

Adequate ventilation is particularly important for darkrooms and other film-processing areas. Without proper ventilation, personnel working with film-processing chemicals may be subject to illness and injury. Specifications provided by equipment manufacturers do not necessarily comply with all local building code requirements. Therefore, both manufacturer's specifications and building code requirements should be carefully reviewed.

Air filtration in film-processing areas also is important to prevent dust particles from settling on the film and either obscuring the image or possibly causing a false reading of the film. The control of dust and other airborne particles is particularly important when renovation or new construction is taking place nearby. (Ventilation and filtration guidelines for darkrooms are listed in table 16-3.)

Table 16-3. Ventilation Requirements for X-Ray Rooms and Darkrooms

Requirement	X-Ray (Surgical/Critical Care and Catheterization)	X-Ray (Diagnostic and Treatment)	Darkrooms
Air movement relationship with adjacent area	Out	—	In
Minimum hourly air changes of outdoor air	3	—	—
Minimum total hourly air changes	15	6	10
All air exhausted directly to outdoors	—	—	Yes
Air recirculated by means of room units	No	—	No
Relative humidity	45–60%	—	—
Design temperature	70–75° F	75° F	—

Note: These guidelines may not take into account recent guidelines or requirements for control of tuberculosis and they may differ from (or even conflict with) various state and local codes and requirements.

Source: The American Institute of Architects. *Guidelines for Construction and Equipment of Hospital and Medical Facilities, 1992–1993 Edition.* Table 2. Washington, DC: AIA, 1993.

Nuclear Medicine

The *Guidelines for Construction and Equipment of Hospital and Medical Facilities, 1992–1993 Edition* also describes requirements for shielding and ventilating of areas in which nuclear medicine is practiced. A sampling of those requirements follows:

> If radiopharmaceutical preparation is performed on-site, an area adequate to house a radiopharmacy shall be provided with appropriate shielding. This area should include adequate space for preparation, dose calibrators, and record keeping. Flooring and walls should be constructed of easily decontaminated materials. Vents and traps for radioactive gases should be provided if such are used. Hoods for pharmaceutical preparation shall meet applicable standards. If pre-prepared materials are used, storage and calculation areas may be considerably smaller than that for on-site preparation. Space shall provide adequately for dose calibration, quality assurance, and record keeping. The area may still require shielding from other portions of the facilities.[22]

Requirements for facilities that handle radioactive substances also are described in NFPA 801, *Facilities for Handling Radioactive Substances.*

Other Requirements

Gas-scavenging systems designed to vent waste gases should be installed in areas routinely used to administer inhalation anesthesia. Waste gases should be directly vented to the outdoors.[23]

Piping and ductwork that penetrate radiation, radio-frequency, or other types of protective barriers must not impair the effectiveness of those barriers.[24] Consultation with qualified specialists is suggested. (See chapter 15, "Physical Properties Influencing Design," for further discussion of similar issues.)

Plumbing

Many forms of medical imaging equipment require substantial amounts of cooling. This is particularly true of computed tomography, magnetic resonance imaging, cardiac catheterization, and angiography equipment. Therefore, an adequate chilled water supply must be available. In addition, because most imaging rooms and many of their associated support spaces contain hand-washing or service sinks, supply and waste lines must be conveniently located throughout the imaging facility.

Darkrooms have special plumbing requirements. Due to the corrosive chemicals used for film processing, drain lines should be made of cast iron or plastic. (Note: Plastic is not permitted in some jurisdictions.) Glass drains are sometimes used, but they are very expensive and usually unnecessary. Floor drains should be provided where overflow or spills are likely to occur. Drain slopes for processors and other lines that carry corrosive chemicals should be steeper than minimum required slopes for other types of drains. Cleanout traps should be provided at easily accessible locations.

Regulations governing disposal of hazardous chemicals and heavy metals have become increasingly strict in recent years and are likely to become more so in the near future. Often, federal regulations are compounded by even stricter local requirements. The Environmental Protection Agency and local regulations governing discharge of heavy metals should be reviewed and strictly followed. Regulations specify maximum allowable concentrations of silver that may be discharged. Mechanisms for monitoring concentrations of silver and other chemicals need to be integrated into radiology film-processing systems.

Recently, "chemicalless" processing systems have been introduced at radiology trade shows. Such systems are likely to become more popular as chemical disposal regulations become increasingly conservative.

References

1. Pile, J. F. *Interior Design.* New York City: Harry N. Abrams, 1988.
2. American National Standards Institute/The Human Factors Society. *American National Standard for Human Factors Engineering of Visual Display Terminal Workstations.* (ANSI/HFS 100–1988, Section 5.3.) New York City: ANSI/HFS, 1988.
3. Rostenberg, B. Unpublished chapter on lighting for IEEE.
4. Rostenberg.
5. Pile, p. 238.
6. Stringfellow, M. F. *Grounding and Power Conditioning of Medical Electronic Equipment.* (ASHE Technical Document Series, No. 055935.) Chicago: American Society for Hospital Engineering, Aug. 1990, pp. 1, 6.
7. Vail, J. D. Protecting digital equipment from power line disturbances—part 1. *MED Medical Electronics* 1, Dec. 1987.
8. Vail.
9. Vail, J. D. Protecting digital equipment from power line disturbances—part 2. *MED Medical Electronics* 2, Feb. 1988.
10. Vail, Protecting digital equipment from power line disturbances—part 2.
11. American National Standards Institute/Institute of Electrical and Electronic Engineers. *IEEE Recommended Practice for Electric Systems in Health Care Facilities (The White Book).* (ANSI/IEEE Standard 602–1986.) New York City: ANSI/IEEE, 1986, p. 129.
12. ANSI/IEEE Standard 602–1986.
13. The American Institute of Architects. *Guidelines for Construction and Equipment of Hospital and Medical Facilities, 1992-1993 Edition.* (Section 7.32.E4.) Washington, DC: AIA, 1993.
14. National Fire Protection Association. *Health Care Facilities 1994.* (NFPA 99, Section 8.3.) Quincy, MA: NFPA, 1985.
15. NFPA 99.
16. NFPA 99.
17. NFPA 99, Appendix A-8-3.2.3.
18. NFPA 99, Section 8.3.
19. ANSI/IEEE Standard 602–1986, p. 199.
20. Office of the State (of California) Healthwide Planning and Development, Spring 1993, follow-up notice on PIN (policy intent notice) 4-TBL 2110-A, dated Nov. 23, 1992.
21. AIA, pp. 52–54.
22. AIA, chapter 7.11.F.
23. AIA, chapter 7.31.
24. AIA, pp. 52–54.

Chapter 17

Renovation versus New Construction

One of the first steps in planning a new imaging service is to decide whether the project will involve new construction, renovation, or both. As cost-containment pressures increase, renovation of health care facilities is becoming more common than new construction. In some cases, however, one or the other option may not be feasible because of site constraints. For example, if adequate site area is unavailable, new construction would be impossible—at least without first demolishing a portion of an existing structure. (Figure 17-1 shows a magnetic imaging unit designed as a renovation to an existing structure, where there was no room for a new construction.) On the other hand, if existing facilities are fully utilized, there might be no suitable location for renovation without displacing existing services. In either case, a site and facility master plan should guide the process of deciding between renovation and new construction.

Other issues to consider when deciding on a construction strategy include:

- Comparative costs and project durations for each type of project
- Evaluation of the remaining useful life of a renovated facility versus that of new construction
- The ability of each type of project to meet functional requirements (for example, providing functional adjacencies between related services such as imaging, surgery, and emergency services)
- The degree to which either renovation or new construction adheres to previously established long- and short-range planning objectives

In addition, the impact of both new construction and renovation must be considered in terms of future growth and flexibility, operational efficiency, longevity, safety, and code compliance.

This chapter examines five key questions that must be considered when deciding whether to renovate an existing imaging facility or to build a new one. It also explores some of the special considerations involved in planning renovation projects.

Key Questions in the Decision on Construction Approach

Renovation often is viewed as a less-expensive alternative to new construction because floors, foundations, exterior walls, and so on already exist. Although renovation sometimes is the most cost-effective approach to construction, this by no means is always the case. If significant building and infrastructure components (which already exist) require extensive modification, renovation may end up requiring more work than new construction. Additionally, some factors such as existing floor-to-ceiling heights cannot be easily changed. Therefore, the resulting renovation project may be less flexible and adaptable to change than new construction because the existing construction may act as a physical constraint limiting size, configuration, and circulation patterns.

Technically demanding programs such as imaging services have rigorous physical requirements. In particular, imaging facilities place significant demands on structural, plumbing, air-handling, and power capacities. Additionally, imaging equipment requires a higher floor-to-floor height than is required by many other types of equipment. Finally, the rapid development of imaging technology demands a facility that will accommodate change easily. Most of these criteria are more difficult to satisfy with renovation than with new construction.

Figure 17-1. MRI Suite Designed as Renovation in an Existing Structure Where Site Constraints Prohibited New Construction

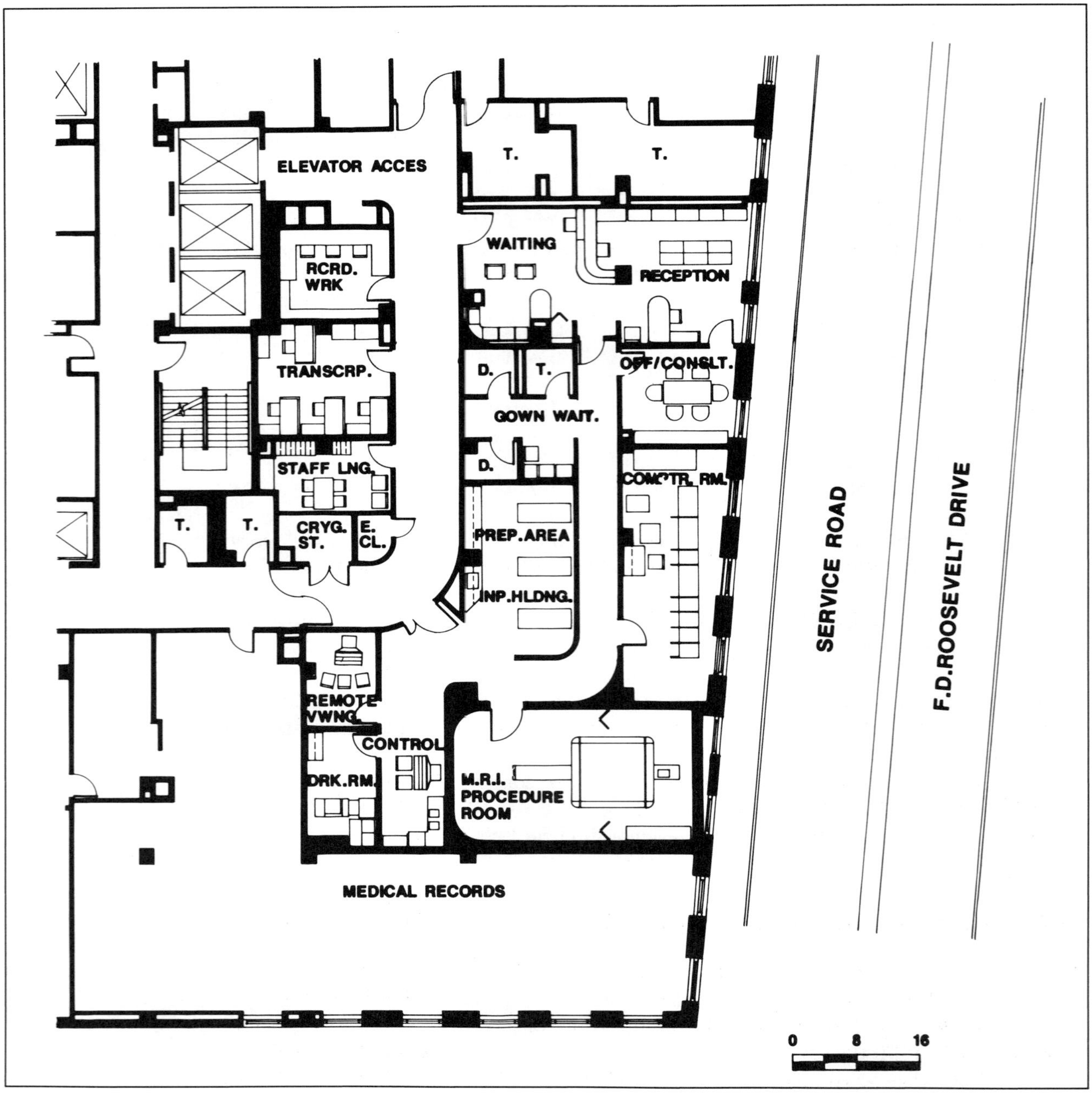

The Hospital for Special Surgery, New York City. Architects: Architecture for Health Science and Commerce, P.C., Tarrytown, New York. Reprinted with permission.

On the other hand, new construction may be inappropriate for small projects or projects consisting solely of minor modifications to existing facilities. For example, a newly built two-room radiology expansion would be expensive relative to its size because the cost of new foundations, roofing, and so on must be amortized over the small area. Furthermore, numerous small additions to an existing campus tend to compromise the effectiveness of campuswide master plans that provide a strategic direction for growth and the location of specific services over time. Finally, renovation may be preferred over new construction if it will enable new services to be made available sooner than will new construction.

Many imaging projects involve expansion or upgrading of existing services, rather than replacement. For this type of project, there may be significant value remaining in portions of the facility that require little or no work. Renovation may be the preferred alternative in such cases. However, numerous hidden costs also may emerge.

In an article in *Health Facilities Management,* Bacher lists five questions that should be asked when assessing the appropriateness of a construction approach for any given project:[1]

1. *Is the project mostly of a cosmetic nature or functional?* Projects whose scope of work involves mostly new finishes and furnishings are good candidates for renovation. On the other hand, projects involving major functional changes usually require replacement of mechanical and electrical systems, as well as relocation of partitions and smoke and fire protection assemblies and increased structural capacities. These projects may be more effective as new construction.

   With the exception of minor administrative remodeling projects or replacement of equipment in a few rooms, renovation of an imaging facility almost always involves major functional changes. "Costs to be saved in a renovation project that involves a functional upgrade are principally those related to the building's core and shell; its foundations, structure, and exterior walls remain, and are used again in the renovated facility. With this type of project, core-and-shell costs are reduced by an average of 80 percent, but savings in other areas are often minimal."[2]
2. *When was the existing facility built?* The age of the existing facility may shed light on the nature of code requirements that were in effect at the time the original facility was built. Although such limitations are likely to have been upgraded, Bacher identifies three significant dates in the regulatory history of health care facilities:

   > In 1947, the Hill–Burton Act, which began to define requirements for hospital environments for the first time, was implemented. Noteworthy among these new requirements was the call for forced ventilation.
   >
   > Health facilities that were built before 1947 provided fresh air through open windows and might have had floor-to-floor heights of just 10 feet; today, new facilities are built with [much higher floor-to-floor heights. Sixteen feet is not uncommon for conventional construction to house an imaging facility. [Most facilities] . . . are hard pressed to accommodate modern ventilation and other above-the-ceiling systems with any less. Although there are methods to mitigate this problem (such as running ventilation vertically rather than horizontally), such solutions limit flexibility or require waivers from current code provisions.
   >
   > Also in 1947, regulations began to mandate minimum room sizes for various health care functions. (These [space guidelines], updated every three years, present problems for even recently built structures!) So a space planning review is critical before committing to renovation.
   >
   > In 1967, an update to the National Electrical Code required for the first time that all power circuits had to be installed with three-prong, green-wire plugs and that emergency electrical distribution systems had to provide three separate emergency-power branches: critical, life safety and emergency. [See chapter 16, "Utility Requirements."] As a result, any health care institution built before 1967 [and not renovated since then] and undergoing renovation today may face the expensive prospect of completely replacing these systems. [For imaging facilities,

> it is almost certain that electrical systems will need to be replaced or substantially upgraded, unless significant reserve capacity has already been provided in a previous renovation project.]
>
> Managers of health facilities constructed before 1972 must look carefully at the extent to which asbestos was integrated into their facilities. At one time, asbestos was widely used in construction of all kinds, [because of] its excellent insulating and heat-resisting qualities; in health facilities, asbestos typically was used in floors, ceilings, walls, doors, laboratory benches, structural system fireproofing and mechanical system insulation.
>
> Although the presence of asbestos doesn't rule out renovation, it will increase construction costs and can delay schedules. An asbestos-abatement contractor or consultant can help . . . sort out the problem and . . . estimate the cost of abatement.[3]

3. *How will the new space be used?* The degree of technical complexity required for the new use has a considerable impact on the ease and expense with which existing construction can be renovated. For low-tech or "soft" space (offices, conference rooms, storage areas, and so on), space and utility system requirements are relatively simple. On the other hand, high-tech uses (which is the category that imaging services fall into) have precise and substantial facility needs. Existing physical constraints are likely to add expense to, and even compromise the usability of, renovation plans.
4. *Do state regulations include a standard for total upgrade?* Bacher writes that many states require institutions desiring to renovate more than a certain percent of a building (for example, 50 percent) to bring the entire institution up to current code requirements, which can have a major impact on costs.[4]
5. *What impact will renovation have on day-to-day operations?* In addition to the basic cost of construction, there are numerous secondary costs related to both new construction and renovation. Many of these costs relate to the ability to maintain operations of existing services during the construction of services.
   - Noise and dirt generated by construction disturb ongoing operations. In particular, airborne dust particles can degrade the quality of film images and excessive vibration can disrupt certain imaging techniques. The temporary disconnection of utility lines also is disruptive.
   - Temporary phasing may be required to provide an interim location for some services while their permanent space is being constructed. In essence, this means more work because some spaces are being built twice.

Special Considerations for Renovation Projects

Renovation projects involve a number of special considerations. The following subsections discuss these considerations in terms of planning, phasing, and cost.

Planning Considerations

An imaging department planned within the shell of an existing facility may be restricted by some of the physical features inherent in the present structure. For example, if the available area is smaller than desired, some spaces may become undersized. If the available area is adequate but its configuration is irregular, ideal room-to-room adjacencies may not be practical and the amount of space devoted to circulation may be excessive. If both the available area and the configuration of space are adequate but the location is remote from other related services, operational efficiencies may suffer.

A thorough analysis of the unique conditions inherent in renovation projects can help reduce the likelihood and impact of unexpected surprises. Such an analysis involves consideration of questions in a variety of categories.

Available Options for New Construction versus Renovation

- Do several options exist? If the proposed plan is to renovate existing space, is there adequate area on the site that provides an option for new construction? Similarly, if the proposed plan is for new construction, is renovation a possible alternative? If feasible alternatives exist, have comparative planning studies and cost estimates been prepared and compared for both renovation and new construction alternatives?
- Has a strategic plan been developed for the organization? Has a site and facility master plan been developed for the existing site or campus? If so, which renovation or new construction options (if any) most successfully achieve the goals set forth in both the strategic plan and the site and facility master plan?

Available Area and Configuration

- How much space is available in the proposed location, and is it of a regular configuration? If the space is oddly shaped, a greater amount of area may be needed to accommodate the desired program. For example, if the space is too narrow, it may not accommodate a core layout with multiple procedure rooms working off a central technologist work core. (See figure 11-8 [p. 196] in chapter 11, "Department Location and Configuration.") If the overall space is too long and narrow, resulting travel distances may become inappropriately long.
- Is the area subdivided by fixed elements such as stairs or shafts? If so, functional adjacencies may be difficult to achieve, resulting in operational inefficiencies such as long travel distances for staff and/or patients.
- What is the spacing of the existing structural columns? If they are closely spaced, it may be difficult to arrange multiple rooms adjacent to each other without having columns projecting into some of the rooms. (See figure 17-2, p. 338.) Shallow structural bays also may limit the depth or width of rooms that have corridors running alongside them. (See figure 17-3, p. 339.)
- What is the floor-to-floor height of the existing structure? Shallow floor-to-floor heights may not allow for an efficient arrangement of mechanical systems above functional areas (such as procedures rooms) and below beams and girders of the structural system. (See figure 8-16 [p. 153] in chapter 8, "Design Concepts.") Inefficient mechanical (and other) system arrangements can lead to significant cost premiums.

Functional Adjacencies

- If the renovation project involves relocating imaging services, is the proposed location near other related services? Does it allow for a separation of inpatient and outpatient traffic (if this is applicable to the project)? Does it allow for easy access to and from the emergency and surgery departments?
- Will the renovated area disrupt the existing horizontal and/or vertical circulation routes serving other parts of the building? Can the required exiting for the renovated area be easily accommodated without modifying corridors and/or exitways beyond the boundary of the renovated area?

Future Flexibility and Adaptability

- What is the useful remaining life of all physical elements that are not being replaced? Will they limit the future use of the renovated area? Are any building systems that are not being replaced approaching their maximum capacities?
- Is the existing facility constructed of a building system that is easy to modify? For example, a steel structural frame accommodates internal modifications more easily than a building with structural concrete walls. (See following section on structure and infrastructure.)

- Was the existing facility specifically designed to easily accommodate future change? For example, are utility systems located in interstitial spaces that are separate from functional areas? Do structural and utility systems have reserve capacity to handle additional loads?
- Is there available "soft" space that could be used for future expansion within the facility? Is external expansion possible in the future? Would it be easy to integrate into the plan a technology dock for relocatable imaging services (such as those housed in trucks or other movable structures)?

Structure and Infrastructure

- What is the loading capacity of the existing floors, walls, and roof area? How much supplemental structural modification will be needed to support the heavily concentrated loads of imaging equipment? Will required structural modifications affect operations in other areas of the building?
- Is the project located in a seismically active area? Does the existing structure conform to current structural requirements (structural code requirements often increase with each new major seismic event)? Is seismic stability provided by a braced frame or by shear walls, either of which system may limit initial or future planning flexibility?
- Does the depth of beams limit vertical clearances and thus compromise the efficient layout of air-handling (and other) systems? (Beam depth should be considered in conjunction with floor-to-floor height.)

Figure 17-2. Structural Bay Spacing Relative to Room Configuration— Two Procedure Rooms within a Bay

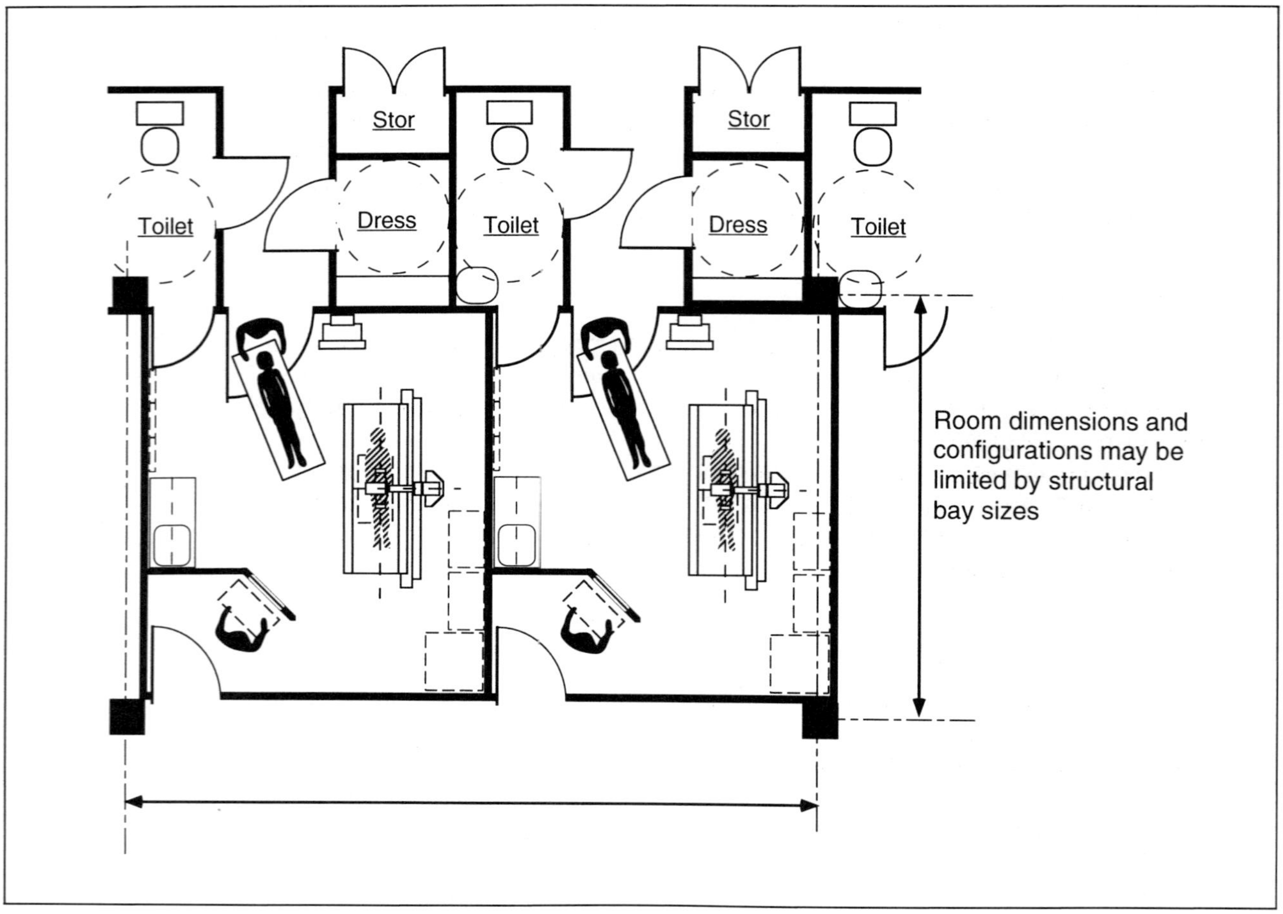

Figure 17-3. Structural Bay Spacing Relative to Room Configuration—Procedure Rooms and a Corridor within a Bay

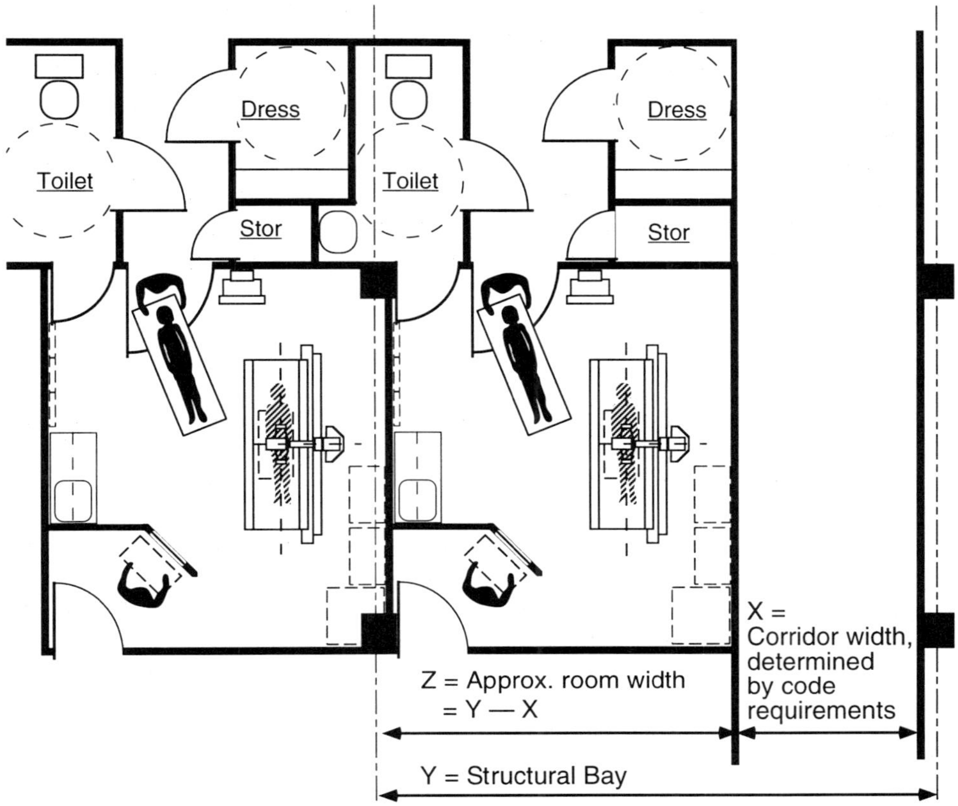

- Is there a convenient location for air-handling units to supply and exhaust air to and from the area of renovation? Will new vertical risers need to be added, thus disrupting functions above the area of renovation? Can the ductwork presently servicing the area of renovation be easily replaced without requiring major modifications to adjacent areas of the building that will remain operational?
- Is asbestos present in the existing facility?
- Does the existing facility have a source of clean, uniform, uninterrupted power? Does the existing facility have adequate power capacity? Can power be efficiently distributed between the main power supply location and its points of use?
- Is an information network or communications system in place that will allow for electronic image management and picture archiving? If not, is it appropriate to install one either throughout the entire facility or in portions of the facility?
- Can the existing fire protection system be easily modified to serve the area of renovation?
- Will the existing structure cause excessive vibration that would be disruptive to vibration-sensitive procedures (interventional imaging and MRI, for example)?

Code Compliance

- To what codes and regulations must the facility conform? Will the renovation project require additional areas of the existing facility to be upgraded so that they conform to current codes? Will this project trigger the need for a more extensive upgrade elsewhere in the facility? (This may vary by regional jurisdiction and by the proposed scope of renovation.)

- How easy will it be to conform to current accessibility requirements? Do special accessibility allowances exist for renovation as compared to new construction? Has the existing facility been assessed for Americans with Disabilities Act compliance?
- Will structural codes require the primary structure to be upgraded?
- Is the intended occupancy different from the occupancy type that the facility was initially designed for? For example, if an existing office building (usually designed for a business occupancy) is renovated to be used as a freestanding outpatient imaging center (the occupancy classification for this use may vary by location and by the particular nature of the proposed imaging procedures), the life safety and exiting code requirements for the new occupancy type might exceed those attained by the building's construction. Furthermore, if patients become "nonambulatory" during some portion of the procedure, yet another level of life safety and exiting criteria might have to be met.

Phasing Considerations

There are many kinds of renovation projects. Some involve only a cosmetic upgrade; others require replacement of everything except the building's exterior skin and structural system. However, almost all renovation projects involve some degree of interim phasing regardless of the scope of renovation.

Renovation often involves adapting a space that is to be used for a new or different purpose. Unless the area to be renovated (and immediately adjoining areas) is already vacated or unless the scope of construction is so minor that it can be accomplished entirely during off-hours, it is likely that some functions will need to be temporarily relocated to enable construction to take place without disrupting existing services. With complex projects, numerous interrelated phases of temporary construction may need to be choreographed in order for these services to be provided throughout the course of construction.

Two types of renovation projects are common. These are:

1. *In-place renovation,* where imaging services are physically upgraded without being moved to a new location
2. *Relocation projects,* where an entire imaging service or department is relocated to an unoccupied portion of an existing building

Each type of renovation has advantages and disadvantages. Some may cause a series of additional projects to occur in order to free up unoccupied space for temporary or long-term relocation of services.

In-place renovation projects may be the sole alternative if adequate vacant space is unavailable elsewhere in the facility. However, even in-place renovation may require temporary relocation of some services. For example, if an existing imaging department is to be remodeled in place, it may be necessary to temporarily relocate some functions during construction (perhaps into a temporary modular structure or a semitrailer unit) and move them back once the work is complete.

Some renovation projects are more appropriately designed as relocation projects. One advantage of relocation is that the old service can usually operate in place until the new area is completed. However, this approach requires that vacant space be available in the new location. As a result, multiple interrelated relocation projects often evolve in an effort to both create a vacant area and then utilize each area that consequently becomes vacant.

Cost Considerations

Often renovation is selected over new construction for either one or all of the following reasons:

1. Adequate space is not available for new construction.
2. Adequate time is not available for new construction.

3. The existing area has a significant remaining useful life, making new construction relatively less appealing and more difficult to justify.
4. It is assumed that renovation is less expensive than new construction.

Although renovation often is (but not always) more affordable than new construction, it is important to consider both the obvious and the less-obvious cost components of renovation before selecting an approach. The obvious cost benefit of renovation is that some elements of a facility already exist and thus do not have to be built again. Some of the less-obvious aspects of cost are discussed in the following subsections.

First Cost versus Life Cycle Costs

Any cost determination should include both initial construction costs and the life cycle costs of maintaining, modifying, and operating the facility during the next decades. Most important, these costs should be amortized over the facility's expected life in order to compare the value of new construction dollars to renovation dollars.

Hidden Construction Costs

Most renovation projects involve myriad hidden conditions. As a result, the likelihood often exists that some previously unknown physical conditions will be discovered during the renovation process. To reduce the potential impact of such surprises, the following steps should be taken:

- Existing conditions should be examined and documented as carefully as possible.
- If available, a set of drawings for the building's initial construction and subsequent modifications should be obtained and verified.
- An ample construction contingency (usually a higher percentage of construction than would be provided for new construction projects) should be provided.

Required Related Work Costs

Renovation work may require interim construction, phasing of work, and demolition. As a result, funds should be allocated for required interim construction, phasing, and demolition, as well as for final construction.

Plan Efficiency and Operational Costs

Several plan layouts that can be accommodated within the space available for renovation should be analyzed. Do physical constraints (such as size and configuration of the area; floor-to-floor height; and column spacing) limit the types of layout that can be accommodated? If optimal adjacencies and circulation routes cannot be achieved, operational inefficiencies may result. All plans should be examined closely to ensure that patient circulation and staff work flow are ideal and that imaging rooms and their associated support spaces are arrayed appropriately. The cost of operational inefficiency—over time—can exceed the cost of construction.

References

1. Bacher, L. C. Deciding between renovation and new construction. *Health Facilities Management* 4(7):20–24, July 1991.
2. Bacher.
3. Bacher.
4. Bacher.

Part 5

The Future

Chapter 18

Future Trends

During the 1970s and much of the 1980s, long-range planning established an integral foundation for the design and construction of most health care facilities. However, as the eighties and nineties progressed, the duration of planning horizons shortened noticeably as health care delivery systems began to reflect changes in health care reimbursement, notably, the advent of managed care and cost containment. At present, even short-term planning forecasts frequently are qualified with great risk and uncertainty.

This uncertainty during an era of rapid change requires that today's planning be done in such a way as to accommodate many possible outcomes. Although the details of tomorrow's health care environment are unclear, it is possible to determine a general direction. This chapter summarizes the key areas in which a managed care environment will affect the design of medical imaging facilities in the future and describes some scenarios that both health care providers and design and planning professionals are likely to encounter.

The New Health Care Environment

The drive toward market reform in the U.S. health care delivery system is likely to result in the eventual replacement of most individual health care providers with integrated health networks. This change will dramatically alter the political, economic, and social setting in which health care services generally and medical imaging services specifically will be provided. The integrated health care environment will probably be characterized by:

- Increased incentives for cost containment and penalties for spending that does not result in overall savings
- More paying patients, as some 37 million individuals who are presently uninsured gain access to the health care system
- Regional and community-based integrated health networks, less duplication of services, and creation of centers of excellence
- The extensive growth of ambulatory care services dispersed throughout a community, with inpatient services focusing on patients with greater acuity than in the past
- The increased importance of information management, outcomes analysis, and communications systems
- Operational restructuring, institutional downsizing, and reduction in the number of physician and support staff per patient
- The proliferation of gatekeeper systems in which primary care physicians monitor referrals to specialized services
- Managed care and other capitated payment systems
- An emphasis on disease and injury prevention

- Less money than in the past to support teaching hospitals and research and more resources devoted to rural health care providers than in the past

The following subsections look at the impact of changes in the health care reimbursement and delivery system on three areas in particular: medical imaging, ambulatory care, and technology.

Medical Imaging

The impact of integrated health care on the future of medical imaging can be characterized by:

- A shakeout or survival of imaging modalities with high-outcome-to-cost ratios, while less efficacious techniques struggle for reimbursement
- Increased requirements to justify the economic value of new modalities
- An increased reliance on predetermined clinical pathways or courses of action for patient care
- The increased volume and complexity of outpatient imaging services
- A decreased cost per imaging procedure
- Improved cost accounting and pricing required by capitation
- The development of telemedicine and teleradiology as integral components of health care delivery
- Volatile political debates surrounding outcome monitoring as a means of directing the future growth of specific imaging modalities
- Cross-trained health care technicians performing technical tasks that previously were performed exclusively by imaging technologists
- An increased development of interventional imaging procedures, including imaging applications in the operating room

As alliances are formed, providers of health care will develop regional networks to deliver services in the most efficient method possible. A prime objective will be to reduce costs by fostering competition. In some regions, providers will be able to avoid the unnecessary duplication of both facilities and expensive equipment. In other locales, duplication of facilities will result. One likely approach is the creation of satellite health facilities offering basic imaging services, as well as selective specialty health centers focusing on particular types of special imaging, such as complex cardiovascular or neurological procedures. Each specialty center also would provide other types of advanced imaging not available at the satellite centers.

Ambulatory Care

In the future, both the volume and complexity of outpatient imaging procedures will continue to grow. There also will be greater regulation of outpatient imaging than there has been in the past. Whereas hospital-based imaging will serve patients with higher acuity than in the past, ambulatory imaging will encompass a broader range of services and yet involve complex techniques. This will vary depending on demographic differences among rural communities and metropolitan areas. Emphasis will be both on diagnostic imaging for early detection and screening and on interventional treatment. As a result, ambulatory imaging facilities will require additional support spaces—for patient preparation and recovery—and thus greater power and air-handling systems than are presently required. Satellite imaging facilities will be electronically linked to nearby imaging centers within the region and to remote centers that provide specialized services and consultations. In some instances, batch reading of radiologic images will be performed at locations distant from where the images are acquired. This approach will be similar to the way that laboratory tests are analyzed in large quantities at regional reference labs, rather than in small quantities at their point of origin.

Satellite facilities will enable health care alliances to distribute services throughout the community. With a broader population base and improved access throughout the community, services can be offered more efficiently and with limited duplication of equipment and staff. Thus, imaging services provided in most ambulatory centers will include modalities having a high demand within a limited catchment area. Imaging services requiring a larger population base for high utilization will tend to be located in larger regional centers.

Following the pattern of health care reimbursement, many outpatient imaging services will be capitated rather than paid per procedure. "The key to control is aligning incentives so that radiologists are paid to take care of a population rather than by procedure. The second part of the equation is educating the primary-care physician. The $56 billion that the nation spends each year on diagnostic imaging now faces heavy scrutiny. Outpatient procedures, reimbursed mostly on a fee-for-service basis, are a popular target for payers that want to reduce costs."[1]

Capitated payment, which is based on a fixed monthly or annual fee per patient or enrollee, replaces incentives for ordering more tests with incentives for reducing overall expenses. "Many health plans see capitating radiologists as the surest way to level imaging expenditures. Still rare, capitation fixes health plan expenses. It encourages providers to carefully watch how medical care is delivered because inappropriate services eat up profit instead of contribute to it."[2]

Referral patterns for imaging services in the future will differ from current models. As health care evolves further into a networked delivery system where (1) fewer primary care physicians are independent providers (and more are aligned with health networks) and (2) more radiologists are paid capitated rates rather than per procedure, referrals will become increasingly prenegotiated, perhaps with each primary care provider having several options for imaging referrals. Education of primary physicians on the appropriate use of imaging services is a key component of the networked delivery system.

> [In several regions throughout the nation] . . . capitated radiology networks are springing up, often preceding integrated delivery networks. . . . The network's radiology groups screen out poor use of imaging by talking with referring physicians, distributing educational material and contributing to the development of utilization guidelines. . . . Some radiologists and hospitals, however, are leery of the risks and benefits of capitation. Many avoid it when they can.[3]

As primary care providers assume broader roles as gatekeepers, satellite health facilities will include a greater mix of primary care and ancillary services (such as imaging) to which they refer. In many centers, some specialty services also will be provided, thus locating imaging equipment and personnel conveniently proximate to those providers likely to make imaging referrals.

Technology

With the emphasis on cost containment, the resources needed to support the invention and refinement of new imaging technologies will become more scarce in the future. This may adversely affect the United States' ability to export technical expertise. However, because the rewards of cost-saving technological advances will remain great, research and development of imaging systems that improve patient outcomes and reduce operational costs will endure. Technologies with both economic and medical promise will be favored over those with medical merit alone. As a result, champions of specific imaging modalities will have to justify the financial value of their requests more than ever before.

The following imaging technologies are likely to see noticeable advancement in the near future:

- Information management and telemedicine
- Interventional procedures
- Imaging and surgery
- Less-invasive diagnostic and treatment procedures
- Smaller, less-expensive imaging equipment

Information Management and Telemedicine

After a decade and a half of false starts, many hospital-based and freestanding imaging facilities are now using electronic alternatives to image acquisition and management. The ability to electronically link various components of imaging facilities to each other and to remote sites has altered many of the traditional functional adjacencies from which imaging facility plans develop.

Information networks will become the backbone of health care facilities, and medical images will continue to be a vehicle essential to the sharing of information and knowledge. Sophisticated communications systems will link radiologic data to comprehensive health care information systems. High-speed transmission of data will reduce both staff and patient travel time and eventually reduce the need for extensive hard-copy storage. As sophisticated information management systems and electronic imaging systems further evolve, imaging services will be able to become increasingly decentralized.

Interventional Procedures

Many diagnostic and treatment procedures that in the past required surgery or other invasive techniques are now routinely performed using less-invasive imaging methods. For example, interventional angiographic procedures, including the placement of vascular stents, sometimes are viable alternatives to surgery. The development of new interventional procedures will continue. In particular, the complexity and variety of interventional procedures performed on an outpatient basis will grow significantly. Additional patient support spaces for patient preparation, observation, and recovery will be part of most imaging facilities—both hospital based and freestanding. As a result, greater electrical power quality and improved air-handling and cooling systems will be necessary.

Imaging and Surgery

Whereas imaging and surgery will continue to compete with each other in some arenas, multispecialty teams composed of radiologists, surgeons, and other medical specialists will collaborate on new treatments that will bring imaging expertise further into the operating room. For example, ultrasound and robotically guided imaging systems will provide new powers of vision for neurosurgeons performing intracranial surgery. Also of particular interest will be the future development of magnetic resonance apparatus designed to be used in the operating environment or interventional imaging suite.

Less-Invasive Diagnostic and Treatment Procedures

Whereas many imaging procedures will compete with invasive surgical treatment, some imaging techniques will replace other invasive imaging techniques. For example, magnetic resonance angiography, although not yet as effective as conventional angiography, is less invasive and potentially safer than its counterpart. As another example, electron beam tomography provides exquisite detail regarding arterial calcification using noninvasive imaging. Finally, the use of ultrasound will become widespread, in some applications because it is noninvasive and in others because it is relatively inexpensive.

Smaller, Less-Expensive Imaging Equipment

Today, many types of imaging services can be performed using small, relatively inexpensive equipment, and this trend will continue. For example, several manufacturers offer computed tomography units that require significantly less environmental conditioning (such as heat dissipation and humidity control) than in the past. Additionally, equipment is getting smaller. Thus, it can be installed within smaller spaces, although this may limit utilization somewhat. As another example, some special low-field MRI instruments, designed specially for imaging extremities, are very compact and lightweight. Some require no external magnetic shielding. The price of these units also is going down. Many manufacturers are designing imaging equipment specifically for use in outpatient facilities and even in physicians' offices. At the same time, the market for reconditioned imaging equipment is growing. This trend suggests that in some facilities many of the challenging environmental and siting requirements characteristic of the 1980s will not disappear immediately.

Design Goals

The architecture of imaging facilities reflects the humanistic, technical, social, and economic characteristics of health care in general and medical imaging in particular. As in the design of any complex facility type, functional concerns must be integrated with the physical image that is intended for the facility. For example, the spatial quality of a healing environment—the use of color and the introduction of natural lighting to enhance a patient's sense of privacy and comfort—must be considered as high a priority as the efficiency of circulation routes and the adaptability of spaces.

Yet health care architecture in the 21st century is certain to have a different emphasis than it has had in the past. As health care functions in an era of cost containment and downsizing, there may be a tendency among some to devaluate the importance of facility image and favor the economic criteria by which facility design is judged. However, a sounder approach is to consider that health care is changing its focus from a treatment-based industry to one of both prevention and treatment. In this regard, image and ambiance are better judged in terms of both their cost and contribution to health and well-being than in terms of cost alone.

Furthermore, as managed health care delivery systems become common in all areas of the country and as medical services begin to be administered more sparingly, it is likely that navigation through the delivery system will, in fact, become more cumbersome and stressful than it is at present. As incentives for medical services focus more on efficacy and frugality, the physical environment will play an even greater role in how patients and staff feel. Indeed, the physical environment contributes to health. However, the quality of that environment must represent an integral value, not an added cost. Achieving a healing environment means enhancing the operational efficiency and ultimate flexibility of the imaging facility, not compromising those qualities.

References

1. Scott, L. Diagnostic imaging targeted for change—common practices challenged; field eyed for cost cutting, capitation. *Modern Healthcare,* Nov. 29, 1993, pp. 34–41.
2. Scott.
3. Scott.

Part 6

Appendixes and Index

Appendix A

Descriptions of Selected Imaging Facilities and Departments

The following descriptions of imaging facilities illustrate a variety of architectural solutions to numerous operational and physical challenges. Every project is different because the needs of every program are unique. Some represent large military installations; some are part of a network of university facilities. Some are located on dense urban sites; others are rural. Some include comprehensive imaging departments based on filmless technology; others include only limited imaging services. One example is not site specific but, rather, represents a template to be used for planning imaging departments for numerous hospitals owned and operated by a large health maintenance organization.

Note: Most of the material in this appendix is based on design reports and other project documentation. The reference citations for direct quotations are given at the beginning of sections where applicable. Commentary from the author is indicated by brackets when it is embedded in direct quotations; whole sections written by the author are preceded by the heading Author's Commentary.

The MDIS System/Madigan Army Medical Center[1-4]

The Medical Diagnostic Imaging Support (MDIS) system is a large project to install Picture Archival and Communications Systems (PACS) and teleradiology across several military medical sites in the United States and overseas. Phased implementation began at Madigan Army Medical Center in Tacoma, Washington, in the spring of 1992, Wright Patterson Air Force Medical Center in Dayton, Ohio, in the fall of 1992, and Brooke Army Medical Center in San Antonio, Texas, in the winter of 1992–1993. Other sites . . . [in progress include] teleradiology in Korea and in the Azores (off the coast of Portugal). The hardware and software components of the system include computed radiology units, central processing unit (CPU) working storage unit (WSU), fiber network, optical disk jukebox (ODJ), radiology information system (RIS), modality interfacing, and physician monitor workstations. . . .

Technology Configuration

The MDIS system is a network of computer based medical devices whose primary function is to work as a single 'super device' to communicate and manage digital radiological examinations for diagnosis and consultation by clinicians in a health care environment. With the MDIS system, the clinician uses a viewing workstation as his [or her] operating platform to access a patient's image and radiological exam report electronically through a centralized Work Storage unit (WSU) host via a high-speed fiber optic network. The patient's image is digitally acquired and gated into the system from the various radiology modalities present in a health care facility; these include Magnetic Resonance Imaging (MRI), Computed Tomography (CT), Ultrasound, and is ultimately archived on Optical Platters within an Optical Disk Juke Box. The hard copy x-rays in the existing film systems are scanned and converted into a digital format, using a Film Digitizer. Both forms are archived, recalled, viewed, and networked within the [Military Treatment Facility] (MTF).

Between MTF's and remote sites, via "Teleradiology", images are transmitted through modems and commercial wide area telecommunication, allowing for interpretation and consultative support to remote, difficult to serve or underserved clinical areas.

The MDIS system accomplishes four primary activities to support diagnostic medical imaging:

1. Acquire diagnostic images in digital format; gate them into the system.
2. Communicate patient demographics and study information into an RIS.
3. Archive and manage images and data in the data base.
4. Display images and patient data on workstations.

The *Acquisition Subsystem* utilizes inherently digital modalities, such as CT, MRI, as well as Computed Radiology (CR) to create filmless, soft-copy diagnostic images. CR technology consists of reusable phosphor plates in cassettes as the image transfer medium, in lieu of conventional film as the imaging medium. Film Digitizers are available to convert existing [X-ray films] to digital format as they are introduced into the system.

The *Communication Subsystem* will allow high speed transfer of diagnostic-quality images and data in a digital format, and is capable of interfacing with a RIS. Both Intra-MTF and Inter-MTF network communication is accomplished by one of several transfer mediums to include: fiber optic media and various long haul telecommunications such as satellite transmissions.

The *Image Storage and Database Subsystem* maintains the information integrity of the system and insures the proper flow of images and data. The images and data flow to a combination of short-term storage on magnetic disks and long-term storage on optical platters, contained in optical juke boxes.

The *Image Display Subsystem* through high resolution computer video terminals, display diagnostic-quality, soft-copy medical images and data. Hard copy digital versions of these same images can also be printed on single-emulsion laser film on an "as required" basis.

System Payoffs

The benefits from MDIS will be realized in both hard dollar cost savings as well as improvements in clinical quality.

Cost Savings

- Film and processing cost savings accrue as immediate near-term savings with a totally implemented system.
- Contract prices for radiologists at small DoD [Department of Defense] medical facilities will be reduced, through the use of Teleradiology. Remote sites can transmit the image to a host, tertiary care military hospital, rather that paying for a contract radiologist to read the image at the remote site. An economy of scale is achieved with this operating technique.
- The potential for sharing resources between services using this approach is unlimited. As an example, the Air Force medical treatment facility at McChord AFB Hospital will have the ability to electronically deliver medical images acquired at their facility to Radiologists at Madigan Army Medical Center, who in-turn provide primary interpretation services.

Improvements in Clinical Quality

- Because of the inherent limitations with film as a hard copy media, lost film is the chronic productivity problem in . . . [most] facilities. MDIS will virtually eliminate this problem with electronic acquisition of images.
- Film room personnel presently needed to file and retrieve existing films can be eliminated or utilized elsewhere within the department.
- The storage space and management requirements for hard copy films will be dramatically reduced as the digital film archive grows.
- Patient waiting time is reduced. The image is ready for interpretation, immediately upon acquisition, as well as being available to the referring physician.
- Additionally, the disposal of film chemicals as hazardous waste will be significantly reduced.

Madigan Army Medical Center (MAMC)

The Madigan Army Medical Center is the largest medical facility built for the Army Corps of Engineers. It has 1.2 million square feet of space, plus an additional 1 million square feet of interstitial floor space, sited on 161 acres. The nine story, 414-bed hospital has a three-story outpatient clinic and a four-story support complex. It will be used by approximately 154,000 people per year.

Interstitial floors seven-and-a-half feet high between each hospital floor contain all building utilities. This innovative design means utilities can be revised or repaired without interruption of hospital functions, thus helping meet the Army's goal of a 100-year life span for the Center.

Hospital Goals

- A therapeutic environment for the healing process
- A 100-year physical life in adapting to changing medical care techniques and equipment
- A cost-effective and durable plant for conservative use of tax dollars
- Significant "passive" planning of the facilities to make them yield the highest economies in the areas of staffing, operations, energy use and change
- A comprehensive facility that will encompass teaching functions and attract the respect of the medical world and the patient population

Features

- 414-bed tertiary care teaching hospital
- Mobilization expansion to 622 beds
- 1.2 million square foot medical center
- 14 operating rooms (10 inpatient and 4 outpatient)
- 10-bed surgical ICU, 10-bed medical ICU, 8-bed CCU
- Cardiac catheterization lab
- Full MRI, CT and nuclear medicine
- Medical digital imaging system
- 65-bassinet nursery, 4 delivery rooms, 2 birthing rooms and 6 labor rooms
- 14 dental treatment rooms
- Full shock trauma emergency with air evacuation
- 36 radiographic rooms
- Medical mall
- 3500 clinic outpatients per day
- [Interstitial building system with] mechanical utility floor above all functional floors

Transition to Filmless Imaging

A major consideration for transition to a "filmless" environment is how to assimilate the large number of historical comparison images into the database. The digitization of more than 3 million films in the [Madigan Army Medical Center (MAMC)] file room would be impractical. The MDIS system solution is to run a "parallel" system for the first year, building up the digital historical image database for all new exams, while printing a hardcopy to be read, filed, and retrieved as in the usual film based system. Additional older comparison images will be selected for digitization by the radiologists and clinicians as patients present to MAMC for treatment. This will provide the vast majority of comparison exams needed from the MDIS system database when all the workstations are installed throughout the hospital.

Changing from a film-based to softcopy diagnosis and review environment requires a period of user familiarization. This will be accomplished by a combination of initial training by the vendor followed by the use of the initial workstations by the radiologists and clinicians on a periodic basis until full implementation. The radiology staff and residents will rotate to the Emergency Radiology workstation at MAMC one or two times per month for a full day of familiarization each time. The clinical staff will have a workstation dedicated for image review in the radiology department as well as one in the ER and MICU. The project manager will work with all the radiology physicians and most clinicians individually, especially the first several months. A major strength of the MDIS system diagnostic and clinical workstation is the [proprietary] computer user interface with adaptations and additions for the medical imaging environment. This [user-friendly interface] allows each new user to quickly become facile and proficient enabling them to train others as well.

Magnetic Resonance Treatment Suite/Brigham and Women's Hospital

Author's Commentary: Brigham and Women's Hospital in Boston was offered the first magnetic resonance treatment (MRT) prototype in the world (developed by General Electric—GE) for installation. This highly specialized magnetic resonance imaging (MRI) system enables medical staff to perform invasive treatment in addition to diagnostic procedures in the MRI suite. (See figure A-1.)

The design team worked closely with GE to determine how to accommodate such a high-tech piece of equipment without any previous example to rely on. Rigging the equipment into place, accessing it for servicing, compensating for the excessive heat gain emitted, and air-conditioning and ventilation requirements had to be considered. In addition, the design team had to address containment of the equipment's magnetic field. The project involved close coordination among medical researchers and equipment developers.

Functionally, the MRT room was treated as a diagnostic and treatment room. A broad range of medical activities is performed within. Ancillary spaces also were designed to support the equipment associated with the MR unit. In addition, a computer room, an equipment room, three patient rooms, a nurse's station, a waiting room, and clean and soiled utility rooms were included in the design. Design parameters were identified by the various team members—architects, structural engineers, mechanical engineers, and electrical engineers.

A special structural system was used during construction to support existing buildings adjacent to the site and to accommodate the 39-foot-deep excavation necessary for the placement of the MRT. The below-grade floors—in addition to the MRT suite—house administrative support, a visiting doctors' office suite, and a 100-seat seminar room, bulk materials storage, and biomechanical shops.

The MR is encased in a room with a thick steel floor, walls, and ceiling to contain the magnetic fields. The space is situated on a 24-inch-thick reinforced concrete footing positioned between two 6-inch-thick reinforced concrete slabs, with the top slab being the MRT floor.

Figure A-1. Brigham and Women's Hospital MRI Suite

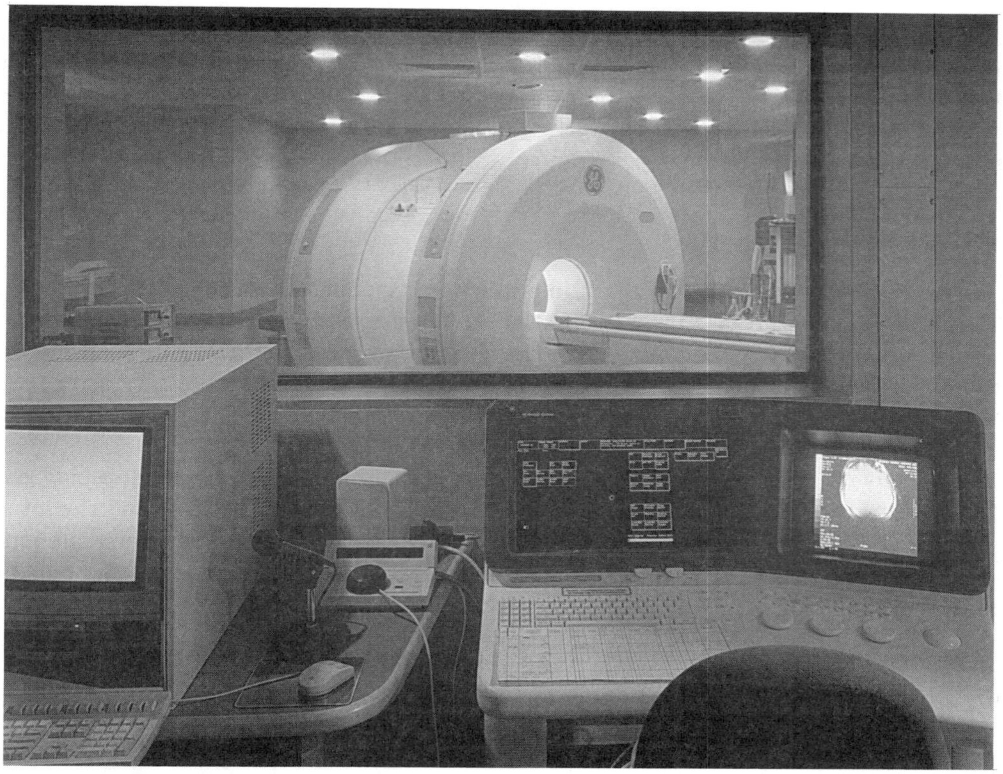

Interventional Magnetic Imaging Suite, Brigham and Women's Hospital, Boston. ©Steve Rosenthal, 1994. Architecture and interior design by Tsoi/Kobus & Associates. Used with permission.

University of California, San Diego/Thornton Hospital

Author's Commentary: As the first phase of the University of California, San Diego's (UCSD's) long-range development plan, Thornton Hospital in La Jolla, California, is one of the first buildings on a new site that is part of the overall UCSD campus. As a result, this 40-acre project sets the architectural character of the new 260-acre East Campus.

The design focus of the 120-bed hospital was to create a health care environment that is contemporary in its relationship to people and yet timeless in design quality. A regional response in architectural detailing and materials establishes the complex within a broader context, utilizing a sandstone-colored upper facade, granite base, and cast stone columns. The interiors of Thornton Hospital reflect a hospitality environment rather than a hospital setting. The building design consists of three building blocks that house nursing units, a diagnostic and treatment center, and an ambulatory care center. (See figure A-2.) A three-story atrium serves as the connecting element for the three blocks. The atrium is anchored by a rotunda entry that marks the arrival point for the three zones of the complex.

Plants, exhibits, and artwork in the atrium, combined with an adjacent inner court, soften and enliven the hospital's public areas. The inner courtyard provides visual relief for staff and patients, and serves as a means of orientation for visitors. (See figure 8-6 in chapter 8, "Design Concepts.")

Diagnostic imaging is located on the first floor of the Diagnostic and Treatment Center. The department is planned with both a perimeter corridor and adjacent soft space to enable expansion and/or conversion that will easily accommodate future changes in imaging services. (See figure 8-10 in chapter 8, "Design Concepts.") The design of Thornton Hospital uses interstitial floors to provide additional flexibility for future building modifications. (See figure 8-15 in chapter 8, "Design Concepts.")

Imaging Research Facility/Mallinckrodt Institute of Radiology

Author's Commentary: The Washington University School of Medicine and the Mallinckrodt Institute of Radiology in St. Louis, Missouri, have created a center of excellence for neurologic imaging research. The impetus for this project came from the desire to provide a world-class facility that would serve as a gathering place for distinct research functions in magnetic resonance imaging (MRI) and positron emission tomography (PET) imaging.

Unique Design Approach

The 48,000-square-foot annex to an existing structure is unique in both content and approach. The facility houses advanced high field MRI, PET instrumentation, electronic laboratories, wet laboratories, and support space. The design solution showcases state-of-the-art medical technology—literally by displaying it for the public—maintaining necessary separations between private and public zones. This duality shapes the major architectural components of the new facility.

The large heavily shielded magnets are displayed to the public through the sweeping glass facade that cuts through the massing elements. (See figure A-3.) The scale and rhythm of the existing East Building facade are carried along the north side of the annex and are replicated as an apparent screen wall along the south elevation—respecting the existing building form while creating a new entity.

Figure A-2. University of California, San Diego, Thornton Hospital

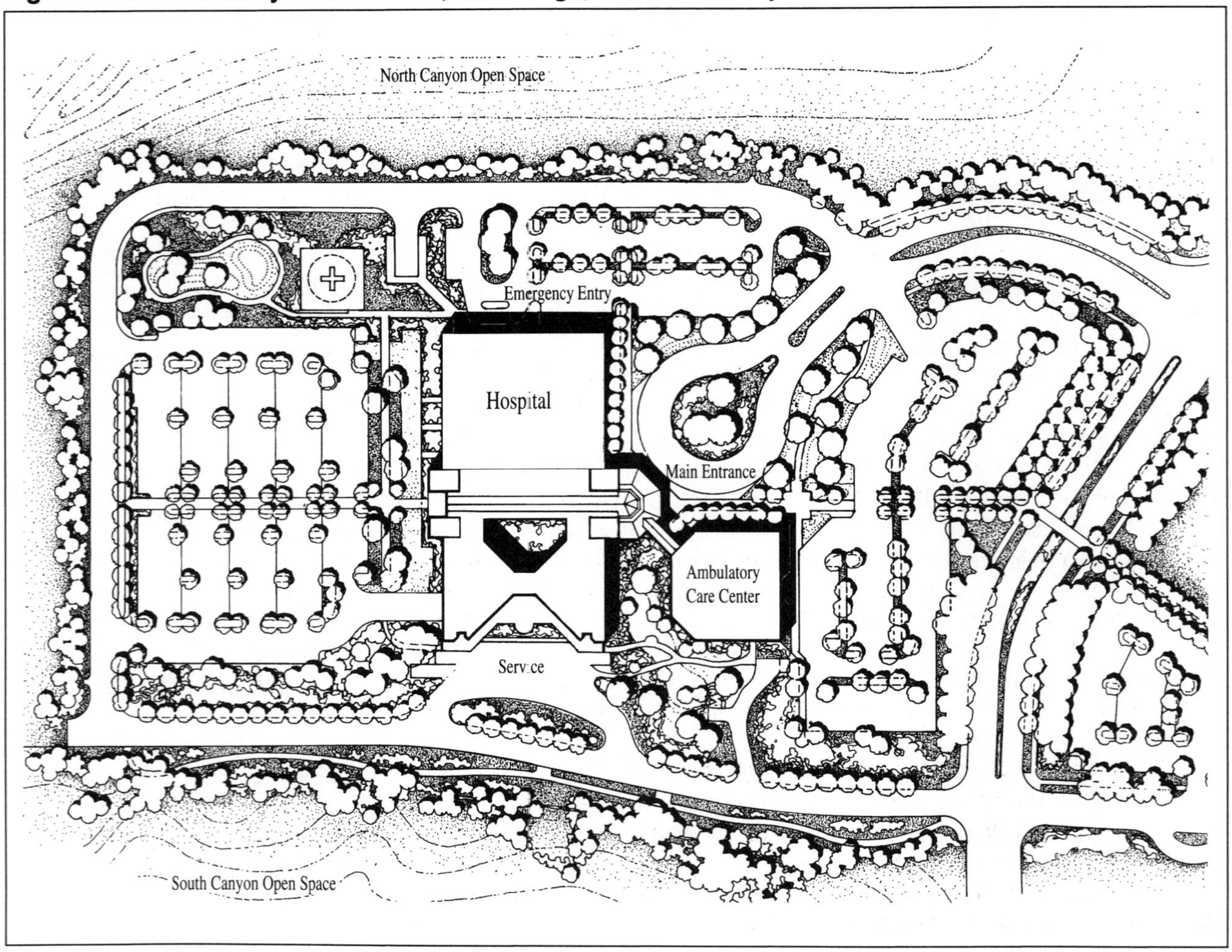

Courtesy of Stone Marraccini Patterson, San Francisco. Used with permission.

Figure A-3. Imaging Research Facility for the Mallinckrodt Institute of Radiology

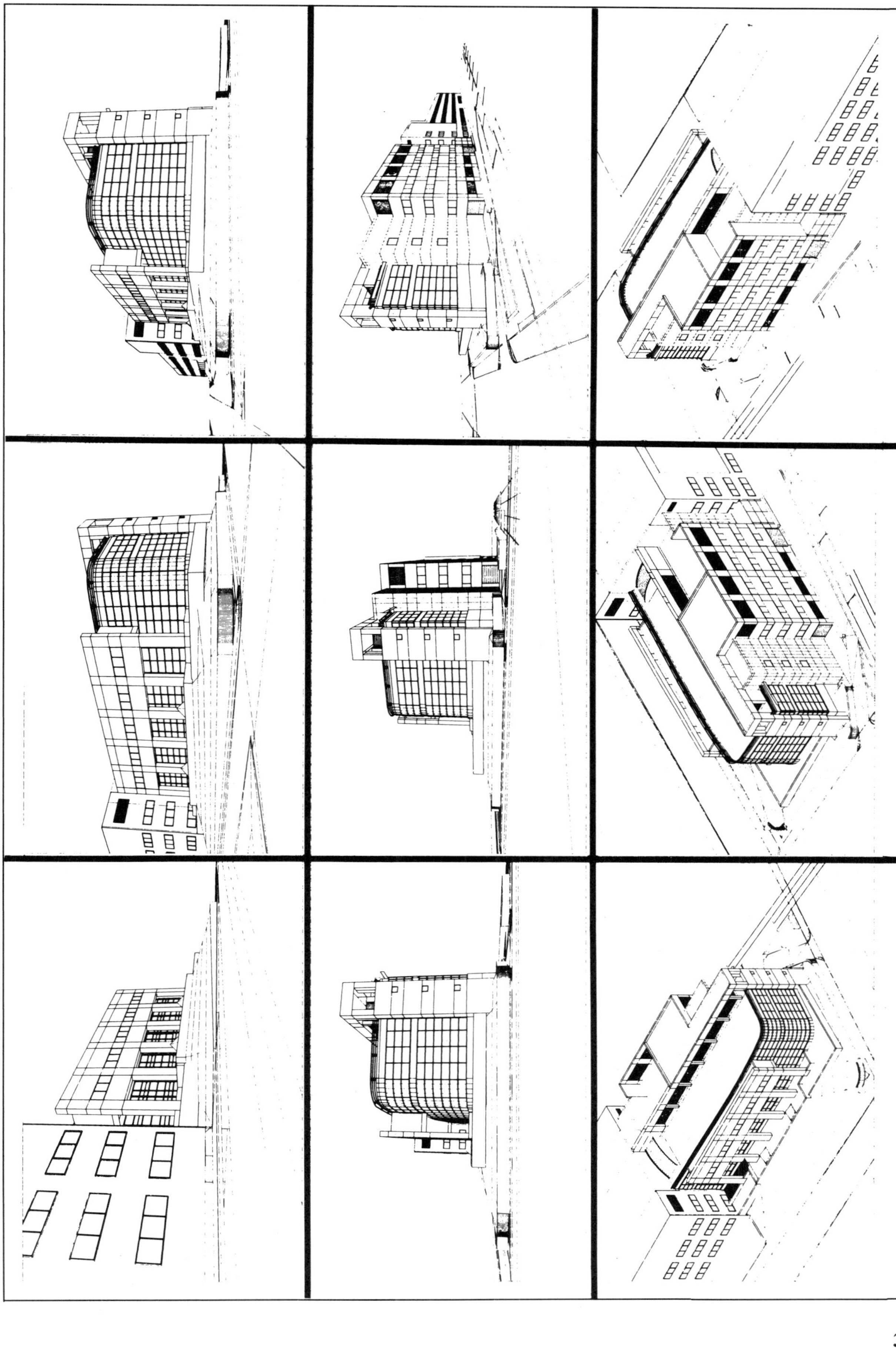

Courtesy of Stone Marraccini Patterson, St. Louis. Used with permission.

Contextual Considerations

Public access into the annex is not required. Therefore, part of the site has been consciously given back to the adjacent streetscape. This, in turn, helps create a viable node for the continued development of the medical center campus. Site walls serve as a visual means of defining the edge of the public domain and the secure zone. They also emphasize the layering of architectural masses that contain the high field magnets.

Technical Challenges

With stringent site constraints and myriad precise physical requirements for equipment placement, a strong planning direction and compositional strategy served as the seed for the development of the architectural concept. The client's desire to publicly display the equipment within the structure added to the articulation of public zones.

Medical School Laboratory Surge and Magnetic Resonance Spectroscopy Facility/Stanford University Medical School[5]

A strong attractive force is quietly drawing together members of usually disparate disciplines from all over campus. With three powerful magnets at its core, it is no wonder that the [Stanford University] Medical School's [Palo Alto, California] new Lucas Center for Magnetic Resonance Spectroscopy and Imaging is luring engineers, chemists and physicists—as well as physicians—through its doors.

The Lucas Center stands at the crossroads of many disciplines. . . . It's an intensely collaborative effort between the schools of medicine and engineering. To achieve its full potential, the technology requires many disciplines working together.

The fundamental mission of the Lucas Center . . . is to gain a basic understanding of magnetic resonance science with the aim of developing tools for medicine and biotechnology. And in order to do that . . . you have to have physics types and medical types rubbing elbows. That's one of the Lucas Center's reasons for being—to foster that kind of interaction. . . . It is particularly appropriate that such a center be located at Stanford University, the site where magnetic resonance in the nuclei of atoms was discovered by Felix Bloch in the 1940s.

Author's Commentary: Stanford University decided to develop the new research facility to help them remain preeminent in medical research and teaching, accommodate multiple departmental research needs, and meet the following objectives:

- Long-term flexibility
- Enhancement of collegial interactions
- Recognizable continuity and enhancement of the medical center's image

The new facility, the Medical School Laboratory Surge (MSLS)/Magnetic Resonance Spectroscopy (MRS) building (also known as the Lucas Center for Magnetic Resonance Spectroscopy and Imaging), combines two distinct programs, each with its own identity. One component houses researchers from numerous medical school departments. The second houses the magnetic resonance spectroscopy program. (See figure A-4 and figure 1-1 in chapter 1, "Design Considerations for Imaging Facilities.") In the spirit of research itself, the design includes spaces and subtle details that evoke a sense of curiosity, experimentation, and surprise.

Long-Term Flexibility

MSLS is a highly adaptable and modular biomedical laboratory. Building systems are planned in an integrated, rational manner to reconfigure individual labs. Backdoor galleys provide temporary storage, access to building systems, and a second means of exiting for increased safety.

Figure A-4. Stanford University Medical School Laboratory Surge/ Magnetic Resonance Spectroscopy Facility

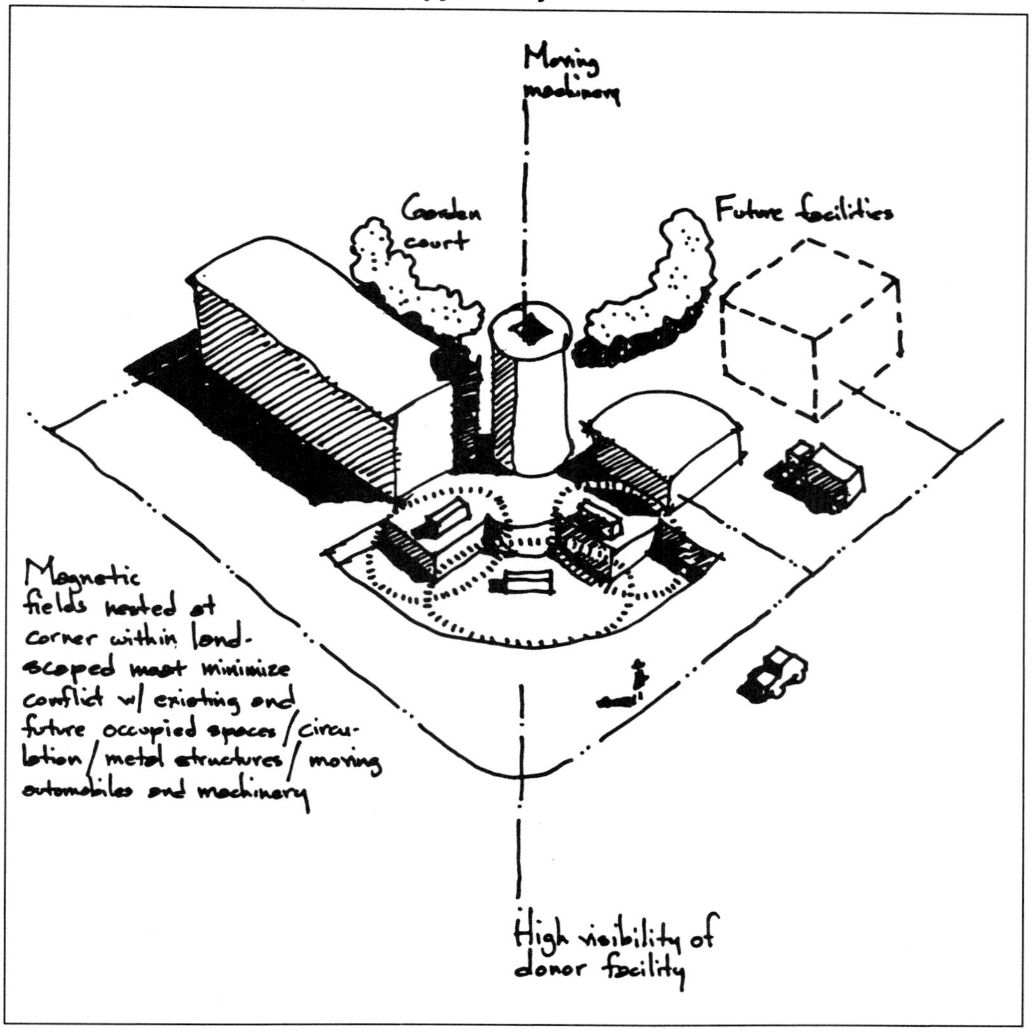

Courtesy of Stone Marraccini Patterson, San Francisco. Drawing by Eric Meub. Used with permission.

Collegial Interaction

The building's atrium is the interactive center of discourse for the resident researchers and their assistants. Offices and conference areas are located at this end, nearest the medical center. To facilitate the informal exchange of ideas, interaction spaces are situated along sunlit personnel corridors.

Design Continuity

The newly constructed MSLS/MRS is visually connected and stylistically harmonic with the original medical center. Its architectural vocabulary evolved from the interpretation key design principles used throughout the existing campus. The facility fulfills the early planning intentions by reinforcing the street grid and entry sequence to the medical center.

Gateways Templates/Kaiser Foundation Health Plan of Northern California[6-7]

[*Author's Commentary:* As part of an effort to efficiently design and build numerous new hospitals and health care facilities in Northern California, Kaiser Foundation Health Plan, Inc., and Anderson DeBartalo Pan Architects and Planners developed a system in which functional and operational criteria are predetermined. The system, named Gateways, includes the following information for each hospital department:

- Purpose of department
- Planning assumptions
- Hours of operation
- Room-by-room standards and special considerations
- Predictions of future trends
- Primary and secondary adjacency and access requirements
- A room-by-room space program
- Departmental templates, including room, equipment, and furniture locations
- Room-by-room medical equipment list
- Room-by-room medical furniture list

The Purpose of Gateways

The purpose of Gateways is not so much to "predesign" each facility as it is to simplify and structure the planning and design process by which numerous architectural and engineering consultants individually design facilities that are functionally similar to those designed by other consultants. The Gateways approach also provides a baseline standard for facility users and health care providers regarding space allocations, inter- and intradepartmental adjacencies, and equipment options. *End of Author's Commentary.*]

The purpose of Gateways is to refine the current planning and design process for Kaiser Permanente [Northern California] and to provide quality facilities in a timely manner. In order to accomplish this, the objective is to create a methodology that will streamline the customized building process into one that is founded on the design of projects using common functional elements. Designing in this manner does not presume a predetermined end result. To allow this to happen, Gateways develops departmental template designs which can be assembled into buildings with the necessary flexibility to meet specific needs while also allowing accurate projection of project schedules and construction costs.

The final product of Gateways are departmental templates that have been refined to a Design Development level with sufficient detail to allow for the implementation into Construction Documents. This project is not a prototype hospital to be site adapted, but a flexible tool to allow each Medical Center to create an individual identity within the Gateways system.

These templates were based upon two different acute care hospital sizes, a 106-bed hospital and a 150-bed hospital. Each of the Gateways hospital templates was designed to meet the OSHPD [Office of State (of California) Healthwide Planning and Development] requirements of the time. A check of OSHPD recent revisions should be made at the initiation of a project.

Gateways is a dynamic process and allows for new templates to be created if they do not exist. This concept of a group of templates used to design rather than a single building design will allow for multiple building configurations and individual architectural expression.

The Gateways Diagnostic Imaging/Nuclear Medicine/EKG/MRI Gateways Templates

Imaging services include general radiography, fluoroscopic and tomographic radiography, mammography, angiography, ultrasound, nuclear medicine, computed tomography (CT), and MRI. Both decentralized and centralized concepts were analyzed. The decentralized approach locates one radiographic imaging unit in a medical office building near the orthopedic clinic. The templates assume that one MRI unit located in hospital space will serve each medical center. A 15-room departmental template is assumed to support the imaging demand for a 106-bed medical center and a 18-room template for a 150-bed medical center. MRI is provided as a separate template. [See figure A-5.]

Figure A-5. MRI Template

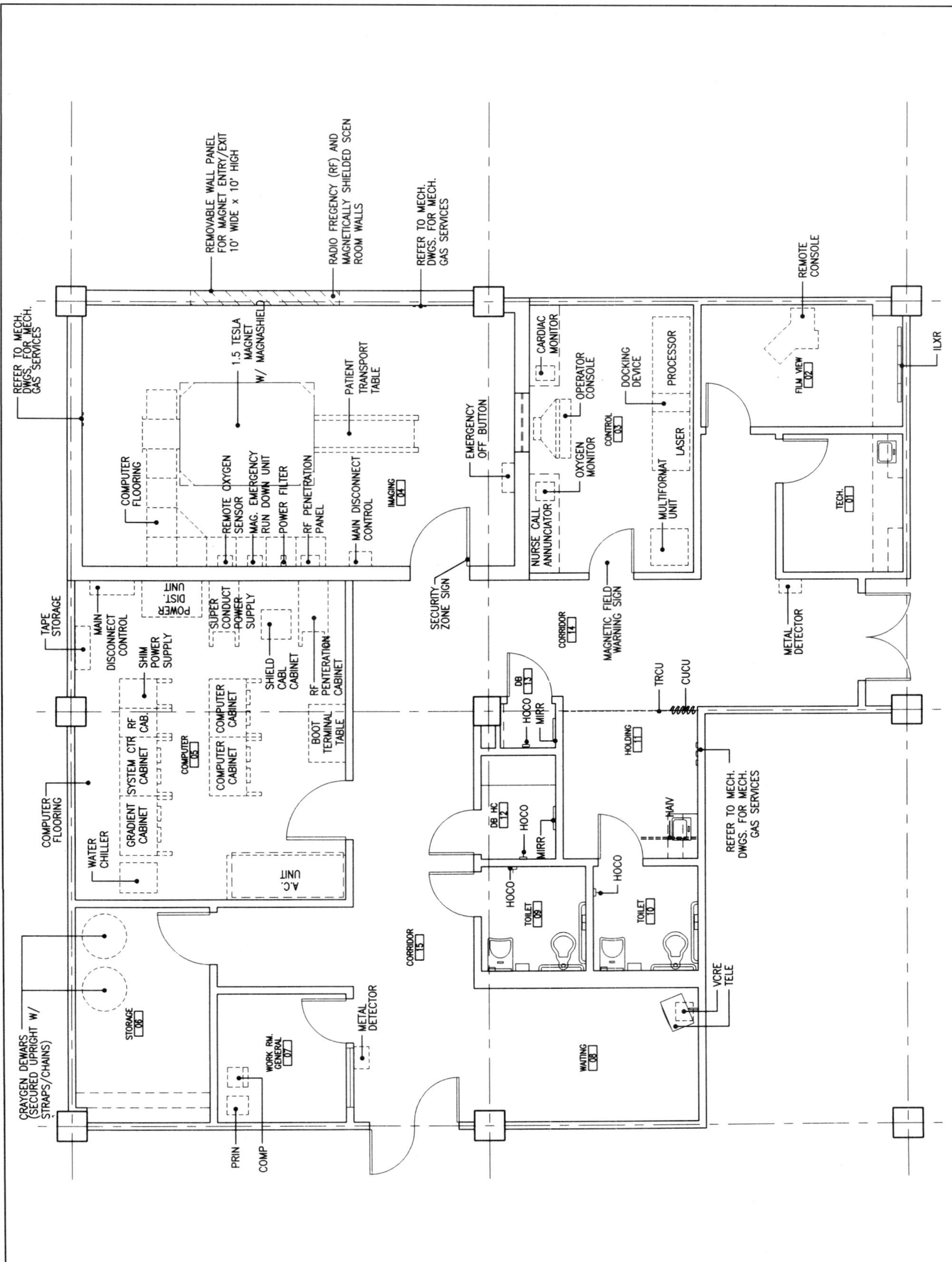

Anderson DeBartalo Pan Architects, Tucson, Arizona. Used with permission.

- Key organizational concepts
  - Flexibility for an exterior mobile technology parking pad for future van/trailer-mounted equipment should be incorporated into the site and building design.
  - A Recovery Area to support the interventional therapeutic practice of Radiology should be incorporated with the Surgical Suite Recovery Area.
  - The department is assumed to have adjacency or close proximity to the Emergency Department.
- Expansion
  - Future expansion is expected to occur at the back or rear of the Department or by relocating Nuclear Medicine and converting Nuclear Medicine space to Diagnostic Imaging functions.
- Nuclear Medicine
  - Film processing/view/sort may be shared between Diagnostic Imaging and Nuclear Medicine.
  - Nuclear Medicine will be integrated with Diagnostic Imaging for the efficiency of shared support spaces.
- MRI
  - Magnetic Resonance Imaging (MRI) is designed to be immediately adjacent to, and accessible from, Diagnostic Imaging, located in [hospital] . . . MRI contains a sub-wait area, but shares main waiting, reception, and scheduling with Diagnostic Imaging.
  - MRI should be located on the exterior of the building, adjacent to Diagnostic Imaging for ease of equipment installation/repair.

Veterans Administration Medical Center, Baltimore[8]

The Baltimore VA Replacement Medical Center is the keystone to the consolidation of all VA facilities in the Baltimore region. [See figure A-6.] Affiliated with the University of Maryland Hospital and School of Medicine, this 324-bed replacement hospital is located adjacent to the University Hospital on a 2.6-acre urban site. The 700,000-square-foot hospital includes inpatient, ambulatory care, diagnostic/treatment, teaching, and major research facilities. A 700-car underground parking structure also is part of the project.

Building System

Designed in accordance with the Veterans Administration Hospital Building System, the project utilizes interstitial space above all functional areas. Mechanical zones are stacked at two ends of the building to further integrate architecture and infrastructure. [See figure A-7, p. 366.]

Blue-gray curtain wall glass of the upper levels establishes a distinct identity for the medical center, while warm-toned reddish-brown granite on the exterior of the service bays and lower floors relates to the brick of the surrounding university buildings.

Filmless Imaging

Completed in 1992 and open to patients in 1993, the VA Medical Center represents one of the most advanced filmless imaging departments of its time and one of the first hospitals in the country with a filmless radiology department. Twenty-three thousand square feet of diagnostic imaging and nuclear medicine are located on the first floor served by a dedicated imaging computer area located on the Ground Floor. [See figure A-8, p. 367.]

Images are stored on optical discs holding tens of thousands of pictures equivalent to about five to seven years of images legal limit for retaining records. Having diagnostic imaging data available on computer rather than on film allows the information to be readily accessible to clinicians throughout the medical center. Rather than going to a different floor to check out an X-ray, a physician can simply call up the images on a PACS work station. The system also allows people in various departments throughout the medical center to look at

Figure A-6. Veterans Administration Medical Center, Baltimore

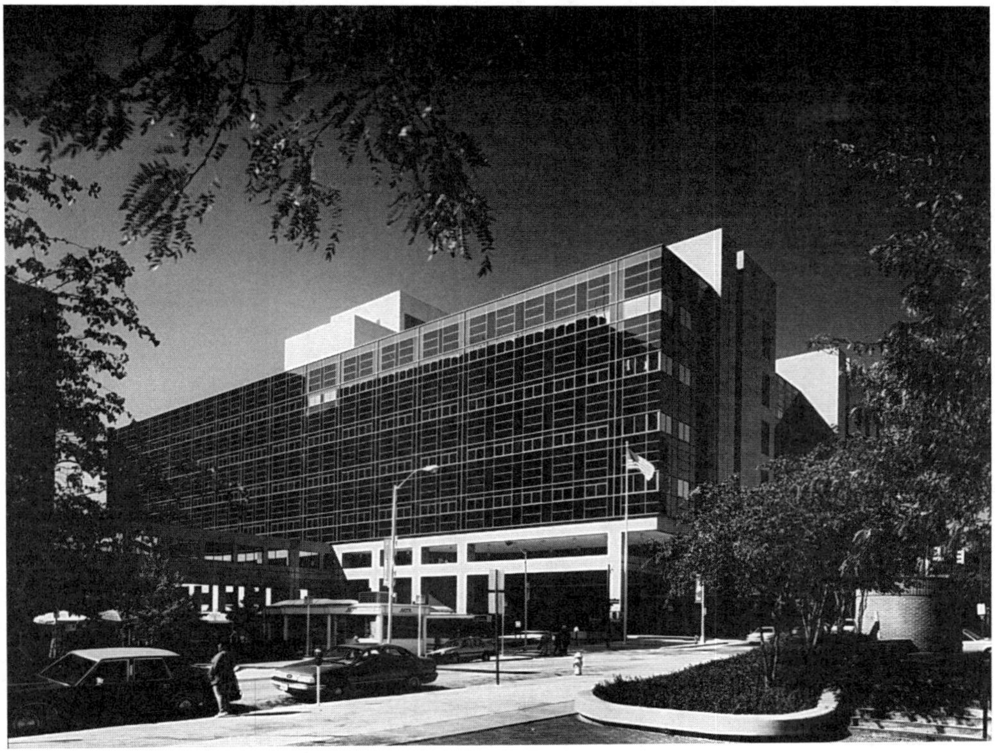

The Baltimore VA Medical Center. ©1992 Maxwell MacKenzie, photographer. Architect: RTKL & Associates. Used with permission.

the same image simultaneously, eliminating the need to wait for films to be available. . . . The all-digital technology will also enable the rapid transfer of images and diagnostic data from [the VA Baltimore Medical] Center to other VA military and civilian facilities. . . . Providing such radiological expertise should enhance (the VA's) ability to serve as a system-wide referral center of excellence.

Imaging services consist of the following procedure rooms and associated support spaces:

- Three general radiography
- Three R/F
- One chest
- One ultrasound
- One mammography
- Two CT
- One MRI
- Two special procedures
- One gamma camera
- One nuclear medicine special procedures
- One stationary imaging
- One cardiac cath lab (located in the cardiology department)
- Two cystoscopy rooms (located in the surgical suite)

References

1. Lemke, H. U. Organizer: Computer Assisted Radiology. CAR '93, Proceedings of the International Symposium; and Leckie, R. G., Smith, C. S., Smith, D. V., Donnelly, J., Cawthon, M., Weiser, J., Willis, C. E., and Goeringer, F. MDIS: A Large PACS and Teleradiology Project, Berlin, Germany.

Figure A-7. VA Medical Center, Baltimore, Building Section

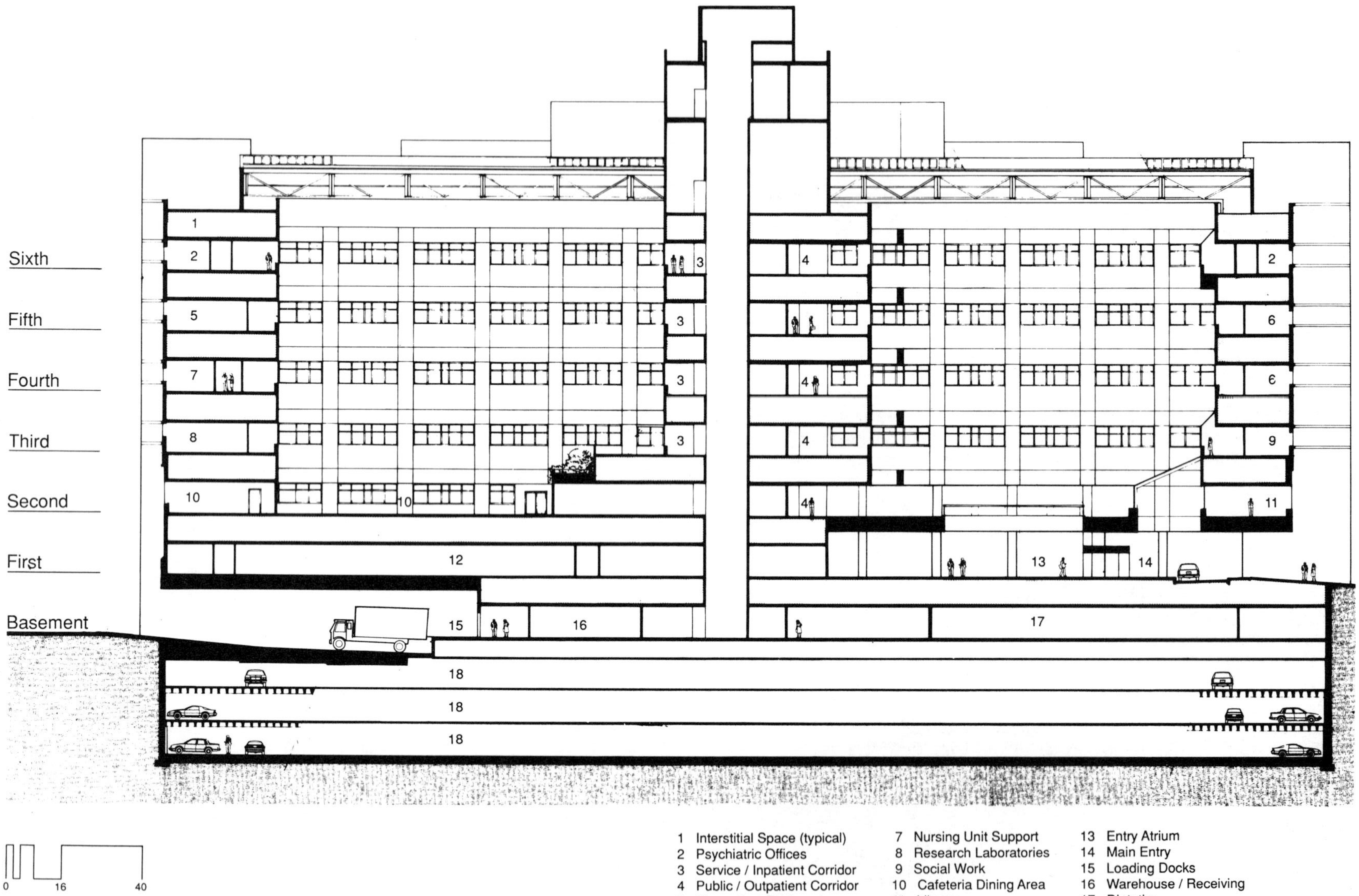

1 Interstitial Space (typical)
2 Psychiatric Offices
3 Service / Inpatient Corridor
4 Public / Outpatient Corridor
5 Biomedical Engineering
6 On-call Rooms
7 Nursing Unit Support
8 Research Laboratories
9 Social Work
10 Cafeteria Dining Area
11 Library
12 Radiology
13 Entry Atrium
14 Main Entry
15 Loading Docks
16 Warehouse / Receiving
17 Dietetics
18 Parking Garage

The Baltimore VA Medical Center. Architect: RTKL & Associates. Used with permission.

2. Communication from U.S. Army Medical Material Agency MDIS Project Office, SGMMA-OMD, Fort Detrick, Frederick, MD, Dec. 1992.

3. Madigan Army Medical Center, Ft. Lewis, Washington—A one-hundred-year hospital investment. U.S. Army Corps of Engineers report, Seattle [no date].

4. Smith, D. V., Smith, S., Sauls, F., Cawthorn, M. A., and Telepak, R. J. Design strategy and implementation of the medical diagnostic image support system at two large military medical centers. Department of Radiology, Madigan Army Medical Center, Fort Lewis, WA; Department of Radiology, Brooke Army Medical Center, Ft. Sam Houston, TX.

5. Miller, M. Images from within. *Stanford Medicine,* winter 1993–1994, p. 19.

Figure A-8. VA Medical Center, Baltimore, First Floor Plan

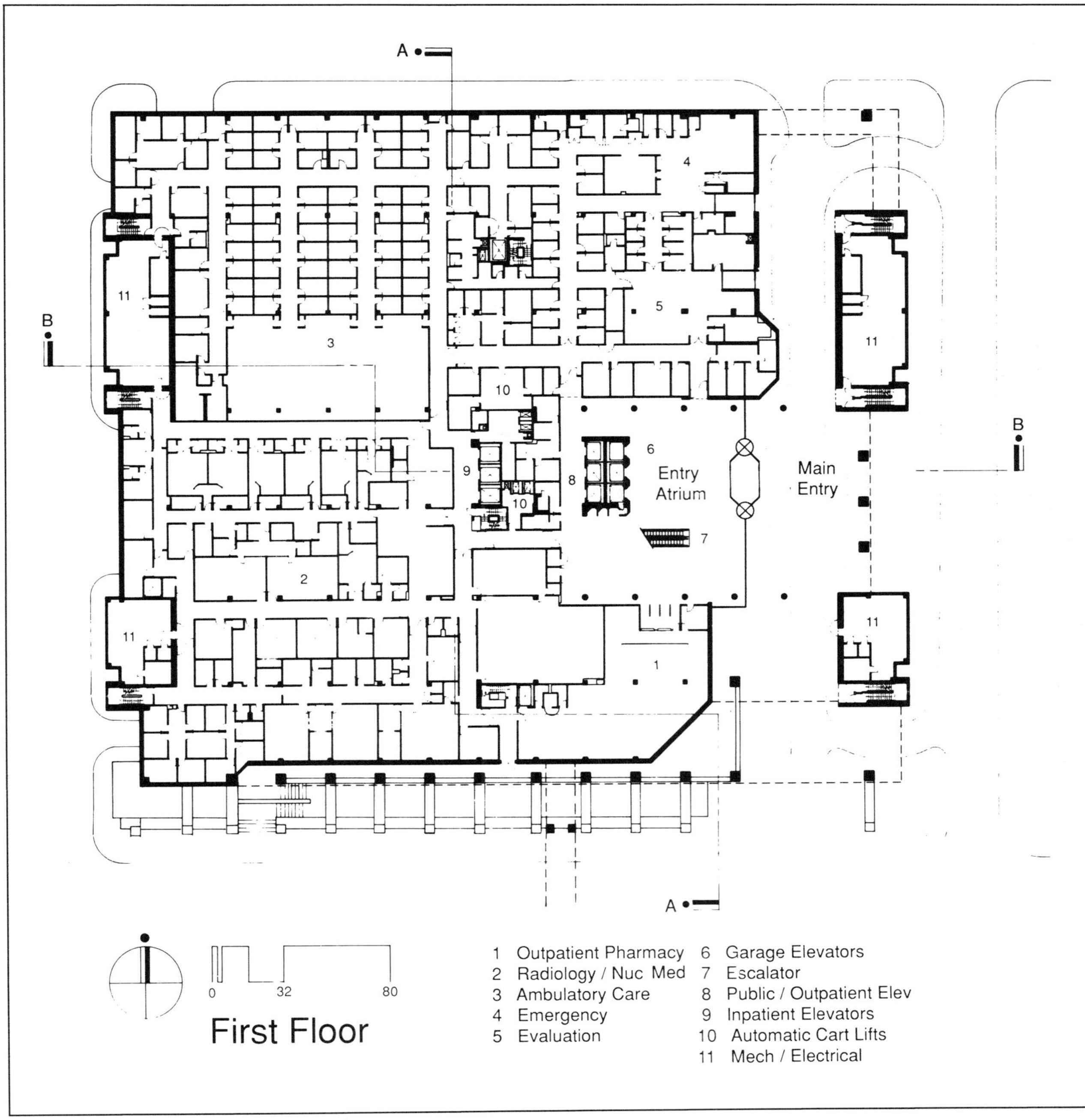

The Baltimore VA Medical Center. Architect: RTKL & Associates. Used with permission.

6. Gateways 106 & 150 Bed Acute Care Hospitals. Vol. 6: Gateways Concept and Application Principles; Section 1: Synopsis. Oakland, CA, Kaiser Foundation Health Plan [no date].
7. Gateways 106 & 150 Bed Acute Care Hospitals. Vol. 4: Ancillary/Clinical Support; Section 15: Diagnostic Imaging/Nulcear Medicine/MRI. Oakland, CA, Kaiser Foundation Health Plan [no date].
8. Internal project description data. Baltimore, RTKL & Associates.

Appendix **B**

Weight and Thickness Equivalents for Commercial Lead Sheets and Commercial Building Materials

Table B-1. Commercial Lead Sheet Thickness Equivalents

Thickness		Weight in Pounds for 1-Square-Foot Section	
Inches	Millimeter Equivalent	Nominal Weight	Actual Weight
1/64	0.40	1	0.92
3/128	0.60	1.5	1.38
1/32	**0.79**	**2**	**1.85**
5/128	**1.00**	**2.5**	**2.31**
3/64	1.19	3	2.76
7/128	1.39	3.5	3.22
N/A	1.50	N/A	3.48
1/16	**1.58**	**4**	**3.69**
5/64	1.98	5	4.60
3/32	**2.38**	**6**	**5.53**
N/A	2.50	N/A	5.80
N/A	3.00	N/A	6.98
1/8	3.17	N/A	7.38
5/32	**3.97**	**8**	**9.22**
3/16	4.76	10	11.06
7/32	5.55	12	12.90
1/4	6.35	14	14.75
1/3	**8.47**	**16**	**19.66**
2/5	10.76	20	23.60
1/2	12.70	30	29.50
2/3	16.93	40	39.33
1	25.40	60	59.00

Notes: The more common thicknesses are highlighted in bold. The density of commercial rolled lead is 11.36 g cm^{-3}. The commercial tolerances are ±0.005 inches for lead up to 7/128 and ±1/32 for heavier sheets. It should be noted that lead sheets less than 1/32 inch thick are frequently more expensive than heavier sheets in cost of materials and cost of installation.

Source: National Council on Radiation Protection and Measurement. *NCRP Report No. 49—Structural Shielding Design and Evaluation for Medical Use of X-Rays and Gamma Rays of Energies of Up to 10 MeV.* Bethesda, MD: NCRP, 1976, p. 87.

Table B-2. Densities of Commercial Building Materials

Material	Range of Density[a]	Average Density[b]	
		g cm^{-3}	lb ft^{-3}
Barium sulfate	N/A	4.5	280
Barytes concrete	3.6 to 4.1	3.6	210
Brick, soft	1.4 to 1.9	1.65	103
Brick, hard	1.8 to 2.3	2.05	128
Earth, dry, packed	N/A	1.5	95
Ferrophosphorus concrete	6.0	4.8	300
Granite	2.6 to 2.7	2.65	165
Ilmenite concrete	4.4 to 4.7	3.85	240
Lead	N/A	11.36	709
Lead glass	N/A	3.27	205
Lead glass, high density	N/A	6.22	387
Limestone	2.1 to 2.8	2.46	153
Marble	2.6 to 2.86	2.7	170
Sand, dry, packed	1.6 to 1.9	N/A	100–120
Sand plaster	N/A	1.54	96
Concrete	2.25 to 2.4	2.35	147
Steel	N/A	7.8	489
Tile	1.6 to 2.5	1.9	118

[a]Density values for the concrete aggregate are given for the aggregate only.

[b]Density values are given for the concrete made from the specified aggregate.

Note: Concrete blocks and cinder blocks vary too much to be listed. (*Mark's Mechanical Engineering Handbook.* 5th ed. New York City: McGraw-Hill, 1941.)

Source: National Council on Radiation Protection and Measurement. *NCRP Report No. 49—Structural Shielding Design and Evaluation for Medical Use of X-Rays and Gamma Rays of Energies of Up to 10 MeV.* Bethesda, MD: NCRP, 1976, p. 86.

Appendix C

Excerpt from *1992–1993 Guidelines for Construction and Equipment of Hospitals and Medical Facilities*

4. Equipment

4.1. General

4.1.A. An equipment list showing all items of equipment necessary to operate the facility shall be included in the contract documents. This list will assist in the overall coordination of the acquisition, installation, and relocation of equipment. The equipment list should include the classifications identified in Section 4.2 below and whether the items are new, existing to be relocated, owner provided, or not-in-contract.

4.1.B. The drawings shall include provisions for the installation of equipment that requires dedicated building services, or special structures, or that illustrate a major function of the space. Adjustments shall be made to the construction documents when final selections are made.

4.1.C. Space for accessing and servicing fixed and building service equipment shall be provided.

4.1.D. Some equipment may not be included in the construction contract but may require coordination during construction. Such equipment shall be shown in the construction documents as owner-provided or not-in-contract for purposes of coordination.

4.2. Classification

Equipment will vary to suit individual construction projects, and therefore will require careful planning. Equipment to be used in projects shall be classified as building service equipment, fixed equipment, or movable equipment.

4.2.A. Building Service Equipment

Building service equipment shall include such items as heating, air conditioning, ventilation, humidification, filtration, chillers, electrical power distribution, emergency power generation, energy management systems, conveying systems, and other equipment with a primary function of building service.

4.2.B. Fixed Equipment (Medical and Non-medical)

4.2.B.1. Fixed equipment includes items that are permanently affixed to the building or permanently connected to a service distribution system that is designed and installed for the specific use of the equipment. Fixed equipment may require special structural designs, electromechanical requirements, or other considerations.

a. Fixed medical equipment includes, but is not limited to, such items as fume hoods, sterilizers, communication systems, built-in casework, imaging equipment, radiotherapy equipment, lithotripters, hydrotherapy tanks, audiometry testing chambers, and lights.

b. Fixed non-medical equipment includes, but is not limited to, items such as walk-in refrigerators, kitchen cooking equipment, serving lines, conveyers, mainframe computers, laundry, and similar equipment.

4.2.C. Movable Equipment (Medical and Non-medical)

4.2.C.1. Movable equipment includes items that require floor space or electrical connections but are portable, such as wheeled items, portable items, office-type furnishings, and monitoring equipment.

a. Movable medical equipment includes, but is not limited to, portable X-ray, electroencephalogram (EEG), electrocardiogram (EKG), treadmill and exercise equipment, pulmonary function equipment, operating tables, laboratory centrifuges, examination and treatment tables, and similar equipment.

b. Movable non-medical equipment includes, but is not limited to, personal computer stations, patient room furnishings, food service trucks, and other portable equipment.

4.3. Major Technical Equipment

Major technical equipment is specialized equipment (medical or non-medical), that is customarily installed by the manufacturer or vendor. Since major technical equipment may require special structural, electromechanical requirements, or other considerations, close coordination between owner, building designer, installer, construction contractors, and others is required.

4.4. Equipment Shown on Drawings

Equipment which is not included in the construction contract but which requires mechanical or electrical service connections or construction modifications shall, insofar as practical, be identified on the design development documents to provide coordination with the architectural, mechanical, and electrical phases of construction.

4.5. Electronic Equipment

Special considerations shall be given to protecting computerized equipment such as multiphasic laboratory testing units, as well as computers, from power surges and spikes that might damage the equipment or programs. Consideration shall also be given to the addition of a constant power source where loss of data input might compromise patient care.

Source: The American Institute of Architects Committee on Architecture for Health, with assistance from the U.S. Department of Health and Human Services. *1992–1993 Guidelines for Construction and Equipment of Hospital and Medical Facilities.* Washington, DC: USDHHS, 1993, pp. 8–9.

Appendix **D**

Imaging Terminology

ACR: American College of Radiology.

AIA/AAH: American Institute of Architects/Academy of Architecture for Health.

AHRA: American Health Care Radiology Administrators.

Backscatter radiation: Photons that are deflected approximately 180° back into the direction of the X-ray beam. Backscatter radiation can leave an imprint of the cassette hinge on radiographic film and can be harmful to staff if radiation protection is not designed and installed properly.

CAR: Computer-assisted radiology.

Certified radiation physicist: Physicist trained in evaluating and calculating radioactive emission from X-ray equipment, and also in prescribing suitable radiation protection for such equipment installations.

Cinefluorography: A fluorographic procedure in which the image is recorded on cinegraphic film and stored for future playback. The radiation dose is higher than that required to store the image electronically or on magnetic tape or disk, but so is the image quality. Cinefluorography frequently is employed with certain angiographic procedures such as cardiac catheterization.

Collimation/collimator: The process of restricting X-ray beam diffusion by attaching a collimating device to the imaging tube. The collimator causes the X rays to be parallel.

Color flow mapping: A vascular imaging technique for ultrasound that uses Doppler shifts to plot the shape of a vessel manually and indicate relative blood flow.

Contrast media: A radiopaque substance used to provide a contrast in density between tissue or organs being examined and surrounding tissue. Contrast media cause soft tissue to absorb X rays and therefore become visible on X-ray film.

Cryogens: Liquids at extremely low temperatures (usually liquid nitrogen and liquid helium) used to cool the coils of superconductive magnets to approximately absolute zero.

Cyclotron: A machine, capable of accelerating charged particles to very high energy levels, used to produce radionuclides for applications in nuclear medicine.

Darkroom: A room from which daylight is excluded so that photographs can be processed. (See *Film processor* and *Safelight.*)

Daylight processing: Radiographic film-processing system that does not require a darkened room. Proponents of daylight film processing suggest that this system can reduce patient examination time because the technician does not have to travel between the exam room and a darkroom. In some installations, daylight processors are placed directly in the procedure room.

Dewar: A vacuumlike container with highly reflective interior surfaces, used to maintain MRI cryogens (typically liquid helium) at near constant temperatures approaching absolute zero.

Digital archiving: A system of storing images in digitized format on magnetic or optical disks rather than storing films. Digital archiving is directly compatible with imaging processes, such as computed tomography and nuclear medicine, whose output is digitized, and it can be compatible with processes whose output relies on developed film, such as basic radiography, if those images are later digitized. (See also *PACS.*)

Digital subtraction: An imaging technique that takes two X-ray images—one with contrast media injected into the area of interest and one without—and subtracts one from the other to mask or suppress surrounding details, thus improving the clarity of the area of interest.

Doppler effect: A principle of light wave physics applied to ultrasound to monitor the movement of tissue interfaces. The doppler effect indicates that light or sound wavelength is higher (frequency is lower) than that emitted when the source and receiver are moving away from each other, and that frequency is higher when they are moving toward each other.

Dosimetry: The detection or measurement of radiation intensity. (See *Rad equivalent man* and *Radiation absorbed dose.*)

Dual photon absorptiometry (DPA): A type of nuclear medicine imaging that precisely measures the calcium content of bone where osteoporosis (softening of the bone) is suspected. Two photons are emitted from a radioactive gadolinium (Gd) isotope source, through the patient, and into a detector where they are analyzed. Radioactive gadolinium has a relatively long half-life and will remain stable for up to a year. A DPA scan is both fast and relatively inexpensive.

Electromagnetic radiation: Visible light; electromagnetic energy radiation by the sun. One of two classifications of ionizing radiation. Nonelectromagnetic ionizing radiation is known as particulate radiation. (See *Ionizing radiation.*)

Exclusion zone: Area where the magnetic flux density is greater than five gauss. Personnel with cardiac pacemakers, neurostimulators, and other biostimulation devices must not enter this zone. Signs are posted outside the 5-gauss line alerting personnel of this requirement. Because the magnetic field is three-dimensional, signs also are posted on floors above and below the exam room in which the 5-gauss line exists. (See *Gauss.*)

Faraday cage: A specially constructed wire mesh cage enclosing the bore of the magnet in an MRI. The cage, usually constructed of closely spaced copper strands, attenuates external sources of radio-frequency signals that would otherwise interfere with the MRI's internal radio signals. (See *Radio-frequency shielding.*)

Field strength: A measure of the amount of magnetic energy present in a magnet used for MR imaging. Field strength is measured in tesla (abbreviated as T).

Film fog: A generalized dulling of the image on a radiograph caused by non-information-carrying, or scattered, X rays absorbed by the film. Special techniques and apparatus are employed to reduce the occurrence of film fog.

Film processor: Equipment used to develop or process film. The four factors affecting traditional film development are: (1) chemical composition, (2) agitation during development, (3) development time, and (4) development temperature. Some film-developing processes require the absence of light. Others, known as daylight processing, do not.

Gamma camera: Used in nuclear medicine, the gamma camera detects and counts photons emitted from radiopharmaceuticals with affinities for specific organs. The gamma camera maps the spatial configuration of the photons, thus creating an image of the organ under examination.

Gamma radiation: A form of electromagnetic radiation. Both X rays and gamma rays, also known as photons, carry no mass and no charge. Gamma rays are emitted from the nucleus of a radioisotope and usually are associated with alpha and beta emission. Both X rays and gamma rays exist only at the speed of light.

Gantry assembly: An equipment component of CT, MRI, and other imaging modalities. In CT, the gantry assembly contains the X-ray tube, the detector array, the high-voltage generator, the patient support and positioning couch, and the mechanical support for each. The gantry assembly receives information electronically from the operating console and transmits information to the computer for image development.

Gauss: An international unit of magnetic flux: 1 gauss = 0.00001 tesla. (See *Tesla.*) Gauss lines of an MRI often are mapped on architectural drawings to locate the area boundaries where public thoroughfare should be excluded. (See *Security zone* and *Exclusion zone.*)

Hot lab: A room designed for handling "hot" radioactive isotopes used in nuclear medicine. The hot lab usually is located near the nuclear medicine exam room(s) and is designed for the temporary containment of "hot" sources.

ICRP: International Council on Radiation Protection.

Image format: The format used for storing an image. Image format is determined by both the media on which the image is stored and the process used to create the image. In conventional radiography, for example, the image usually is stored on film. CT images, which often are stored on magnetic disks or magnetic tapes, sometimes are recorded on multiformat film for later viewing. Multiformat cameras can record up to six images on a single 8×10-inch film. However, 11×14-inch multiformat film will allow for larger, and therefore clearer, images. Magnetic disks often contain data from a single patient. Magnetic tapes have a greater storage capacity and can store multiple scans from many patients. (See *Digital archiving* and *PACS.*)

Image intensifier: A complex electronic vacuum tube used to convert radiant energy from the X-ray beam into visible light photons. The result is an image with an increased illumination level that is thousands of times brighter than without intensification. The image intensifier provides tremendous flexibility in manipulation of fluoroscopic information and permits the use of cine and spot film cameras as well as other accessories. Brightness gain of image intensifier tubes decreases with age and use.

Image subtraction: A number of computer-assisted techniques in which one image is superimposed and subtracted from another image resulting in visible information that would otherwise be obstructed. Image subtraction methods include temporal subtraction in which an earlier image is subtracted from a later one, energy subtraction in which two different X-ray beams are alternated, and hybrid subtractions which combine both temporal and energy subtraction techniques. (See *Digital subtraction.*)

Ionizing radiation: Any form of radiation that is capable of ionization (removing an orbital electron from an atom with which it interacts). Nonionizing radiation can be harmless, but ionizing radiation is very dangerous to man. (See *Radiation absorbed dose* and *Rad equivalent man.*) Ionizing radiation is classified as either particulate radiation or electromagnetic radiation. Alpha, beta, and other particles are forms of particulate radiation. Gamma rays and X rays are forms of electromagnetic radiation and often are called photons or visible light. Gamma rays are used in nuclear medicine. X rays are used in different forms of radiography, fluoroscopy, and tomography.

Irradiation: Therapeutic application of roentgen rays, radium rays, ultraviolet rays, or other radiation to a patient.

Isocenter: Center of the imaging volume ideally located at the magnet center.

Isotope: One of a series of chemical elements that have nearly identical chemical properties but that differ in their atomic weights and electric charge. Many isotopes are radioactive, and many radioactive isotopes are used as tracer elements in nuclear medicine and related imaging techniques.

Kilovolt (kV): A unit of electrical energy potential: 1 kV = 1,000 volts (V). High voltage and adequate electric current are required to produce X rays. X-ray voltage is measured in kilovolt peak (kVp); X-ray current is measured in milliamperes (mA), where 1 mA = 0.001 amperes (A) of electric current. Transformers are used to convert V to kVp and A to mA.

Laser: Acronym for *light amplification by stimulated emission of radiation.*

Lead shielding: Radiation protection in the form of thin lead sheets usually applied in conjunction with gypsum board. Lead shielding protection is specified in terms of pounds per square foot and is determined by a certified radiation physicist who calculates the average amount of exposure in the exam room relative to the estimated occupancies of adjacent rooms. (See *Radiation protection.*)

Linear array scanning (ultrasound): Use of an assembly containing several ultrasound transducers electronically connected in series. Sequential operation of each transducer (sequential linear array) allows for real-time monitoring. Segmented operation, where groups of four or five transducers are activated simultaneously but each group is activated sequentially (segmented linear array), provides increased image line density over sequential linear array scanning. (See *Phased array scanning.*)

Magnetic shielding: The use of material, such as steel, to redistribute a magnetic field or to reduce a fringe field. Some magnets are self-shielded and require no additional magnetic shielding.

Magnetic source imaging: A noninvasive imaging technique that maps electrical activity of the brain, heart, and neuromuscular system, and converts the data into a three-dimensional image.

Mammography: X-ray study of the breast, often used in cancer diagnosis.

Mobile imaging facility: Freestanding imaging facility that can be relocated to numerous sites. Mobile facilities allow capital expenditures to be shared by multiple owners or users.

This can be advantageous where single-site workloads cannot justify the installation of expensive imaging equipment.

Monoclonal antibodies (MoAbs): Radiolabled tracer elements used in nuclear medicine to both detect certain diseases and deliver drugs to specific affected sites. Some MoAbs "piggyback" onto white blood cells, enabling quicker and more effective treatment for certain diseases than was previously possible.

Multiformat camera: Output device used to record multiple images on a single sheet of film. All computer-assisted images are ultimately displayed on a CRT and are directly compatible with multiformat cameras. (See *Image format.*)

NCRP: National Council on Radiation Protection and Measurement.

Nonionizing radiation: Energy emitted and transferred through matter without causing ionization or the removal of an orbital electron from the atom with which the radiation interacts. Nonionizing radiation generally is not harmful to man. (See *Ionizing radiation.*)

Orthovoltage X rays: X rays with accelerated electrons having an energy of 125 to 500 KeV (kiloelectron volts). Orthovoltage rays, sometimes referred to as conventional X rays, are common for many X-ray machines compared to megavoltage or supervoltage energies (above 1 MeV), which are common for linear accelerators.

PACS: See *Picture archiving and communications systems.*

Permanent magnet: A permanently magnetized material providing the magnetic field for MRI. Permanent magnets do not require electric sources or cryogens and presently are limited to about 0.5-T field strength.

Phased array scanning (ultrasound): Use of an assembly similar to linear array scanning except that operation of each transducer is controlled by a special electronic circuit that incorporates precisely timed delays to create a wider or "sector" scan. (See *Linear array scanning.*)

Phased contrast magnetic resonance angiography: A noninvasive method of imaging the circulatory system using magnetic resonance imaging. The method eliminates the use of potentially harmful contrast media. A sensitive image processor records signals from resonating hydrogen atoms in the bloodstream. The resulting three-dimensional image shows the rate of blood flowing through veins and arteries.

Picture archiving and communications systems (PACSs): In contrast to traditional radiographic storage systems, which store individual hard copies of X-ray films, PACSs allow multiple users to simultaneously receive, file, and display images via computer systems. Users have access to CT, ultrasound, MR, and other digital images, as well as plain film images that have been digitized. PACS images, which can be transported over cable or via satellite and are stored on magnetic or optical disks, have a tremendous potential for reducing the storage problems associated with traditional image storage systems.

Positron: A particle having the same mass as a negative electron, but having a positive charge.

Primary beam: Radiation beam originating directly from X-ray source prior to being scattered. Primary radiation is more intense and therefore more difficult to protect against than secondary (scattered or leaked) radiation.

Quench: Condition occurring when a superconductive magnet becomes resistive and quickly boils off liquid helium.

Rad equivalent man (Rem): Unit of dose equivalent (DE) used to express the quantity of radiation received by a radiation worker. Personnel-monitoring badges worn by such workers record cumulative radiation exposure.

Radiation absorbed dose (Rad): Unit of radiation absorbed dose most often used when describing the quantity of radiation received by a patient or experimental animal. One rad = 100 ergs/g, where the erg is a unit of energy and the gram is a unit of mass.

Radiation protection: Means of protecting against the harmful effects of radiation exposure; minimizing radiation exposure to staff and patients. Methods of radiation protection include: filtration, collimation, intensifying screen cassettes, protective apparel, gonadal shielding, and protective barriers.

Radiation therapy: The application of ionizing radiation to kill cancerous cells. Radiation therapy, also known as therapeutic radiation, often is performed in conjunction with other treatment modalities such as chemotherapy, surgery, or hyperthermia.

Radio-frequency shielding: The use of material such as copper or brass to reduce interference from external radio frequencies.

Radioactive half-life: Time required for the nucleus of a radioactive substance to lose its activity by undergoing radioactive decay.

Radioisotopes: Radioactive forms of chemicals. Although a few elements have naturally occurring radioisotopes, artificial radioisotopes have been produced for nearly all chemical elements.

RSNA: Radiological Society of North America.

Radionuclide: Atoms that disintegrate by emission of electromagnetic radiation.

Resistive magnet: A type of magnet used in magnetic resonance imaging that produces a magnetic field by passing an electric field through wire coils. Heat is produced due to the electrical resistance of the wire. Resistive magnets are more simple to produce and maintain than superconductive magnets, but require continuous power and water cooling. Also, resistive magnets are not able to produce magnetic field strengths as great as those produced by superconductive magnets.

Roentgenography: The process of obtaining pictures by use of roentgen rays (X rays). Roentgenography is a synonym for radiography.

Safelight: Light source providing illumination in a darkroom without fogging or exposing daylight-sensitive film.

SCAR: Society for Computer Applications in Radiology.

Scatter radiation: Form of secondary radiation occurring when the primary beam intercepts any object, thus causing some X rays to bounce or scatter.

Scintillation: The emissions that come from radioactive substances. A nuclear medicine scan.

Security zone: Area within an MRI exam room where the magnet is located. Signs are posted outside the room warning personnel of the high magnetic field existing in the room and the possibility of ferrous objects becoming dangerous projectiles within this zone. (See *Gauss.*)

Shimming: Correction of inhomogeneity of the main magnetic field due to imperfections in the magnet or to the presence of external ferromagnetic objects. Shim coils are used when shimming is required.

Slice thickness: The width of the X-ray beam, usually measured in mm, that passes through the patient. Smaller slices provide greater spatial resolution but require a larger radiation dose.

Soft tissue radiography: Radiographic techniques designed to enhance differential absorption of muscle and fat, which have similar mass densities.

Sonar: Device for detecting objects under water by reflection of sound waves. Acronym for sound navigation and ranging. Ultrasound is based on sonar techniques.

Spectroscopy, MR: The ability to accurately measure the amount of elements in specific chemical states. In vivo spectroscopy generally requires a magnet with a field strength of at least 1.5 T.

Spot film: A single frame exposure, often used in conjunction with a fluoroscopic examination. Spot films can be made from conventional cassette-loaded film or from a spot film "movielike" camera that exposes only one frame when activated. The latter process is less disruptive to the examination and requires a lower radiation dose.

Superconductive quantum interference device (SQUID): An experimental form of imaging consisting of tiny magnetometers that measure the minute biomagnetic fields of electrical energy flowing throughout the entire human nervous system. In SQUID, small superconductive rings image this electrical flow. Some applications show promise in the treatment of epilepsy.

Superconductive magnet: A magnet containing coils made from a superconducting metal alloy. Because superconductive materials have no electrical resistance, electrical energy is not dissipated as heat. Such magnets must be cooled to a temperature approaching absolute zero to maintain their superconducting properties.

Teleradiology: A delivery system in which diagnostic images are electronically transported via cables, wires, local area networks, and so on to various remote locations. Teleradiology is one component of telemedicine.

Tesla (T): An international unit of magnetic force that is used to describe the strength of magnets used in magnetic resonance imaging: 1 T = 10,000 gauss (G). The earth's magnetic force is approximately 0.5 G, or 0.00005 T. A 1.0-T MRI magnet is 20,000 times stronger than the earth's average magnetic force.

Tomography: Any of several special techniques of roentgenography designed to show detailed images of structures in a selected plane by blurring images of structures in all other planes. Tomography is also applied to some nuclear medicine procedures.

Ultrasonography: Use of inaudible sound in the frequency range of 20,000 to 10,000,000,000 cycles per second to produce an image or photograph of an organ or tissue. Ultrasonic echoes are recorded as they strike tissue of different densities. (See *Sonar.*)

Xeroradiography: In contrast to conventional radiography, which is based on wet chemistry processing to produce a visible image, xeroradiography is based on a dry processing technique where an electrostatic latent image is formed by a photoconductive material. Xeroradiography was first invented in 1939. The inventor's rights were passed on to the Hayloid Corporation, which later became the Xerox Corporation.

Zonography: A tomographic process in which a relatively small tomographic angle (1 to 5 degrees) is employed, resulting in a large "zone" of tissue being brought into focus. Zonography, which is employed when thin-section tomography would result in a poor image, is mostly used in chest examinations.

Appendix E

Bibliography

Design

American Institute of Architects, Committee on Architecture for Health. *A Generic Process for Projecting Health Care Space Needs.* Washington, DC: AIA, 1985.

American Institute of Architects, Academy on Architecture for Health. *Guidelines for Construction and Equipment of Hospital and Medical Facilities.* Washington, DC: AIA, 1992.

Aldrich, J. E., and Berkey, J. Access control systems for radiotherapy treatment rooms. *Medical Physics* 15(6):930–31, Nov.–Dec. 1988.

American College of Radiology. *Planning Guide for Radiologic Installation.* Fascicle 8: CT Facilities. Chicago: ACR, 1981.

Brocke, J. E. Solving difficult site problems for MRI and PET. *European Journal of Radiology* 16(1):30–34, Dec. 1992.

Brovold, R. Imaging department designs that bridge the film/digital gap. *European Journal of Radiology* 16(1):40–42, Dec. 1992.

Brovold, R., and Farah, J. William Beaumont Hospital Imaging Center design update. *European Journal of Radiology* 16(1):35–39, Dec. 1992.

Condon, P. M., and Robertson, A. R. Magnetic resonance imaging: project planning and management of a superconductive MRI installation. *Australasian Radiology* 33(1):40–46, Feb. 1989.

Conoley, P. M., Lenker, M. D., and Harwood, H. Radiology on the move—phase II: planning of a new outpatient specialty center radiology department. *European Journal of Radiology* 16(1): 13–16, Dec. 1992.

Cory, D. A., and Cohen, M. D. Laser cameras and radiology department design. *Applied Radiology* 18(3):30–32, Mar. 1989.

D'Alessio, A. Flint, MI, institutions join forces to build, operate MRI center. *Health Facilities Management* 2(11):12–13, Nov. 1989.

Delany, D. J., Scatliff, J. H., and Thompson, B. G. A multimodality projection console for the radiology conference room. *Investigative Radiology* 22(4):336–37, Apr. 1987.

Einstein, S. G., and Hilal, S. K. Site planning design: influences and implementation. *Magnetic Resonance Annual* 1985, pp. 267–311.

Eldar, R., and Inbar, A. Diagnostic radiology in disaster medicine: implications for design, planning and organization of X-ray departments. *Injury* 18(4):247–49, July 1987.

Elliot, A. T., Hilditch, T. E., Murray, T., and McNulty, H. The design and construction of a central radiopharmacy. *Nuclear Medicine Communications* 14(4):328–34, Apr. 1993.

Galvin, J. M., Claytor, N., Cedrone, B., and Graff, R. L. A guide to design of radiation therapy facilities. *Applied Radiology* 14(1):86–90, Jan.–Feb. 1985.

Gardner, D. K. Diagnostic imaging centers. *Journal of Healthcare Interior Design* 2:159–66, 1990.

Gothlin, J. H. Planning departments of radiology. *European Journal of Radiology* 16(1):vii–viii, Dec. 1992.

Herman, J. G. Interior and exterior design of mobile imaging units. *Applied Radiology* 15(3):93–98, May–June 1986.

Horii, S. C., Horii, H. N., Mun, S. K., Benson, H. R., and Zeman, R. K. Environmental designs for reading from imaging work stations: ergonomic and architectural features. *Journal of Digital Imaging* 2(3):156–62, Aug. 1989.

James, A. E., Kaye, J. J., Partain, C. L., Heller, R. M., and others. Facility report: Department of Medical Imaging and Radiological Sciences at Vanderbilt University. *Applied Radiology* 13(4):108–12, July–Aug. 1984.

Johnson, K. 2 MRI centers: 10 design mistakes to avoid. *Hospitals* 61(7):82, Apr. 5, 1987.

Keenan, L. Design and architecture in radiology. *Administrative Radiology* 9(6):43, 45, 47–48, June 1990.

Keenan, L. A., and Goldman, E. F. Positive imaging: design as marketing tool in diagnostic centers. *Administrative Radiology* 8(2):36–41, Feb. 1989.

Lambert, R., Keane, B., and Rahim, B. Computer aided design of the X-ray room. *Radiography* 52(603):149–51, May–June 1986.

Lindsey, M. S. "Landlocked" hospital finds room for its MRI unit under the ground. *Health Facilities Management* 5(9):14–15, Sept. 1992.

Malkin, J. *The Design of Medical and Dental Facilities.* New York City: Van Nostrand Reinhold, 1982.

Malkin, J. *Hospital Interior Architecture.* New York City: Van Nostrand Reinhold, 1984.

Malkin, J. *Medical and Dental Space Planning for the 1990's.* New York City: Van Nostrand Reinhold, 1990.

Meadow, M. Management brief: thinking about building. *Applied Radiology* 18(1):12–13, Jan. 1989.

Milner, S. H., Feig, S. A., and McArdle, G. H. A successful breast imaging center: design to reality. *Administrative Radiology* 7(3):35–38, Mar. 1988.

Monteleoni, P. Imaging adjacencies: three recent projects illustrate central vs. dedicated specialty planning considerations. *European Journal of Radiology* 16(1):26–29, Dec. 1992.

Powills, S. Imaging centers get bigger (and better). *Hospitals* 62(21):66, Nov. 1988.

Roebuck, E. J., Manton, D. J., and Fordham, G. L. Building or extending a hospital department: radiology. A path through the planning minefield. *Journal of the Royal Society of Medicine* 80(1):40–46, Jan. 1987.

Roebuck, E. J., Manton, D. J., and Fordham, G. L. Building or extending a hospital department: radiology. A path through the planning minefield. *Journal of the Royal Society of Medicine* 80(2):107–13, Feb. 1987.

Roebuck, E. J., Manton, D. J., and Fordham, G. L. Building or extending a hospital department: radiology. A path through the planning minefield. *Journal of the Royal Society of Medicine* 80(3):173–79, Mar. 1987.

Roebuck, E. J., Manton, D. J., and Fordham, G. L. Building or extending a hospital department: radiology. A path through the planning minefield. *Journal of the Royal Society of Medicine* 80(5):308–13, May 1987.

Roebuck E. J., Manton, D. J., and Fordham, G. L. Building or extending a hospital department: radiology. A path through the planning minefield. *Journal of the Royal Society of Medicine* 80(7):449–55, July 1987.

Roebuck, E. J., Manton, D. J., and Fordham, G. L. Building or extending a hospital department: radiology. A path through the planning minefield. *Journal of the Royal Society of Medicine* 80(8):512–22, Aug. 1987.

Roebuck, E. J., Manton, D. J., and Fordham, G. L. Building or extending a hospital department: radiology. A path through the planning minefield. *Journal of the Royal Society of Medicine* 80(9):577–83, Sept. 1987.

Roebuck, E. J., Manton, D. J., and Fordham, G. L. Building or extending a hospital department: radiology. A path through the planning minefield. *Journal of the Royal Society of Medicine* 80(10):640–46, Oct. 1987.

Schwartz, B. Soft neutrals: creating a warm envelope for radiation patients. *Interiors* 151(12):68–69, Dec. 1992.

Seago, K. Transport design considerations in mobile imaging trailers. *Applied Radiology* 16(7):38, 42–43, July 1987.

Seelye, A. Planning for magnetic resonance imaging units. *New Zealand Hospital* 39(5):12–14, July 1987.

Sixth International Symposium on Planning of Radiological Departments, Bergen, Norway, June 10–13, 1992. *European Journal of Radiology* 16(1):1–73, Dec. 1992.

Slater, J. M., Miller, D. W., and Archambeau, J. O. Development of a hospital-based proton beam treatment center. *International Journal of Radiation, Oncology, Biology, Physics* 14(4):761–75, Apr. 1988.

Thiele, J. The sharper image. . . . Kaiser Permanente/San Diego's new MRI unit. *Contract Design* 34(7):70–71, July 1992.

Timms, W. E. Interference problems and screening in NMR and MRI. *Journal of Medical Engineering and Technology* 16(2):69–78, Mar.–Apr. 1992.

Williams, C. O., and Groce, K. A. The importance of appropriate medical suite designs in the era of computerized imaging. *Radiologic Clinics of North America* 24(3):337–46, Sept. 1986.

Williams, R. C., Choplin, R. H., Boehme, J. M., Park, W. C., and Maynard, C. D. Site planning for radiology computer systems. *American Journal of Roentgenology* 145(5):1087–88, Nov. 1985.

Imaging

Advances in radiology at Dunedin Hospital. *New Zealand Health and Hospital* 41(2):14, Mar.–Apr. 1989.

American Hospital Assocation. Cine CT: progress and opportunities. *Hospital Technology Series: Guideline Report* 5(20), 1986.

American Hospital Assocation. CT scanners. *Hospital Technology Series: Guideline Report* 3(8), 1984.

American Hospital Association. Diagnostic and therapeutic applications of radiolabeled monoclonal antibodies. *Hospital Technology Series: Executive Briefing* 8(12), May 1989.

American Hospital Association. Mobile MRI—issues to consider. *Hospital Technology Series: Special Report* 6(24):1–18, Sept. 1987.

American Hospital Association. Nonsurgical options grow as technology and techniques improve. *Hospital Technology Series: Meditrends* 8(3), Feb. 1989.

American Hospital Association. Picture archiving and communications. *Hospital Technology Series: Guideline Report* 4(16), 1985.

American Hospital Association. Positron emission tomography (PET): progress and opportunities. *Hospital Technology Series: Guideline Report* 6(8), 1987.

American Hospital Association. Projecting MRI utilization: two new approaches. *Hospital Technology Series: Guideline Report* 6(13):1–37, 1987.

American Hospital Association. SPECT/magnetic source imaging. *Hospital Technology Series: Executive Briefing* 9(1), Jan. 1990.

American Hospital Association. SPECT/magnetic source imaging. *Hospital Technology Series: Technology Scanner* 9(2), Jan. 1990.

American Hospital Association. Superconductivity research produces a new neuroimaging device: SQUID. *Hospital Technology Series: Executive Briefing* 8(20), 1989.

American Hospital Association. A view of the inner workings of the body. *Hospital Technology Series: Meditrends* 8(22), Sept. 1989.

American Hospital Association. What's new in radiology–measurable progress. *Hospital Technology Series: Meditrends* 8(1), Jan. 1989.

Ayton, V. T., Smith, M. A., and Bingham, J. B. Practical considerations for patient investigation using a high field (1.5T) magnetic resonance system. *Radiography Today* 55(620):12–15, Jan. 1989.

Biggs, P. J. Calculation of shielding door thickness for radiation therapy facilities using the ITS Monte Carlo program. *Health Physics* 61(4):465–72, Oct. 1991.

Biggs, P. J. An interactive computer graphics program for determining the shielding for a megavoltage radiotherapy facility. *Health Physics* 43(4):601–7, Oct. 1982.

Biggs, P. J. Shielding design for the ceiling of a 6-MV accelerator in an existing facility. *Health Physics* 52(4):491–93, Apr. 1987.

Bishop, K. O. Improving patient throughput in an MRI center. *Administrative Radiology* 7(2):36–38, Feb. 1988.

Bragg, D. G., Putman, C. E., and Hendee, W. R. Oncological imaging: state of the art and research priorities. *American Journal of Clinical Oncology* 11(3):394–403, June 1988.

Bronzino, J. D., Smith, V. H., and Wade, M. L. *Medical Technology and Society: An Interdisciplinary Perspective.* Cambridge, MA: MIT Press, 1990.

Broody, W. R. Does MRI belong in the hospital? *Radiology Management* 9(2):16, Spring 1987.

Brovold, R. Bridging the film–digital gap. *Administrative Radiology* 10(11):57, 59–61, Nov. 1991.

Brown, S. E., and English, R. J. *SPECT Single Photon Emission Computed Tomography: A Primer.* New York City: The Society of Nuclear Medicine, 1986.

Bushong, S. C. *Radiologic Science for Technologists.* 5th edition. St. Louis: Mosby-Year Book, 1993.

Council on Scientific Affairs. Magnetic resonance imaging. *JAMA* 258:3283–85, 3417–23, 1987.

Davis, G. Cost analysis: self-shielding vs. magnetic room shielding. *Administrative Radiology* 7(11):98–102, Apr. 1988.

Dean, M. H., and Stedeford, B. Leakage through gaps around shielding windows in radiotherapy treatment rooms. *Physics in Medicine and Biology* 29(6):711–18, June 1984.

Fordham, G. L. Health building note 6. *Radiography* 51(600):316–18, Nov.–Dec. 1985.

Future improvements in magnetic imaging. *Health Technology* 2(1):12–19, Jan.–Feb. 1988.

Gitterman, M., and Webster, E. W. Shielding hospital rooms for brachytherapy patients: design, regulatory and cost/benefit factors. *Health Physics* 46(3):617–25, Mar. 1984.

Glenn, A. L., King, P., and Moen, P. Checklist for efficient operation of MRI. *Radiology Management* 9(4):63–65, Fall 1987.

Gunn, T. W. Image, architecture, and costs of ambulatory care. *Michigan Hospitals* 26(3):14–16, 18, 20–22, Mar. 1990.

Hanafee, W. N. Imaging with a permanent magnet system. In: *Magnetic Resonance Annual.* Los Angeles: UCLA School of Medicine, Department of Radiology, 1985, pp. 217–29.

Health Care Strategic Management. New, less costly "open-air" MRI will scan more types of patients. *Health Care Strategic Management* 6(8):15, Aug. 1988.

Hendee, W. R. *The Selection and Performance of Radiologic Equipment.* Baltimore: Williams and Wilkins, 1985.

Herman, J. G. Interior and exterior design of mobile imaging units. *Applied Radiology* 15(3):93–98, May–June, 1986.

Ho, B. K. Automatic acquisition interfaces for computed radiography, CT, MR, US, and laser scanner. *Computerized Medical Imaging Graphics* 15(3):135–45, May–June 1991.

Jonsson, E. Methods of assessing medical technology. *World Hospitals* 23(3–4):29–33, Oct. 1987.

Johnsson, J., and others. Technology acquisition: trends in imaging. *Hospitals* 65(21):26–30, 32–34, 36, Nov. 5, 1991.

Karlik, S. J., Heatherley, T., Pavan, F., Stein, J., and others. Patient anesthesia and monitoring at a 1.5-T MRI installation. *Magnetic Resonance in Medicine* 7(2):210–21, June 1988.

Kaufman, L., and Crooks, L. E. Field strength issues in MRI. *Administrative Radiology* 6(8):17–19, Aug. 1987.

Kohn, D. Refined imaging technologies spark urgent interest. *Computers in Healthcare* 12(10):23–24, 26, Oct. 1991.

Lee, J. K. Magnetic resonance imaging. *Health Facilities Management* 1(3):18, 20–22, Nov. 1988.

Lehr, J. L. Diagnostic radiology at the University of Chicago. *Applied Radiology* 14(4):73–77, July–Aug. 1985.

Levine, B., and Mun, S. K. Image management and communication systems: a new challenge in radiology. *Medical Progress through Technology (West Germany)* 15(3–4):199–216, 1989.

Lim, B. MRI: a sensitive tool of unseen potential. *Australian Hospital* 6(1):13–25, Oct. 1988.

Lumsdon, K. Hospitals move toward image management, but pace is slow. *Hospitals* 66(11):58, 60, 62, June 5, 1992.

Magnetic resonance imaging. *JAMA* 259(14):2134–38, Mar. 1988.

McAfee, J. G., Kopecky, R. T., and Frymoyer, P. A. Nuclear medicine comes of age: its present and future roles in diagnosis. *Radiology* 174(3)1:609–20, Mar. 1990.

Medical imaging and radiation oncology resources. 1992 organization directory. *Administrative Radiology* 11(1):55–61, Jan. 1992.

Mellenger-Blouch, J. New diagnostic center brings radiology, lab services into the '90s. *Health Facilities Management* 5(7):16–17, July 1992.

MRI field strength: how important a criterion? *Health Technology* 2(1):20–23, Jan.–Feb., 1988.

MRI—magnetic resonance imaging. *Medical Electronics* 18(5):144–49, Oct. 1987.

MRI: what are its applications; what will it replace? *Health Technology* 2(1):3–11, Jan.–Feb., 1988.

Naylor, A. F. Radiology department design to accommodate the future introduction of global PACS. *European Journal of Radiology* 16(1):51–53, Dec. 1992.

Nickoloff, E. L., and Donnelly, E. M. Use of gypsum drywall as shielding material for mammography. *Health Physics* 54(4):465–68, Apr. 1988.

Ottes, F. P. Methodology for the evaluation of diagnostic image quality. *International Journal of Biomedical Computing* 30(3–4):221–27, May 1992.

Protection of the patient in nuclear medicine. *Annals of the ICRP* 17(4):1–37, 1987.

Rejger, V. S., Cohn, B. F., Vielvoye, G. J., and de Raadt, F. B. A simple anaesthetic and monitoring system for magnetic resonance imaging. *European Journal of Anaesthesiology* 6(5):373–78, Sept. 1989.

Remanufactured equipment "as good as new." *Health Facilities Management* 5(2):58, 60, Feb. 1992.

Romeo, M. A., Skrtich, P., and Alexander, J. An imaging department for the 90s: 3 years of experience. *European Journal of Radiology* 16(1):10–12, Dec. 1992.

Rossi, R. P., and Hendee, W. R. New equipment for room 2210: the critical path method. *American Journal of Roentgenology* 134(5):1084–88, May 1980.

The safety of MRI: considerations for site planning and clinical use. *Health Technology* 2(1):24–32, Jan.–Feb. 1988.

Seago, K. Equipment focus: shielding systems for MRI installations. *Applied Radiology* 16(10):25, 28–30, Oct. 1987.

Seeyle, A. Planning for magnetic resonance imaging units. *New Zealand Hospital* 39(5):12–14, July 1987.

Snopek, A. M. *Fundamentals of Special Radiographic Procedures.* Philadelphia: W. B. Saunders, 1984.

Sochurek, H. *Medicine's New Vision.* Easton, PA: Mack Publishing Co., 1988.

Sochurek, H. Medicine's new vision. *National Geographic* 171(1):2–41, Nov. 1987.

Thiele, J. Scanning the crowd. *Contract Design* 33(8):56–59, Aug. 1991.

Thompson, G. The Bristol MRI centre. *Bristol Medico-Chirurgical Journal* 103(2):5–6, May 1988.

Thompson, J. L. Experiences at the new magnetic resonance imaging centre at Bristol. *British Journal of Radiology* 62(734):134–37, Feb. 1989.

Thompson, T. T., Radford, E. L., and Key, J. F. Cost effectiveness of automated radiographic equipment. *Applied Radiology* 10(2):51–52, 54–56, Mar.–Apr. 1981.

Weck, E. P. A primer on medical imaging—part one. *FDA Consumer* 23(3):23–27, Apr. 1989.

Weck, E. P. A primer on medical imaging—part two. *FDA Consumer* 23(4):12–15, May 1989.

Index